ACSM's Certification Review

THIRD EDITION

SENIOR EDITORS

Khalid W. Bibi, PhD
Professor and Chair, Department of Sports Medicine, Health & Human Performance
Professor, Graduate School of Education
Canisius College
Buffalo, New York

Michael G. Niederpruem, MS
Vice President of Certification
American Health Information Management Association
Chicago, Illinois

ACSM's Certification Review

THIRD EDITION

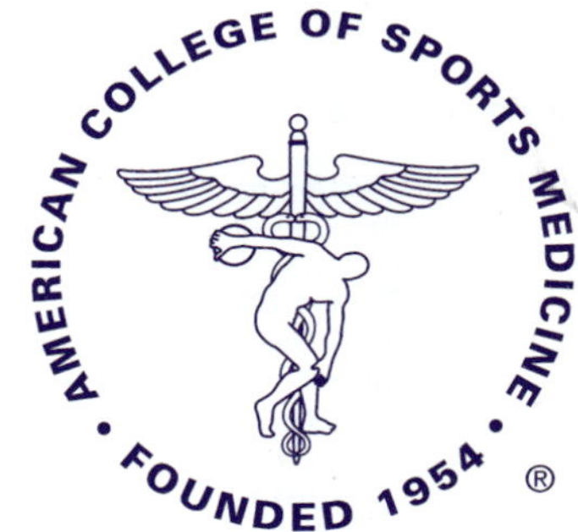

AMERICAN COLLEGE OF SPORTS MEDICINE

Wolters Kluwer Health | Lippincott Williams & Wilkins

Philadelphia • Baltimore • New York • London
Buenos Aires • Hong Kong • Sydney • Tokyo

Acquisitions Editor: Emily Lupash
Managing Editor: Andrea M. Klingler
Marketing Manager: Christen Murphy
Production Editor: Mary Kinsella
Manufacturing Coordinator: Margie Orzech
Creative Director: Doug Smock
Compositor: Aptara, Inc.

ACSM Publication Committee Chair: Jeffrey L. Roitman, EdD, FACSM
ACSM Group Publisher: Kerry O'Rourke

3rd Edition

351 West Camden Street
Baltimore, MD 21201

530 Walnut Street
Philadelphia, PA 19106

Printed in China

Library of Congress Cataloging-in-Publication Data

ACSM's certification review / senior editors, Khalid W. Bibi, Michael G. Niederpruem.—3rd ed.
p. ; cm.
Includes bibliographical references and index.
ISBN 978-0-7817-6901-3
1. Sports medicine—Outlines, syllabi, etc. 2. Sports medicine—Examinations, questions, etc. 3. Personal trainers—Outlines, syllabi, etc. 4. Personal trainers—Examinations, questions, etc. I. Bibi, Khalid W. II. Niederpruem, Michael G.
[DNLM: 1. Sports Medicine—Examination Questions. 2. Sports Medicine—Outlines. 3. Exercise—Examination Questions. 4. Exercise—Outlines. 5. Physical Fitness—Examination Questions. 6. Physical Fitness—Outlines. QT 18.2 A1864 2010]
RC1213.A268 2010
617.1′027076—dc22

2008041285

The publishers have made every effort to trace the copyright holders for borrowed material. If they have inadvertently overlooked any, they will be pleased to make the necessary arrangements at the first opportunity.

To purchase additional copies of this book, call our customer service department at **(800) 638-3030** or fax orders to **(301) 223-2320**. International customers should call **(301) 223-2300**.

Visit Lippincott Williams & Wilkins on the Internet: http://www.lww.com. Lippincott Williams & Wilkins customer service representatives are available from 8:30 am to 6:00 pm, EST.

For more information concerning American College of Sports Medicine Certification and suggested preparatory materials, call **(800) 486-5643** or visit the American College of Sports Medicine web site **www.acsm.org**.

9 8 7 6 5

CCS0410

Chapter Authors

CHAPTER 1

Jeffrey J. Betts, PhD
Health Sciences Department
Central Michigan University
Mt. Pleasant, Michigan

Elaine Filusch Betts, PhD, PT, FACSM
Physical Therapy
Central Michigan University
Mt. Pleasant, Michigan

Chad Harris, PhD
Department of Kinesiology
Boise State University
Boise, Idaho

CHAPTER 2

Michael Deschenes, PhD, FACSM
Kinesiology Department
College of William & Mary
Willamsburg, Virginia

CHAPTER 3

Deborah Riebe, PhD, FACSM
Department of Kinesiology
University of Rhode Island
Kingston, Rhode Island

Robert S. Mazzeo, PhD, FACSM
Department of Integrative Physiology
University of Colorado
Boulder, Colorado

David S. Criswell, PhD
Department of Applied Physiology and Kinesiology
University of Florida
Gainesville, Florida

CHAPTER 4

Carol Ewing Garber, PhD, FFAHA, ACSM
Department of Biobehavioral Sciences
Teachers College
Columbia University
New York, New York

CHAPTER 5

Andrea Dunn, PhD, FACSM
Klein Buendel Inc.
Golden, Colorado

Bess H. Marcus, PhD
Community Health and Psychiatry and Human Behavior
Brown University
Providence, Rhode Island

David E. Verrill, MS, FAACVPR
Presbyterian Hospital
Presbyterian Center for Preventive Cardiology
Charlotte, North Carolina

CHAPTER 6

Stephen C. Glass, PhD, FACSM
Department of Movement Science
Grand Valley State University
Allendale, Michigan

CHAPTER 7

Frederick S. Daniels, MS, MBA
CPTE Health Group
Nashua, New Hampshire

Nancy J. Belli, MA
Physical Activity Department
Plus One Holdings, Inc.
New York, New York

Kathy Donofrio
Swedish Covenant Hospital
Chicago, Illinois

CHAPTER 8

Kathleen M. Cahill, MS, ATC
Sugar Land, Texas

John W. Wygand, MA
Adelphi University
Human Performance Laboratory
Garden City, New York

Julie J. Downing, PhD, FACSM
Central Oregon Community College
Health and Human Performance
Bend, Oregon

CHAPTER 9

Janet R. Wojcik, PhD
Department of Health and Physical Education
Winthrop University
Rock Hill, South Carolina

R. Carlton Bessinger, PhD, RD
Department of Human Nutrition
Winthrop University
S. Rock Hill, South Carolina

CHAPTER 10

Frederick S. Daniels, MS
CPTE Health Group
Nashua, New Hampshire

Gregory B. Dwyer, PhD, FACSM
Department of Exercise Science
East Stroudsburg University
East Stroudsburg, Pennsylvania

CHAPTER 11

Khalid W. Bibi, PhD
Sports Medicine, Health and Human Performance
Canisius College
Buffalo, New York

Dennis W. Koch, PhD
Human Performance Center
Canisius College
Buffalo, New York

CHAPTER 12

Theodore J. Angelopoulos, PHD, MPH
Center for Lifestyle Medicine
University of Central Florida
Orlando, Florida

Joshua Lowndes, MA
Center for Lifestyle Medicine
University of Central Florida
Orlando, Florida

Chapter Contributors

CHAPTER 1

John Mayer, PhD, DC
Spine and Sport Foundation
San Diego, California

Brian Undermann, PhD, ATC, FACSM
Department of Exercise and Sports Science
University of Wisconsin-La Crosse
La Crosse, Wisconsin

CHAPTER 10

Neal I. Pire, MA
Plus One Fitness
New York, New York

Kathy Donofrio
Swedish Covenant Hospital
Chicago, Illinois

CHAPTER 11

Stephen C. Glass, PhD, FACSM
Department of Movement Science
Grand Valley State University
Allendale, Michigan

Manuscript Reviewers

Joseph Hamill, PhD, FACSM
University of Massachusetts - Amherst
Amherst, MA
Chapter 1

William Simpson, Ph.D., FACSM
Department of Health and Human Performance
University of Wisconsin-Superior
Superior, WI
Chapters 1 & 7

Stephen Glass, Ph.D., FACSM
Grand Valley State University
Allendale, MI
Chapter 2

Janet Wallace, Ph.D., FACSM
Indiana University
Bloomington, IN
Chapter 3

Ray Squires, Ph.D., FACSM
Mayo Cardiovascular Health Clinic
Rochester, MN
Chapter 4

Dalynn Badenhop, Ph.D., FACSM
University of Toledo Medical Center
Toledo, OH
Chapter 4

Steven Edwards, Ph.D., FACSM
Oklahoma State University
Stillwater, OK
Chapter 5

Michelle Miller, MS
Indiana University
Bloomington, IN
Chapters 5 & 11

Jason Conviser, Ph.D., MBA, FACSM
President, JMC & Associates
Glencoe, IL
Chapter 6

Jacalyn Robert/McMcomb, Ph.D., FACSM
Texas Tech University
Lubbock, TX
Chapter 6

Sue Beckham, Ph.D., FACSM
Dallas VA Medical Center
Dallas, TX
Chapter 7

Gregory Hand, Ph.D., FACSM
University of South Carolina
Columbia, SC
Chapter 8

Gregory Dwyer, Ph.D., FACSM
East Stroudsburg University
East Stroudsburg, PA
Chapter 8

Christopher Berger, Ph.D., CSCS
University of Kentucky
Lexington, KY
Chapter 9

Dino Costanzo, MA, FACSM
The Hospital of Central Connecticut
New Britain, CT
Chapter 10

Benjamin F. Timson, Ph.D., FACSM
Missouri State University
Springfield, MO
Chapter 11

Julianne Frey, MS
Kronodynamics
Bloomington, IN
Chapter 12

Examination Reviewers

Sandra Billinger, PT, PhD
University of Kansas Medical Center
Kansas City, Kansas
ACSM Certified Clinical Exercise Specialist

Anthony Clapp, MED, MPE
Ausburg College
Minneapolis, Minnesota
ACSM Certified Health Fitness Specialist

Carol Cole, MS
Sinclair Community College
Dayton, Ohio
ACSM Health/Fitness Director

Heidi Greenhalgh, MS
JUNTOS Coordinator, YMCA
Los Alamos, New Mexico
ACSM Certified Health Fitness Specialist

Jon Herting, BS
Health Fitness Corporation
Chalfont, Pennsylvania
ACSM Certified Health Fitness Specialist

Jeffrey Kazmucha, MS
Lucile Packard Children's Hospital at Stanford
Palo Alto, California
ACSM Certified Clinical Exercise Specialist

Roslyn McLean, MD
Royal Hobart Hospital
Hobart Tasmania, Australia
ACSM Certified Clinical Exercise Specialist

Teresa Merrick, MA
Master Trainer, 24 Hour Fitness
Bellevue, Nebraska
ACSM Certified Health Fitness Specialist

Carolyn Petersen, BS
Mayo Clinic
Rochester, Minnesota
ACSM Certified Health Fitness Specialist

Karin Richards, MS
University of the Sciences
Philadelphia, Pennsylvania
ACSM Certified Personal Trainer

Stacey Scarmack, MS
Exercise Physiologist
Lancaster, Ohio
ACSM Certified Clinical Exercise Specialist

Chet Zelasko, Ph.D.
Grand Rapids, Michigan
ACSM Certified Health Fitness Specialist

Foreword

This third edition of ACSM's *Certification Review* is an important step up from the previous edition. Dr. Khalid Bibi and Mr. Michael Niederprum have produced an excellent revision of this important resource. Once again, *ACSM's Certification Review* is both health/fitness and clinical Knowledge, Skills and Abilities (KSAs) combined into a single publication. The previous edition of this book was a first-time attempt at combining these certifications. That edition was very well-received; thus, it has become the standard for review texts in ACSM's certification resources. This is the definitive review resource for health professionals preparing to take either an ACSM Health Fitness or Clinical certification examination.

ACSM's stable of certifications has undergone significant change in the four years since the publication of the seventh edition of ACSM's *Guidelines for Exercise Testing and Prescription. Certification Review* has been updated in concert with those changes and is a reflection of the current state of ACSM's certification process, the KSAs that accompany the Health/Fitness and Clinical Certifications, and the latest information that supports these publications.

Additionally, for the first time, ACSM is publishing *ACSM's Resource Manual for Guidelines for Exercise Testing and Prescription, 6th Edition; ACSM's Resources for Clinical Exercise Physiology, 3rd Edition; ACSM's Certification Review, 3rd Edition; and ACSM's Exercise Management for Persons with Chronic Diseases and Disabilities, 2nd Edition*, simultaneously with the industry's gold standard, *Guidelines for Exercise Testing and Prescription*, 8th Edition. These four resources, all revised and published at the same time, are an invaluable addition to the reference library for Exercise Professionals and for those aspiring to ACSM certification. This *Certification Review* provides an excellent outline-style document of the critical information in the accompanying *Guidelines and Resource Manual* texts. My most sincere congratulations and thanks go out to the editors and contributors who successfully completed this difficult and daunting task.

The project editors of the ACSM books serve as the backbone for the Guidelines-related publications. The efforts of many volunteers that came together under the capable leadership of the two editors of *Certification Review*, as well as the Literally dozens of contributors, writers, and reviewers came together to produce this review book. Those volunteers, as well as the literally hundreds of others that comprise the entire group that produced the three accompanying volumes, is a tribute to the dedication and loyalty of ACSM's membership who worked continuously for the past three years to complete these books.

Health and fitness professionals, as well as rehabilitation professionals, should aspire to an appropriate level of ACSM certification. The certifications are "mature" enough to have achieved a level of consistency in outcomes and in actually validating a base level of knowledge for the various levels. ACSM-certified exercise professionals don't merely demonstrate to their employers or prospective employers that they have a base level of information, they confirm for themselves that their knowledge and practice is at a level expected of the most accomplished exercise professionals. I encourage all of those professionals to aspire to ACSM certification and to use this excellent resource to aid in your success.

Jeffrey L. Roitman, EdD, FACSM
Director, Sports Science Program
Rockhurst University
Kansas City, MO

Preface

This edition of the ACSM's Certification Review has been revised and updated to cover most of the **Knowledge, Skills and Abilities** (KSAs) related with the ACSM Certified Health Fitness Specialist (HFS), the ACSM Clinical Exercise Specialist (CES), and the ACSM Certified Personal Trainer (CPT) certifications.

This text provides the reader with an easy-to-read review book that covers many of the ACSM KSAs. Each chapter ends with certification-type questions to test your knowledge on select KSAs in that chapter. The book ends with a full-length comprehensive practice examination to help you prepare for the actual examination, and answers and explanations are provided to all questions to help you better understand the material. A searchable version of the full text is available on line at http://thepoint.lww.com.

This book was written with the assumption that the reader has met the minimal requirements set by ACSM to qualify to sit for the examination. Hence, this book is not intended to be the sole text for preparing for the ACSM certifications. Rather, it will help you **review** for the examination. In the process, the book should help you identify your strengths and weaknesses, which will guide you to areas where you might require more in-depth review. Readers seeking a more detailed examination of the KSAs addressed in this book should refer to the 6th edition of the ACSM's Resource Manual (RM6).

The Clinical Exercise Specialist certification encompasses all HFS KSAs. Hence, individuals who intend to use this book to review for the CES certification are responsible for all KSAs covered therein. Individuals preparing for the HFS or CPT certification should refer to their relevant KSAs, as outlined in the RM6 or the 8th edition of the *ACSM's Guidelines for Exercise Testing and Prescription* (GETP8), and review from that book accordingly.

We are aware that facts, standards, and guidelines change on a regular basis in this ever growing field of knowledge. Hence, in the event that conflict may be noted between this book and the GETP8, the latter text should be used as the **definitive and final resource**. In such cases where an update is needed on where conflict or error is identified, we will make every effort to provide further explanations or corrections online. The web address is http://www.acsm.org/bookupdates.com

Khalid Walid Bibi
Mike Niederpruem

Acknowledgments

A special thank you is due to my co-editor, Dr. Khalid Bibi, for both his patience and commitment. I also want to thank the literally hundreds of exceptional ACSM professionals and volunteers that I had the pleasure of working with during my tenure as ACSM's National Director of Certification. Without your collective involvement, many of the recent accomplishments for ACSM's certification programs simply would not have been possible. I am also very grateful to the following individuals specifically for their personal support during my tenure, and especially thankful for their significant contributions to ACSM's organizational accomplishments in certification between 2004 and 2007: Dino Costanzo, Julie Downing, Steven Keteyian, Neal Pire, Traci Rush, Walt Thompson, and last but definitely not least, my dear friend Hope Wood.

— Mike G. Niederpruem

A very special thanks goes to my mother Ghada and father Walid for their unconditional love and ardent support throughout my life, my wonderful sisters Rula, Deema, and Rana for their trust and respect, my wife Lana for her patience and many sacrifices, and my wonderful children Tala and Walid for making it all worthwhile. To a very special friend, Dr. Jeffrey Roitman, with whom I have had the pleasure and honor to work with in most rewarding ways over the past 17 years, my greatest gratitude. To my students and colleagues at Canisius, I am forever and always indebted to you for making coming to work so rewarding. I am also grateful to Adrienne Beggs for her help in reviewing the references. A special "Thank You" goes to my colleague and co-editor, Mike Niederpruem, for his patience and hard work. Hats-off to all the dedicated and hard working ACSM employees who make it all come together. Finally, this book represents the efforts of many volunteers who wrote, reviewed, and contributed to the text. Thank you all.

— Khalid W. Bibi

Contents

Anatomy and Biomechanics

CHAPTER 1

I. INTRODUCTION

A. GROSS ANATOMY

1. Can be learned as **regional or topographic anatomy** organized according to regions, parts, or divisions of the body (e.g., hand, mouth).
2. Can be learned as **systemic anatomy** organized according to organ systems (e.g., respiratory system, nervous system). **This chapter uses the systemic anatomy approach,** and it discusses the anatomy of the following systems only: skeletal, muscular (skeletal muscles), cardiovascular, and respiratory.

B. BIOMECHANICS

1. Is the field of study concerned with the principles of physics related to energy and force as they apply to the human body.
2. Is discussed in this chapter as it applies to specific movements or activities.

C. ORIENTATION *(FIGURE 1-1)*

1. **Proximal**: nearest to the body center, joint center, or reference point.
2. **Distal**: away from the body center, joint center, or reference point.
3. **Superior (cranial)**: above, toward the head.
4. **Inferior (caudal)**: lower than, toward the feet.
5. **Anterior (ventral)**: toward the front.
6. **Posterior (dorsal)**: toward the back.
7. **Medial**: closer to the midline.
8. **Lateral**: away from the midline.

D. BODY PLANES AND AXES

Segmental movements occur around an axis and in a plane. Each plane has an associated axis lying perpendicular to it.

1. The body has **three cardinal planes** (*Figure 1-2*). Each plane is perpendicular to the others.
   a. The **sagittal plane** makes a division into right and left portions.
   b. The **frontal plane** makes a division into anterior (front) and posterior (back) portions.
   c. The **transverse plane** (or horizontal plane) makes a division into upper (superior) and lower (inferior) portions.
2. These planes can be applied to the whole body or to parts of the body.
3. The body has three axes.
   a. The **mediolateral axis** lies perpendicular to the sagittal plane.
   b. The **anteroposterior axis** lies perpendicular to the frontal plane.
   c. The **longitudinal axis** lies perpendicular to the transverse plane.

II. MOVEMENT

Depending on the type of articulation between adjacent segments, one or more movements are possible at a joint (*Figure 1-3*).

A. **FLEXION** is movement that decreases the joint angle. It occurs in a sagittal plane around a mediolateral axis.

B. **EXTENSION**, a movement opposite to flexion, increases the joint angle. It occurs in a sagittal plane around a mediolateral axis.

C. **ADDUCTION** is movement toward the midline of the body in a frontal plane around an anteroposterior axis.

D. **ABDUCTION** is movement away from the midline of the body in a frontal plane around an anteroposterior axis.

E. **ROTATION** is movement around a longitudinal axis and in the transverse plane, either toward the midline (internal) or away from the midline (external).

F. **CIRCUMDUCTION** is a combination of flexion, extension, abduction, and adduction. The segment moving in circumduction describes a cone.

G. **PRONATION** is rotational movement at the radioulnar joint in a transverse plane about a longitudinal axis that results in the palm facing downward.

H. **SUPINATION** is rotational movement at the radioulnar joint in a transverse plane around a longitudinal axis that results in the palm facing upward.

I. **PLANTARFLEXION** is extension at the ankle joint.

J. **DORSIFLEXION** is flexion at the ankle joint.

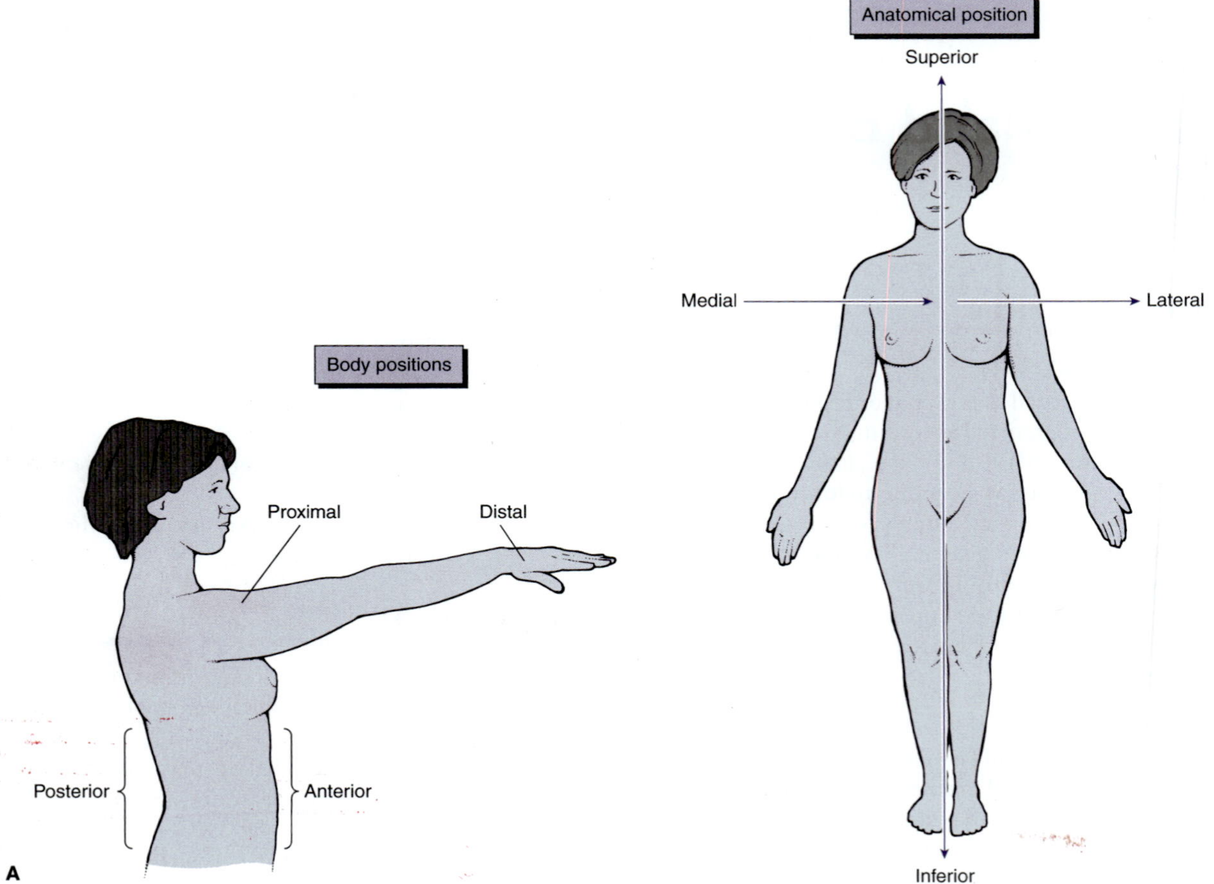

FIGURE 1-1. Terms of orientation. (Adapted from Figure 1-1 of *ACSM's Resource Manual for Guidelines for Exercise Testing and Prescription,* 6th ed. Baltimore, Williams & Wilkins, 2010, p. 3.)

K. EVERSION is turning the sole of the foot away from the midline (outward).

L. INVERSION is turning the sole of the foot toward the midline (inward).

III. THE SKELETAL SYSTEM

A. DIVISIONS *(FIGURE 1-4)*

1. Axial Skeleton

The axial skeleton includes the bones of the skull, vertebral column, ribs, and sternum. It forms the longitudinal axis of the body, supports and protects organ systems, and provides surface area for the attachment of muscles.

a. Skull

Of the 29 bones of the skull, the most significant in terms of exercise testing is the mandible, which may serve as an orienting landmark for palpating the carotid artery to assess pulse.

b. Spine

Also called the vertebral column *(Figure 1-5)*, the spine serves as the main axial support for the body.

1) Vertebrae

The human spine commonly has 33 vertebrae: 7 cervical, 12 thoracic, 5 lumbar, 5 sacral (fused into one bone, the sacrum), and 4 coccygeal (fused into one bone, the coccyx).

2) Intervertebral Disks

Intervertebral disks are round, flat, or platelike structures composed of fibrocartilaginous tissue.

a) The outer, fibrocartilaginous portion of the disk is the annulus fibrosus.

b) The inner gelatinous portion is the nucleus pulposus.

c) Disks unite the vertebral bodies and serve to absorb shock and bear weight.

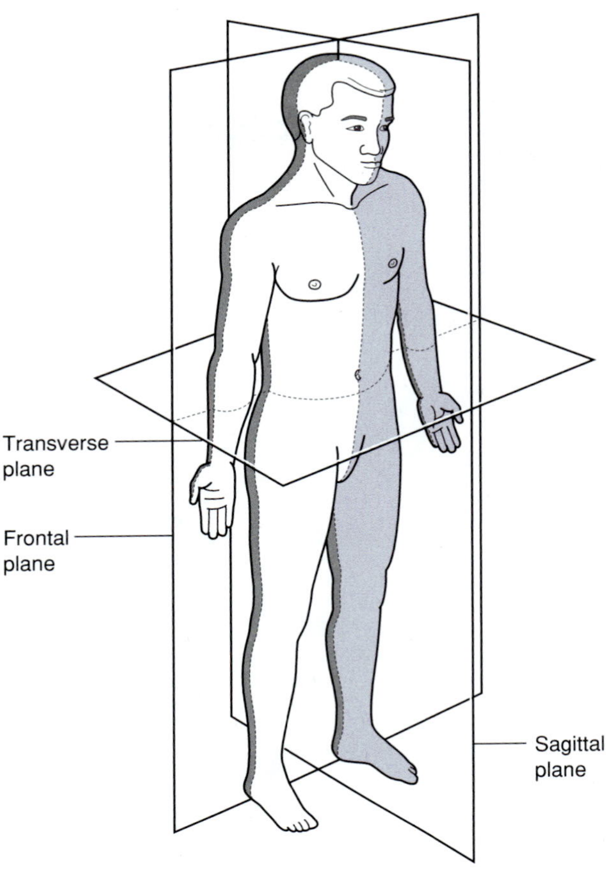

FIGURE 1-2. Planes of the human body.

3) Adult vertebral column
The adult vertebral column has **four major curvatures** in the sagittal plane *(Figure 1-5)*.
   a) **Normal spinal curves** in the sagittal plane are present in the major regions of the vertebral column.
      (i) The curves of the **thoracic** and **sacral** regions are defined as **kyphosis**, because the convexity of the curve is posteriorly directed. These are **primary curves**, because they retain the same directional curvature as the spine in the fetus.
      (ii) The curves of the **cervical** and **lumbar** regions are defined as **lordosis**, because the convexity of the curve is anteriorly directed. These are **secondary curves**, because they develop after birth as the infant progresses in weight bearing.
   b) **Commonly found abnormal curves** in the **sagittal plane** *(Figure 1-6)* include **hyperkyphosis** (exaggerated posterior thoracic curvature) and **hyperlordosis** (exaggerated anterior lumbar curvature).
   c) **Commonly found abnormal curve** in the frontal plane *(Figure 1-6)* includes **scoliosis** (lateral deviation in the **frontal plane**).

c. Ribs
   1) The body has **12 pairs of ribs: 7 pairs of true ribs**, in which the costal cartilage articulates directly with the sternum, and 5 pairs that do not articulate directly with the sternum.
   2) The costal cartilage of ribs 8, 9, and 10 articulates with the costal cartilage of the adjacent superior rib. The cartilaginous ends of ribs 11 and 12 are free from articulation.
   3) The spaces between the ribs are called **intercostal spaces. Palpation of the intercostal spaces of the true ribs** is important for correct placement of **electrocardiography (ECG) electrodes** (in the fourth and fifth intercostal spaces).

d. Sternum
The **sternum** lies in the midline of the chest and has three parts: the **manubrium** (superior), the **body** (middle), and the **xiphoid process** (inferior).
   1) The **sternal angle** is a slightly raised surface landmark where the manubrium meets the body of the sternum.
   2) The **xiphoid process** is also a surface landmark, situated at the bottom of the sternum and in the middle of the inferior border of the rib cage. **Palpation of the xiphoid** is necessary for cardiopulmonary resuscitation (CPR).
   3) **Palpation of the manubrium** helps to determine **proper paddle placement in defibrillation.**

2. Appendicular Skeleton

a. Includes the bones of the arms and legs and the pectoral and pelvic girdles.
b. Functions to attach the limbs to the trunk.
   1) Clavicles
      a) Clavicles articulate with the sternal manubrium proximally and

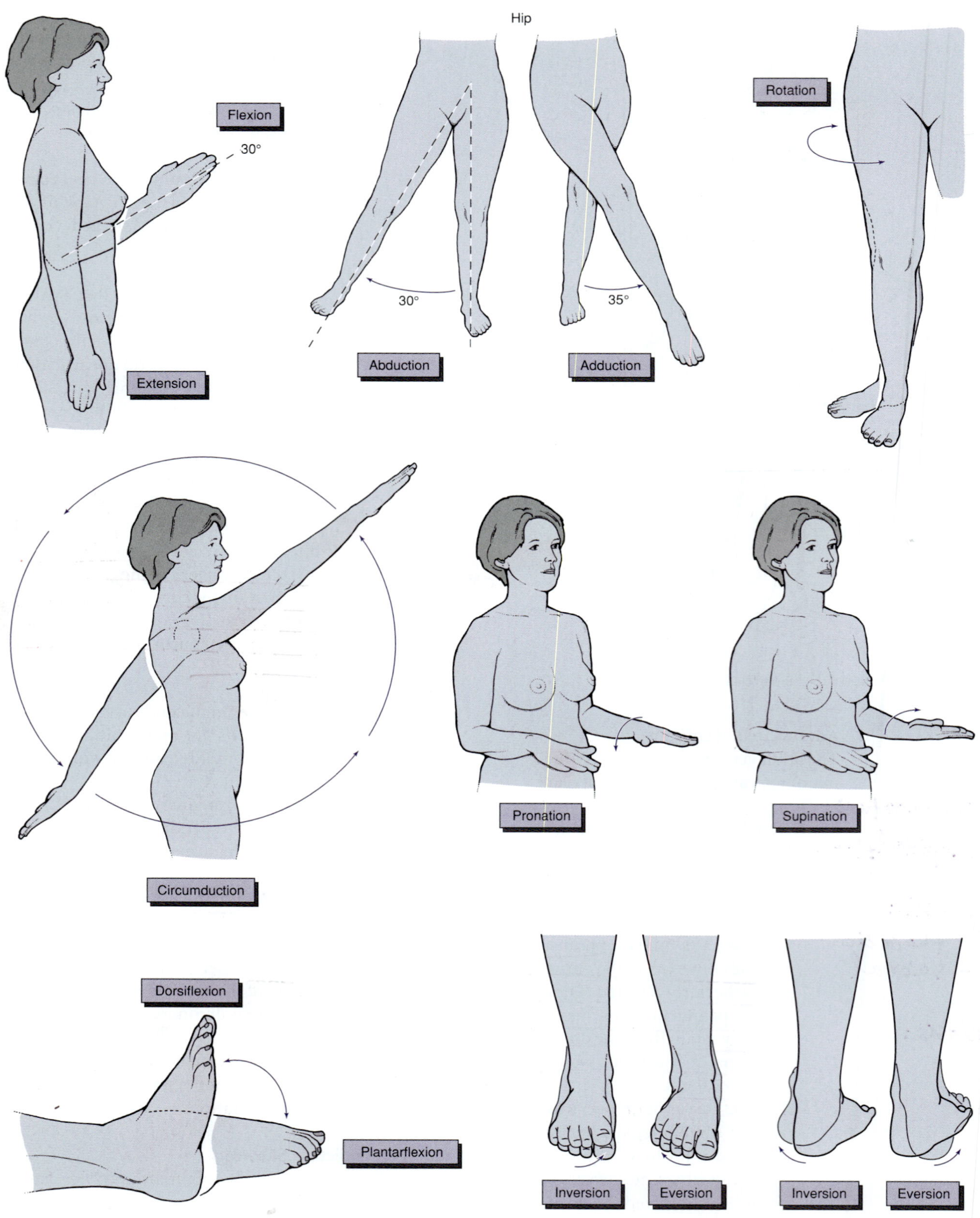

FIGURE 1-3. Body movements at joints. (Adapted in part from Figure 1-26 of *ACSM's Resource Manual for Guidelines for Exercise Testing and Prescription*, 6th ed. Baltimore, Williams & Wilkins, 2010.)

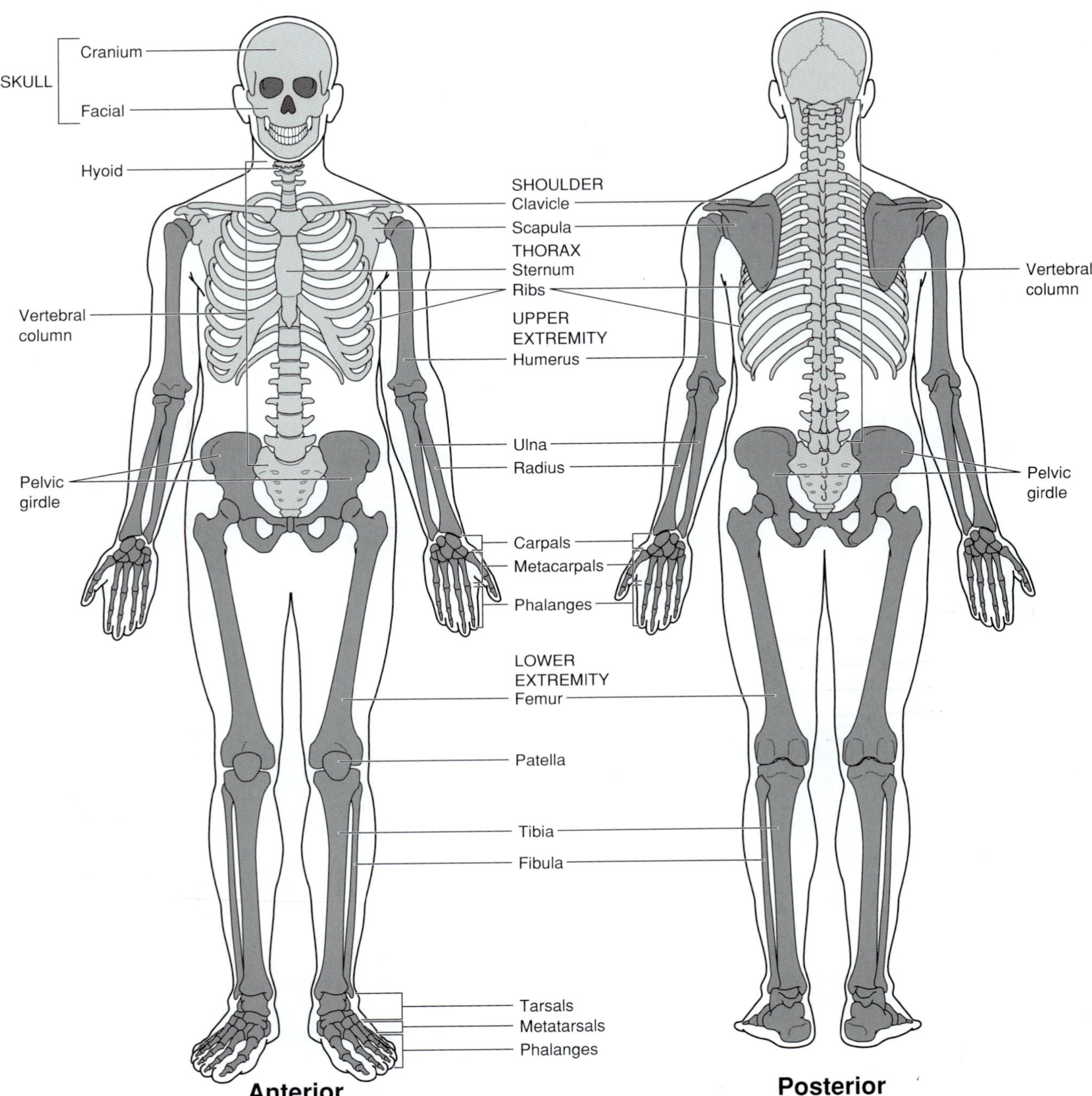

FIGURE 1-4. Divisions of the skeletal system.

the scapulae distally and are positioned just superior to the first rib.

b) Palpation of the clavicles helps to determine electrode placement for ECG and defibrillation.

2) Scapulae

a) Scapulae are situated on the posterior side of the body in the region of the first seven ribs.

b) Each scapula has two important landmarks:

(i) The **inferior angle** (used for skinfold site location) at the bottom of the scapulae, forming the junction between the medial and lateral borders.

(ii) The **acromion process** (used for shoulder breadth

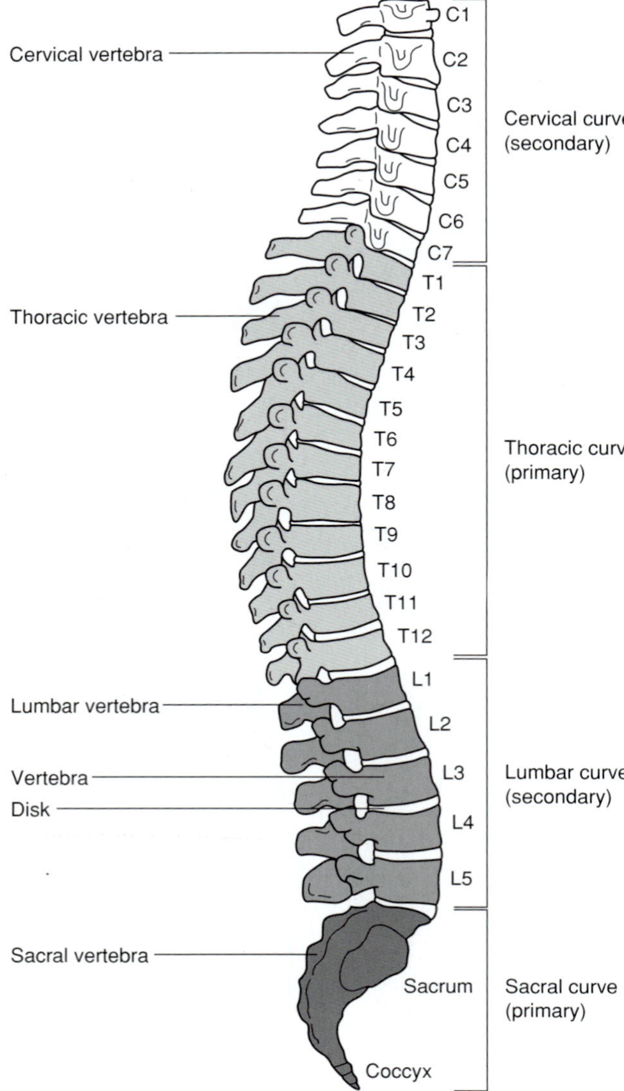

FIGURE 1-5. Lateral view of the spine, showing the vertebrae and disks.

measurement), the bony process at the most lateral part of the shoulder.

3) Upper Arm
   a) The **humerus** proximally articulates with the glenoid fossa of the scapula and distally articulates with the ulna and radius.
   b) The most easily palpable aspects of the humerus are the **medial and lateral epicondyles** at its distal end. The epicondyles are located for elbow width measurement in estimating frame size.

4) Forearm
   The forearm includes two bones: the **ulna**, and the **radius.**
   a) The most prominent bony landmark of the proximal forearm is the **olecranon process** on the posterior ulna.
   b) At the distal end of the forearm are the **radial styloid process** laterally and the **ulnar styloid process** medially. These areas help to identify the proper location for assessing radial pulse.

B. LOWER BODY

The **appendicular skeleton** comprises the bones of the pelvic girdle, thigh, leg, and foot.

1. Pelvic Girdle

a. The pelvic girdle is formed by the hip bones (**ilium, ischium,** and **pubis**), **sacrum,** and **coccyx.**
b. The superiormost aspect of the **ilium** is the **iliac crest,** and the anteriormost structure is the **anterosuperior iliac spine.**
c. These structures are easily palpated and serve as landmarks for skinfold measurements.

2. Thigh

a. The thigh is formed by the **femur.** The most easily palpable landmark is the **greater trochanter** on the proximal lateral side.
b. Distally, the **patella** is located anterior to the knee joint. It serves as a landmark for locating the thigh skinfold.

C. BONE

Bone is an **osseous tissue.** It is a supporting connective tissue composed of calcium salts. Bone is relatively resistant to tensile and compressive forces compared with soft tissues. It is covered by a **periosteum** that isolates it from the surrounding tissues and provides for circulatory and nervous supply. Types include **compact** (cortical, dense) and **cancellous** (trabecular, spongy) bone.

1. Functions

a. Provide structural support for the entire body.
b. Protect organs and tissues of the body.
c. Serve as levers that can change the magnitude and direction of forces generated by skeletal muscles.
d. Provide storage for calcium salts to maintain concentrations of calcium and phosphate ions in body fluids.
e. Produce blood cells.

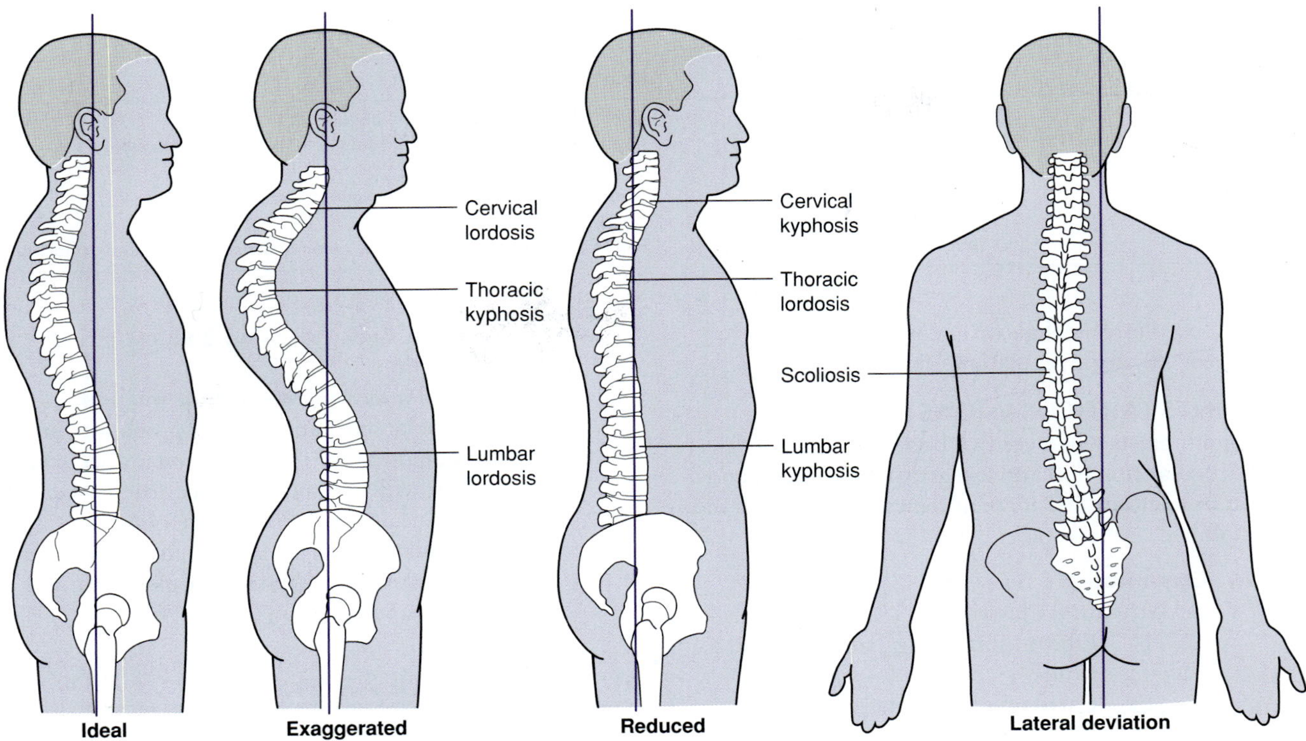

FIGURE 1-6. Ideal and abnormal spinal curvatures.

2. General Bone Shapes

a. Long Bones
   1) Found in the appendicular skeleton.
   2) Consist of a central cylindrical shaft, or diaphysis, with an epiphysis at each end (e.g., femur).
      a) Diaphysis
      The diaphysis consists of compact bone surrounding a thin layer of cancellous bone, within which lies the medullary cavity, which is filled with yellow bone marrow.
      b) Epiphysis
      The epiphysis consists of cancellous bone surrounded by a layer of compact bone. Red bone marrow is contained in the porous chambers of spongy bone; hematopoiesis (production of red blood cells, white blood cells, and platelets) occurs within red bone marrow. Epiphyses articulate with adjoining bones and are covered with articular (hyaline) cartilage, which facilitates joint movement.
   3) Epiphyseal Plate
   In immature long bones, the junction between the epiphysis and the diaphysis is the location of the epiphyseal plate, where growth of long bone occurs.

NB

b. Short Bones
   1) Are almost cuboidal in shape (e.g., bones of the wrist and ankle).
   2) Are often covered with articular surfaces that interface with joints.

c. Flat Bones
   Flat bones are thin and relatively broad (e.g., bones of the skull, ribs, and scapulae).

d. Irregular Bones
   Irregular bones have mixed shapes that do not fit easily into other categories (e.g., vertebrae).

D. CONNECTIVE TISSUES

Connective tissues are not generally exposed outside the body.

1. Basic Components

a. Specialized cells (e.g., in blood, bone, cartilage).
b. Extracellular protein fibers (e.g., elastin, collagen, fibrin).
c. Ground substance.

2. Functions

a. Provide support and protection.
b. Transport materials.

TABLE 1-1. TYPES OF SYNOVIAL JOINTS

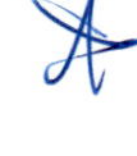

TYPE	EXAMPLE	MOVEMENTS
Ball and socket	Hip, shoulder	Circumduction, rotation, and angular in all planes
Condyloid	Wrist (radiocarpal)	Circumduction, abduction, adduction, flexion, and extension
Gliding	Ankle (subtalar)	Inversion and eversion
Hinge	Knee, elbow	Flexion and extension in one (talocrural) plane
Pivot	Atlas/axis	Rotation around central axis
Saddle	Thumb	Flexion, extension, abduction, adduction, circumduction, and opposition

c. Store mechanical energy reserves.
d. Perform regulatory functions.

E. JOINTS (ARTICULATIONS)

A joint exists wherever two bones meet. The particular function and integrity of a joint depends on its anatomy and its requirement for strength or mobility.

1. Classification

a. Structural Classes
   1) **Fibrous joints** (e.g., sutures of the skull).
   2) **Cartilaginous joints** (e.g., disk between vertebrae).
   3) **Synovial joints** (e.g., hip, elbow).

b. Functional Classes
   1) **Immovable joints**: synarthroses.
   2) **Slightly movable joints**: amphiarthroses.
   3) **Freely movable joints**: diarthroses or synovial joints.

2. Types of Synovial Joints

See *Table 1-1*.

3. Characteristics of Synovial Joints (*Figure 1-7*)

a. Bony surfaces are covered with **articular cartilage**.
b. Surrounding the joint is a **fibrous joint capsule**.
c. **Ligaments** join bone to bone.
d. Inner surfaces of the **joint cavity** are lined with **synovial membranes**.
e. Synovial fluid from the membrane provides lubrication to the joint.
f. Some synovial joints, such as the knee, contain **fibrocartilaginous disks** (e.g., menisci).
g. **Bursae** reduce friction and act as shock absorbers.

4. Movements at Synovial Joints (*Table 1-1* and *Figure 1-3*)

Movements are determined by the structure of the joint and the arrangements of the associated muscles and bone.

a. **Angular movements** (decrease or increase of the joint angle) include flexion, extension, hyperextension, abduction, and adduction.
b. **Circular movements** include rotation (medial or lateral, supination or pronation) and circumduction. These movements occur at joints with a rounded surface articulating with the depression of another bone.
c. **Special movements** include inversion, eversion, protraction, retraction, elevation, and depression.

IV. THE MUSCULAR SYSTEM

The muscular system includes skeletal, cardiac, and smooth muscle. Skeletal muscles are controlled voluntarily.

A. GROSS ANATOMY OF SKELETAL MUSCLES

Skeletal muscle contains three layers of connective tissue.

1. The **epimysium** is the outer layer that separates the muscle from surrounding tissues and organs.

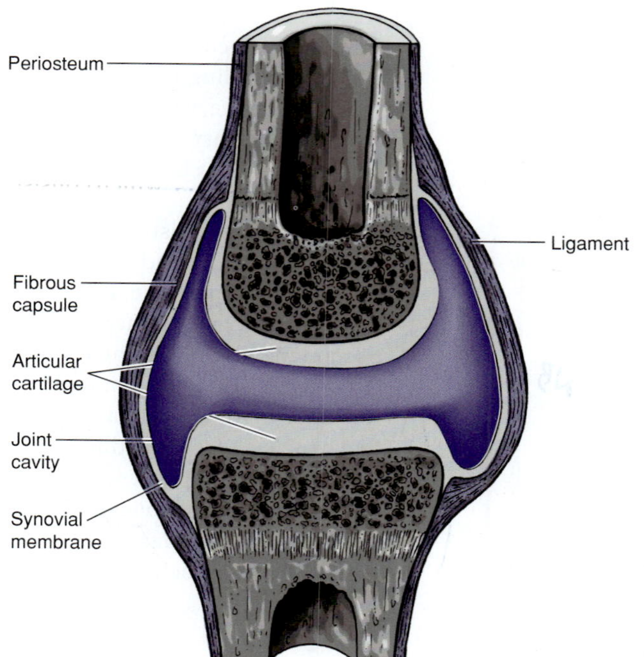

FIGURE 1-7. Synovial joint characteristics.

The epimysium converges at the end of the muscle to form the tendon that attaches muscle to bone.

2. The **perimysium** is the central layer that divides the muscle into compartments called **fascicles** that contain skeletal muscle cells (muscle fibers).
3. The **endomysium** is the inner layer that surrounds each muscle fiber.

B. MUSCLE CONTROL

1. A **motor neuron** controls each skeletal muscle fiber.
2. The cell bodies of the motor neurons lie within the central nervous system.
3. A motor neuron and all the muscle fibers that it innervates comprise a **motor unit**.
4. Motor units are recruited separately for muscle contraction.
5. **Communication** between a motor neuron and a skeletal muscle fiber occurs at the **neuromuscular junction**.
6. Each axon of the motor neuron ends at a **synaptic knob** containing the neurotransmitter **acetylcholine (ACh)**.
7. The **synaptic cleft** separates the synaptic knob from the sarcolemma of the skeletal muscle fiber.
8. The **sarcolemma** of the motor end plate contains chemically gated sodium channels and membrane receptors that bind ACh.

C. MICROANATOMY OF THE MUSCLE CELL

1. The cytoplasm of the muscle cell is called **sarcoplasm**.
2. Extensions of the **sarcolemma** form a network of tubules called **transverse or T-tubules**.
3. The T-tubules extend into the sarcoplasm and communicate with the **sarcoplasmic reticulum**, which stores calcium in special sacs called **terminal cisternae**.
4. **Myofibrils** contain **myofilaments**, which consist of the contractile proteins **actin** and **myosin**.
5. Myofilaments are organized in repeating functional units called **sarcomeres**.
6. Actin and myosin form **crossbridges** and slide past one another during muscle contraction, thus shortening the sarcomeres.
7. **Tropomyosin** covers the actin bridging site during resting condition. Tropomyosin is attached to **troponin**.
8. Tropomyosin and troponin regulate bridging of actin and myosin for **muscle contraction and relaxation**.

D. MUSCLE CLASSIFICATION

Each muscle begins at a proximal attachment (**origin**), ends at a distal attachment (**insertion**), and contracts to produce a specific **action**.

1. A prime mover, **or agonist**, is responsible for producing a particular movement. Prime movers and their associated joints and movements are outlined in *Table 1-2* and *Figures 1-8* and *1-9*.
2. An **antagonist** is a prime mover that opposes the agonist.
3. A **synergist** assists the prime mover but is not the primary muscle responsible for the action.

E. CLINICAL IMPORTANCE

1. Identification of the superficial landmarks of some skeletal muscles and other anatomic structures is important for body composition and exercise testing.
2. In the upper body, identification and palpation of the **sternocleidomastoid**, **pectoralis major**, **biceps brachii**, and **triceps brachii** are of particular importance to exercise testing.
3. In the lower body, identification and palpation of the **gluteus maximus**, **quadriceps femoris**, and **gastrocnemius** are of particular importance to exercise testing.
4. An important landmark for skinfold measurement is the **inguinal crease**, which is a natural, diagonal crease in the skin formed where the musculature of the thigh meets the pelvic girdle.

V. THE CARDIOVASCULAR SYSTEM

A. HEART

The heart receives blood from the veins and propels it into the arteries. It is located near the center of the thoracic cavity and is divided into four chambers: right and left atria, and right and left ventricles. It is enclosed by connective tissues of the pericardium in the mediastinum.

1. Anatomy

a. The **atria** lie superior to the **ventricles**.
b. The **coronary sulcus** marks the border between the atria and the ventricles.
c. The atria have thin muscular walls and, when not filled with blood, are called **auricles**.
d. The ventricles have thicker muscular walls.
e. The **interventricular sulcus** marks the boundary between the left and right ventricles.
f. The great veins and arteries of the circulatory system are connected to the base of the heart.
g. The **apex** lies inferiorly at the tip of the heart.

2. Internal Anatomy

a. The right atrium receives blood from the systemic circulation through the **superior and inferior venae cavae**.

TABLE 1-2. MUSCLES THAT ARE PRIME MOVERS

JOINT	MOVEMENT	MUSCLE(S) (PORTION)
Shoulder	Abduction	Deltoid (middle), supraspinatus
	Adduction	Latissimus dorsi, pectoralis major, teres major, posterior deltoid
	Extension	Latissimus dorsi, pectoralis major (sternal), teres major, deltoid (posterior)
	Horizontal extension	Deltoid (posterior), infraspinatus, latissimus dorsi, teres major, teres minor
	Hyperextension	Latissimus dorsi, teres major
	Flexion	Deltoid (anterior), pectoralis major (clavicular)
	Horizontal flexion	Deltoid (anterior), pectoralis major
	Lateral rotation	Infraspinatus, teres minor
	Medial rotation	Latissimus dorsi, pectoralis major, teres major, subscapularis
Shoulder girdle	Abduction (protraction)	Pectoralis minor, serratus anterior
	Adduction (retraction)	Rhomboids, trapezius (middle fibers)
	Depression	Pectoralis minor, subclavius, trapezius (lower fibers)
	Elevation	Levator scapulae, rhomboids, trapezius (upper fibers)
Scapula	Upward rotation	Serratus anterior, trapezius (upper and lower fibers)
	Downward rotation	Pectoralis minor, rhomboids
Elbow	Flexion	Biceps brachii, brachialis, brachioradialis
	Extension	Triceps brachii
Radioulnar joint	Supination	Supinator, biceps brachii
	Pronation	Pronator quadratus, pronator teres
Wrist	Abduction (radial flexion)	Flexor carpi radialis, extensor carpi radialis longus, extensor carpi radialis brevis
	Adduction (ulnar flexion)	Flexor carpi ulnaris, extensor carpi ulnaris
	Extension/hyperextension	Extensor carpi radialis longus, extensor carpi radialis brevis, extensor carpi ulnaris
	Flexion	Flexor carpi radialis, flexor carpi ulnaris, palmaris longus
Trunk	Flexion	Rectus abdominus, internal oblique, external oblique
	Extension	Erector spinae, multifidus
	Lateral flexion	Internal oblique, external oblique, quadratus lumborum
	Rotation	Internal oblique, external oblique, multifidus, rotatores
Hip	Abductors	Gluteus medius, piriformis
	Adductors	Adductor brevis, adductor longus, adductor magnus, gracilis, pectineus
	Extensors	Biceps femoris, gluteus maximus, semimembranosus, semitendinosus
	Flexors	Iliacus, pectineus, psoas major, rectus femoris
	Lateral rotation	Gemelli, gluteus maximus, obturator externus, obturator internus
	Medial rotation	Gluteus medius, gluteus minimus
Knee	Extension	Rectus femoris, vastus intermedius, vastus lateralis, vastus medialis
	Flexion	Biceps femoris, semimembranosus, semitendinosus
Ankle	Extension (plantarflexion)	Gastrocnemius, soleus
	Flexion (dorsiflexion)	Extensor digitorum longus, peroneus tertius, tibialis anterior
Foot (intertarsal)	Eversion	Peroneus brevis, peroneus longus, peroneus tertius
	Inversion	Flexor digitorum longus, tibialis anterior, tibialis posterior

b. **Coronary veins** return venous blood from the myocardium to the **coronary sinus**, which opens into the right atrium.

c. Each atrium communicates with the ventricle on the same side by way of an **atrioventricular (AV) valve**. The right AV valve is a **tricuspid valve**; the **left AV valve** is a **bicuspid (mitral) valve**.

d. Each cusp is braced by **chordae tendineae, which are connected to papillary muscles.**

e. Unoxygenated blood leaving the right ventricle flows through the right semilunar **(pulmonic)** valve to the pulmonary artery.

f. Oxygenated blood leaving the left ventricle flows through the left semilunar **(aortic)** valve to the aorta.

3. Circulation Through the Heart (Physiology)

a. **Blood from the periphery** flows through the heart according to the following sequence: superior and inferior venae cavae, right atrium, tricuspid valve, right ventricle, pulmonic semilunar valve, pulmonary arteries, and lungs.

b. **Blood from the lungs** flows through the heart according to the following sequence: left pulmonary vein, left atrium, bicuspid valve, left ventricle, aortic semilunar valve, ascending aorta, and systemic circulation.

B. CIRCULATORY SYSTEM

1. Blood Vessels

a. Arteries

Arteries are muscular-walled vessels that carry blood away from the heart, decrease

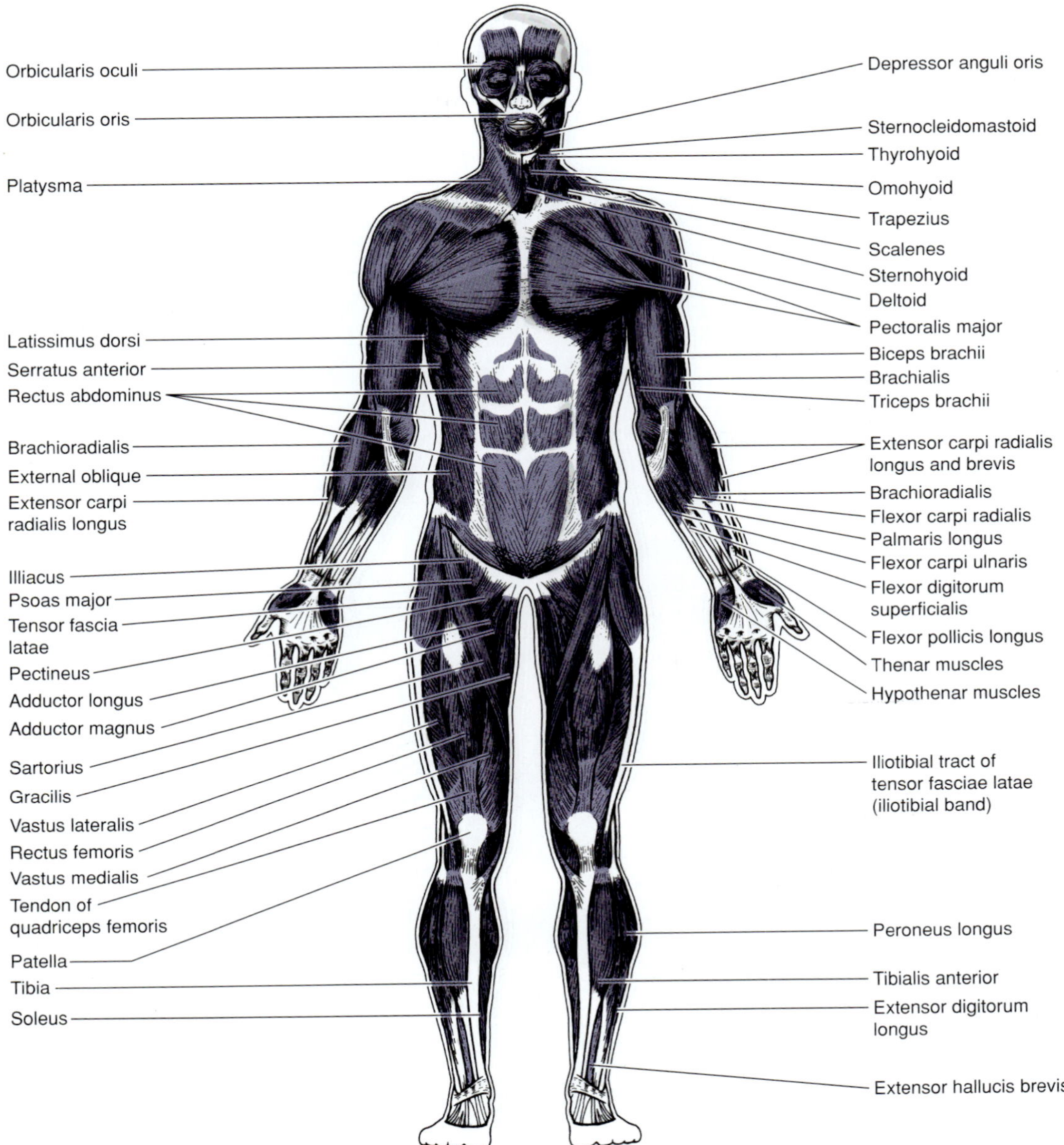

FIGURE 1-8. Anterior superficial muscles of the human body.

progressively in size to become **arterioles**, and then connect to capillaries.

b. Capillaries
Capillaries are vessels composed of one cell layer that functions to exchange nutrients and waste materials between the blood and tissues.

c. Veins
Veins are vessels that carry blood toward the heart, and they are classified according to size.

1) **Venules** are small veins that carry blood from the capillaries to medium-sized veins.
2) Medium-sized veins are larger in diameter than small veins and they empty into large veins.
3) Large veins include the two **venae cavae**.

2. Blood flow

a. The heart circulates oxygenated blood through arteries to arterioles to capillaries.
b. At the capillaries, blood delivers oxygen and nutrients to the tissues and carries waste products away.
c. Deoxygenated blood returns to the capillaries and travels to venules and then to veins, which return blood to the heart.

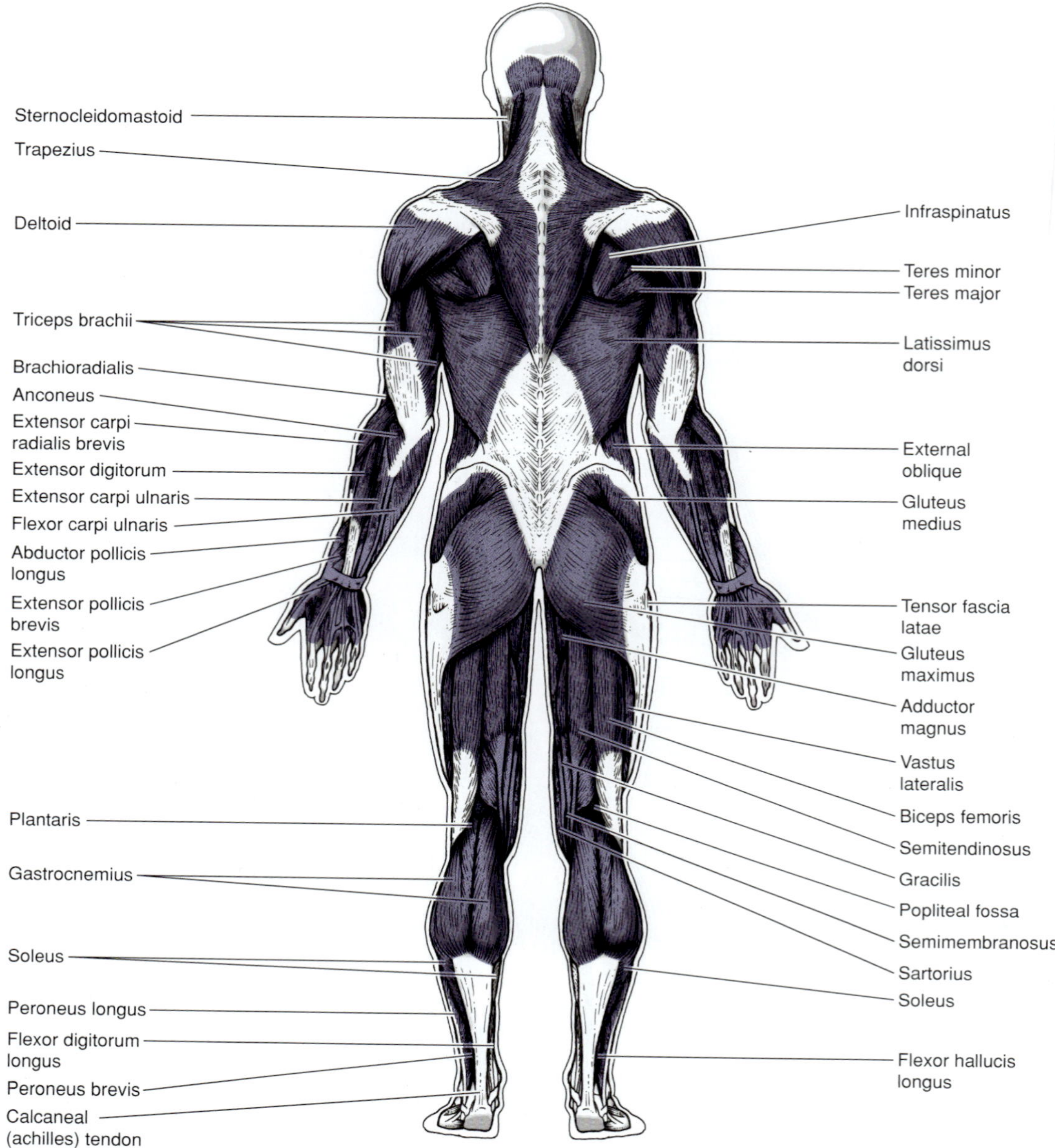

FIGURE 1-9. Posterior superficial muscles of the human body.

VI. THE RESPIRATORY SYSTEM

A. DIVISIONS

1. The **upper respiratory tract** consists of the **nose** (including the nasal cavity) and paranasal sinuses, the **pharynx**, and the **larynx**.
2. The **lower respiratory tract** consists of the **trachea** and the **lungs**, which include the **bronchi**, **bronchioles**, and **alveoli**.

B. LUNGS

Lungs are organs of respiration where oxygenation of blood occurs. They occupy the **pleural cavities** and are covered by a **pleural membrane**.

1. The **right lung** has three distinct lobes: superior, middle, and inferior.
2. The **left lung** has two lobes: superior and inferior.
3. The **apex** of each lung extends into the base of the neck above the first rib.
4. The **base** of each lung rests on the **diaphragm**, which is the respiratory muscle that separates the thoracic from the abdominopelvic cavities.

C. AIR FLOW AND GAS EXCHANGE

1. Air enters the respiratory system through two external **nares** and proceeds through the **nasal cavity** and **sinuses**.

   a. Air is **warmed, filtered, and moistened** before entry into the nasopharynx at the internal nares.
   b. **Cilia** line the nasal cavity and function to sweep mucus and to trap microorganisms.
2. The incoming air then passes through the **pharynx.**
   a. The pharynx extends between the internal nares and the entrances to the **larynx and esophagus.**
   b. The pharynx is shared by the digestive and respiratory systems.
3. Incoming air leaving the pharynx passes through a narrow opening in the larynx called the **glottis.** Air movement causes the vocal cords to vibrate, generating sound.
4. From the larynx, incoming air enters the **trachea.**
   a. The trachea extends from the larynx into the lungs.
   b. **C-shaped cartilages** of the trachea perform several functions.
      1) Protect, support, and maintain an open airway.
      2) Prevent overexpansion of the respiratory system.
      3) Allow large masses of food to pass along the esophagus.
5. Air enters the **lungs** via the **tracheobronchial tree,** which consists of the **bronchi, bronchioles, and alveoli.**
   a. The trachea branches to form the right and left **primary bronchi.**
   b. Each primary bronchus enters a lung and branches into **secondary bronchi.**
   c. Further branching forms smaller, narrower passages that terminate in units called **bronchioles. Variation in the diameter of the bronchioles** controls the resistance to air flow and ventilation of the lungs.
   d. **Terminal bronchioles,** the smallest branches, supply air to the **lobules** of the lung.
   e. The lobules consist of **alveolar ducts and alveoli,** where actual **gas exchange** occurs. **Alveoli** are one-cell-layer thick and have an abundance of capillaries on the outer surface.

VII. APPLIED ANATOMY

Knowledge of basic surface anatomy is essential in assessing pulse rate and blood pressure, obtaining anthropometric measurements, determining ECG lead placements, and performing CPR and emergency defibrillation.

A. ASSESSMENT OF PULSE RATE

Pulse is a measurement of heart rate. It can be palpated on any large- or medium-sized artery (most commonly the carotid, brachial, or radial) by using a fingertip to compress the vessel and sense the pulse *(Figure 1-10).*

1. The **carotid artery** runs along the trachea as the **common carotid.** At approximately the level of the mandible, the common carotid bifurcates to the **external and internal carotid arteries.** The carotid artery can be palpated inferior to the mandible and lateral to the larynx in the groove between the trachea and the sternocleidomastoid muscle.
2. The **brachial artery** runs along the medial side of the upper arm between the biceps brachii and triceps brachii muscles to a point just distal of the elbow joint. The artery can be palpated in the groove between the biceps and triceps or, more commonly, at the medial antecubital space on the frontal aspect of the elbow.
3. The **radial artery** divides from the brachial artery and continues distally along the forearm on the radial (thumb) side. The radial artery is palpable at the distal lateral wrist immediately superior to the thumb.

B. ASSESSMENT OF SYSTEMIC ARTERIAL BLOOD PRESSURE

1. Reflects hemodynamic factors (e.g., cardiac output, peripheral vascular resistance, blood flow).
2. Is **an indirect measurement of the pressure inside an artery** caused by the force exerted (by the blood) against the vessel wall.
3. Is usually measured in the arm over the brachial artery, medial to the biceps tendon, **using a sphygmomanometer and a stethoscope.**
4. In **blood pressure measurement,** the arterial reference indicator on the cuff is placed over the brachial artery. The bottom of the cuff is located approximately 1 inch above the antecubital space, and the stethoscope is positioned in the medial antecubital space *(Figure 1-11).*

C. ASSESSMENT OF ANTHROPOMETRIC MEASURES

1. Skinfold Measurements

Because of the assumed relationship between subcutaneous fat and total body fat, skinfold measurements are a common method of **estimating body fat percentage.** Various skinfold sites may be measured using skinfold calipers *(Figure 1-12).*

   a. **Chest/pectoral**: diagonal fold, half the distance between the anterior axillary line and

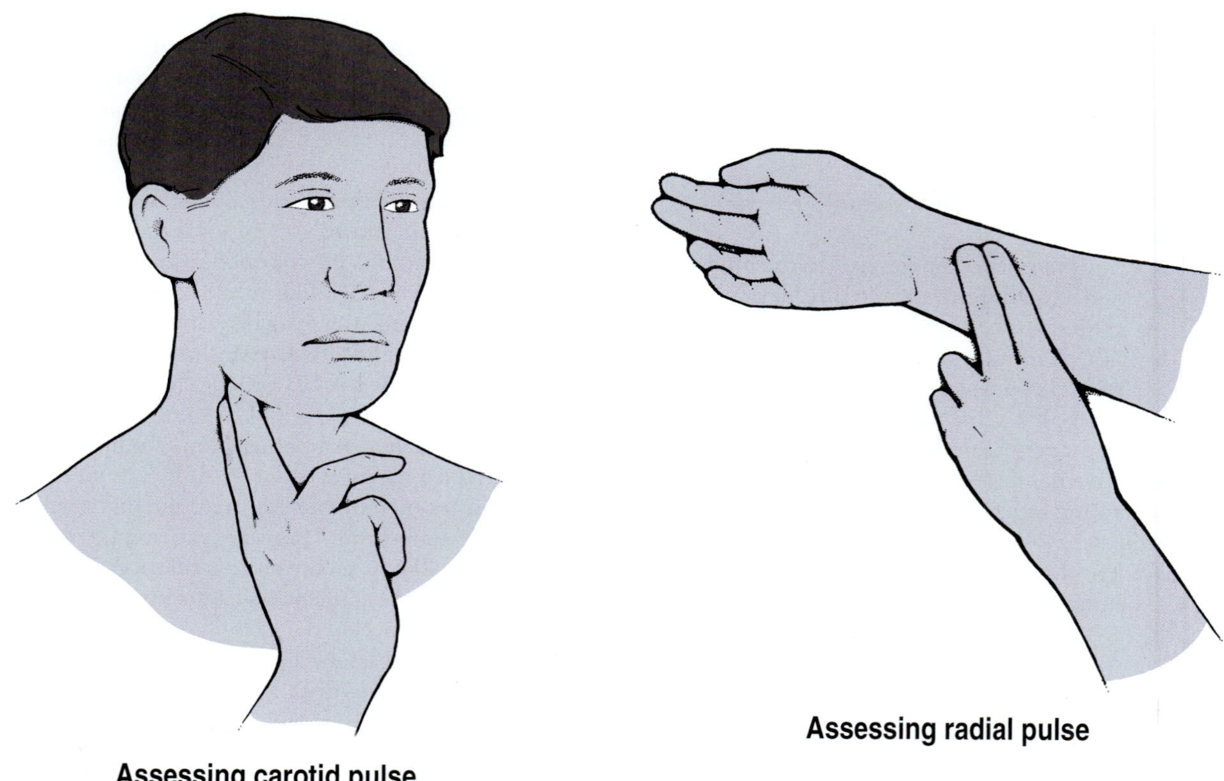

FIGURE 1-10. Assessing carotid and radial pulses. (Adapted from *ACSM's Resource Manual for Guidelines for Exercise Testing and Prescription,* 6th ed. Baltimore, Williams & Wilkins, 2010, p. 287.)

the nipple in men or a third of this distance in women.

b. **Midaxillary**: vertical fold, on the midaxillary line at the level of the xiphoid process.
c. **Abdominal**: vertical fold, 2 cm to the right of the umbilicus.
d. **Suprailiac**: diagonal fold, on the anterior axillary line immediately superior to the natural line of the iliac crest.
e. **Subscapular**: diagonal fold (45° angle), 1 to 2 cm inferior to and along the line of the inferior angle of the scapula.
f. **Triceps brachii**: vertical fold, on the posterior midline of the upper arm midway between the acromion and olecranon processes.
g. **Biceps brachii**: vertical fold, on the anterior arm over the belly of the muscle, 1 cm above the triceps brachii site.
h. **Thigh**: vertical fold, on the anterior midline of the thigh midway between the inguinal crease and superior patellar border.
i. **Calf**: vertical fold, at the midline of the medial border of the calf at the greatest circumference.

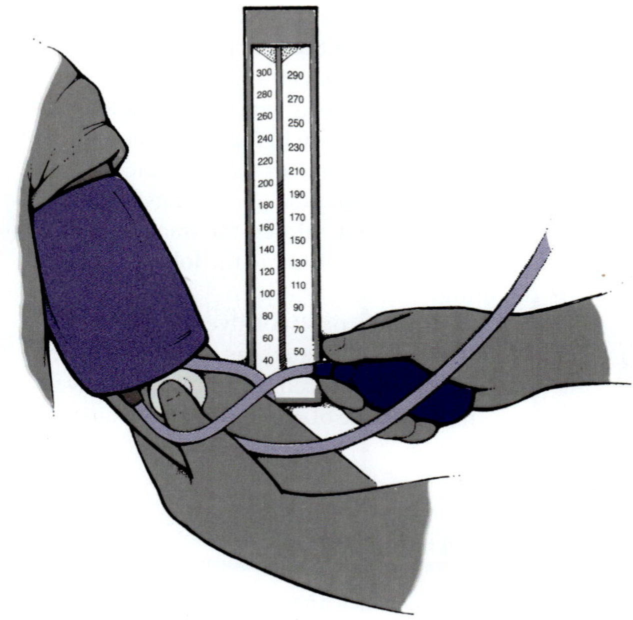

FIGURE 1-11. Measurement of blood pressure. (Adapted from *ACSM's Resource Manual for Guidelines for Exercise Testing and Prescription,* 6th ed. Baltimore, Williams & Wilkins, 2010, p. 287.)

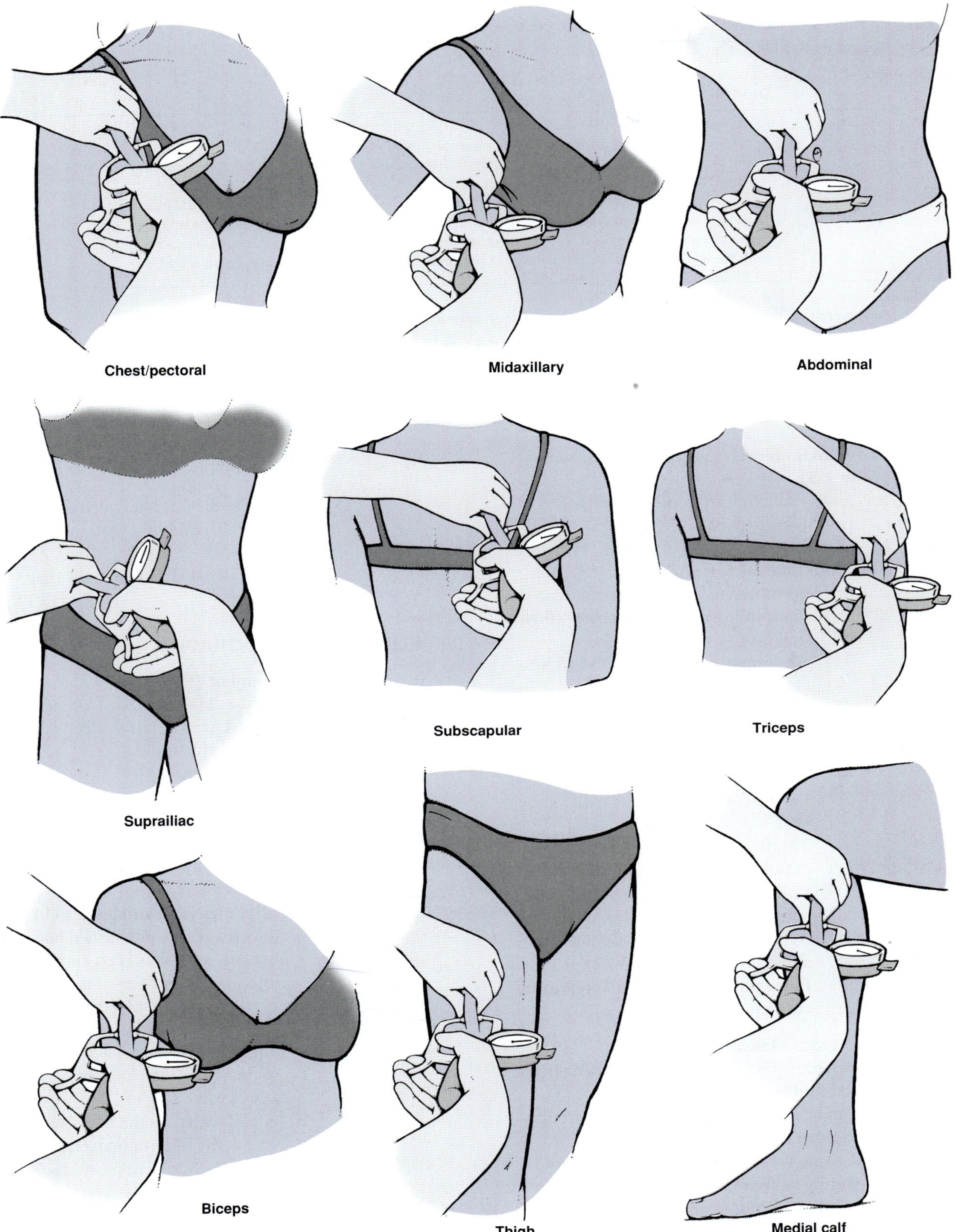

FIGURE 1-12. Obtaining skinfold measurements. (Adapted from *ACSM's Resource Manual for Guidelines for Exercise Testing and Prescription,* 6th ed. Baltimore, Williams & Wilkins, 2010, p. 288.)

TABLE 1-3. STANDARDIZED DESCRIPTION OF CIRCUMFERENCE MEASUREMENT SITES AND PROCEDURES

CIRCUMFERENCE SITE	DESCRIPTION
Abdomen	At the level of the umbilicus
Calf	Between the knee and the ankle, at the maximal circumference
Forearm	At the maximal forearm circumference, palms facing forward with the arms hanging downward, but slightly away from the trunk
Hips	Above the gluteal fold, at the maximal circumference of the hips or buttocks, whichever is larger
Arm	Midway between the acromion and olecranon processes, with the arm to the side of the body
Waist	At the narrowest part of the torso (superior to the umbilicus and inferior to the xiphoid process)
Thigh	With the legs slightly apart, at the maximal circumference of the thigh (below the gluteal fold)

Procedures

- All limb measurements should be taken on the right side of the body using a tension-regulated tape
- The subject should stand erect but relaxed
- Place the tape perpendicular to the long axis of the body part in each case
- Pull the tape to proper tension without pinching skin
- Take duplicate measures at each site and retest if duplicate measurements are not within 7 mm or 0.25 inch

(Modified from *ACSM's Guidelines for Exercise Testing and Prescription, 8th ed.*, Baltimore, Williams & Wilkins, 2010, Box 4.1, p. 65.)

2. **Body Circumferences or Girth Measurements *(Table 1-3)***
   a. Assess the **circumferential dimensions** of various body parts.
   b. Provide an indication of **growth, nutritional status, and fat patterning.**
   c. Are determined using a **tape measure.**
   d. Involve the following common sites (*Figure 1-13*):
      1) **Abdomen:** at the level of the umbilicus.
      2) **Waist:** at the narrowest part of the torso, inferior to the xiphoid process and superior to the umbilicus.
      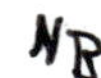
      3) **Hip:** at the maximal circumference of the hips or buttocks, above the gluteal fold.
      4) **Thigh:** at the maximal circumference of the thigh, below the gluteal fold.
      5) **Calf:** at the maximal circumference between the knee and ankle joint.
      6) **Arm:** midway between the acromion and olecranon processes.
      7) **Forearm:** at the maximal forearm circumference.

3. **Body Width Measurements**
   a. Provide information for determining **frame size and body type.**
   b. Can be used **to estimate desirable weight** based on stature.
   c. Are measured using **spreading calipers, sliding calipers, or an anthropometer.**
   d. Involve the following common sites:
      1) **Elbow:** the distance between the lateral and medial epicondyles, with the elbow flexed to 90°.
      2) **Biacromial:** the distance between the acromion processes.
      3) **Knee:** the distance between the lateral and medial condyles, with the knee flexed to 90°.
      4) **Bi-iliac:** distance between the iliac crests.

D. ELECTROCARDIOGRAPHY

1. **ECG Lead Placement *(Figure 1-14)***
   a. The **standard or Mason-Likar 12-lead system** uses 10 electrodes: 4 limb electrodes and 6 precordial electrodes.
      1) Limb Electrodes
         a) **Right arm (RA) and left arm (LA) electrodes** are positioned just inferior to the distal ends of the right and left clavicle, respectively.
         b) **Right leg (RL) and left leg (LL) electrodes** are positioned just superior to the iliac crest along the midclavicular line.
      2) **Precordial (or "V") Electrodes**
         a) **V_1 and V_2** are positioned at the fourth intercostal space on the right and left sternal border, respectively.
         b) V_4 is located on the midclavicular line at the fifth intercostal space.
         c) V_3 is positioned at the midpoint between V_2 and V_4.
         d) **V_5 and V_6** are positioned on the anterior axillary line and midaxillary line, respectively, both at the level of V_4.

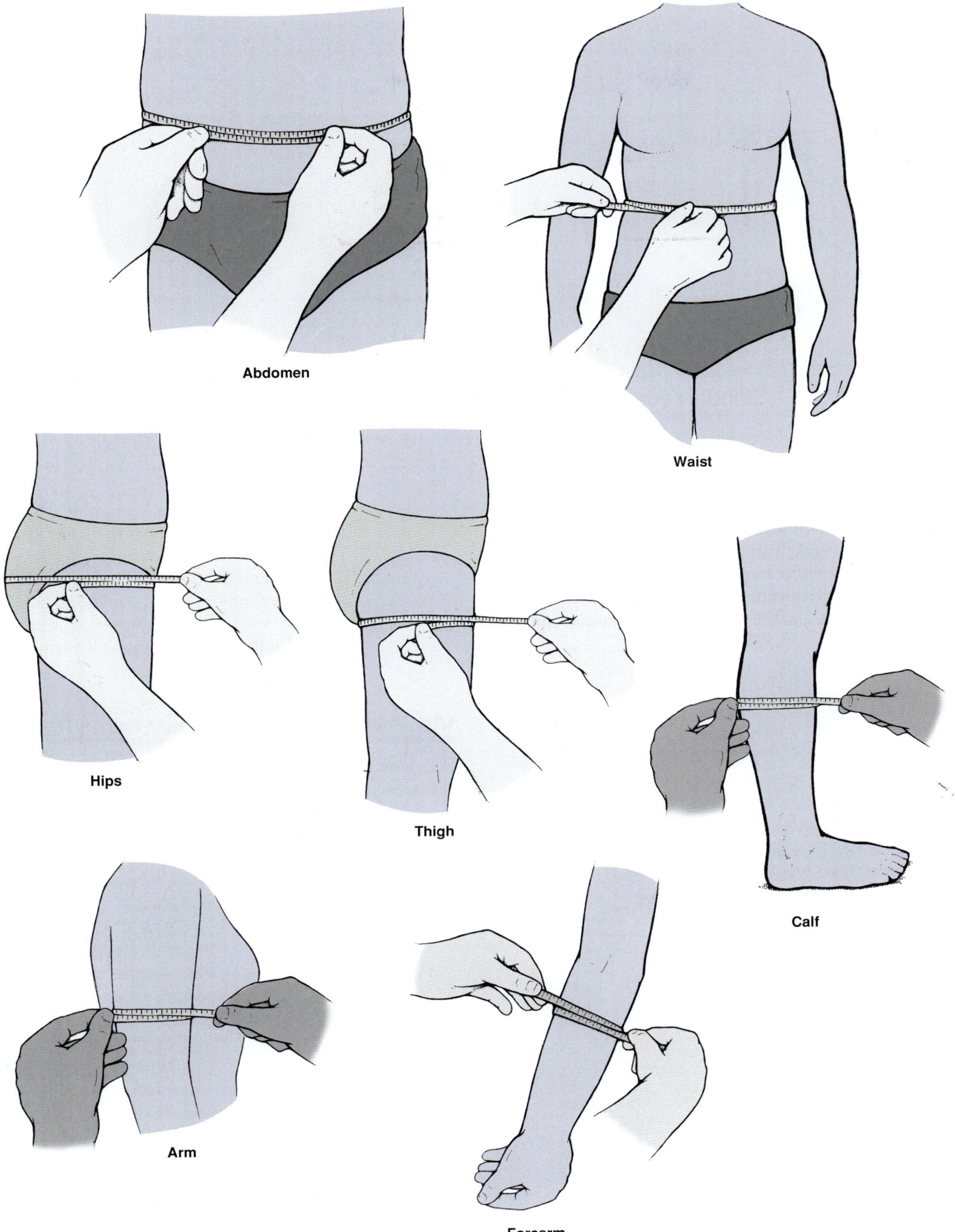

FIGURE 1-13. Measuring body circumferences. (Adapted from *ACSM's Resource Manual for Guidelines for Exercise Testing and Prescription,* 3rd ed. Baltimore, Williams & Wilkins, 1998, pp. 97–99.)

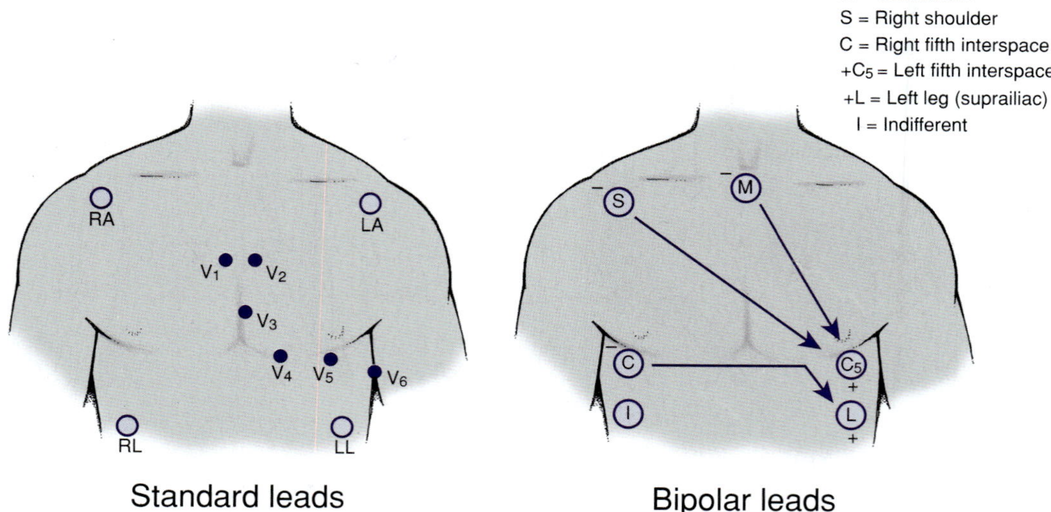

FIGURE 1-14. ECG lead placement. (Adapted from *ACSM's Resource Manual for Guidelines for Exercise Testing and Prescription,* 6th ed. Baltimore, Williams & Wilkins, 2010.)

b. **Bipolar Electrodes**
Electrode placement for the bipolar leads can take various configurations. Electrodes may be placed at the manubrium, the right fifth intercostal space at the anterior axillary line, and the standard electrode placements of RA, RL, LL, and V_5.

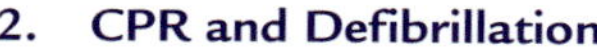

2. **CPR and Defibrillation**
   a. In **CPR**, chest compressions are done with the hand on the sternal body, at the xiphoid. The middle finger is placed on the xiphoid notch with the index finger next to it. The heel of the opposite hand is then placed superior to the index finger *(Figure 1-15)*.

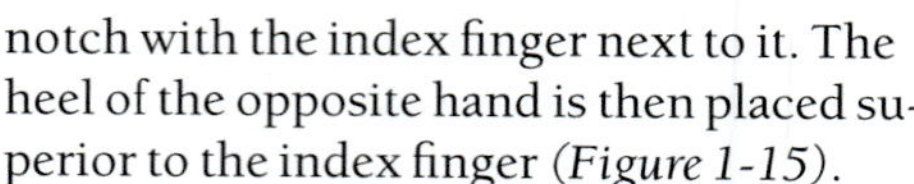

   b. The upper electrode for **defibrillation** is placed just inferior to the clavicle and to the right of the sternum. The lower electrode is located at the midaxillary line just lateral to the left nipple *(Figure 1-16)*.

VIII. PRINCIPLES OF BIOMECHANICS

For movement to occur, a net force must be present. **Biomechanics** is the study of the forces and torques affecting movement and the description of the resulting movement.

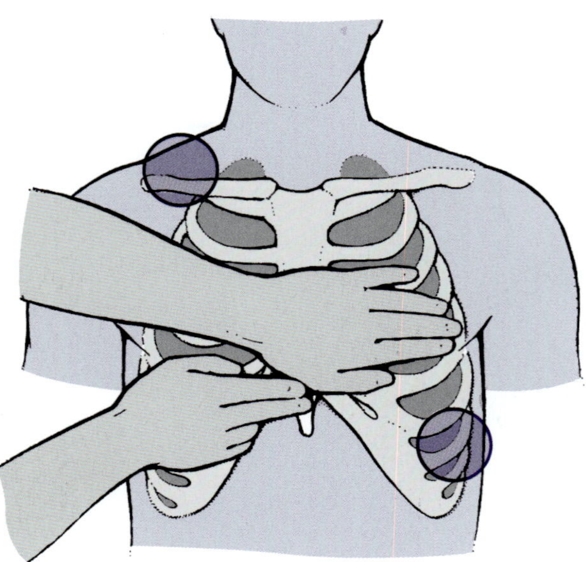

FIGURE 1-15. Hand positions for cardiac compression in CPR. (Adapted from *ACSM's Resource Manual for Guidelines for Exercise Testing and Prescription,* 6th ed. Baltimore, Williams & Wilkins, 2010.)

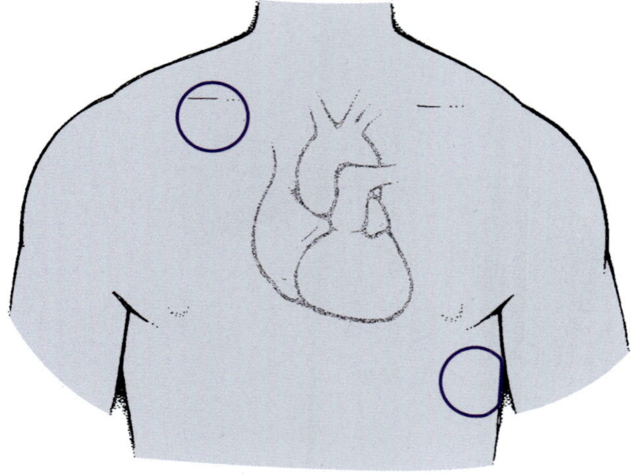

FIGURE 1-16. Standard placement for defibrillation electrodes. (Adapted from *ACSM's Resource Manual for Guidelines for Exercise Testing and Prescription,* 6th ed. Baltimore, Williams & Wilkins, 2010.)

A. FORCES

1. A **force** can be thought of as a push or a pull that either produces or has the capacity to produce a change in motion of a body.
2. Multiple forces from multiple directions can act on a body. The sum of these forces, or the **net force**, determines the resulting change in motion.

B. NEWTON'S LAWS

The relationships between forces, torques, and the resulting movements were described by Sir Isaac Newton (1642–1727). Three laws describe the interactions:

1. The **law of inertia** states that a body will maintain its state of rest or uniform motion in a straight line unless acted on by an external force.
2. The **law of acceleration** states that the acceleration of a body resulting from an applied force will be proportional to the magnitude of the applied force, in the direction of the applied force, and inversely proportional to the mass of the body. The formula for acceleration is

$$a = F/m$$

where

F = force
m = mass
a = acceleration

3. The **law of reaction** states that when two bodies interact, the force exerted by the first body on the second is met by an equal and opposite force exerted by the second body on the first. In other words, **for every action, there is an equal and opposite reaction.**

C. FORCES AFFECTING MOVEMENT

The forces influencing movement can be classified as reaction, friction, and muscular.

1. Ground Reaction Force

a. In accordance with **Newton's law of reaction**, as a body applies a force to the ground, the ground applies an equal and opposite force to the body.
b. Ground reaction forces are measured with a force plate in **three directions**: vertical, anteroposterior, and mediolateral. The net effect of the three-dimensional forces determines the resulting movement.
c. **Typical patterns** of ground reaction force are seen in **walking and running** (*Figure 1-17*).
d. **Abnormalities in gait** can be assessed by evaluating ground reaction force patterns.

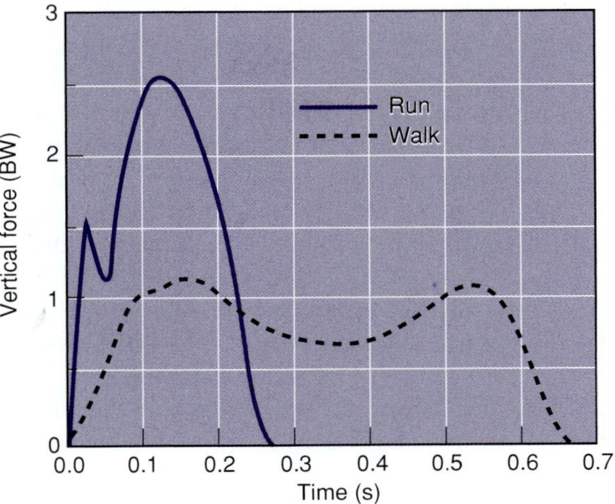

FIGURE 1-17. Vertical ground reaction forces during walking and running.

2. Frictional force

a. When two objects interact, **friction** acts parallel to the surface contact of the objects in a direction opposite the motion or impending motion (*Figure 1-18*).
b. **Frictional force** (Ff) is influenced by the nature and interaction of the contacting surfaces (the coefficient of friction, m) and the force pressing the surfaces together (the normal force, N). The formula for frictional force is

$$Ff = mN$$

3. Muscular Force

a. To move body segments, muscular forces must be present. Muscles provide a **pulling force on bone**. Across any joint, the net

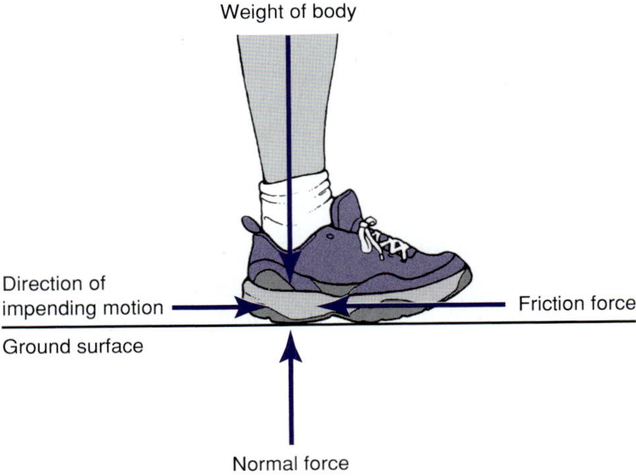

FIGURE 1-18. Friction force during foot contact of a running stride. (Adapted from *ACSM's Resource Manual for Guidelines for Exercise Testing and Prescription*, 6th ed. Baltimore, Williams & Wilkins, 2010.)

effect of individual muscle forces acting across the joint determines the joint movement.

b. Because all segmental movement is rotational, both the net muscular force and **the distance the force acts from the rotational axis of the joint** influence movement. **Torque** is the rotary effect of force produced by a muscle or a group of muscles.

c. Also affecting movement are the **length of the muscle at the time of contraction** and the **velocity of muscle shortening.**

d. **Normal movement patterns** result from the coordinated actions of the muscles acting across a joint.

e. **Abnormal movement patterns** result from disruptions in the coordinated muscular actions because of the application of inappropriate force, co-contraction of musculature, muscular weakness, or neurologic disorders affecting muscular recruitment.

D. PRINCIPLES OF BALANCE AND STABILITY

Each segment of the body is acted on by the **force of gravity** and has a **center of gravity.**

1. Line of Gravity (LOG)

Line of gravity is the downward direction of the force of gravity on an object (vertically, toward the center of the earth).

2. Center of Gravity (COG)

a. Is the **point of exact center around which the body freely rotates.**

b. Is the **point around which body weight is equal on all sides.**

c. Is the **point of intersection of the three cardinal body planes.**

d. Lies approximately anterior to the second sacral vertebra when all segments of the body are combined and the body is considered to be a single, solid object (in **anatomic position**).

e. Changes as the segments of the body move away from the anatomic position.

3. Base of Support (BOS)

Base of support is the area of contact between the body and the supporting surface.

4. Balance and Stability

a. **Balance** is maintained when the COG remains over the BOS.

b. **Stability** is firmness of balance; the COG must fall within the BOS.

1) **Increased stability** occurs when COG is closer to the BOS.

2) For **maximal stability**, the COG should be placed over the center of the BOS.

E. APPLIED WEIGHTS AND RESISTANCES

1. The ability of any force to cause rotation of a lever is known as **torque.**

2. **Rotation** of a segment of the body is dependent on:

a. The magnitude of force exerted by the **effort force and the resistance force.**

b. The **distance of these two forces from the axis of rotation.**

3. Moving the COG of segments alters resistive torque. **Changing the torque provides a method for altering the difficulty of an exercise when weight is applied** (*Figure 1-19*).

a. Weight applied at the end of an extended arm changes the COG of the arm to a more distal position, requiring greater muscular support to maintain the arm in a horizontal position. Conversely, by shifting the mass of the weight proximally, less muscular effort is required.

b. Some externally applied forces (e.g., exercise pulleys) do not act in a vertical direction, and those **forces exert effects that vary according to the angle of application.**

c. Weights applied to the extremities frequently exert traction **(distractive force)**

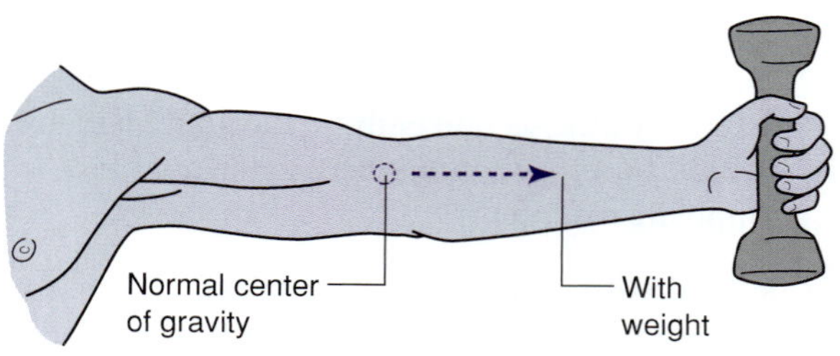

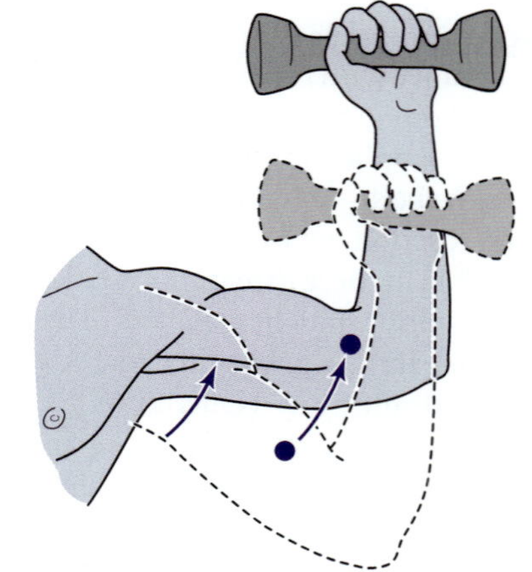

FIGURE 1-19. A change in center of gravity changes the torque.

on joint structures. A distractive force is sometimes used to promote normal joint movement in rehabilitation exercise, but distractive force can also be injurious or undesirable.

F. MOTION

1. Translatory Motion

a. Occurs when a freely movable object moves in a straight line when a force is applied on the center of the object.
b. Occurs when, regardless of where the force is applied, the object is free to move in a rectilinear or a curvilinear path.

2. Rotary Motion

a. Occurs when a force is applied off center to a freely movable object.
b. Occurs when, regardless of where the force is applied, the object is free to move only in a rotary path.

3. Velocity

a. **Velocity** represents the distance traveled in a period of time.
b. **Acceleration** refers to increasing velocity.
c. **Deceleration** refers to decreasing velocity.

4. Momentum

Momentum is the mathematical product of the mass and velocity of a moving object.

G. LEVERS

A lever is a rigid bar that **revolves around a fixed point or axis (fulcrum)**. Levers are **used with force to overcome a resistance**.

1. Parts of a Lever

a. The **axis** is the pivot point between the force and the resistance.
b. The **force arm** is the distance from the axis to the point of application of force.
c. The **resistance arm** is the distance from the axis to the resistance.

2. Classes of Levers *(Figure 1-20)*

a. In a **first-class lever**, the axis is between the force and the resistance arm, and the force arm may be greater than, smaller than, or equal to the resistance arm.
b. In a **second-class lever**, the resistance lies between the effort force and the axis of rotation, and the force arm is greater than the resistance arm.
c. In a **third-class lever**, the effort force lies closer to the axis of the lever than the resistance, and the force arm is smaller than the resistance arm.
d. When the principles of levers are actually applied in the body, the joint serves as the axis, the contraction of skeletal muscles around the joint serves to generate the force, and the moving segment (including anything supported by that segment) is the resistance.

IX. APPLICATION OF BIOMECHANICAL PRINCIPLES TO ACTIVITY

A. WALKING

1. Normal Walking Gait

a. **Locomotion** occurs from repetition of the **gait cycle**, which is the time between successive ground contacts of the same foot *(Figure 1-21)*.
   1) A **stride** is the time between ground contacts of the right heel. **Stride length** is measured from initial contact of one lower extremity to the point at which the same extremity contacts the ground again.
   2) Half of a stride is a **step**, defined as the time from ground contact of one heel to ground contact of the other heel.
   3) Normally, 60% of the gait cycle is in **stance** (foot in contact with the ground), and 40% is in **swing** (foot not in contact with the ground).
b. Typical **walking speed** in adults is approximately 1.5 m/s. Decreases in walking speed occur with aging, injury, and disease.
c. A typical stride length, or **cycle length (CL)**, is approximately 1.5 m, and a typical stride rate, or **cycle rate (CR)**, is approximately 1 cycle/s. With increasing gait speed, CL and CR increase.
d. In the frontal plane, **pelvic movement** during walking is approximately 5 cm on each side, alternating as each leg assumes a support role. In the transverse plane, the pelvis rotates a total of 8° , half of it anteriorly and half of it posteriorly.
e. In a normal walking gait, the vertical **ground reaction force** pattern is bimodal in shape and of maximal magnitude on the order of 1- to 1.2-fold the body weight. The two peaks represent heel contact to midstance and midstance to push-off.

2. Phases of the Gait Cycle

During a single gait cycle, each extremity passes through two phases.

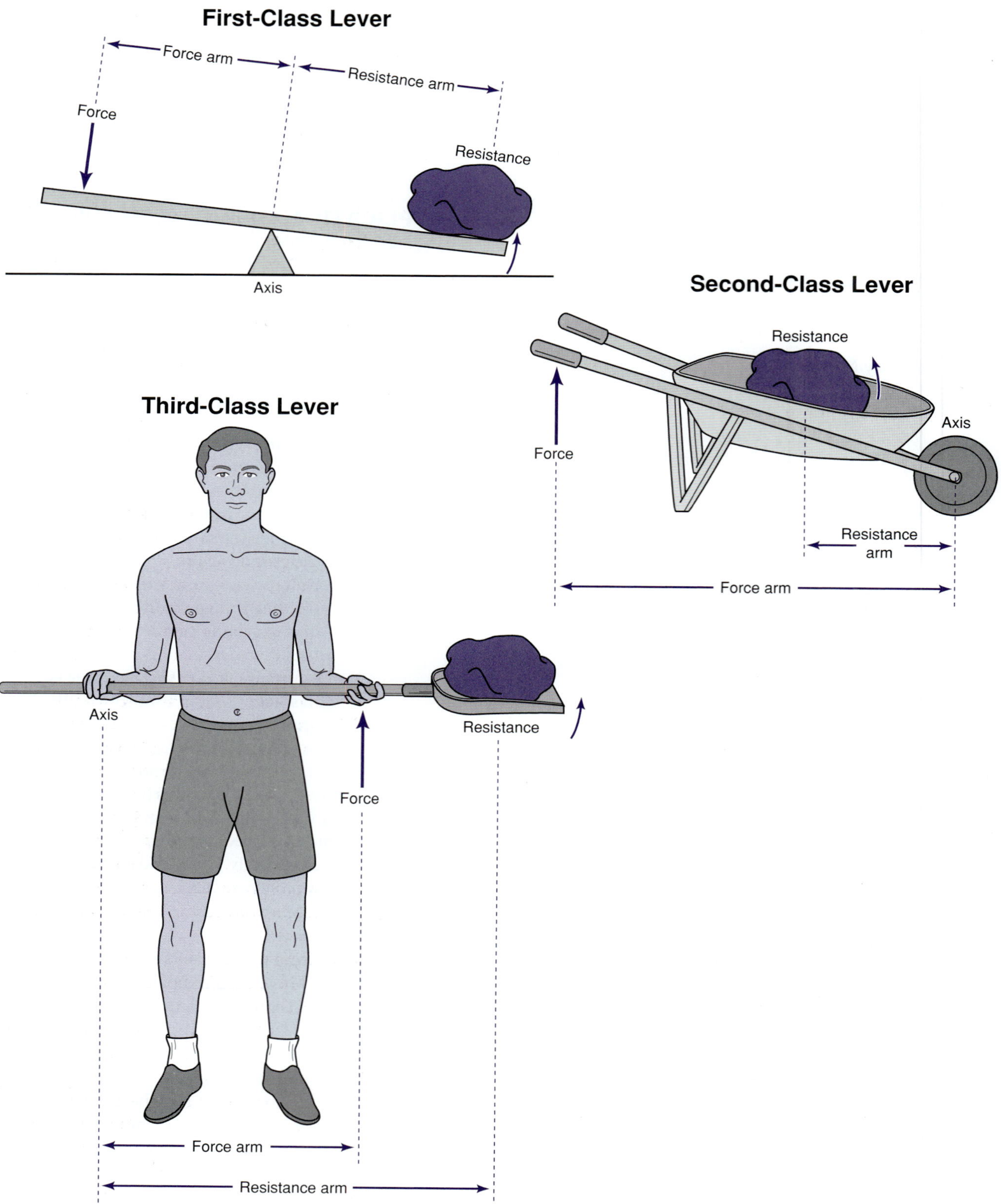

FIGURE 1-20. Lever systems.

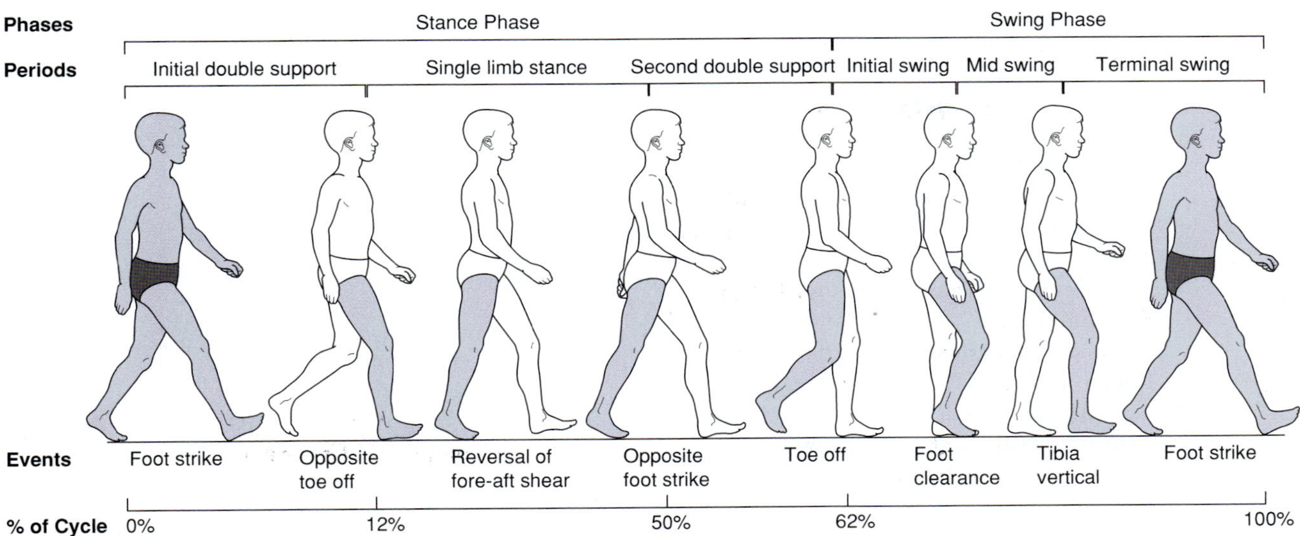

FIGURE 1-21. Normal walking gait cycle. (Adapted from Rose J, Gamble JG [eds]: *Human Walking*, 2nd ed. Baltimore, Williams & Wilkins, 1994, p. 26.)

a. Stance Phase
   1) Begins when one extremity contacts the ground (heel strike).
   2) Continues as long as some portion of the foot is in contact with the ground (toe off).
   3) Subdivisions of the Stance Phase
      a) **Heel strike.**
      b) **Foot flat.**
      c) **Midstance.**
      d) **Heel off.**
      e) **Toe off.**

b. Swing Phase
   1) Begins when the toe of one extremity leaves the ground.
   2) Ends just before heel strike or contact of the same extremity.
   3) Subdivisions of the Swing Phase
      a) **Initial swing (acceleration).**
      b) **Midswing.**
      c) **Terminal swing (deceleration).**

3. Abnormal Walking Gait

Deviations from a normal walking gait occur for various reasons (e.g., pain from injury, decreased flexibility or range of motion) and take many different forms. **Common causes of gait abnormalities** include muscular weakness and neurologic disorders.

a. Muscular Weakness
   1) **Weakness in the gluteus maximus** can contribute to an anterior lean of the upper body at heel strike.
   2) **Weakness in the gluteus medius and minimus** decreases their stabilizing function during the stance phase of gait, possibly leading to an increased lateral shift in the pelvis (increased frontal plane movement) and side-to-side movement during gait.
   3) Severe **weakness in the plantarflexors** reduces push-off and thus step length on the affected side.
   4) **Dorsiflexor insufficiency** results in slapping of the foot during heel contact (foot drop) and increased knee and hip flexion during the swing phase.
   5) Because of the inability to adequately support loads or control knee extension, **weakness of the quadriceps femoris** can lead to forward lean of the trunk or hyperextension of the knee joint (genu recurvatum).

b. Neurologic Disorders
   1) In **hemiplegia**, the affected leg is often circumducted during the swing phase and the affected arm is held across the upper body with flexion in the elbow, wrist, and hand.
   2) **Parkinsonism** can produce a characteristic gait pattern of increased hip and knee flexion, forward trunk lean, and shuffling step.

B. RUNNING

1. Normal Running Gait

Running differs from walking in several ways.

a. **Running requires greater balance** because of the absence of a double support period and the presence the "flight phase" when both feet are out of contact with the supporting surface.

b. **Running requires greater muscle strength** because of many muscles contracting more rapidly and with greater force.

c. **Running requires greater range of motion** because of greater joint angles at the extremes of the movement.

d. The **direction of the driving force is more horizontal** and the **stride is longer.**

e. The body has a **greater forward incline.**

f. **Rotary actions** of the spine and pelvic regions **are increased.**

g. **Arm actions are higher and more vigorous.** (The arms should move in an anterior/posterior direction to improve efficiency.)

h. **Stride length and frequency are increased** with increasing speed.

i. The normal running gait is similar to the walking gait but with the addition of a **flight phase**, during which both feet are off the ground.

j. **CL** and **CR** are related to running speed:

$$\text{velocity} = \text{CL} \times \text{CR}$$

Up to approximately 5 m/s, CL increases with speed, and CR stays relatively constant or increases slightly. Increases in speed beyond 5 m/s generally result from increased CR.

k. At running speeds up to 6 m/s, vertical **ground reaction forces** are between two- and threefold the body weight. These forces are realized at heel strike as an impact peak and during push-off as an active peak.

2. Abnormal Running Gait

As with walking, running gait disorders are difficult to generalize because of their complexity and varying manifestations. Most common problems associated with running involve rear foot motion during heel strike and push-off.

a. Pronation
   1) A combination of abduction, eversion, and dorsiflexion, pronation is greatest at midstance and can be affected by running speed and by shoe hardness and design.
   2) Some degree of pronation is helpful in reducing impact forces, but excessive and very rapid pronation is undesirable. Shoe wear patterns in overpronators show medial wear.

b. **Supination**
   1) Supination is a combination of adduction, inversion, and plantarflexion.
   2) Excessive supination (marked by excessive shoe wear on the lateral side) at take-off may impair running performance because of misdirection of propulsive forces.

C. SWIMMING

1. Buoyancy

a. Is the tendency of a body to float when submerged in a fluid.

b. Is **dependent on the percentage of weight composed of bone and muscle**, because these tissues are more dense (and, therefore, less buoyant) than other body tissues such as fat.

c. According to **Archimedes' principle**, a body immersed in fluid is buoyed up with a force equal to the weight of the displaced fluid.

2. Propelling Forces

a. Result from the **stroke and kick.**

b. Should contribute to **forward progress**, not to vertical or lateral movement.

c. During the propelling phase, the arms, hands, and feet should present a large

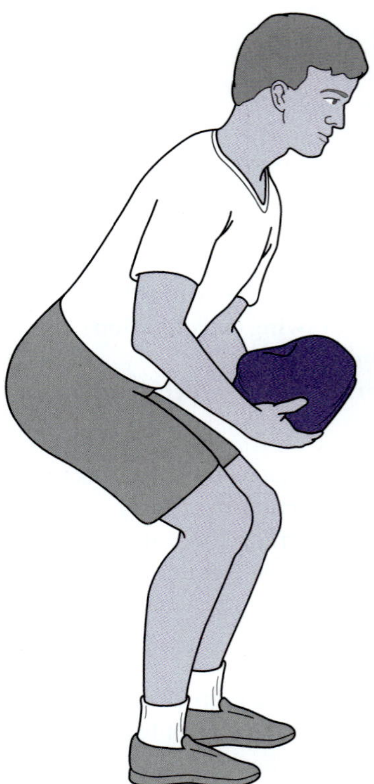

FIGURE 1-22. Power position of the body.

surface to the water and should push against the water.

3. **Resistive Forces**
   Resistive forces result from:
   a. Skin resistance (friction).
   b. Wave-making resistance caused by up-and-down body movement.
   c. Eddy current resistance.

D. LIFTING AND BODY MECHANICS

1. In applying the laws of motion to lifting, reaching, pushing, pulling, and carrying of objects, the effects of gravity, friction, muscular forces, and external resistance are important.
2. The **basic principles of good body mechanics** are:
   a. **Assume a position close to the object**, or move the position of the object closer to the COG, allowing the use of upper extremities in a shortened position (short lever arms). Lower torque is required, thus allowing muscles to function more efficiently.
   b. **Likewise, position COG as close to the object's COG as possible**, reducing torque and energy requirements.
   c. **Widen the BOS** by lowering the COG and maintaining the COG within the BOS.
   d. **Position the feet according to the direction of movement** required to perform the activity, thus increasing stability.
   e. **Avoid twisting** when lifting.
   f. When possible, **push, pull, roll, or slide an object** rather than lift it.
   g. **Use the "power position"** (*Figure 1-22*).
      1) Knees slightly bent.
      2) Body bent forward from the hips.
      3) Back straight.
      4) Chest and head upright.

Review Test

DIRECTIONS: Carefully read all questions, and select the BEST single answer.

1. The maintenance of an open airway during esophageal distention is provided by what structure?
   A) Trachea.
   B) Pharynx.
   C) Larynx.
   D) Epiglottis.

2. Producing red blood cells, protecting organs and tissues, and providing support for the body are all functions of what tissue?
   A) Collagen.
   B) Muscle.
   C) Tendon.
   D) Bones.

3. Which of the following is a contractile protein in skeletal muscle?
   A) Myosin.
   B) Fascicle.
   C) Myofibril.
   D) Muscle fiber.

4. Which type of bone consists of a central cylindrical shaft, or diaphysis, and has an epiphysis at each end?
   A) Short bone.
   B) Long bone.
   C) Flat bone.
   D) Irregular bone.

5. Which of the following movements decreases the joint angle and occurs in a sagittal plane around a mediolateral axis?
   A) Circumduction.
   B) Rotation.
   C) Flexion.
   D) Extension.

6. Which of the following muscle groups is a prime mover for extension of the knee?
   A) Biceps femoris.
   B) Biceps brachii.
   C) Quadriceps femoris.
   D) Gastrocnemius.

7. A baseball pitcher complains of weakness in the lateral rotation motions of the shoulder. Which of the following muscles would you advise him to strengthen?
   A) Subscapularis.
   B) Teres major.
   C) Latissimus dorsi.
   D) Teres minor.

8. Cartilage is categorized as which of the following types of connective tissue?
   A) Loose.
   B) Dense.
   C) Fluid.
   D) Supporting.

9. Through which valve in the heart does blood flow when moving from the right atrium to the right ventricle?
   A) Bicuspid valve.
   B) Tricuspid valve.
   C) Pulmonic valve.
   D) Aortic valve.

10. Which of the following is considered an abnormal curve of the spine with lateral deviation of the vertebral column in the frontal plane?
    A) Lordosis.
    B) Scoliosis.
    C) Kyphosis.
    D) Primary curve.

11. Which of the following is considered to be a "ball-and-socket" joint?
    A) Ankle.
    B) Elbow.
    C) Knee.
    D) Hip.

12. Which of the following terms describes the ability of a force to cause rotation of a lever?
    A) Center of gravity.
    B) Base of support.
    C) Torque.
    D) Stability.

13. Which of the following is a standard site for the measurement of skinfolds?
    A) Medial thigh.
    B) Biceps.
    C) Infrailiac.
    D) Forearm.

14. Which of the following is a standard site for the measurement of circumferences?
    A) Abdomen.
    B) Neck.
    C) Wrist.
    D) Ankle.

15. Which of the following is the most common site used for measurement of the pulse during exercise?
    A) Popliteal.
    B) Femoral.
    C) Radial.
    D) Dorsalis pedis.

16. Blood flows from the peripheral anatomy to the heart through the superior and inferior venae cavae into which of the following chambers?
    A) Right atrium.
    B) Left atrium.
    C) Right ventricle.
    D) Left ventricle.

17. Which blood vessel is composed of one cell layer and functions to exchange nutrients and waste materials between blood and tissues?
    A) Capillary.
    B) Arteriole.
    C) Venule.
    D) Vein.

18. Which of the following statements most accurately represents the law of inertia?
    A) A body at rest tends to remain at rest, whereas a body in motion tends to continue to stay in motion with consistent speed and in the same direction unless acted on by an outside force.
    B) The velocity of a body is changed only when acted on by an additional force.
    C) The driving force of the body is doubled and the rate of acceleration is also doubled.
    D) The production of any force will create another force that will be opposite and equal to the first force.

19. Why does running require greater muscular strength as compared with walking?
    A) Because of the absence of the double support period.
    B) Because of greater joint angles at the extremes of movement.
    C) Because of the greater forward incline that occurs during running.
    D) Because of greater number of muscles contracting more rapidly and with greater force.

20. Who first described that a body immersed in fluid is buoyed up with a force equal to the weight of the displaced fluid?
    A) Einstein.
    B) Freud.
    C) Whitehead.
    D) Archimedes.

21. Which of the following bones articulates proximally with the sternal manubrium and distally with the scapula and is helpful to palpate in electrode placement?
    A) Scapula.
    B) Sternum.
    C) Clavicle.
    D) Twelfth rib.

22. In regard to lifting and proper body mechanics, what position is described when the knees are slightly flexed and the body is bent forward from the hips with the back remaining straight and the chest and head up?
    A) Ready position.
    B) Power position.
    C) Center of gravity position.
    D) Base of support position.

23. The intervertebral disks have which of the following characteristics?
    A) Calcified outer ring.
    B) Gelatinous inner nucleus portion.
    C) Gray matter surrounding the neural cell bodies.
    D) Actin and myosin proteins.

24. Which of the following will increase stability?
    A) Lowering the center of gravity.
    B) Raising the center of gravity.
    C) Decreasing the base of support.
    D) Moving the center of gravity farther from the edge of the base of support.

25. Which type of musculoskeletal lever is most common?
    A) First-class.
    B) Second-class.
    C) Third-class.
    D) Fourth-class.

26. What type of motion occurs when a force is applied off center to a freely movable object?
    A) Rotary.
    B) Translatory.
    C) Angular.
    D) Transverse.

27. Which of the following is a characteristic of a second-class lever?
    A) Axis is located between the effort force and the resistance.
    B) Resistance is located between the effort force and the axis.
    C) Effort force is located between the resistance and the axis.
    D) Force arm may be greater than, or equal to the resistance arm.

28. Which of the following muscle groups is most likely weak when slapping of the foot during heel strike and increased knee and hip flexion during swing are observed?
   A) Gluteus medius and minimus.
   B) Quadriceps femoris.
   C) Plantarflexors.
   D) Dorsiflexors.

29. Which of the following is characteristic of running versus walking?
   A) Less vigorous arm action.
   B) Decreased stride length.
   C) Period of nonsupport.
   D) Period of double-support.

30. The rear-foot motion called **pronation** results from a combination of
   A) Abduction, eversion, and plantarflexion.
   B) Adduction, inversion, and plantarflexion.
   C) Abduction, eversion, and dorsiflexion.
   D) Adduction, inversion, and dorsiflexion.

ANSWERS AND EXPLANATIONS

1–A. The C-shaped cartilages of the trachea provide a certain rigidity to support the trachea and maintain an open airway so that collapse does not occur. In addition, the rigidity caused by these cartilages prevents overexpansion of the trachea when pressure changes occur in the respiratory system. The proximity of the trachea to the esophagus (the esophagus is posterior to the trachea) could cause obstruction to the airway if a large bolus of food is passed in the esophagus. This is remedied by the arrangement of the C-shaped cartilages of the trachea, with the open end of the C being posterior. Distention of the esophagus can occur without compromise to the airway.

2–D. The bones of the skeletal system act as levers for changing the magnitude and direction of forces that are generated by the skeletal muscles attaching to the bones. The bones of the skeletal system provide structural support for the body through their arrangement in the axial and appendicular skeletal divisions. The axial skeleton forms the longitudinal axis of the body and it supports and protects organs as well as provides attachment for muscles. The appendicular skeleton provides for attachment of the limbs to the trunk. Blood cells are formed in bone marrow.

3–A. The skeletal muscle consists of bundles of muscle fibers called muscle fascicles, or fasciculi. Each fasciculus contains muscle cells. Within the muscle cells are cylinders called myofibrils, which are responsible for the contraction of the muscle fiber. The myofibrils have this ability because they contain myofilaments, which are the contractile proteins, actin and myosin. Actin is a thin filament that is twisted into a strand. Myosin is a thick filament that has a tail and a head. During activation of the muscle, actin and myosin interact, causing crossbridging between the two filaments. The myosin pulls the actin, which shortens the muscle and causes tension development.

4–B. Most bones of the appendicular (rather than the axial) skeleton are long bones. Long bones have a central shaft (called the diaphysis) that is made of compact (dense) bone. The shaft forms a cylinder around a central cavity of the bone, which is called the medullary canal.

5–C. Angular movements decrease or increase the joint angle and include flexion, extension, abduction, and adduction. Circular movements can occur at joints having a bone with a rounded surface that articulates with a cup or depression on another bone. Included in circular movements are circumduction and rotation, including the specialized rotational movements of supination and pronation.

6–C. The quadriceps femoris muscle is the major muscle responsible for knee extension, as dictated by its proximal and distal attachments. The muscle has four heads (quad), three of which originate from the anterior portion of the ilium and one of which originates on the shaft of the femur. All four heads converge and insert on the tibia via a common tendon (patellar). Contraction of the muscle causes the knee to extend. The biceps brachii is found in the upper body and is an elbow flexor. Although the biceps femoris and gastrocnemius muscles cross the knee joint, they do so posteriorly and are primarily active in knee flexion and ankle plantarflexion, respectively.

7–D. The subscapularis, teres major, and latissimus dorsi are all medial rotators of the arm. They function as antagonists to the teres minor, which is a lateral rotator of the arm.

8–D. Cartilage and bone are found in the supporting connective tissue category. Connective tissues of the body are categorized according to specific characteristics of their ground substance. Connective tissue has many types of cells and fibers in a somewhat syrupy ground substance. Loose and dense connective tissues are of this type. Fluid connective tissue cells are suspended in a watery ground substance; included in this category are blood and lymph. Supporting connective tissues have a dense ground substance, with very closely packed fibers.

9–B. Blood from the peripheral anatomy flows to the heart through the superior and inferior venae cavae into the right atrium. From the right atrium, the blood passes through the tricuspid valve to the right ventricle, then out through the pulmonary semilunar valve to the pulmonary arteries, and then to the lungs to be oxygenated. The tricuspid valve is so named because of the three cusps, or flaps, of which it is made. The bicuspid valve is a similar valve, having only two cusps; it is found between the left atrium and left ventricle. Blood leaving the left ventricle will pass through the aortic semilunar valve to the ascending aorta and then out to the systemic circulation.

10–B. The vertebral column serves as the main axial support for the body. The adult vertebral column exhibits four major curvatures when viewed from the sagittal plane. Scoliosis is an abnormal lateral deviation of the vertebral column. Kyphosis is an abnormal increased posterior curvature, especially in the thoracic region. Lordosis is an abnormal, exaggerated anterior curvature in the lumbar region. A primary curve refers to the thoracic and sacral curvatures of the vertebral column that remain in the original fetal positions.

11–D. The ankle is a gliding joint that allows flexion, extension, inversion, and eversion. The shoulder and hip are both ball-and-socket joints, allowing circumduction, rotation, and angular motions. The knee is a hinge joint, allowing flexion and extension in only one plane.

12–C. Torque is the ability of any force to cause rotation of the lever. It is calculated as the product of the force and the perpendicular distance from the axis of rotation at which the force is applied. The center of gravity is the point of exact center around which the body freely rotates, the point around which the weight is equal on all sides, and the point of intersection of the three cardinal planes of the body. Balance is maintained when the center of gravity stays over the base of support, and stability is the firmness of balance.

13–B. The standard sites for the measurement of skinfold thicknesses include the abdominal, triceps, biceps, chest, medial calf, midaxillary, subscapular, suprailiac, and thigh (a measurement taken on the anterior midline of the thigh).

14–A. The standard sites for the measurement of body circumferences are the abdomen, calf, forearm, hips, arm, waist, and thigh.

15–C. The most common sites for measurement of the peripheral pulse during exercise are the carotid and radial arteries. These sites are more easily accessible during exercise than the femoral, popliteal, posterior tibial, or dorsalis pedis arteries.

16–A. Blood from the peripheral anatomy flows to the heart through the superior and inferior venae cavae into the right atrium. From the right atrium, blood passes through the tricuspid valve to the right ventricle and then out through the pulmonary semilunar valve to the pulmonary arteries and to the lungs to be oxygenated.

17–A. Arteries are large-diameter vessels that carry blood away from the heart. As they course through the body, they progressively decrease in size until they become arterioles, the smallest vessels of the arterial system. From the arterioles, blood enters the capillaries, which are one layer thick and function to exchange oxygen, nutrients and waste materials between the blood and tissues. Venules and veins return blood back to the heart.

18–A. The law of inertia states that a body at rest tends to remain at rest whereas a body in motion tends to continue in motion, with consistent speed and in the same direction, unless acted on by an outside force. The law of acceleration states that the velocity of a body is changed only when acted on by an additional force, that the driving force of the body is doubled, and that the rate of acceleration is also doubled. The law of counterforce states that the production of any force will create another force that will be opposite and equal to the first force.

19–D. Running is a locomotor activity similar to walking, but with some differences. In comparison with walking, running requires greater balance, muscle strength, and range of motion. Balance is necessary because of the absence of the double-support period and the presence of the float period in which both feet are out of contact with the supporting surface. Muscle strength is necessary because many muscles are contracting more rapidly and with greater force during running as compared with walking. Joint angles are at greater extremes with the running gait.

20–D. Archimedes first described the principle of buoyancy. If a body displaces water weighing more than itself, the body will float. When the lungs are filled with air, most individuals float in water. However, the ability to float is dependent on the percentage of weight that is composed of bone and muscle, because these tissues are denser than other body tissues.

21–C. The clavicle articulates with the sternum and scapula, which the twelfth rib does not do. Also, the location of the clavicle is helpful in placing electrodes for some ECG lead placements and defibrillation to avoid the large muscle mass in the area and to apply the shock in an appropriate location for effect.

22–A. The power position does not indicate a slouching of the shoulders; rather, it focuses on stabilization of the low back. The power position is to maintain a stable center of gravity and keep the load distributed effectively, which is why the head and neck are up, and so forth.

23–B. The intervertebral disk acts to absorb shock and bear weight for the spinal column and, therefore, has the gelatinous inner portion to absorb the forces experienced.

24–A. Lowering the center of gravity will increase stability. Stability would also be increased by increasing the size of the base of support, by moving the center of gravity closer to the center of the base of support, or both.

25–C. Third-class lever systems are those most commonly found in the musculoskeletal system. An example would be the arrangement of the biceps femoris: The insertion of the biceps femoris, which provides the effort force, is between the elbow joint (the axis) and center of gravity of the forearm (the resistance). Examples of first- and second-class levers can be found in the musculoskeletal system, but they are not common. There is no such thing as a fourth-class lever.

26–A. Rotary motion will occur with a freely movable object when a force is applied off-center; it will also result when a force is applied to an object that is free to move only in a rotary path. A force applied on-center to a freely movable object, or to an object that is free to move only on a linear path, will result in linear motion.

27–B. In a second-class lever system, the resistance is located between the effort force and the axis; thus, the effort force moment arm is greater than the resistance moment arm, providing an advantage for force. When the axis is between the effort force and the resistance, the result is a first-class lever. When the effort force is between the resistance and the axis, the result is third-class lever.

28–D. Dorsiflexor weakness leads to foot drop during heel strike. To ensure that the toe does not catch the walking surface, knee and hip flexion increases during swing. Weakness in the plantarflexors reduces push-off and, thereby, step length. Weakness in the gluteus medius and minimus decreases their stabilizing function during stance and can lead to increased lateral shift in the pelvis. Quadriceps weakness can lead to forward lean of the trunk or knee hyperextension.

29–C. Only running has a period of nonsupport, when both feet are off the ground. Walking has a period of double-support, when both feet are in contact with the ground. In addition, running has a more vigorous arm action and increased stride length compared with walking.

30–C. Pronation is a type of rear-foot motion that occurs during heel strike and push-off in running. Pronation results from a combination of abduction, eversion, and dorsiflexion. Although a certain amount of pronation is normal and helpful in reducing impact forces, excessive and very rapid pronation can lead to injury. The rear-foot motion called supination results from a combination of adduction, inversion, and plantarflexion.

Exercise Physiology

CHAPTER 2

I. BIOENERGETICS

The term "bioenergetics" refers to the body's ability to acquire, convert, store, and utilize energy. The immediate source of energy for all cellular activities, including muscle contraction, is **adenosine triphosphate (ATP)**. In releasing its energy, ATP is broken down to **adenosine diphosphate (ADP)**. Because only a limited amount of ATP is stored in the cell, ATP is replenished via other energy pathways, to replace ATP as it is utilized (e.g., during exercise).

A. PHOSPHAGEN SYSTEM

1. This energy pathway is composed of the ATP and **phosphocreatine (PCr)** stored in muscle fibers.
2. Through the activity of the enzyme **creatine kinase**, PCr yields its phosphate group so that it can be added to ADP to synthesize ATP.
3. Although immediately available for use by the working muscle, the phosphagen system is limited in its capacity to supply energy. During exercise of all-out effort, for example, stored ATP and PCr can sustain activity for no more than 30 seconds.

B. NONOXIDATIVE SYSTEM

1. This system is sometimes referred to as the "**anaerobic**" pathway because oxygen is not required for it to produce ATP.
2. In this system, only carbohydrates (glucose, glycogen) can be used to produce ATP.
3. In the absence of oxygen, the breakdown of carbohydrates yields **lactic acid**—more accurately referred to as lactate—which can contribute to muscle fatigue as it accumulates.
4. The nonoxidative system is the main provider of energy to the working muscle in athletic events lasting from 30 seconds to 3 minutes.

C. OXIDATIVE SYSTEM

1. This ATP-producing pathway is also called the "**aerobic**" system because oxygen is required for it to proceed.
2. Both carbohydrates and lipids (fats)—and even to a limited extent proteins—can be used to synthesize ATP by this pathway.
3. The metabolic by-products that result from **oxidative phosphorylation** are water and carbon dioxide, which have no fatiguing effects on working muscle.
4. In activities lasting more than 3 minutes, and where intensity is limited, muscles primarily rely on oxidative metabolism to produce ATP.
5. Although a prolific producer of ATP, this system is disadvantaged because it is relatively slow in synthesizing the ATP demanded by exercising muscle.
6. Moreover, should inadequate oxygen be delivered to the working muscle, it will also depend on the nonoxidative system to produce energy resulting in lactate accumulation.
7. The exercise intensity at which this occurs is referred to as the "**anaerobic threshold**" or the "**lactate threshold.**"

D. LONG-TERM EFFECTS OF EXERCISE TRAINING ON BIOENERGETIC PATHWAYS

1. Endurance training has been shown to increase the capacity of the oxidative system to produce ATP.
2. This is directly attributed to the increased mitochondrial density noted in muscle that has undergone prolonged endurance training. Indeed, it appears that as much as a doubling of mitochondrial content can occur in trained muscle, leading to a similar increase in the enzymes and other proteins involved in the oxidative synthesis of ATP.
3. Although endurance training does not increase the phosphagen content of muscle, it does amplify the storage of energy substrates (carbohydrates and lipids) used in the oxidative pathway. Glycogen, the form in which the body stores carbohydrates, is deposited in greater amounts both in the muscle and in the liver of well-trained athletes. In addition, lipid depots are more pronounced in aerobically trained muscle. In contrast, resistance training improves the capacity of the muscle to produce ATP anaerobically by increasing glycolytic enzymes used in that pathway along with the amount of glycogen stored in muscle.

II. SKELETAL MUSCLE

Skeletal muscle tissue has been specialized to move the bony levers of the skeletal system, thus enabling mobility—or movement—of the body. Other types of muscle in the body include **cardiac muscle**, which will be discussed later, and **smooth muscle**, which among other things assists in regulation of blood flow to various parts of the body. Among the three types, however, skeletal muscle is the most abundant; it accounts for nearly 50% of the human body's mass. As with all types of tissue, skeletal muscle is composed of individual cells. Skeletal muscle cells are typically termed "**myocytes**" or "**myofibers.**" The structure of these cells, and the manner in which they are arranged, yields insight into the mechanism of muscle function.

A. CONNECTIVE TISSUE

1. The **endomysium** is a layer of connective tissue that is found wrapped around each myofiber.
2. A group of as many as 150 myofibers lying in parallel are bundled together to form a **fasciculus**, which is encased by a layer of tissue called the **perimysium**.
3. The layer of connective tissue that surrounds the entire muscle is referred to as the **epimysium** (*Figure 2-1*).

B. MAJOR ORGANELLES

1. Unlike most cells, an individual myofiber contains more than one nucleus. Indeed, these multinucleated cells may possess 200–300 nuclei/mm of fiber length.
2. The endoplasmic reticulum—in muscle, termed the **sarcoplasmic reticulum**—is richly developed in the myofiber as the **calcium** it stores is needed to stimulate muscle contraction.
3. The plasma membrane of the myofiber is referred to as the **sarcolemma.** The voltage-gated sodium channels regularly distributed along the sarcolemma allow electrical stimulation of the myofiber via the generation of **action potentials.** As a result, myofibers are considered "excitable" cells.
4. Because muscle tissue demonstrates a high degree of metabolic activity, mitochondrial content is substantial in myofibers, providing much ATP via the oxidative pathway.

C. PROTEIN FILAMENTS

1. The contractile filaments **myosin** and **actin** account for approximately 60% of the protein content of the myofiber.
2. Myosin is the larger protein and is sometimes called the "thick filament."
3. Actin is the smaller of the contractile proteins and is termed the "thin filament."
4. In addition, regulatory filaments, **troponin** and **tropomyosin**, are essential in triggering the contractile event.

D. TYPES OF MUSCLE FIBERS

1. Although several different methods are used to classify myofibers, the most commonly one used is based on the isoform of myosin expressed by the cell.
2. In humans, the three myosin isoforms are type I, IIA, and IIX, which correspond to the fiber types of I, IIA, and IIB.
3. **Type I** fibers have slow twitch properties, but high oxidative capacity.
4. **Type IIB** myofibers are fast twitch with low oxidative potential.
5. **Type IIA** fibers are intermediate, both in twitch velocity and oxidative capacity.
6. Exercise of high intensity and short duration (e.g., sprinting) is principally powered by type II myofibers, whereas activities featuring low intensity and long duration (e.g., marathon running) are almost exclusively dependent on type I myofibers.

E. MECHANISM OF THE MYOFIBER TWITCH

1. Both regulatory and contractile filaments are essential to the generation of the myofiber twitch.
2. The force generated by the whole muscle is a function of both the number of myofibers within that muscle that are twitching and the rate at which these twitches occur.
3. The **sliding-filament theory** of muscle contraction explains how these protein filaments interact to produce a twitch of the fiber. The sequence of events is as follows:
   a. As the nervous system excites the myofiber's sarcolemma and its **transverse tubules** (T tubules), calcium stored within the sarcoplasmic reticulum is released into the cell's cytosol.
   b. Calcium binds to troponin, causing the associated tropomyosin to undergo a conformational shift (a change in shape).
   c. Because of this shift, "**active sites**" on the actin filament are exposed.
   d. **Cross-bridge** heads located on the myosin molecule bind to the exposed active sites of actin.
   e. The enzyme adenosine triphosphatase (**ATPase**), which is found on the cross-bridge head, cleaves ATP, resulting in the "power stroke" that pulls actin toward the center of the myosin molecule. This sliding action of the actin over myosin results in the fiber shortening and the force generation.

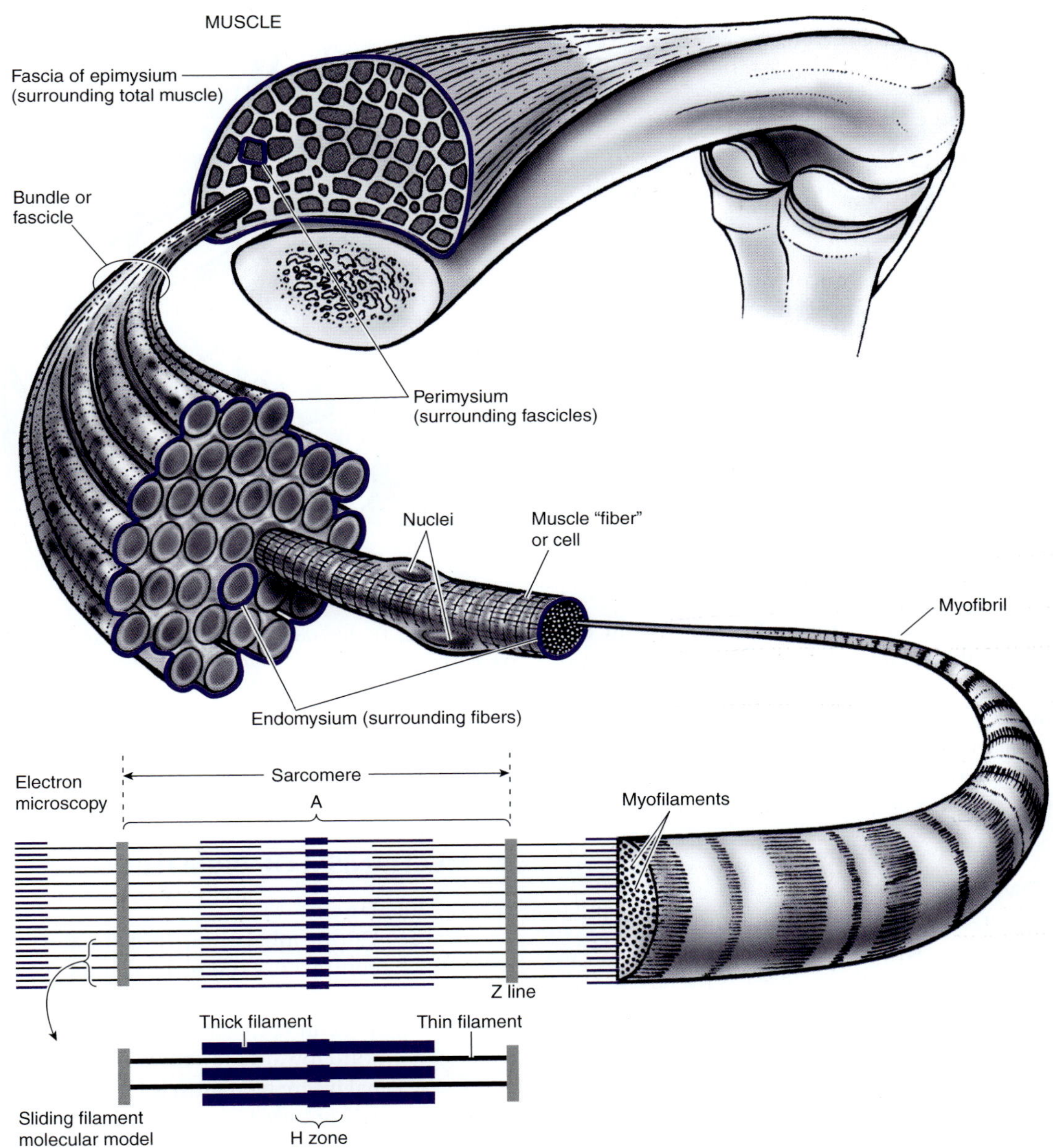

FIGURE 2-1. Cross-section of skeletal muscle and the arrangement of its connective tissue wrappings. (From *ACSM's Resource Manual for Guidelines for Exercise Testing and Prescription*, 5th ed. Baltimore, Lippincott Williams & Wilkins, 2006.)

f. When a new molecule of ATP binds to the myosin cross-bridge head, the link between myosin and actin is broken, allowing the entire process to repeat itself so long as cytosolic calcium levels remain elevated. The "**calcium pump**" is responsible for delivering cytosolic calcium back into the sarcoplasmic reticulum, thus returning the myofiber to a state of relaxation.

F. EXCITATION OF MYOFIBERS

1. Myofibers will contract only on stimulation by the nervous system. A single motor neuron and all of the myofibers that it innervates comprise what is referred to as a "**motor unit.**"
2. When stimulated, all of the myofibers of a motor unit contract simultaneously and at maximal force ("all or none").
3. All myofibers of a single motor unit are of the same type (i.e., I, IIA, or IIX).
4. A whole muscle is able to regulate its force production during contraction either by controlling the number of motor units that are activated or by varying the firing rate of neural impulses delivered by the motor neuron to its myofibers.

5. During maximal force output by a muscle, all of its motor units have been recruited and each one is firing at its highest possible rate.

G. LONG-TERM EFFECTS OF TRAINING ON MYOFIBERS

1. Any type of training, whether it is resistance or endurance training, will cause a conversion of type IIX fibers to type IIA.
2. In contrast, neither form of training (endurance or resistance) is capable of the more dramatic conversion between type I and type II myofibers. Prolonged resistance training will result in a significant increase in the size (hypertrophy) of myofibers, particularly those of the type II category. Endurance training, on the other hand, does not bring about myofiber hypertrophy.

III. THE PULMONARY SYSTEM

The pulmonary system allows the body to breathe by exchanging gases with the environment. During **inspiration** (inhalation), air is taken into the lungs and, during **expiration** (exhalation), air leaves the lungs to re-enter the environment. The purpose of inspiration is to bring needed oxygen into the body, whereas expiration serves to eliminate carbon dioxide—a by-product of metabolism—from the body.

A. ANATOMY

1. Air enters the pulmonary system through the mouth and nose.
   a. Inhaling through the nose has the advantages of warming the air and removing many air-borne particles that may cause irritation or infection.
   b. During exercise, however, breathing through the mouth is generally required to accommodate the increased rate and depth of ventilation.
2. Passageways through the nose and mouth join at the **pharynx** (throat).
3. Inhaled air then passes through the **larynx** before entering the cartilage-lined **trachea** (windpipe). The trachea then branches off to form two *bronchi*, each leading into one of the two lungs located within the thoracic cavity.
4. Within the lungs, the bronchi divide to form numerous **bronchioles**.
5. Located at the end of each bronchiole is a cluster of **alveoli**. Within these tiny air sacs gases are exchanged between the lungs and the blood traveling through the capillaries surrounding each alveolus (Figure 2-2).

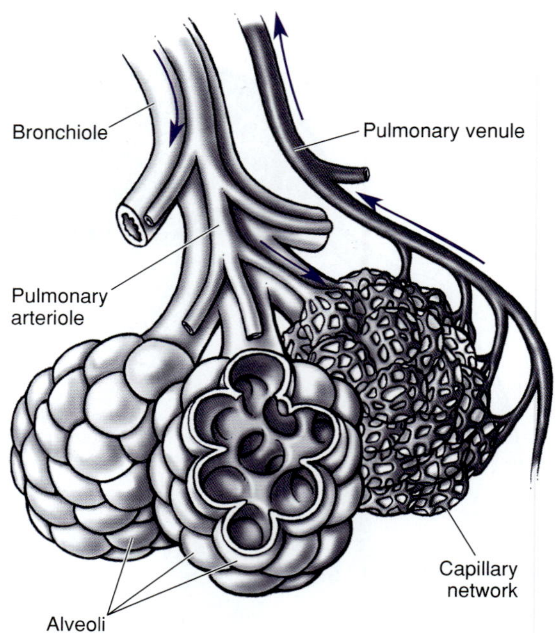

FIGURE 2-2. The functional respiratory unit. It consists of a bronchiole and corresponding blood supply; the pulmonary arteriole carries deoxygenated blood, and the pulmonary venule carries oxygenated blood. The rich capillary network supplies the alveoli for the purpose of gas exchange. (From *ACSM's Resource Manual for Guidelines for Exercise Testing and Prescription*, 5th ed. Baltimore, Lippincott Williams & Wilkins, 2006.)

B. MECHANISM OF BREATHING

1. Inhalation

a. During inhalation, the inspiratory muscles contract to expand the volume of the thoracic cavity.
b. To achieve this, the **diaphragm** moves downward toward the abdomen, while the external **intercostal muscles** pull the rib cage up and outward.
c. During exercise, when the depth of breathing increases, accessory inspiratory muscles (sternocleidomastoid, scalenus) also contribute to the expansion of the rib cage by lifting upward.

2. Exhalation

a. Under resting conditions, expiration is a passive process that involves the relaxation of the inspiratory muscles and consequent recoil of the thoracic cavity returning the lungs back to their original dimensions. This increases the pressure of the gases inside the lungs, forcing air out of the body through the nose and mouth.
b. During exercise, however, exhalation becomes an active process where the

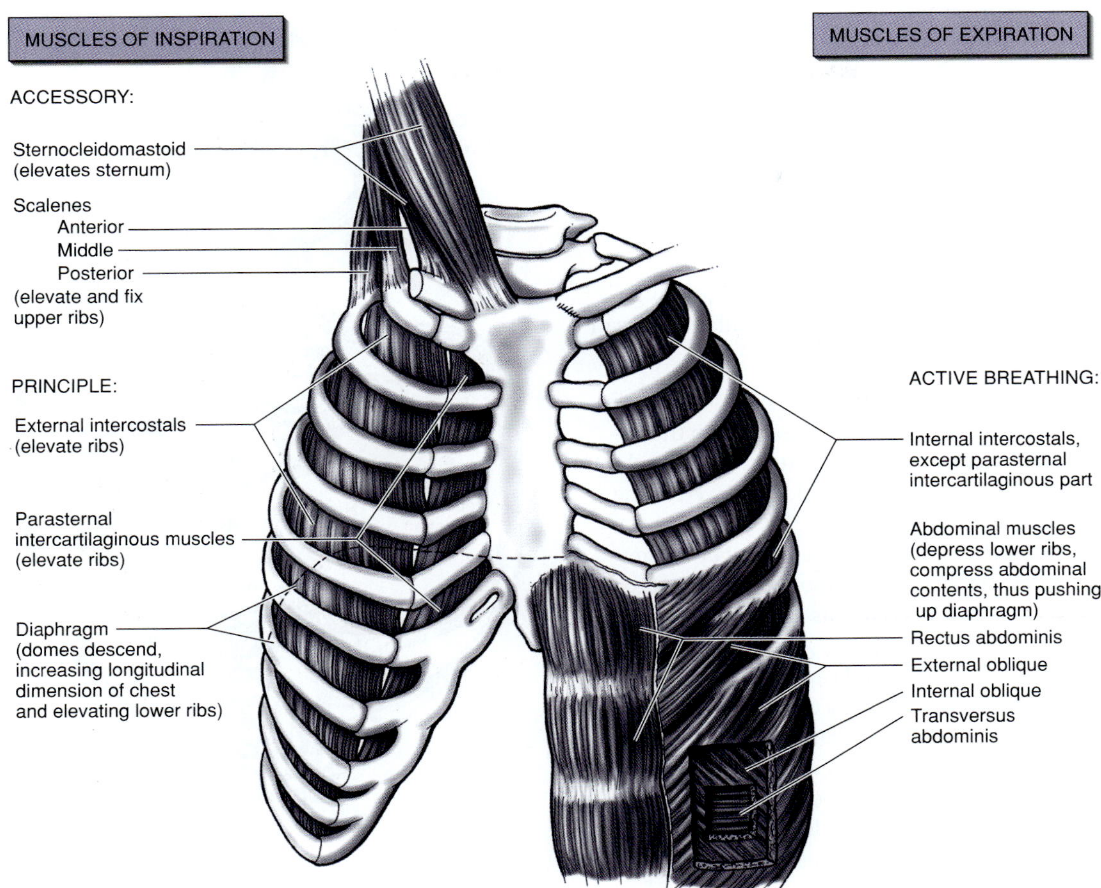

FIGURE 2-3. The major muscles of respiration. The principal inspiratory muscles, shown on the *left*, include the diaphragm, external intercostal muscles, and parasternal muscles. The principal expiratory muscles, shown on the *right*, include the internal intercostal muscles and the abdominal muscles (rectus, transverse, and internal and external oblique muscles). (From *ACSM's Resource Manual for Guidelines for Exercise Testing and Prescription*, 5th ed. Baltimore, Lippincott Williams & Wilkins, 2006.)

abdominal and internal intercostals muscles contract to more forcefully collapse the size of the thoracic cavity and drive air out of the lungs (Figure 2-3).

C. RESPONSES TO EXERCISE AND TRAINING

1. Minute ventilation ($\dot{V}_E$)

a. $\dot{V}_E$ is the volume of air either inspired, or expired over the course of 1 minute.

b. At rest, $\dot{V}_E$ is about 6 L/min.

c. Exercise results in an elevation of $\dot{V}_E$, and exercise intensity determines the degree of this increase. This increase in $\dot{V}_E$ occurs in two phases:

   1) Initially, there is a sharp increase in the depth of breathing (increased tidal volume).

   2) As the exercise stimulus becomes more intense, the rate of breathing substantially increases. A secondary, less pronounced increase in the depth of breathing becomes apparent.

d. During maximal intensity exercise, minute ventilation may be 20- to 25-fold higher than the typical 6 L/min that is observed under resting conditions.

   1) This response is a consequence of both an increment in **tidal volume**—the amount of air entering or leaving the lungs in a single breath—from 0.5 L to about 4 L, as well as an increase in **respiratory rate** from 12/min to almost 50/min.

   2) Accordingly, the relative energy demand required to support this exercise-induced increase in ventilation also rises. At rest, about 3% of the body's energy expenditure is accounted for by breathing, and during moderate intensity exercise

this figure varies between 3% and 5%.

3) At maximal intensity exercise, however, the work of breathing accounts for approximately 10% of total oxygen consumption among untrained individuals, and it may be as high as 15% in highly trained athletes.

e. In healthy individuals, exercise capacity is not limited by ventilation, nor does long-term exercise training induce adaptations in ventilatory capacity.

2. Ventilatory Adaptations

a. Training adaptations are evident in the exercise intensity at which anaerobic threshold occurs. This threshold is viewed as the exercise intensity at which ATP demand by working muscles can no longer be met solely by aerobic metabolism, and anaerobically produced ATP is needed to satisfy demand.

b. Anaerobic threshold can be indirectly assessed by identifying a disturbance in the typically linear relationship between exercise-induced increments in expired carbon dioxide ($\dot{V}CO_2$) and minute ventilation.

c. In untrained individuals, anaerobic threshold as determined by this "ventilatory breakpoint," occurs at approximately 55% of a person's maximal aerobic capacity ($\dot{V}O_{2max}$). In contrast, the anaerobic threshold of well-trained endurance athletes occurs at a much greater exercise intensity, perhaps 80%–85% of their $\dot{V}O_{2max}$.

d. This variable is an important predictor of performance because anaerobic threshold is the exercise intensity at which blood lactate levels rise and muscle fatigue sets in. This intensity is also referred to as the "onset of blood lactate accumulation" (**OBLA**).

IV. THE CARDIOVASCULAR SYSTEM

The cardiovascular system is composed of the heart and the blood vessels that carry blood throughout the body. The heart is a powerful, fatigue-resistant organ that acts as a pump (via the contraction of its muscle, the **myocardium**) to drive blood returning from all parts of the body, first to the lungs where it can be oxygenated, and then the newly oxygenated blood is pumped out to the rest of the body. Blood vessels are responsible for delivering the oxygen- and nutrient-rich blood ejected from the heart to all the needy tissues of the body, and for returning oxygen-depleted blood carrying metabolic by-products from those tissues back to the heart (Figure 2-4).

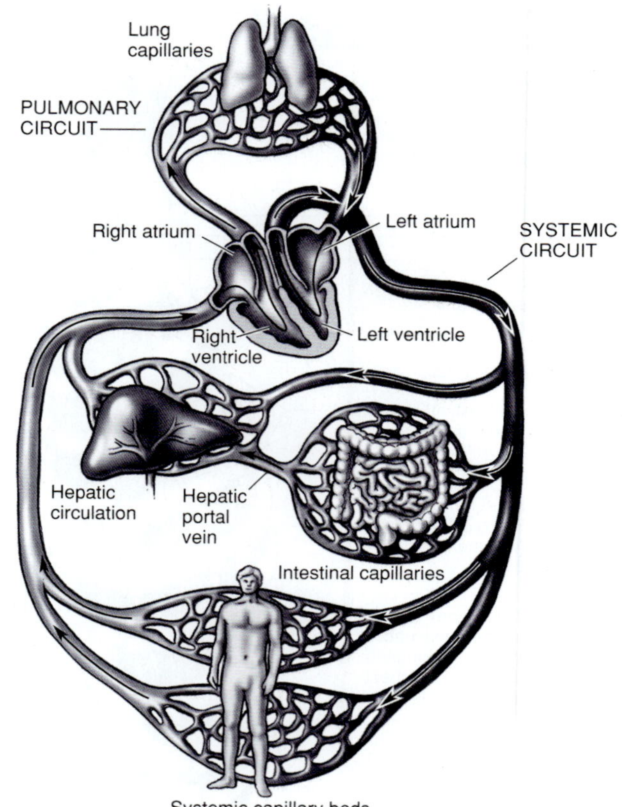

FIGURE 2-4. Schematic diagram of blood circulation. (From *ACSM's Resource Manual for Guidelines for Exercise Testing and Prescription*, 5th ed. Baltimore, Lippincott Williams & Wilkins, 2006.)

A. THE HEART

1. Anatomy

a. The human heart is composed of four separate chambers. The two upper chambers are referred to as the **atria** (singular, atrium); the two lower chambers are called **ventricles** (Figure 2-5).

b. The left atrium receives blood from the lungs whereas the right atrium from all other parts of the body.

c. The atria pump blood into the right and left ventricles which, respectively, drive blood to the lungs and the rest of the body. The right and left sides of the heart are separated by the **septum**.

d. The right and left atria contract in unison, as do the right and left ventricles.

e. The contractions of the atria and ventricles are staggered so that while blood is being delivered to the ventricles, those chambers are in their resting phase, and during contraction of the ventricles, the atria are at rest.

f. The heart receives its oxygen needs through a specialized circulation, called the coronary

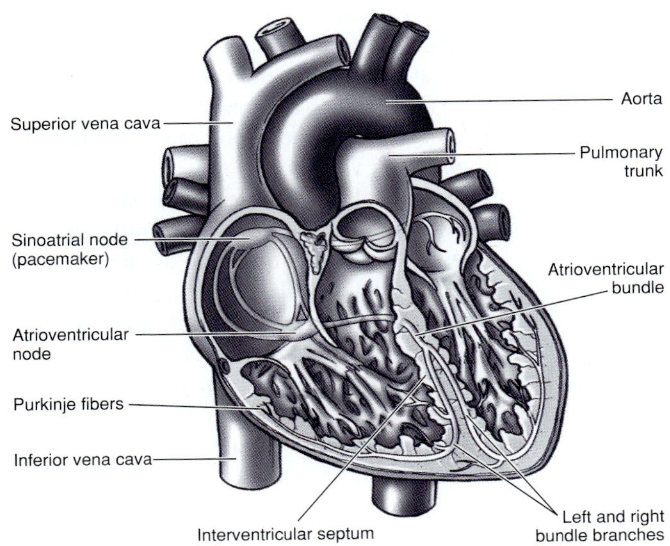

FIGURE 2-5. The electrical conduction system of the heart. (From *ACSM's Resource Manual for Guidelines for Exercise Testing and Prescription*, 5th ed. Baltimore, Lippincott Williams & Wilkins, 2006.)

circulation, which feeds the highly oxidative myocardium with oxygen-rich blood.

2. **Physiology**
   a. The sequence of events during the heart's pumping action is described as the **cardiac cycle**.
   b. **Systole** refers to the contractile phase of the **myocardium**, and **diastole** is the relaxation phase between contractions.
   c. **Stroke Volume** (SV) is the volume of blood ejected with each ventricular contraction. At rest, SV is typically 70 mL.
   d. **Heart Rate** (HR) is the number of times the heart contracts per minute. Under resting conditions, HR is about 72 beats/min.
   e. **Cardiac Output** ($\dot{Q}$) is the amount of blood pumped from the heart by each ventricle per minute. In turn, cardiac output is a function of stroke volume and heart rate, where

$$\dot{Q} = HR \times SV.$$

   Using normal resting values of HR (72 beats/min) and SV (70 mL/beat), cardiac output as rest is about 5 L/min.

   f. **End-diastolic Volume** (EDV) is the amount of blood in each ventricle at the end of the resting phase (diastole) of the cardiac cycle. According to the **Frank-Starling Law**, EDV will significantly affect SV because the greater the volume of blood in the ventricle, the greater the stretch imparted on the myocardium. As stretch increases, so does contractile force, both by elastic recoil of the muscle and by optimizing the length of the fibers comprising the myocardium. At rest, a normal EDV would be approximately 125 mL.
   g. **End-systolic Volume** (ESV) is the volume of blood remaining in each ventricle following its contraction. At rest, ESV equals about 55 mL.
   h. **Ejection Fraction** (EF) is the percentage of the blood in the ventricle during diastole that is actually pumped out during systole. Sometimes EF is defined as the ratio of stroke volume to end-diastolic volume, or EF = SV/EDV. Under resting conditions, EF is typically 60%, although in healthy adults, it can range between 50% and 75%.

3. **Acute Effects of Endurance Exercise on Cardiac Function**
   a. The greater demand for blood that is evident as exercise begins results in increased cardiac output.
      1) This acute response in cardiac function is directly linked to exercise intensity. At maximal effort, cardiac output can be five- to sixfold higher (25–30 L/min) than at rest (5 L/min). This elevated pumping capacity is brought about by increments in both HR and SV.
      2) SV increases until exercise intensity reaches approximately 50% of $VO_{2\,max}$, at which point it levels off. Consequently, further elevations in cardiac output are accounted for solely by increased heart rate.
      3) A linear relationship exists between HR and exercise intensity. As a result, monitoring HR is a common method of assessing exercise intensity during submaximal efforts.
   b. As greater amounts of blood are pumped to the working muscle, the amount of blood returning to the heart is similarly enhanced.
      1) This leads to elevations in EDV, which can be as high as 160 mL when SV is at its peak value.
         a) As EDV increases during exercise so does SV.
         b) In young, untrained men, SV may increase from 70 mL at rest to 100 mL during exercise.
      2) Another method the heart uses to amplify its pumping ability during exercise is to increase its contractility. This increased force of contraction results

in a change in EF from about 60% at rest to as high as 70%.

4. **Cardiac Adaptations**
   a. Chronic aerobic training has no impact on maximal HR.
   b. In contrast, resting HR is significantly lowered following a prolonged training program.
   c. Because resting cardiac output remains unchanged (about 5 L/min) in those who are trained, SV increases to counter this reduction in HR. At rest, SV is almost 85 mL following training. During high-intensity exercise, SV of aerobic trained athletes may be as high as 170 mL, contributing to the elevated maximal cardiac output (35–40 L/min) observed in those athletes.
   d. During exercise of any submaximal intensity, cardiac output remains unaltered with exercise training. However, among trained individuals, this cardiac output is sustained with lower HR and higher SV values than are noted in untrained individuals.

5. **Effects of Posture**
   a. During normal upright posture, gravity greatly affects blood return to the heart.
   b. In the supine or prone positions, blood return from the legs is more efficient. Because of these postural influences, SV during exercise in a supine position (swimming) is greater at any given intensity than it is during upright exercise (running or cycling).
   c. Because cardiac output is unaffected by posture, the greater SV occurring during supine exercise is accompanied by a lower HR than would be seen during exercise of the same intensity in the upright position.
      1) This lowering of HR during exercise in the supine position must be borne in mind when monitoring exercise intensity with HR response.
      2) Specifically, HR may underestimate exercise intensity during exercise performed in a prone position.

B. THE VASCULATURE

1. **Anatomy**
   Five types of vessels make up the vascular system.
   a. Arteries are thick walled, large-diameter vessels that carry blood away from the heart. The largest artery is the aorta, which directly receives blood from the left ventricle. Because of their proximity to the heart, blood pressure, or the force exerted by the blood on the walls of the vessels, is highest in the arteries.
   b. Each artery then branches off to form several arterioles, which are smaller, and which demonstrate a lower blood pressure than their feeder vessels.
   c. Each arteriole then gives rise to two to five capillaries. The diameter of a capillary is very small, barely larger than the size of a red blood cell. Similarly, the walls of the capillary are very thin—only a single cell in thickness—thus allowing the exchange of nutrients and gases with the tissue.
   d. Several capillaries then join together to form a venule, and these venules then begin the return of blood to the heart.
   e. A number of venules form a single larger vein, and these low-pressure, large-diameter vessels ultimately return blood to the heart.

2. **Physiology**
   a. The main function of the vascular system is to satisfy the demand of active tissue for blood, both to provide nutrients and oxygen, as well as to remove metabolic by-products and carbon dioxide.
   b. One-way valves located at regular intervals throughout the vasculature ensure unidirectional blood flow through this network and allow for the circulation of blood within the entire body.
   c. Proper function of the vasculature entails not only providing direction for the delivery of blood, but also regulating flow rates that are appropriate for the needs of the tissue. In effect, the greater the metabolic activity displayed, the greater the flow rate of blood to the specific tissue.
   d. The blood supply required by skeletal muscle can vary dramatically, thus challenging the vascular system. In meeting the increased demand for blood that occurs in exercising muscle, that tissue undergoes vasodilation of the arterioles. To satisfy working muscle, however, blood flow to other tissue, especially the viscera, is reduced as a result of vasoconstriction within those internal organs (e.g., kidneys, liver, spleen).
   e. Vasodilation is elicited by a relaxation of the smooth muscle layered around the walls of the arterioles, whereas contraction of the smooth muscle causes vasoconstriction and restriction of blood flow.

3. **Blood Pressure**
   a. The force exerted by the blood on the walls of the vessel as it flows through that vessel is

referred to as blood pressure. Because the heart pumps blood in a pulsatile, rather than a constant fashion, blood pressure oscillates.

b. The degree of this pulsatility differs throughout the vascular network. For example, it is most pronounced at the arteries, where blood exits the heart, but is greatly muted as blood travels within the capillaries, and is no longer evident as the blood moves through the venules and veins on its return to the heart.

c. As blood is pumped from the heart, the resistance imposed by the vessels to its flow is termed **afterload**. Along with **preload**, or the amount of blood in the ventricle immediately before contraction, SV is greatly affected.

d. Enhanced preload imparts a positive effect on stroke volume, but increased afterload negatively affects stroke volume. That is, significant afterload creates greater resistance to the ejection of blood from the heart and, as a result, stroke volume is reduced.

e. Afterload is directly related to the **compliance** of the vessel.
   1) The greater the compliance, the more easily the walls of the vessel can be stretched to accommodate the surge of blood during systole, thus allowing for greater stroke volume.
   2) Healthy blood vessels demonstrate high compliance, easing the burden of the heart to overcome vascular resistance.
   3) Atherosclerosis decreases arterial compliance and increases blood pressure.

f. Blood Pressure Measurements
   1) **Systolic Blood Pressure** (SBP) is the pressure exerted on arterial walls during the contraction of the left ventricle. This value can be used to estimate contractile force generated by the heart. In healthy individuals, systolic pressure under resting conditions is about 120 mm Hg. **Resting values above 140 mm Hg indicate hypertension.**
   2) **Diastolic Blood Pressure** (DBP) is the pressure exerted on arterial walls during the resting phase between ventricular beats. This value reflects peripheral resistance or health of the vasculature. In healthy adults, resting diastolic pressure is approximately 80 mm Hg. **Resting values above 90 mm Hg are considered hypertensive.**
   3) **Pulse Pressure** (PP) is the difference between systolic and diastolic pressures. Assuming a healthy person at rest, it is approximately 40 mm Hg (i.e., 120 mm Hg SBP; 80 mm Hg DBP).
   4) **Mean Arterial Pressure** (MAP) is the average pressure exerted throughout the entire cardiac cycle, and it reflects the average force driving blood into the tissue.

$$MAP = DBP + 1/3\,(SBP - DBP)$$

   Therefore, in a healthy person resting MAP is about 93 mm Hg.
   5) **Rate-Pressure Product** (RPP) is also called the **double product** and is a correlate of myocardial oxygen uptake and hence the workload of the left ventricle. Alterations in heart rate and blood pressure contribute to changes in RPP because it is a function of SBP multiplied by HR,

$$\text{or } RPP = SBP \times HR$$

   At rest, a healthy individual displays a double product of 8,640 (120 mm Hg × 72 beats/min).

4. Acute Vascular Responses to Exercise

The vascular system undergoes two major modifications during exercise to increase efficacy of oxygen delivery to active tissue.

a. The first is to redistribute blood flow to meet the increased demand of the working muscles.
   1) This "**shunting**" of blood away from the visceral organs to the active skeletal muscles occurs via vasoconstriction of arterioles located within the viscera, and vasodilation of arterioles found in the muscle tissue.
   2) Shunting has a dramatic effect on the distribution of blood. For example, at rest only about 20% of cardiac output is directed toward muscle, but at high-intensity exercise, perhaps 85% of the blood ejected from the heart is delivered to skeletal muscle.

b. The second major vascular response to exercise is an overall vasodilation that results in decreased (to one-third resting values) total peripheral resistance, which accommodates the rise in cardiac output that occurs during exercise. In fact, vasodilation enables the exercise-induced increase in pumping capacity of the heart.

1) Despite this vasodilation, however, the several-fold increase in cardiac output during exercise still results in elevated systolic pressure.
2) Also, as with cardiac output, increases in systolic pressure are dependent on exercise intensity.
   a) During maximal effort rhythmic exercise, such as running, systolic pressure may exceed 200 mm Hg.
   b) During sustained submaximal exercise, systolic pressure is generally maintained at 140–160 mm Hg.
3) Diastolic pressure either remains steady or decreases slightly even during maximal effort exercise.
4) A sudden, significant drop in systolic pressure, an increase in diastolic pressure (>15 mm Hg), or systolic pressures elevated beyond 260 mm Hg should lead to the immediate cessation of exercise because these responses indicate cardiovascular failure or disease.

5. Long-Term Effects of Training on Vascular Function

a. A prolonged endurance training program results in several beneficial vascular adaptations.
   1) Under resting conditions, trained individuals display reduced systolic, diastolic, and mean arterial pressures.
   2) As a therapeutic measure in treating hypertension, however, it appears that exercise is effective only among those who are mildly hypertensive.

b. During submaximal exercise at any given intensity, those who are trained demonstrate lower SBP, DBP, and MAP. Maximal SBP is typically higher among the well conditioned (indicating greater myocardial contractility), whereas maximal DBP and MAP are attenuated compared with untrained individuals.

c. Endurance training also improves the ability of the vascular system to redistribute blood flow during the onset of exercise so that the "shunting" of blood to working muscles occurs more quickly.

d. Another well-documented adaptation to endurance training is an improved capillarity within the muscle. As a result of this—along with increased mitochondrial density of myofibers—trained muscle shows an enhanced capacity to extract oxygen ($a\text{-}vO_{2\ difference}$) from the blood delivered to it.

6. Effects of Mode of Exercise

a. At any given submaximal intensity, rhythmic upper body endurance exercise (arm cranking) elicits higher SBP and DBP than those values evident during more conventional endurance exercise, such as running or cycling.
   1) This effect is probably owing to the smaller muscle mass involved and greater resistance to blood flow that occurs during arm cranking exercise in nonexercising muscles.
   2) The additional cardiovascular strain associated with upper body exercise should be considered when making exercise recommendations, particularly for those who may have cardiovascular disease.

b. Resistance exercise (e.g. weightlifting) features forceful contractions of myofibers that impede blood flow through the muscle, thus elevating blood pressure. The degree of this increased peripheral resistance and the concomitant pressure elevations are proportionate to the force exerted by the muscle, and the total muscle mass that is contracting.
   1) The amplification of blood pressure during resistance exercise is even more pronounced when **isometric** (no movement) contractions are performed. Systolic pressures greater than 450 mm Hg have been recorded during maximal intensity isometric contractions while weightlifting.
   2) These blood pressure responses should be accounted for when prescribing exercise programs for those with cardiovascular disease, or those who are unfit. Moderate intensity resistance exercise featuring repetitions with full range of motion (combined concentric and eccentric contractions) should be recommended to those who may have cardiovascular limitations.

V. BLOOD

The blood performs a host of functions, only one of which is to carry oxygen throughout the body. Because of the many tasks performed by the blood, both at rest and during exercise, numerous cellular and noncellular constituents can be identified.

A. COMPOSITION

Blood, which accounts for about 8% of a person's body weight, is composed of fluid **(plasma)** along with several types of cells **(erythrocytes, leukocytes, platelets)**.

1. Plasma

a. Plasma comprises about 55% of the blood's volume in men and 58% in women.

b. The main component of plasma is water (90%–93%). However, it also contains dissolved substances such as proteins (albumins, globulins, fibrinogen), electrolytes (sodium, potassium, calcium, etc.), gases (oxygen, carbon dioxide, nitrogen), nutrients (glucose, lipids, amino acids, vitamins), waste products (urea, creatinine, uric acid, bilirubin), and various hormones.

2. Cells

a. Only small amounts of oxygen are dissolved in the plasma. Most (98.5%) of the oxygen transported in the blood is bound to hemoglobin, a protein that is found only in the **erythrocytes**, or red blood cells. Erythrocytes are the most abundant of the cell types in the blood, accounting for more than 99% of the blood's cells.

b. **Hemoglobin** also carries some (30%) of the carbon dioxide transported by the blood.

c. "**Hematocrit**" is a measure of the percentage of the blood's volume that is composed of erythrocytes. In men, the average hematocrit is about 45%, whereas in women it is usually 42%. This gender difference exists because the male hormone testosterone affects production of erythrocytes. Because of lower hematocrit levels, women also have a reduced hemoglobin content, about 14 g/100 mL of blood compared with 16 g/100 mL of blood in men.

d. **Leukocytes** are also called white blood cells and, as components of the body's immune system, their primary function is to destroy potentially infectious agents that enter the body.

e. **Platelets** are actually fragments of much larger cells. The main function of platelets is to accumulate and form a plug where damage has occurred to the wall of the blood vessel to prevent loss of blood.

B. ACUTE EFFECTS OF EXERCISE ON BLOOD

1. The most obvious effect of exercise is to induce "**hyperemia,**" or an increase in the volume of blood delivered to the working muscles. This allows a greater delivery of oxygen and nutrients, as well as a more efficient removal of carbon dioxide and metabolic by-products such as lactate.
2. Another response that is commonly observed during prolonged endurance exercise is the movement of plasma out of the blood vessels and into the surrounding tissue. This "**cardiovascular drift**" serves to prevent overheating of the body by having more water available for sweating and it is more pronounced during exercise in hot environments. However, this drift decreases the total volume of blood in the vasculature, resulting in decreased stroke volume, and increased heart rate even though exercise intensity remains constant.
3. The movement of plasma out of the blood also leads to "**hemoconcentration,**" which is apparent in elevations in hematocrit and hemoglobin values.

C. LONG-TERM EFFECTS OF TRAINING ON BLOOD

Endurance training is associated with several favorable adaptations of the blood.

1. Production of erythrocytes significantly increases, leading to a greater oxygen-carrying capacity.
2. Plasma volume, however, increases to an even greater extent than that of erythrocytes. As a result, relative measures of hemoglobin and hematocrit (i.e., per unit volume of blood) are actually decreased in well-conditioned athletes. This has been termed "**runner's anemia,**" but it should not be considered a negative adaptation.
3. Because the total amount of red blood cells and hemoglobin is enhanced by training, so is the oxygen-carrying capacity of the blood.
4. Increased plasma volume in trained individuals has several advantageous effects.
   a. At rest, it results in a higher SV and lower HR. During exercise, an increased availability of plasma enhances the trained individual's capacity for thermoregulation; recall the effect of cardiovascular drift (see section V.B.2).
   b. Similar to resting conditions, a trained person's SV is higher and HR is lower during submaximal exercise than that of an untrained individual.

c. Maximal stroke volume and cardiac output are also more impressive in the trained individual largely because of their greater plasma volumes.

VI. HEALTH BENEFITS

Regular exercise training can bestow a host of health benefits, affecting numerous systems of the participant's body.

A. Regular endurance training decreases the risk of cardiovascular disease (e.g., heart attack, hypertension, stroke), obesity, and some forms of cancer (e.g., breast, prostate, colon).

B. It can also improve blood lipid profiles by lowering total cholesterol while elevating HDLs, or the "good cholesterol."

C. Resistance training provides significant protection against type II diabetes, osteoporosis, and the loss of muscle mass that accompanies aging (sarcopenia).

D. Convincing evidence also indicates that regular exercise training is associated with a decrease in the symptoms of depression, particularly among the aging.

E. As a result of the many health benefits gained from exercise training and regular physical activity, virtually every major health organization in the United States, including the American College of Sports Medicine, the American Heart Association, the Centers for Disease Control and Prevention, the National Institutes for Health, and the Surgeon General's Office recommends exercise for just about everyone.

F. In general, these organizations suggest daily activity on most, if not every, day of the week for a total of 30 min/day.

G. If weight loss is the primary objective of the exercise program, then it is suggested that the individual accumulate 60 min/day of physical activity. These activities should be of a moderate intensity, such as brisk walking in order to achieve most of the health benefits associated with exercise.

H. Additional benefits can be gained by increasing either the duration or the intensity of the exercise sessions. It is also recommended that resistance training and flexibility activities (stretching) should be regularly included in an exercise regimen.

Review Test

1. The immediate source of energy for all cellular activity, including the contraction of muscle fibers is
   A) Phosphocreatine (PCr).
   B) Adenosine triphosphate (ATP).
   C) Adenosine diphosphate (ADP).
   D) Glucose.

2. Which bioenergetic pathway is sometimes called the "anaerobic" pathway?
   A) Phosphagen.
   B) Oxidative.
   C) Nonoxidative.
   D) Aerobic.

3. The primary advantage of which bioenergetic pathway is that it can produce large amounts of ATP to sustain prolonged exercise, without producing fatiguing by-products?
   A) Oxidative.
   B) Nonoxidative.
   C) Anaerobic.
   D) Phosphagen.

4. Within a skeletal muscle fiber, large amounts of calcium are stored in the
   A) Nuclei.
   B) Mitochondria.
   C) Myosin.
   D) Sarcoplasmic reticulum.

5. During long duration exercise of submaximal intensity (e.g., marathon running), which type of muscle fibers are primarily recruited?
   A) Type I.
   B) Type IIA.
   C) Type IIX.
   D) Type IIB.

6. The ATPase that is used to produce a muscle fiber twitch by way of sliding filaments is found
   A) On actin.
   B) On myosin cross-bridge heads.
   C) Within the sarcoplasmic reticulum.
   D) Within nuclei.

7. The capacity of endurance training to increase the amount of ATP produced by oxidative phosphorylation is owing to
   A) Increased mitochondrial content.
   B) Increased muscle fiber size.
   C) Increased size of the sarcoplasmic reticulum.
   D) Decreased capillarity.

8. A single motor neuron and all the muscle fibers it innervates comprise a
   A) Muscle unit.
   B) Motor unit.
   C) Fascicle.
   D) Sarcomere.

9. Both resistance training and endurance training result in which of the following conversions of muscle fiber type?
   A) Type II $\rightarrow$ Type I.
   B) Type I $\rightarrow$ Type II.
   C) Type IIX $\rightarrow$ Type IIA.
   D) Type IIA $\rightarrow$ Type IIX.

10. Within the pulmonary system, the actual exchange of gasses with the blood occurs at the
    A) Trachea.
    B) Bronchi.
    C) Alveoli.
    D) Bronchioles.

11. During maximal intensity exercise, minute ventilation can increase by
    A) 50%.
    B) 100%.
    C) 5-fold.
    D) 20–25-fold.

12. Under resting conditions, stroke volume in a typical male (70 kg) is about
    A) 70 mL.
    B) 40 mL.
    C) 100 mL.
    D) 120 mL.

13. The amount of blood ejected from the heart per minute is referred to as
    A) Stroke volume.
    B) Heart rate.
    C) Cardiac output.
    D) End-diastolic volume.

14. The Frank-Starling mechanism plays a vital role in determining
    A) End-diastolic volume.
    B) Stroke volume.
    C) Heart rate.
    D) Myocardial oxygen consumption.

15. During maximal intensity aerobic exercise, cardiac output increases by ______ in an untrained individual.
    A) 50%.
    B) 2-fold.
    C) 5- to 6-fold.
    D) 10- to 12-fold.

16. Which of the following adaptations would NOT be expected to occur as a result of long-term aerobic training?
    A) Decrease in resting heart rate.
    B) Increase in resting stroke volume.
    C) Increase in resting cardiac output.
    D) Increase in maximal heart rate.

17. While performing a running workout of submaximal intensity, which of the following responses would be expected to occur?
    A) Increase in end-diastolic volume.
    B) Decrease in end-diastolic volume.
    C) Decrease in ejection fraction.
    D) Decrease in cardiac output.

18. Compared with running, swimming will result in ________ even if exercise intensity is the same.
    A) A higher heart rate.
    B) A lower heart rate.
    C) A lower cardiac output.
    D) A higher cardiac output.

19. The exchange of gases between the blood and the surrounding tissue (e.g., muscle) takes place at these vessels.
    A) Arteries.
    B) Arterioles.
    C) Capillaries.
    D) Veins.

20. The processes of vasoconstriction and vasodilation, which regulate blood flow to a given muscle mass, occur at the
    A) Arteries.
    B) Arterioles.
    C) Venules.
    D) Veins.

21. During aerobic exercise, which of the following responses would NOT be considered normal?
    A) Increased systolic blood pressure.
    B) Increased pulse pressure.
    C) Increased mean arterial pressure.
    D) Increased diastolic blood pressure.

22. Which of the following statements regarding blood pressure and resistance exercise (weightlifting) is correct?
    A) People with even mild cardiovascular disease should never perform resistance exercise.
    B) Blood pressure elevations are highest during isometric muscular actions.
    C) Blood pressure elevations during resistance exercise are independent of the muscle mass involved.
    D) Typically, blood pressure elevations seen during maximal resistance exercise are less than those observed during maximal aerobic exercise.

23. The reason that men have higher hematocrit and hemoglobin levels than women is
    A) Men produce more testosterone than women.
    B) Men have greater muscle mass than women.
    C) Unlike men, women experience menstrual blood loss.
    D) Men generally train harder than women.

24. The cells of the blood that are often referred to as "white" blood cells are the
    A) Platelets.
    B) Erythrocytes.
    C) Plasmacytes.
    D) Leukocytes.

25. Many of the major health organizations in the United States recommend a minimum of ____ minutes of physical activity on most days of the week to achieve significant health benefits and protection from chronic diseases, such as coronary heart disease.
    A) 30.
    B) 60.
    C) 10.
    D) 90.

ANSWERS AND EXPLANATIONS

1–B. Adenosine triphosphate (ATP) provides the energy directly used for all cellular activity when it is hydrolyzed by the enzyme ATPase into adenosine diphosphate (ADP) and inorganic phosphate (Pi). The energy found in the chemical bonds of the food substrates that we eat is used by cells to synthesize ATP.

2–C. The "nonoxidative" pathway is sometimes called the "anaerobic" pathway. The term nonoxidative is more accurate because the enzymes comprising this ATP-generating pathway do not require oxygen to function. The term anaerobic suggests an inadequate supply of oxygen; however, rather than a shortage of oxygen, this pathway simply does not need oxygen to function.

3–A. The main advantages of the oxidative pathway are its high capacity—the total amount of ATP that it can produce far exceeds that of the phosphagen and nonoxidative systems—and that nonfatiguing by-products (water, carbon dioxide) result from its action. The main disadvantage of the oxidative pathway is that the rate at which it produces ATP is considerably slower than what is observed in the phosphagen and nonoxidative systems. Moreover, the oxidative pathway is dependent on adequate blood flow to the working tissue.

4–D. Within skeletal muscle fibers, the endoplasmic (sarcoplasmic) reticulum is particularly well developed so that it can store large amounts of calcium. When the motor neuron excites the membrane (sarcolemma) of the fiber, calcium is released from the sarcoplasmic reticulum, which triggers the fiber to twitch, or contract.

5–A. Type I fibers are primarily recruited during long endurance events of submaximal intensity. These fibers are designed to produce large amounts of ATP via the oxidative pathway, so they are fatigue resistant, and they have a slow rate of contraction that is well suited for long-term, submaximal activity.

6–B. The myosin cross-bridge head includes both ATP and the ATPase enzyme that hydrolyzes ATP to provide the energy used during cross-bridge cycling. When calcium is released from the sarcoplasmic reticulum, it exposes "active" sites on the actin to which myosin cross-bridge heads, resulting in the power stroke and muscle shortening.

7–A. By increasing mitochondrial content (numbers and volume), the muscle fiber increases the number of enzymes of the Krebs cycle and the electron transport chain, thus enhancing the fiber's capacity to produce ATP via oxidative phosphorylation.

8–B. The motor unit is composed of a single alpha motor neuron and all the fibers it is in contact with and innervates. All fibers of any single motor unit are of the same type because they are innervated by the same motor neuron.

9–C. Any exercise training program, whether it be endurance or resistance training, results in the conversion of Type IIX muscle fibers to Type IIA fibers. Conversely, a decrease in activity, such as detraining, is accompanied by a conversion of Type IIA fibers to Type IIX fibers. The stimulus of exercise does not appear able to convert Type I fibers to Type II fibers, or vice versa, however.

10–C. The alveoli are the thin walled sacs at the end of the ventilatory tract. Because of these thin walls, and the fact that they are richly supplied with capillaries, the alveoli are where the exchange of gases (oxygen, carbon dioxide) occurs between the lungs and blood.

11–D. In normal healthy individuals, the amount of air inhaled (and exhaled) by the lungs each minute is 6 L. During all-out exercise, this "minute ventilation" can be as high as 120–150 L/min. This results from both an increased respiratory rate (number of breaths/min) and depth of breathing (tidal volume).

12–A. Stroke volume, or the amount of blood ejected from the heart with each beat, is 70 mL in an untrained person under resting conditions. This value, multiplied by a normal resting heart rate of 72 beats/min, accounts for a cardiac output of 5 L/min. In a trained individual, resting stroke volume is increased, resting heart rate is decreased, and resting cardiac output remains unchanged at 5 L/min.

13–C. Under resting conditions, cardiac output, the amount of blood ejected by the heart per minute, is 5 L/min. As described above, cardiac output is a function of stroke volume multiplied by heart rate. In an untrained person, cardiac output can increase to 25–30 L/min during maximal effort exercise. In a well-trained endurance athlete, maximal cardiac output can be as high as 35–40 L/min.

14–B. During exercise, the Frank-Starling mechanism affects stroke volume both by stretching the myocardium greater than at rest, thus increasing force produced by elastic recoil, and by optimizing the degree of overlap between myosin and actin filaments resulting in greater contractile force.

15–C. In untrained individuals, a cardiac output of 25–30 L/min (up from 5 L/min at rest) during maximal effort exercise is common. In endurance-trained athletes, cardiac output during maximal intensity exercise can be as high as 35–40 L/min. This training-induced elevation in maximal cardiac output is attributed to a greater maximal stroke volume, because training does not affect maximal heart rate.

16–C. At rest, cardiac output is not affected by training status. The amount of blood needed to sustain the body's functions at rest does not differ between those who are trained and those who are sedentary.

17–A. As the rate of blood flow increases during exercise, so does the rate of blood return to the heart. Accordingly, end-diastolic volume—the amount of blood in the ventricles following the diastolic (resting) phase of the cardiac cycle—is enhanced during exercise. In turn, this enhanced end-diastolic volume accounts for the greater stroke volume observed during exercise.

18–B. At any given intensity, heart rate will be lower during swimming than exercise performed in a standing position, such as running, because of postural differences. While swimming, the body is in a prone position so that the heart's pumping action does not have to overcome the full effects of gravity. Thus, even at rest, stroke volume is at its maximal value. Because of the higher stroke volume evident during submaximal swimming compared with running, the same cardiac output can be achieved with a lower heart rate during swimming.

19–C. Numerous anatomic features of the capillaries make them unique among blood vessels. These include walls that are the thickness of only a single endothelial cell, a diameter so small that red blood cells can pass only one at a time, and "loose" junctions joining endothelial cells, resulting in high permeability of capillary walls. It is because of these features that the exchange of gases (oxygen, carbon dioxide) and nutrients (e.g., glucose, amino acids) occurs only at the capillary level.

20–B. Unlike the capillaries, the walls of the arterioles are surrounded by smooth muscle. These smooth muscle cells are responsive to local tissue conditions, such as oxygen concentration, carbon dioxide concentration and pH level, as well as the influence of the autonomic nervous system. As a result of this sensitivity, the smooth muscle cells of arterioles can either contract or relax, leading to vasoconstriction (decreased blood flow) or vasodilation (increased blood flow), respectively.

21–D. Because of the vasodilation associated with exercise-induced stimulation of the sympathetic nervous system, diastolic pressure remains unchanged, or even slightly decreased, during exercise.

22–B. During isometric contractions, constant—rather then rhythmic—force is generated by the skeletal muscle fibers. This constant force exerts pressure on the blood vessels that results in occlusion (or blocking) of blood flow through the vessels. Owing to this vascular resistance and the heart's efforts to overcome it, blood pressure is highest during isometric contractions. Because of the associated cardiovascular challenges, isometric contractions should be avoided, particularly among those with known cardiovascular disease.

23–A. The hormone erythropoietin stimulates the production of red blood cells in the bone marrow. In turn, the hormone testosterone enhances the synthesis of erythropoietin by the kidneys. Because men have higher testosterone levels than women, they also have higher hematocrit and hemoglobin concentrations.

24–D. Leukocytes are also called "white" blood cells. They are vital components of the immune system that protects us from infectious illnesses.

25–A. Research has shown that 30 minutes of moderate intensity physical activity per day, when performed on most if not all days of the week, will convey significant protection against the major killers in modern society (e.g., cardiovascular disease, some forms of cancer).

Human Development and Aging

CHAPTER 3

I. OVERVIEW OF HUMAN GROWTH AND DEVELOPMENT

A. AGE GROUPS are typically defined as follows:
  1. Neonatal: birth to 3 weeks.
  2. Infancy: 3 weeks to 1 year.
  3. Childhood
     a. Early: 1 to 6 years.
     b. Middle childhood: 7 to 10 years.
     c. Later/Prepuberty: girls, 9 to 15 years; boys, 12 to 16 years.
  4. Adolescence: the 6 years following puberty.
  5. Adulthood
     a. Early: 20 to 29 years.
     b. Middle: 30 to 44 years.
     c. Later: 45 to 64 years.
  6. Senescence
     a. Young-old: 65 to 74 years.
     b. Old: 75 to 84 years.
     c. Old–old: 85 to 99 years.
     d. Oldest–old: 100 years and older.

B. SIGNIFICANT VARIABILITY EXISTS IN GROWTH AND DEVELOPMENT for a given chronological age group.

C. AGING IS A COMPLEX PROCESS that involves the interaction of many factors, including genetics, lifestyle, and disease.

D. THE AGING POPULATION in the United States is increasing. It is estimated that by 2030, 20% of our population will be 65 years or older. The fastest growing age category is the centenarians, those more than 100 years of age (*Figure 3-1*).

E. AGE AND EXERCISE
  1. A person's age must be considered when designing an exercise program. Children, adolescents, and older adults have special physiologic and behavioral characteristics that must be considered in program design to ensure safety and effectiveness. A medical history and proper screening are recommended and, in some cases, are required by the American College of Sports Medicine (ACSM) Guidelines.
  2. Guidelines by The National Association for Sport and Physical Education state that children ages 5–12 years accumulate at least 60 minutes, and up to several hours, of age-appropriate physical activity on all or most days of the week.
  3. Both aerobic and resistance training are recommended for older adults to improve health, functional capacity, and overall quality of life.

II. AGE-RELATED PHYSIOLOGIC CHANGES IN CHILDREN

A. CARDIOPULMONARY FUNCTION

1. Both resting heart rate and exercise heart rate are higher in children, most likely as compensation for the lower stroke volume and cardiac output relative to body mass. Additionally, hemoglobin concentration is lower in children than in adults.
2. Cardiac output at any given submaximal oxygen consumption ($\dot{V}O_2$) is lower in adults than in children. Children compensate for this by increased oxygen extraction, which is achieved by increased blood flow through skeletal muscle.
3. Maximal oxygen consumption ($\dot{V}O_2$ max) is determined by the capacity of the cardiovascular system to deliver oxygen to the working muscles and the capacity of the muscles to extract oxygen for oxidative metabolism. $\dot{V}O_2$ max, a function of maximal cardiac output and maximal arteriovenous oxygen difference, remains relatively unchanged throughout childhood and adolescence.
4. Blood pressure at rest and during exercise is lower in children compared with adults.
5. Changes during growth and development
   a. A general increase in exercise capacity and absolute $\dot{V}O_2$ max (L/min) occurs during childhood. This increase is dramatically accelerated during puberty, especially in boys, before leveling off after maturity.
   b. The large increase in absolute $\dot{V}O_2$ max in adolescent boys corresponding to the growth spurt, which results from androgen-induced hypertrophy of the heart and stimulation of red blood cell and hemoglobin production, facilitates oxygen delivery.

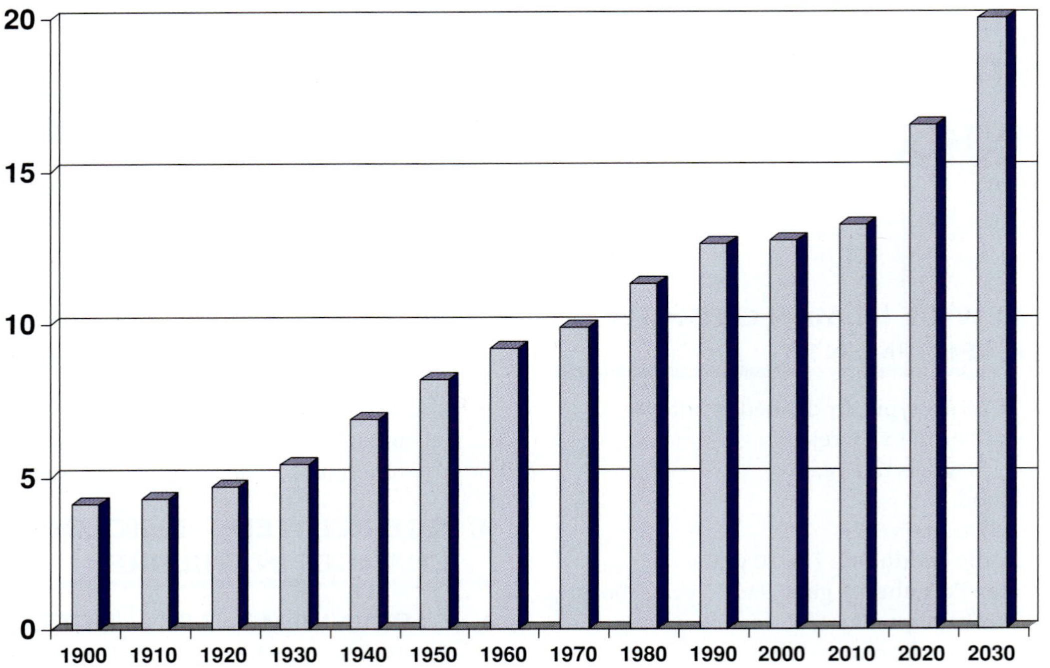

FIGURE 3-1. Estimation of the number of individuals who will be 65 years of age and older by the year 2010 and beyond. Note the exponential growth rate in this age group, making them the fastest-growing population segment in the United States. Data from Older Americans 2000 (2000): Administration on Aging. www.aoa.gov.

Furthermore, increased skeletal muscle mass associated with male adolescence increases the capacity for oxygen extraction.

c. Despite the large increase in absolute $\dot{V}O_2$ max, **relative $\dot{V}O_2$ max ($mL \cdot kg^{-1} \cdot min^{-1}$) plateaus in boys, and shows a slight decline in girls, during puberty.** Whether this represents inadequate physical conditioning of this age group or some other physiologic factor is unclear.

6. **$\dot{V}O_2$** max is not related to endurance fitness in children and preadolescents.

B. MUSCULOSKELETAL FUNCTION

1. Changes in Muscle Mass
   a. An individual's **total number of muscle fibers** becomes fixed before adolescence; however, large changes in muscle mass remain possible via the mechanisms of **muscle fiber hypertrophy.**
   b. At **adolescence,** males exhibit more rapid muscle growth (**hypertrophy**) than females do. Females do not exhibit disproportionate muscle growth during adolescence. Adolescent and postadolescent females have approximately 30%–60% less muscle mass compared with males, both because of smaller stature and because of a smaller average muscle fiber size.
2. Muscular strength can be increased with training in both boys and girls before the age of puberty.
3. Bone Formation During Growth and Development
   a) The human skeleton begins to develop in the embryo as the process of **endochondral ossification** gradually replaces the cartilage with bone tissue.
   b) In long bones, the ossification begins in the **diaphysis.** Secondary ossification occurs at the ends of the long bone, or **epiphysis,** and remains separated from the primary ossification by **epiphyseal plates.**
   c) The epiphyseal plates are regions of cartilage that continue to produce chondrocytes that undergo ossification and, thereby, add bone tissue to the shaft of the bone.
   d) Through this process, long bones continue to grow in length until **the epiphyseal plates close in response to hormonal changes at approximately 16–18 years of age,** following the adolescent growth spurt. Bone mass reaches its peak for both men and women by 25–30 years of age. Problems with bone growth can develop in children as a result of strenuous exercise, because the epiphysis is not yet united with the bone shaft.

1) **Epiphysitis** can occur with overuse.
2) **Fractures** can pass through the epiphyseal plate, disrupting normal bone growth.

C. REACTION TIME, MOVEMENT TIME, AND COORDINATION

1. Performance of tasks requiring **motor skills** improves consistently throughout the preadolescent and adolescent years. This improvement results from growth, the associated increases in strength and endurance, the progress of motor learning, and the development of greater coordination.
2. **Reaction time** decreases (improves) with maturational development. An abrupt decrease in reaction time occurs around 8 years of age, followed by a more progressive improvement throughout the remainder of childhood and adolescence.
3. **Speed of movement** also improves with age.
4. **Improvement of skill following a practice session** increases with age during childhood, indicating an increase in the capacity to integrate feedback during learning.
5. Gender Differences in Skill Performance
   a. Gender differences in skill performance are minimal before adolescence.
   b. During **adolescence**, the gap widens. The performance of girls in skills requiring strength and gross motor patterns (e.g., running, jumping) plateaus, whereas that of boys continue to improve.
   c. Girls often outperform boys in skills requiring fine motor patterns.
   d. Wide individual variations in quantitative skill performances are found at all ages in both genders.

D. BODY COMPOSITION

1. During puberty, **females experience smaller increases in stature and muscle mass** but a greater accumulation of body fat compared with males. Muscle mass represents 42% of an average 17-year-old female but 53% of the weight of an average male of the same age. In the prepubertal years, the values are 43% and 45%, respectively.
2. **Body fat percentage** generally increases from childhood to early adulthood. Acceptable body fat percentages for prepubescent children are between 10% and 15%.
3. Typical gains in fat mass **during puberty in females** are twice those in males because of hormonally induced accumulation of fat in the breasts and around the hips. At age 17, female body fat percentage is twice that of males.

E. THERMOREGULATION

1. Children are less efficient than adults are at temperature regulation because of the **anthropometric and functional differences** of their immature thermoregulatory system.
   a. Children tolerate exercise in the heat more poorly than adults.
2. Children consistently sweat less than adults. Thus, children may have difficulty making thermoregulatory adaptations during extreme temperature conditions.
   a. **Sweating rate** for children (at least in boys) is much lower than that for adults. This causes children to rely more on convective heat loss from increased cutaneous blood flow.
   b. Although the number of **sweat glands** in children equals the number in the adult, the rate of **sweat production** for each gland is half that of the adult glands.
   c. The threshold for sweating is higher in children than in adults.
3. The **surface area** of a child, relative to body mass, is greater than that of an adult, allowing a **greater rate of heat exchange** between the skin and the environment.
   a. In neutral or warm climates, the increased surface area may facilitate heat dissipation.
   b. In **climatic extremes**, this increased surface area becomes a major handicap by increasing unwanted heat transfer from the body to the environment during cold exposure (e.g., swimming in an unheated pool) and vice versa during exposure to heat (e.g., exercising when the ambient temperature exceeds the body temperature).
4. Children **acclimatize** to hot environments less efficiently and **at a slower rate** than adults. Children, therefore, require a **longer and more gradual program** of exposure to a hot environment for acclimatization.
5. **Hypohydrated children** are at increased risk for heat-related illness, because the rise in core temperature in proportion to the degree of dehydration occurs at a greater rate. However, children might be expected to be less susceptible to dehydration because of their smaller fluid losses through sweating.
6. **Heat Disorders in Children**
   a. **Children at highest risk** for heat-related illness include:

1) Children with diseases affecting the sweating mechanism (e.g., cystic fibrosis, diabetes mellitus).
2) Children with diseases affecting the cardiovascular system (e.g., congenital heart diseases, diabetes mellitus).
3) Children with obesity.
4) Children with a history of heat stroke.

b. Prevention of heat-related illness can be achieved by ensuring that children who participate in physical activities, especially in hot, humid environments, are properly hydrated, acclimatized, and conditioned for the exercise.

7. Cold Injuries in Children
   a. Cold injuries are much less common than heat-related injuries.
   b. Cold injuries may be superficial (e.g., frostbite) or systemic (e.g., hypothermia).
   c. Little acclimatization occurs following repeated exposure to cold.
   d. Physical fitness does not appear to decrease the risk of cold injury.
   e. Prevention of cold-related injuries during exercise is dependent on proper clothing and limitation of exposure to cold.
   f. The greater ratio of body surface area to mass in children results in greater heat loss in the cold, especially during swimming. For this reason, children exercising in cool water should exit and warm up at least every 15 minutes.

III. AGE-RELATED PHYSIOLOGIC CHANGES IN OLDER ADULTS

A. CARDIOPULMONARY FUNCTION

1. Maximal heart rate decreases by approximately 6 to 10 bpm per decade with advancing age.
2. Resting stroke volume remains relatively unchanged with advancing age, but maximal stroke volume decreases with advancing age.
3. Decreases in both maximal heart rate and stroke volume cause a significant decline in maximal cardiac output with age. Maximal heart rate and stroke volume are probably decreased because of increased stiffness of the left ventricle, causing decreased diastolic filling.
4. Other Cardiovascular Changes
   a. Decreased arterial compliance and increased arterial stiffness with age can result in elevated systolic and elevated diastolic blood pressures both at rest and during exercise.

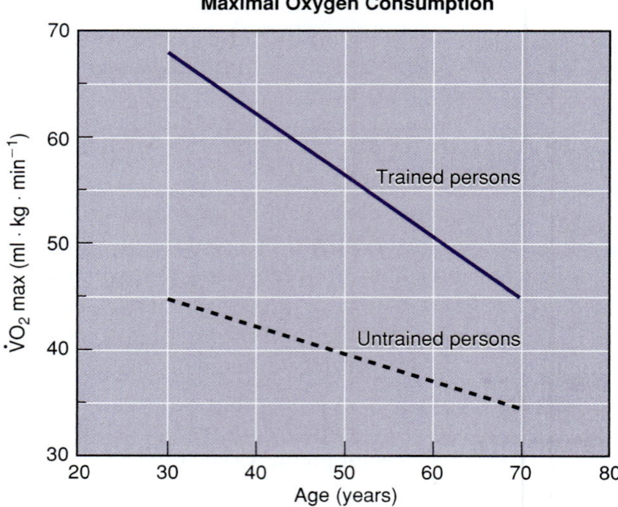

FIGURE 3-2. Changes in maximal oxygen consumption ($\dot{V}O_2$ max) as a function of age in both conditioned and unconditioned individuals.

   b. Skeletal muscle capillary density decreases with age, resulting in decreased muscle blood flow and oxygen extraction.
   c. Left ventricular hypertrophy increases with aging, apparently related to increased afterload associated with increased peripheral resistance.
   d. Early left ventricular diastolic function, both at rest and during exercise, decreases with age.
5. $\dot{V}O_2$ max typically declines by 5%–15% per decade after age 25; this decline is related to decreases in both maximal cardiac output and maximal arteriovenous oxygen difference. The rate of decline can be slowed by regular physical activity (*Figure 3-2*).
6. Changes in Pulmonary Function
   a. Residual volume increases and vital capacity decreases with aging.
   b. Lung compliance increases with aging, as the lungs lose elastin fibers and elastic recoil.
   c. Aging brings a 20% increase in the work of respiratory muscles but a decrease in the strength of these muscles.

B. MUSCULOSKELETAL FUNCTION

1. A decline in muscle mass (atrophy) occurs with advancing age because of a progressive decrease in the number and size of muscle fibers. This sarcopenia directly contributes to an age-related decline in muscle strength. Fast-twitch fibers (especially type IIB fibers) are particularly susceptible to atrophy in aging humans.

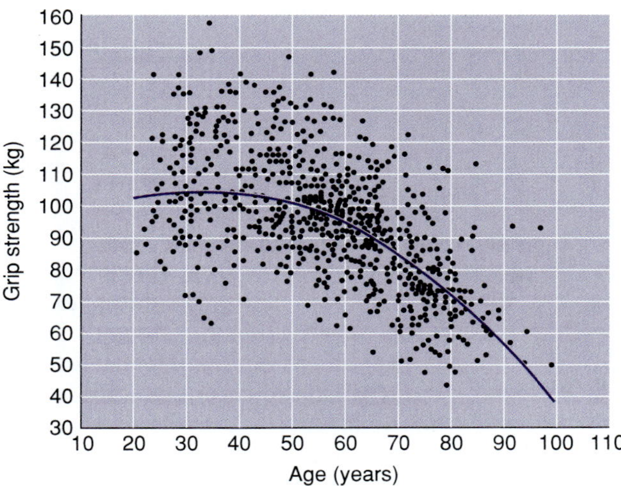

FIGURE 3-3. Grip strength of 847 males from 20 to 100 years of age. (Reprinted, by permission, from Kallmanb DA, Platon CC, and Tobin JD. The role of muscle loss in the age-related decline of grip strength: Cross sectional and longitudinal perspectives. *J Gerontol* 1990;45:M83.)

a. Sedentary individuals lose 20%–40% of their muscle mass over the course of adult life.

2. Changes in Muscle Strength (*Figure 3-3*)
   a. **Muscle strength typically peaks in the mid-20s** for both sexes and remains fairly stable through the mid-30s.
   b. **Muscle strength declines** by approximately 15% per decade in the fifth, sixth, and seventh decades and by approximately 30% per decade thereafter.
3. Bone
   a. **Bone is specialized connective tissue** composed of cells embedded in an extracellular organic matrix impregnated with an inorganic component. This inorganic component, primarily calcium phosphate crystals called hydroxyapatite, makes up approximately 65% of the dry weight of bone. Mature bone continuously undergoes a process called **bone remodeling**, in which bone matrix is reabsorbed and replaced by new matrix. **This process becomes unbalanced with advancing age such that bone formation does not keep pace with reabsorption.**
   b. Bone Loss During Aging and Development of Osteoporosis
      1) **Osteoporosis** is a condition characterized by a decrease in bone mass and bone density, producing bone porosity and fragility. The efficiency of osteoblasts appears to decline with age, resulting in the inability of bone synthesis to keep pace with bone reabsorption. In women, this loss is accelerated immediately after menopause.
      2) As a result, **older individuals are more susceptible to bone fractures**, which are a significant cause of morbidity and mortality in the elderly. Osteoporosis is responsible for more than 1.5 million fractures annually. **Hip fractures** account for a large share of the disability, death, and medical costs associated with falls. Additionally, both wrist and vertebral fractures are common among those with osteoporosis.
      3) Sex-Related Differences in Bone Loss
         a) The average woman attains a peak bone mass that is about 10% below that of a man.
         b) The age at which bone loss begins and the rate at which it occurs vary greatly between men and women.
            (i) Normally, **men** generally begin to lose bone mass between 50 and 55 years of age.
            (ii) Bone loss in **women** may begin as early as age 30–35, and the rate of bone loss is greatly accelerated following menopause.
         c) Some studies suggest that the **overall age-related loss of bone** mineral content in men is proportional to the loss of lean body tissue with aging. Women, however, exhibit a disproportionate loss of bone tissue after menopause.
         d) The rate of bone loss increases in the eighth and ninth decades in men and women.
         e) Of those affected by osteoporosis, 80% are women.
      4) Risk Factors
         Many of the risk factors for age-related bone loss and, hence, the risk for developing osteoporosis can be modified. The risk factors are:
         a) Being **Caucasian** or **Asian.**
         b) Being **female.**
         c) Being **thin-boned** or petite.
         d) Having a **low peak bone mass** at maturity.
         e) **A family history** of osteoporosis.
         f) Premature or surgically induced **menopause.**
         g) **Alcohol abuse.**
         h) **Cigarette smoking.**
         i) **Sedentary lifestyle.**

j) Inadequate **dietary calcium intake.**
k) **Chronic steroid use** (especially for males under the age of 70 years).
l) **Vitamin D deficiency.**
m) **Advanced age.**

C. FLEXIBILITY

1. Joint stiffness and loss of flexibility are common in the elderly. It is difficult to separate the effects of aging on joint flexibility from those of injury and wear-and-tear that occur over the lifespan.
   a. Connective tissue (fascia, ligaments, tendons) **becomes less extensible** with age. Aging is associated with **degradation and increased crosslinkage of collagen fibers,** which comprise much of the connective tissue in the joints. This increases the stiffness and decreases the tensile strength of collagen fibers.
   b. **Degeneration of joints,** especially in the spine, occurs with advancing age, perhaps largely because of **trauma to joint cartilage** causing the formation of scar tissue, which makes the connective tissue stiff and less responsive to stress, thus facilitating the loss of flexibility that is seen with aging.
      1) **Range-of-motion exercises and static stretching** may increase flexibility in persons of all ages.
      2) It is unlikely, however, that any exercise could undo the extensive degenerative damage that is sometimes seen with osteoarthritis in the elderly.
   c. A **progressive loss of flexibility** begins during young adulthood that relates to disuse, deterioration of joints, and degeneration of collagen fibers. **Osteoarthritis** can severely restrict range of motion. This disease occurs primarily in areas of the body that receive the greatest mechanical stress, thereby suggesting that **it may be caused by repeated trauma** rather than by aging.

D. MOTOR CONTROL, MOTOR COORDINATION, AND BALANCE

1. Balance and Postural Stability

a. Balance and postural stability are **affected** by sensory and motor system changes.
b. **Poor balance** is one **risk factor for falling.** (Other risk factors include medication use, muscle weakness, diminished cognitive status, postural hypotension, and impaired vision). Of individuals over the age of 65 years, 30% will experience at least one fall per year. This number increases to 50% for those more than 75 years of age.
c. **Age-related changes in the vestibular, visual, and somatosensory systems** result in diminished feedback to the postural centers.
d. The **muscle effectors** may lack the capacity to respond appropriately to disturbances in postural stability.

2. Age-Associated Changes in Gait

a. Healthy older adults walk at a preferred speed that is 20% slower than the preferred speed of younger adults.
   1) The reduced gait speed is largely attributable to a decrease in stride length.
   2) The reduction in stride length negatively affects other aspects of gait (e.g.; reduced arm swing; reduced rotation of the ankles, knees, and hips; and increased double support time).
   3) Over time, these changes can affect a person's ability to remain an independent ambulator and increase the risk for falls in time-constrained situations.

3. Adulthood and Changes with Aging

a. Many **neurophysiologic changes** occur with aging that **affect motor performance.**
   1) Decreased **visual acuity.**
   2) **Hearing loss.**
   3) Deterioration of **short-term memory.**
   4) Inability to handle several pieces of information simultaneously.
   5) Decreased **reaction time.**
b. The ability to maintain performance of a motor skill at a given level throughout middle and older adulthood depends on the type of skill in question.
c. **Skills requiring accuracy of movement** may be maintained at the level attained as a young adult.
d. Performance of **skills requiring speed and strength of movement** declines with age.
e. **Movement patterns** of older adults are generally well maintained from younger adulthood. **Decreases in performance** during adulthood result from decreases in range of motion, reaction time, movement time, and coordination.
f. It is often difficult to separate the effects of aging from those of disease or deconditioning resulting from inactivity. Nevertheless, **individuals who remain active and continue to practice motor skills can minimize the decline in performance** that occurs with aging.

E. BODY COMPOSITION

1. **Aging is associated with considerable changes in body composition.** With age, fat free mass steadily declines in both men and women, whereas fat mass increases. These changes have important implications for the health and functioning of older adults because of their association with chronic diseases, mobility impairment, falls, and functional decline.
   a. A **gradual decrease in basal metabolic rate is associated with aging.** Coupled with a more sedentary lifestyle, this typically results in a loss of lean (metabolically active) muscle mass and a concurrent increase in the less metabolically active fat mass.
2. Changes in body composition with aging **are increasingly recognized as modifiable.** Although age-related changes in body composition have a strong genetic component, it is also influenced by physical activity, diet, and disease.
3. Fat Mass Changes With Age
   a. **Inactivity is a primary factor in the increase of fat mass with age.** Energy expenditure from physical activity declines with age, and body fat mass increases when an imbalance occurs between caloric intake and energy expenditure.
   b. The **age-related increase in fat mass** accumulates primarily in central areas (**abdominal areas**) as opposed to peripheral areas. **Increased** measurements of **central-to-peripheral adiposity**, such as the ratio of waist to hip circumference, have been linked to an **increased risk for cardiovascular disease and they are associated with insulin resistance, glucose intolerance, and abnormal lipoprotein profiles.**
   c. **Exercise training** can reduce the percentage body fat at any age. However, longitudinal studies of highly competitive athletes suggest that exercise does not prevent an age-related increase in body fat.
4. Fat-Free Mass Changes With Aging
   a. Fat-free mass (FFM) peaks during the third to fourth decades of life, followed by a steady decline with advancing age, especially after age 65 years.
   b. Skeletal muscle mass begins to decline noticeably at approximately 45 years of age. This is caused by a number of underlying mechanisms, including intrinsic changes in the muscle and central nervous system, changes in hormonal stimuli, and lifestyle factors.
   c. Some research suggests that sarcopenia occurs to a greater extent in the lower extremities compared with the upper extremities, although this may be related to changes in physical activity.
   d. **After 70 years of age,** body mass begins to decline, typically by 1–2 kg in the eighth decade and accelerating thereafter. This decline in body mass represents a **loss of FFM,** which exceeds the continued rise in fat mass.
   e. Exercise can increase muscle mass, even in very old, frail persons.
5. Caution must be used when using body mass index (BMI) to classify older adults into the categories of normal, overweight, or obese because it can underestimate body fat in persons who have lost muscle mass.

F. THERMOREGULATION

1. The **primary determinants of sweating rate are acclimation, fitness, hydration, and genetics.** Subtle age differences in sweat gland function exist, but age per se is a minor influence compared with the other factors in changes of sweating rate with aging. The same number of sweat glands are activated, but with less sweat output per gland, when stimulated pharmacologically.
2. Numerous factors can impair thermoregulation in older adults, including:
   a. **Reduced total body water** predisposes the older adult to a more rapid dehydration.
   b. **Elderly men** exposed to prolonged heat stress exhibit lower subcutaneous blood flow values compared with young men.
   c. Heart rate, blood pressure, and oxygen consumption, expressed as a percentage of maximum, are higher in the older adult exercising at a submaximal workload in the heat.
   d. The **decreased tolerance for exercising in hot environments** with aging appears to relate primarily to decreases in **cardiovascular responses** to the heat stress and to a **compromised aerobic capacity.**
3. Initial studies suggest that regular aerobic exercise may attenuate the decrease of peripheral sweat production known to occur with aging.

G. HORMONES

1. **Loss in circulating growth hormone** levels begins in the early thirties and continues throughout life. This contributes to the loss of muscle mass and strength associated with aging.
2. In men, **loss in circulating testosterone** levels begins in the early thirties and continues throughout life. This also contributes to the loss

of muscle mass and strength associated with aging.

3. In women, during perimenopausal and postmenopausal conditions, a dramatic drop in circulating levels of estrogen and progesterone occurs. This contributes to the increased risk for heart disease and osteoporosis.

IV. SPECIAL CONSIDERATION FOR EXERCISE TRAINING IN CHILDREN AND ADOLESCENTS

A. BENEFITS AND RISKS

1. Children and adolescents tend to be more active than adults, but many fail to meet health-related standards for physical fitness.
2. Exercise programs for youths should increase physical fitness in the short term and lead to adoption of a physically active lifestyle in the long term.

B. STRENGTH TRAINING

1. Strength can be increased in boys and girls before puberty. Strength training in preadolescents, as compared with that in adolescents and adults, probably results in smaller absolute strength gains but equal relative increases in strength.
2. If proper instruction, exercise prescription, and supervision are provided, strength training in children and adolescents carries no greater risk of injury than comparable strength training programs in adults.
3. Overly intense or maximal (1 repetition maximum [1-RM]) resistance training should be avoided. The focus should be on participation and proper technique rather than the amount of the resistance.

C. CARDIOVASCULAR CONSIDERATIONS

Most children with cardiovascular disorders can participate in physical activities. Each child with known or suspected heart disease should be carefully evaluated and his or her limits of physical activity set by the health-care provider or exercise professional.

1. Heart Murmurs

a. Heart murmurs are commonly heard in children.

b. Usually, these murmurs are functional murmurs and do not impair normal cardiovascular function.

c. A diagnosis of heart murmurs caused by anatomic defects does not necessarily exclude children from physical activity. Such exclusion should be considered individually and an exercise prescription designed according to the primary physician's recommendations.

2. Dysrhythmias

a. Suspected dysrhythmias should be referred to a physician.

b. Common symptoms associated with dysrhythmias include:
   1) Sensation of "skipped beats."
   2) Headache.
   3) Vomiting.
   4) Loss of vision.
   5) Syncope.
   6) Near-syncope.

c. Different types of dysrhythmias exist. Some are benign, whereas others may preclude participation in physical activity. The appropriate level of activity should be determined by a physician.
   1) Syncope is the loss of muscle tone and consciousness caused by diminished cerebral blood flow. Types of syncope include:
      a) Vasopressor syncope, which is caused by external stimuli (e.g., anxiety or emotion).
      b) Orthostatic syncope, which is caused by pooling of blood in the lower extremities of the body.
      c) Cardiovascular syncope, which is caused by some form of heart disease.
   2) Symptoms of presyncope include:
      a) Dizziness.
      b) Cold and clammy appearance.
      c) Diaphoresis.
      d) Significantly decreased blood pressure.
   3) Following an episode of syncope or presyncope, children should be referred to a physician before participating in vigorous physical activity.

D. ORTHOPEDIC CONSIDERATIONS

1. Bone Mass

During growth, overall bone mass and bone mineral density increase significantly. Weight-bearing physical activity during this time augments this process.

a. Humans have increased capacity to add bone in response to exercise.

b. Weightlifting and compressive exercises (e.g., gymnastics) have the greatest effect for enhancing bone mass in children.

c. The beneficial effects of exercise on bone mass do not appear to occur if **dietary calcium intake** is inadequate.

2. **Orthopedic Injuries (Overuse Injuries)**
Orthopedic injuries (overuse injuries) result from repetitive microtrauma of articular cartilage, bone, muscle, or tendon. They are commonly seen in children and adolescent athletes, particularly those specializing in one organized sport that involves cyclic forces applied to an anatomic structure.
   a. **Overuse injuries of bone (stress fractures)** commonly occur in the:
      1) Tibia, fibula, or foot in running sports.
      2) Femur, pelvis, or patella in jumping sports.
      3) Humerus, first rib, or elbow in overhand throwing and racquet sports.
   b. Risk Factors.
      1) Training Error.
         a) **Increased total volume** of training.
         b) **Increased rate of progression** of training intensity beyond approximately 10% per week.
      2) Muscle-Tendon Imbalance.
      Growth can cause changes in relative strength and flexibility across major joints, especially during the adolescent growth spurt. Repetitive techniques at this age can result in asymmetric stresses on bones and joints.
      3) Anatomic Malalignments.
      Malalignments (e.g., discrepancies of leg length, abnormalities of hip rotation) can result in excessive stress on skeletal units during repetitive exercise.
      4) High-Impact Forces During Running and Jumping Sports.
      These high-impact forces can be reduced by the use of proper footwear but are exacerbated by hard playing surfaces.
      5) Growth.
      Cartilage in growing children is more susceptible to repetitive trauma.

E. ONSET OF PUBERTY IN GIRLS AND AMENORRHEA

The age at which puberty begins in American girls varies from 9 to 14 years.

1. **Delayed menarche and the abnormal absence or suppression of menses (amenorrhea) have been associated with chronic endurance training.**
   a. No single underlying cause has been identified.
   b. **Young competitive athletes** have a higher incidence of amenorrhea than either their nonathletic counterparts or older athletic women.
   c. Blood levels of estradiol, progesterone, and follicle-stimulating hormone are lower in adolescent and **young adult women** involved in intense exercise training.
   d. Recent evidence suggests that **excessive training can interfere with the normal menstrual cycle** in some women by inhibiting the release of gonadotropin-releasing hormone.
2. The **hormonal imbalances associated with long-term secondary amenorrhea** in young female athletes can have deleterious effects on the normal accumulation of bone tissue during growth, which in turn **can increase the risk of both skeletal fragility and osteoporosis later in life**.
3. Obesity is associated with an earlier onset of puberty.

F. EXERCISE-INDUCED ASTHMA (EIA)

1. Asthma is the most common chronic illness in childhood, affecting between 5% and 15% of children in the United States.
2. Exercise-induced asthma consists of **cough, wheeze, chest tightness, chest pain, breathlessness**, or any combination of these during or, more often, immediately after exercise.
3. Exercise-induced asthma has been reported to occur in approximately 80% of patients with asthma and in as many as 10%–15% of apparently healthy children and adolescents.
4. The type of exercise affects the likelihood and severity of EIA episodes. Typically, **short and intense bouts of exercise are more likely to elicit EIA**.
5. **Ambient conditions** (e.g., cold, low humidity, polluted air) **can also exacerbate EIA**.
6. Children with EIA are often physically unfit because of restriction of activity, either self-imposed or imposed by parents or physicians.
7. **Control of EIA** may be through pharmacologic intervention or nonpharmacologic approaches (e.g., use of a mask or scarf during exercise in cold weather). Once EIA symptoms are controlled, most children can safely engage in normal physical activity.
8. **Increasing the duration of warm-up** may help to prevent EIA by mitigating the mechanism causing bronchoconstriction within the airways at the onset of exercise that promotes EIA.

G. UNIQUE RESPONSES OF CHILDREN DURING EXERCISE AND RECOVERY

The basic physiologic responses to exercise are similar in healthy individuals of any age. However, age-related quantitative differences are seen during exercise and recovery.

1. Metabolic Responses

a. **Submaximal, relative oxygen consumption** at a given workload in children is similar to that in adults for cycling exercise, but is 10%–20% higher for running or walking. This is owing to a lower exercise economy in children during running and walking.

b. **Anaerobic capacity is lower in children** than in adults because of the lower concentration and rate of utilization of muscle glycogen as well as the low levels of phosphofructokinase in children.

c. On initiation of exercise, **children reach metabolic steady state more quickly** than adults, which results in lower oxygen deficit.

d. Children exhibit a much more rapid recover of heart rate and blood pressure following exercise testing.

2. Cardiovascular Responses

a. **Cardiac output** at a given oxygen consumption **is slightly lower** in children than in adults.

b. **Heart rate** at a submaximal load **is higher** in children than in adults because of the smaller heart size and stroke volume in children.

c. **Maximal heart rate is higher in children** than in adults, but this does not fully compensate for the smaller heart size, **causing decreased maximal cardiac output**, in children.

d. **Arterial blood pressure**, especially systolic blood pressure, at submaximal and maximal workloads **is lower** in exercising children than in adults.

3. Pulmonary Responses

a. **Absolute maximal minute ventilation** is lower in children than in adults because of body size.

b. **Relative minute ventilation during maximal exercise** in children is similar to that in adults, but is considerably higher than that in adults during submaximal exercise at a fixed $\dot{V}O_2$.

c. Typically, children breathe at a higher frequency than adults and have decreased ventilatory volume compared with adults during exercise.

4. Exercise at a given relative intensity (i.e., percentage of $\dot{V}O_2$ max or maximum heart rate) is perceived to be easier by children.

H. TRAINABILITY OF CHILDREN AND ADOLESCENTS

1. Skeletal Muscle Strength

a. **Resistance training** during preadolescence and adolescence **causes relative strength gains** (percentage improvements) similar to those found in young adults with adequate intensity and volume of training.

b. **Strength gains** associated with resistance training are consistently associated with **muscle hypertrophy in adolescents** and **young adults.** However, muscle hypertrophy is rarely reported following resistance training in preadolescent children despite the increases in strength.

c. **Neurologic adaptations** resulting in an **increase in motor unit activation** have been measured following strength training in preadolescents and adolescents. Increased motor unit activation has been inferred to mediate strength gains in young children.

d. Resistance training in **prepubescent children** should focus on proper mechanics and form to help prevent injury.

2. Functional Capacity

a. Children and adolescents respond to endurance training in a manner similar to that of adults.

b. For preadolescents, the **magnitude of change in relative $\dot{V}O_2$ max** is lower than would be expected from changes in endurance performance. It appears that the cardiovascular system of preadolescents is trainable, but to a lesser extent than that of adolescents and adults. Improvements in performance by endurance-trained children may result, in part, from increases in biomechanical efficiency.

V. EXERCISE IN OLDER ADULTS

A. GENERAL CONSIDERATIONS

1. Older adults who are inactive can greatly benefit from regular participation in a well-designed exercise program.

   a. Adults become less physically active with age, however, so that by 75 years of age, 54% of men and 66% of women report no physical activity (*Figure 3-4*).

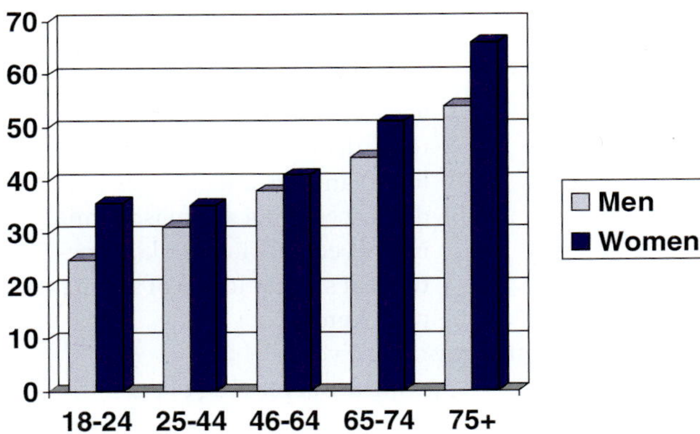

FIGURE 3-4. Percentage of U.S. adults 18 years of age and older who were physically inactive during their leisure time. Note that physical inactivity increases with advancing age. (Data from Schoenborn CA, Barnes PM. Leisure-time Physical Activity Among Adults: United States 1997–98. Advance data from vital and health statistics: no. 325. Hyattsville, Maryland: National Center for Health Statistics, 2002.)

   b. A minimum $\dot{V}O_2$ max of 13 $mL \cdot kg^{-1} \cdot min^{-1}$ is considered necessary for independent living.
2. Benefits of regular exercise include:
   a. Improved functional capacity and increased ability to perform activities of daily living (ADLs) and instrumental ADL (IADLs).
   b. Improved health status (because of reduction in risk factors associated with various diseases).
   c. Increased independence.
   d. An overall improvement in the quality of life.
3. Because of the age-related alterations in cardiovascular capacity, muscle mass and strength, flexibility, and balance, **a well-rounded program should incorporate aerobic, resistance, balance, and flexibility training.**
4. **Older individuals** with age-related limitations in range of motion, orthopedic problems, restricted mobility, arthritis, or other diseases may need an exercise program focusing on **minimal or non–weight-bearing, low-impact activities** (e.g., swimming).
5. Older adults may have a fear of falling. **Strength training and balance training can ameliorate the frequency of falls in older adults.**

B. MEDICAL SCREENING

1. The ACSM recommends screening for adults who are initiating exercise programs based on age and risk status.
   a. Screening requirements for initiating an exercise program are specified in the eighth edition of *ACSM's Guidelines for Exercise Testing and Prescriptions*.
   b. Refer to the eighth edition of *ACSM's Guidelines for Exercise Testing and Prescriptions* for methods and procedures associated with the screening process. Persons with **preexisting medical problems** (e.g., heart disease, arthritis, diabetes) or those who take medications that can affect response to exercise **should be referred to their physician** for guidance before initiating an exercise program.
2. **Evaluation by an exercise professional** is beneficial to document initial measurements of muscle strength, aerobic fitness capacity, flexibility, and range of motion. Any impairment in cardiopulmonary, musculoskeletal, or sensory function should be identified.

C. EXERCISE PRESCRIPTION

1. Guidelines for exercise prescription are found in the eighth edition of *ACSM's Guidelines for Exercise Testing and Prescription*. The ACSM general principles apply to adults of all ages.
   a. Initiating exercise programs in older adults at the lower end of the recommended guidelines for exercise prescription (see above) may be a prudent course of action in newly exercising older adults.
2. Cardiorespiratory Exercise Prescription Considerations For Older Adults
   a. The **exercise modality** should not impose excessive orthopaedic stress.
   b. **Frequency** of exercise can be increased in deconditioned older adults. Frequencies of 5–7 days/week are appropriate if adjustments in duration and intensity are also prescribed.
   c. **Duration** of exercise sessions can range from 20 to 60 minutes of continuous or intermittent aerobic activity.
   d. **Intensity** should be prescribed according to ACSM guidelines.
      1) Duration and intensity of exercise are interdependent and should be modified and adapted to individual functional capacity and interest.
      2) Exercise intensity for deconditioned older adults should start low. Initiating a program at less than 40% $\dot{V}O_2R$ or heart rate reserve (HRR) is not unusual.
      3) Generally, **light- to moderate-intensity exercise** of extended duration is recommended for older adults engaging in aerobic training programs.
3. Exercise Prescription Considerations for Resistance Training in Older Adults

a. Begin with minimal resistance to allow for adaptations of connective tissue.
b. Allow ample time to adjust to postural changes and balance during the transition between resistance training exercises.
c. Discourage participation in strength training exercises during active periods of pain or inflammation for persons with arthritis.
d. A **higher relative intensity** produces optimal training adaptations in muscle mass and strength.

D. BENEFITS AND PRECAUTIONS

1. Cardiovascular Endurance Benefits and Precautions

a. Cardiovascular Function
   1) Numerous studies have documented similar **increases in the $\dot{V}O_2$ max** of older (>60 years) compared with younger subjects following programs of endurance training.
   2) Depending on initial fitness levels, high-intensity exercise training **increases functional capacity** in the older adult as much as or more than that observed in young adults.
   3) **Improvements in $\dot{V}O_2$ max and endurance in men** result from central cardiovascular adaptations (e.g., increased cardiac output) and increased arteriovenous oxygen difference. **In older women,** the increased **$\dot{V}O_2$ max** appears to result primarily from increased arteriovenous oxygen difference.
   4) Moderate physical activity in older adults augments tolerance for daily activities and is associated with **less fatigue and dyspnea** (shortness of breath) and with **lower ratings of perceived exertion.**
b. Coronary Artery Disease and Hypertension
   1) The prevalence of hypertension and coronary artery disease increases with advancing age. The **incidence** of these conditions and the **morbidity and mortality** associated with heart disease are **greatly reduced in physically active individuals.**
   2) Benefits of Low-Intensity Endurance Training
      a) Effectively **lowers systolic and diastolic blood pressure** 8–10 mm Hg in normotensive and moderately hypertensive older adults.
      b) **Reduces myocardial oxygen demand** as a result of peripheral adaptations (e.g., increased oxygen extraction, increased vagal tone, decreased catecholamine release) and central changes (e.g., decreased myocardial ischemia, improved left ventricular function) at similar levels of submaximal exercise.
c. Cardiovascular Events
   1) **Appropriate screening** of exercise program participants (according to ACSM guidelines) is important, because the incidence of cardiovascular disease (both diagnosed and undiagnosed) increases with aging.
   2) The **incidence of cardiac events** during supervised adult fitness programs for apparently healthy older adults **is very low,** with nonfatal cardiac events reported to occur at a rate of approximately 1 per 800,000 hours of supervised exercise and fatal events at a rate of approximately 1 per 1.1 million hours of supervised exercise.
   3) **High-intensity exercise** training increases the risk for cardiac events.

2. Strength Training

a. Muscle strength, power, and endurance begin to decline in middle adulthood.
b. This decline accelerates after 50–60 years of age and is attributable to a number of changes. These changes include:
   1) Decreased muscle fiber size (especially type II).
   2) Decreased muscle fiber number.
   3) Decreased mitochondrial proteins and glycolytic, anaerobic, and oxidative enzyme activities.
   4) Decreased impulse conduction velocity.
   5) Loss of motor units.
   6) Increased intramuscular fat, especially in women.
c. **Regular physical activity seems to slow this decline.** One exception, however, is the loss of muscle fibers, which results from age-related loss of motoneurons and appears to be unaffected by exercise.
d. **Older adults exhibit strength gains from resistance training** that are similar to or even greater than those seen in younger adults (because of lower initial strength levels). These strength gains are related to improved

neurologic function and, to a lesser extent, increased muscle mass.

e. Both strength and power decrease with age, but power decreases to a greater extent.

3. Balance

a. Decreased balance and an associated increased occurrence of falls in the elderly can be attributed to many factors. These factors include:
   1) Muscle weakness.
   2) Inflexibility.
   3) Degradation of neuromotor function.
   4) Obesity.
   5) Visual and vestibular deterioration.

b. Substantial evidence suggests that physically active individuals maintain better balance during old age.
   1) Regular exercise improves muscle strength and flexibility, which has a positive influence on speed and agility of walking as well as on static balance.
   2) Regular exercise also appears to have positive effects on central nervous system functions, such as attention, short-term memory, and information processing speed, all of which commonly deteriorate with age and greatly impact balance and coordination.
   3) The risk of falling is reduced in older adults through an exercise program that incorporates resistance exercise, balance training, and stretching.

4. Preservation of Bone Mass

a. Bone mass peaks in early adulthood and declines slowly thereafter.

b. Regular weight-bearing exercise can slow the loss of bone mass with aging.
   1) The stimulation of osteoblastic bone formation on the periosteal surface of long bones following a given load is greater in the young than in the old, but it does occur in older adults if the stimulus is sufficient.
   2) The type of loading placed on the bone affects the degree of osteogenic stimulation. The magnitude of the load during an exercise session seems to be of greater importance than the number of loading cycles.

c. No consensus exists with regard to the precise intensity, frequency, duration, and type of exercise that most benefits bone.
   1) Regular aerobic exercise enhances bone health, particularly in postmenopausal women.
   2) Resistance training can offset the normal, age-related declines in bone health by maintaining and, sometimes, even improving bone mineral density.

d. Individuals with advanced osteoporosis should not engage in high-impact activities or deep forward flexion exercises, such as rowing.

5. Immune Function

a. The immune system deteriorates significantly with advancing age. This is evidenced by the increased incidence of malignancy, infectious disease, and autoimmune disorders in the elderly.

b. Numerous studies have indicated that lack of physical fitness and improper nutrition is also associated with compromised immune function. It remains unclear how much of the age-related loss of immune function is directly caused by physical inactivity; however, available data suggest that immune function is better in the elderly who are active compared with those who are sedentary.

6. Obesity

a. Longitudinal and cross-sectional studies have indicated that weight gain during adulthood is not caused by aging but, rather, by an increasingly sedentary lifestyle in older adults. Secondarily, older adults who continue the caloric consumption of their more active years also gain weight.
   1) Regular aerobic exercise has an obvious impact on energy balance by increasing energy expenditure.

b. Physical activity plays an important role in the prevention and treatment of obesity as age progresses. Programs of physical activity must be continued for months or even years to reduce and control body mass effectively.

c. Regular resistance training has positive anabolic effects in older individuals, leading to the preservation of skeletal muscle mass, which can help to slow the age-related decline in basal metabolic rate.

d. Older adults at the greatest risk for disability are those who are simultaneously sarcopenic and obese.

7. Insulin Resistance

a. Insulin resistance, a condition leading to type 2 diabetes, is characterized by high

TABLE 3-1. THE ROLE OF PHYSICAL ACTIVITY FOR QUALITY OF LIFE BY AGE CATEGORIES

DESCRIPTION	ROLE OF PHYSICAL ACTIVITY
Infant	Mobility
Child	Mobility, developing identity, self-esteem, recreation, social interaction
Adolescent	Developing identity
Early Adulthood	Self-esteem, recreation, social interaction
Middle Adulthood	Recreation, self-esteem, social interaction
Later Adulthood	Self-esteem, maintenance (job function)
Young-old	Maintenance (mobility, job), recreation, social interaction
Old	Mobility, ADL (eating, bathing, dressing, walking, social interaction), IADL (cooking washing clothes)
Old-old	Mobility, ADL, independent living
Oldest-old	Mobility, ADL, independent living

ADL, activities of daily living; IADL, instrumental ADL.
(Adapted with permission from Spirduso WW, Francis KL, MacRae PR. *Physical Dimensions of Aging*. Champaign, IL: Human Kinetics, 2005, p 28.)

levels of circulating insulin and reduced ability to maintain blood glucose concentration at a constant value.

b. Well-controlled studies have indicated that physical inactivity and obesity, but not aging, are related to increased risk for insulin resistance.

c. **Regular exercise can decrease abdominal fat and increase insulin sensitivity, which may normalize glucose tolerance.**

8. Psychological Benefits *(Table 3-1)*

a. Life Satisfaction
Older adults who exercise regularly have a more positive attitude toward work and are **generally healthier** than sedentary individuals.

b. Happiness
Strong correlations have been reported between the activity level of older adults and their self-reported happiness.

c. Self-Efficacy
1) Self-efficacy refers to the concept of or capability to perform a variety of tasks.
2) Older adults taking part in exercise programs commonly report that they are **able to do daily tasks more easily** than before they began the exercise program.

d. Self-Concept
Older adults improve their scores on self-concept questionnaires following participation in an exercise program.

e. Psychological Stress
Exercise is effective in reducing psychological stress.

f. It is highly probable that physical fitness has beneficial effects on cognitive functioning. Executive functioning may be particularly sensitive to fitness status.

9. Orthopedic Injury

a. The **incidence of musculoskeletal injury among regularly exercising older adults is considerably higher** than that in younger populations.

b. **Factors related to orthopedic injuries in older adults include:**
1) Inadequate warm-up.
2) Muscle weakness.
3) Sudden violent movements.
4) Rapid increases in exercise prescription.

10. Thermoregulatory Concerns

a. Older adults have **lower maximal cardiac output and compromised subcutaneous blood flow** during exercise. Furthermore, total body water is reduced, which decreases maximal capacity for sweating.

b. **Exercise training improves thermoregulation** in older adults. Nevertheless, leaders of exercise programs involving older adults should ensure the **availability of fluids** for the participants, and they should **avoid exercising outdoors in hot and humid conditions.**

11. Osteoarthritis

a. Osteoarthritis affects about 50% of adults over age 65 and 85% of those 75 years of age and older.

b. Exercise training does not affect the pathologic process of osteoarthritis.

c. Exercise training does not exacerbate pain or disease progression and can decrease pain and increase function.

E. UNIQUE RESPONSES OF OLDER ADULTS DURING EXERCISE AND RECOVERY *(TABLE 3-2)*

1. Cardiovascular and Hemodynamic Responses to Exercise

a. The **increase in heart rate** in response to a given increase in relative exercise intensity **is blunted** in older adults.

TABLE 3-2. EXERCISE RESPONSES COMMONLY OBSERVED IN OLDER ADULTS AND SUGGESTED TESTING MODIFICATIONS

CHARACTERISTIC	SUGGESTED MODIFICATION
1. Low aerobic capacity	Begin test at a low intensity (2–3 metabolic equivalents [METs]).
2. More time required to reach metabolic steady state	Increase length of warm-up (3+ min) and stages (2–3 min).
3. Poor balance	Bike preferred over treadmill or step test.
4. Poor leg strength	Treadmill preferred over bike or step test.
5. Difficulty holding mouthpiece with dentures	Add support or use face mask to measure $\dot{V}O_2$ max.
6. Impaired vision	Bike preferred over treadmill or step test.
7. Impaired hearing	Use electronic bike or treadmill to avoid the necessity of following a cadence.
8. Senile gait patterns or foot problems	Bike preferred; if treadmill is used, increase grade rather than speed.

(Adapted with permission from Skinner JS. Chapter 5: Importance of aging for exercise testing and exercise prescription. In: Skinner JS, ed: *Exercise Testing and Exercise Prescription for Special Cases.* Malvern, PA: Lea & Febiger, 1993, p. 79.)

b. It appears that stroke volume and cardiac output at a fixed submaximal workload are similar in healthy young and old adults. **Maximal stroke volume and cardiac output are decreased** in older adults, however, because of decreased blood volume and maximal heart rate.

c. Age-related **reductions in arterial compliance and left ventricular contractile reserve** combine to increase blood pressure and attenuate the increase in ejection fraction during exercise in the older adult.

d. The response of arterial blood pressure to submaximal exercise appears unchanged with advancing age. Because blood volume is reduced, the **maintenance of blood pressure response** in the older person **requires systemic vascular resistance to be elevated** above that found in young adults.

2. **Pulmonary Regulation During Exercise**
   a. **Expiratory flow limitation occurs at lower exercise intensities** with aging because of a loss of lung elastic recoil. This change can compromise inspiratory muscle function and increase ventilatory work. Older adults reach expiratory limitation at lower exercise intensities than do younger adults.
   b. **Dead space is increased** in the older adult from approximately 30% of tidal volume in the young to 40%–45% in the aged. This requires that total ventilatory response be elevated during exercise in the older adult to maintain alveolar ventilation and arterial P_{CO_2}.
   c. The reduction in pulmonary arteriolar compliance with aging **elevates blood pressures in the pulmonary artery and capillaries during exercise.** This may contribute to a **diffusion limitation of gas exchange** in the older adult during moderate-to-intense exercise.

F. TRAINABILITY OF OLDER ADULTS

1. The precise decrements in trainability of older adults remain controversial, because training programs for the elderly rarely employ the same absolute workloads as programs for young adults.
2. **Older adults can adapt to exercise training** and significantly improve health and mobility.
3. When planning an exercise program for older adults, keep in mind the following:
   a. Aging is associated with a **reduced adaptability to physiologic stimuli.**
   b. Exercise programs for older adults require **more time to produce improvements** in variables such as muscle strength, $\dot{V}O_2$ max, and muscle oxidative capacity.
   c. The **goals** of most exercise programs for older adults should include the maintenance of functional capacity for independent living, reduction in the risk of cardiovascular disease, retardation of the progression of chronic disease, promotion of psychological well-being, and opportunity for social interaction.

Review Test

DIRECTIONS: Carefully read all questions, and select the BEST single answer.

1. In terms of chronological age, early childhood is usually described as
   A) Birth to 3 weeks.
   B) 3 weeks to 1 year.
   C) 1 to 6 years.
   D) 7 to 10 years.

2. Which of the following age groups define the fastest-growing segment of the U.S. population?
   A) Preadolescents.
   B) Adolescents.
   C) Adults aged 65 to 85 years.
   D) Adults 100 years of age and older.

3. Which of the following best describes the increase in blood pressure that accompanies aging?
   A) Left ventricular hypertrophy.
   B) Kidney failure.
   C) Liver damage.
   D) Liver failure.

4. An increase in both systolic and diastolic blood pressure at rest and during exercise often accompanies aging. Blood pressure usually increases because of
   A) Increased arterial compliance and decreased arterial stiffness.
   B) Decreased arterial compliance and increased arterial stiffness.
   C) Decrease in both arterial compliance and arterial stiffness.
   D) Increase in both arterial compliance and arterial stiffness.

5. The $\dot{V}O_2$ max remains relatively unchanged throughout childhood. After age 25, it typically decreases by
   A) 0% to 5% each decade.
   B) 5% to 15% each decade.
   C) 15% to 20% each decade.
   D) 15% to 20% each year.

6. Which of the following explains a higher resting and exercise heart rate in children?
   A) Stroke volume is directly related to how much left ventricular stiffness reduces diastolic filling.
   B) Cardiac output is regulated more by peripheral resistance than by any other variable.
   C) Children typically have a lower stroke volume compared with adults.
   D) Children typically have a more elevated peripheral resistance compared with adults.

7. At age 17
   A) Boys and girls have similar levels of body fat.
   B) Boys have more body fat than girls.
   C) Girls have twice as much body fat as boys.
   D) Body fat is not routinely measured in children.

8. The total number of muscle fibers is fixed at an early age, although
   A) At adolescence, males exhibit rapid hypertrophy of muscle.
   B) In comparison to males, females exhibit a more rapid hypertrophy of muscle.
   C) Males lose muscle mass faster at an early age when they remain sedentary.
   D) Males tend to exhibit muscle hypertrophy at a later age than females.

9. Strenuous exercise can predispose children to which of the following?
   A) Osteoporosis.
   B) Osteoarthritis.
   C) Malignant tumors.
   D) Epiphysitis.

10. Which condition is commonly associated with a progressive decline in bone mineral density and calcium content in postmenopausal women?
    A) Osteoarthritis.
    B) Osteoporosis.
    C) Arthritis.
    D) Epiphysitis.

11. All of the following musculoskeletal changes typically occur with advancing age EXCEPT
    A) Decreased flexibility.
    B) Impaired balance.
    C) Inhibited range of motion.
    D) Skeletal muscle hypertrophy.

12. All of the following regarding thermoregulation in children are true EXCEPT
    A) Adults have a greater number of sweat glands compared with children.
    B) The rate of sweat production is lower in children compared with adults.
    C) Children acclimatize to hot environments at a slower rate than adults.
    D) Sweat rate for children is lower than for adults.

13. Which of the following factors does NOT impair an older individual's ability to thermoregulate?
    A) Reduced total body water.
    B) Decreased renal function.
    C) Decreased vascular peripheral responsiveness.
    D) Enhanced sweat response.

14. Healthy older adults walk at a preferred speed that is _____ slower than the preferred speed of younger adults
    A) 10%.
    B) 20%.
    C) 40%.
    D) 50%.

15. Which of the following is a result of an older person participating in an exercise program?
    A) Overall improvement in the quality of life and increased independence.
    B) No changes in the quality of life but an increase in longevity.
    C) Increased longevity but a loss of bone mass.
    D) Loss of bone mass with a concomitant increase in bone density.

16. Which of the following would generally be the preferred mode of exercise for an elderly person?
    A) Jogging.
    B) Calisthenics.
    C) Swimming.
    D) Archery.

17. An exercise program for elderly persons generally should emphasize increased
    A) Frequency.
    B) Intensity.
    C) Duration.
    D) Intensity and frequency.

18. Which of the following statements regarding osteoarthritis in older adults is FALSE?
    A) Exercise training improves function.
    B) Osteoarthritis is common in older adults.
    C) Exercise training slows down the progression of osteoarthritis.
    D) Exercise training does not exacerbate pain.

19. In response to regular resistance training,
    A) Older men and women demonstrate similar or even greater strength gains when compared with younger individuals.
    B) Younger men have greater gains in strength than older men.
    C) Younger women have greater gains in strength than older women.
    D) Younger men and women demonstrate similar or greater strength gains compared with older persons.

20. Hormonal imbalances associated with long-term secondary amenorrhea increases the risk of
    A) Extreme muscle hypertrophy.
    B) Osteoporosis.
    C) Osteoarthritis.
    D) Obesity.

ANSWERS AND EXPLANATIONS

1–C. Typical age groupings or distinctions are as follows: neonatal, birth to 3 weeks; infancy, 3 weeks to 1 year; early childhood, 1 to 6 years; middle childhood, 7 to 10 years; late childhood or prepuberty, 9 to 15 years in females and 12 to 16 years in males; adolescence, the 6 years following puberty; adulthood, 20 to 64 years; older adulthood, 65 years and older.

2–C. It is estimated that by the year 2030, 20% of the population of the United States will be 65 years or older. The fastest growing age category is centenarians, those more than 100 years of age.

3–A. Left ventricular hypertrophy increases with age, apparently related to increased afterload associated with increased peripheral vascular resistance.

4–B. A decrease in arterial compliance and an increase in arterial stiffness with age can result in elevated systolic and diastolic blood pressure, both at rest and during exercise.

5–B. A function of cardiac output and arteriovenous oxygen difference, $\dot{V}O_2$ max can remain relatively unchanged throughout adulthood. Without any exercise intervention, however it decreases 5%–15% each decade after age 25. Both cardiac output and arteriovenous oxygen difference decline with age; regular physical activity will help reduce these effects.

6–C. At rest and during exercise, heart rate is higher in children because of compensation for a lower stroke volume. Maximal heart rate and maximal stroke volume both decrease with age, causing a significant decline in maximal cardiac output.

7–C. Typical gains in fat mass during puberty in females are twice those in males because of hormonally induced accumulation of fat in the breasts and around the hips. At age 17, female body fat percentage is twice that of males.

8–A. At adolescence, males exhibit a rapid hypertrophy of muscle that is disproportionately greater than that observed in females. The total number of muscle fibers seems to be fixed at an early age in both genders. Muscle mass declines (atrophy) with advancing age because of a progressive decrease in the number and size of fibers, with a greater selective loss of type II fibers.

9–D. Because in children the epiphysis is not yet united with the bone shaft, strenuous exercise can cause problems with bone growth. Epiphysitis can occur with overuse. Also, fractures can pass through the epiphyseal plate, leading to disruption in normal bone growth.

10–B. Advancing age brings a progressive decline in bone mineral density and calcium content. This loss is accelerated in women immediately after menopause. As a result, older adults are more susceptible to osteoporosis and bone fractures.

11–D. Connective tissue (fascia, ligaments, tendons) become less extensible with age. Degeneration of joints, especially the spine, occurs with advancing age, causing decreased range of motion along with a progressive loss of flexibility. Balance and postural stability are also affected because of age-related changes in both sensory and motor systems.

12–A. Adults and children have the same number of sweat glands. Children, however, consistently sweat less than adults because the sweat rate and the rate of sweat production for each gland are lower in children.

13–D. A number of factors can impair an older individual's ability to thermoregulate, including reduced total body water, decreased renal function, decreased vascular peripheral responsiveness, rapid dehydration, and blunted sweat response.

14–B. Healthy older adults walk at a preferred speed that is 20% slower than the preferred speed of younger adults. The decrease in gait speed is largely because of a decrease in stride length as opposed to a decrease in stride frequency.

15–A. Most older adults are not sufficiently active. This population can benefit greatly from regular participation in a well-designed exercise program. Benefits of such a program include increased fitness, improved health status (reduction in risk factors associated with various diseases), increased independence, and overall improvement in the quality of life.

16–C. For older adults, who often suffer from limited range of motion, orthopedic problems, restricted mobility, arthritis, and other disorders, an emphasis on minimal or non–weight-bearing, low-impact activities (e.g., swimming) is generally most appropriate.

17–A. Increased frequency of exercise is generally recommended for older adults to optimize cardiovascular as well as balance and flexibility adaptations. The recommended duration of exercise depends on the intensity of the activity; higher-intensity activity should be conducted over a shorter period of time.

18–C. Little scientific evidence suggests that regular exercise slows down the progression of osteoarthritis. Physical activity can lead to the same benefits observed in the general population. Further, exercise improves strength, balance, and postural stability, which may reduce falls in this at risk population.

19–A. Muscle strength peaks in the mid-20s for both genders and remains fairly stable through the mid-40s. Muscle strength declines by approximately 15% per decade in the sixth and seventh decades and by approximately 30% per decade thereafter. However, older men and women demonstrate similar or even greater strength gains when compared with younger individuals in response to resistance training. These strength gains are related to improved neurologic function and, to a lesser extent, increased muscle mass.

20–B Hormonal imbalances associated with long-term secondary amenorrhea may affect the normal accumulation of bone tissue during growth, which may in turn increase the risk of bone fragility and osteoporosis later in life.

Pathophysiology/Risk Factors

CHAPTER 4

I. CHRONIC OBSTRUCTIVE PULMONARY DISEASE (COPD)

A. This is a preventable and treatable disease state characterized by limitations in airflow that are not fully reversible.

B. This limitation in airflow is generally progressive and associated with abnormal inflammatory responses in the lung to noxious particles or gases. **Tobacco smoking is the main risk factor**, although other inhaled noxious particles and gases may contribute to the risk.

C. COPD affects the lungs and has accompanying systemic effects as well.

D. The symptoms of COPD include cough, sputum production, and **dyspnea** (shortness of breath).

E. COPD involves pathophysiologic changes in four lung compartments: central airways, peripheral airways, lung parenchyma (endothelium of the alveoli and pulmonary capillaries, and the alveolar–capillary interspaces), and the pulmonary vasculature. These compartments may be differentially affected.

F. COPD involves an inflammatory response in the lungs causing characteristic lesions. Imbalance between proteinases (enzymes involved in the breakdown of protein) and antiproteinases (enzymes that block the effect of proteinases) and oxidative stress are also part of the pathogenic processes of COPD.

G. The processes of COPD result in hypersecretion of mucus and dysfunction of the cilia of the lung, airflow limitation and hyperinflation of the lung, abnormalities of gas exchange, pulmonary hypertension, and systemic effects.

H. The airflow obstruction characteristic of COPD is caused by a mixture of obstructive bronchiolitis (small airway disease), and **emphysema** (destruction of the parenchyma). The degree to which an individual is affected by these two diseases varies.

I. COPD is diagnosed by pulmonary function testing. A postbronchodilator ratio of **FEV_1** (forced expiratory volume in 1 second)/**FVC** (forced vital capacity) of ≤ 0.7 is indicative of nonreversible airflow limitation.

J. The severity of COPD is categorized by the degree of impairment in the FEV_1:FVC ratio and the FEV_1.

II. ASTHMA

A. Asthma is a common complex chronic disorder of the airways characterized by variable and recurring symptoms, airflow obstruction, hyperresponsiveness of the bronchioles, and underlying inflammation.

B. Genetic and environmental interactions are important in the development and expression of asthma.

C. Airflow limitations, the cause of the asthma symptoms, and result from bronchoconstriction or bronchospasm, edema of the airways, airway hyperresponsiveness, and remodeling of the airways resulting from acute and chronic inflammatory processes.

D. Allergies, respiratory infections, and environmental exposures to tobacco smoke, air pollution, and possibly dietary factors have been associated with the emergence of asthma.

E. Common symptoms include coughing, wheezing, chest tightness, shortness of breath, and faster or noisy breathing. Symptoms of asthma can vary in an individual and between individuals. Frequency and severity of symptoms also can vary.

F. The pathophysiologic processes associated with asthma can be progressive.

III. RESTRICTIVE LUNG DISEASE

A. Restrictive lung disease includes a large group of disorders that restrict or reduce lung volume and tidal volume. These disorders are caused by diseases that affect the thorax, respiratory muscles, nerves, pleura, or parenchyma.

B. Diseases in this category share one or more features: loss of functioning of the alveoli–capillary unit (impairment in gas exchange), altered mechanical function of the thorax and pulmonary system, and secondary cardiovascular dysfunction.

C. Causes of restrictive lung disease include neuromuscular diseases (e.g., muscular dystrophy, spinal cord injury), disorders of the chest wall (e.g., scoliosis, ankylosing spondylitis, morbid obesity), pleural diseases (e.g., fibrosis, effusion), parenchymal diseases (e.g., malignancy, pulmonary edema, immunologic diseases).

D. Symptoms of restrictive lung disease include effort intolerance and dyspnea.
E. Pulmonary function tests in restrictive lung diseases are notable for reduced total lung capacity (TLC) in the presence of a normal ratio of the FEV_1 to FVC.
F. **Hypoxia** becomes a significant problem with progressive disease. Ventilation-perfusion ($\dot{V}/Q$) mismatching is the primary mechanism responsible for the hypoxia.

IV. CARDIOVASCULAR DISEASES (CVD)

A. Cardiovascular diseases are a category of diseases affecting the heart and blood vessels.
B. The most common cardiovascular diseases include the **atherothrombotic** diseases (coronary heart disease [CHD], acute coronary syndromes, hypertension, peripheral arterial disease, and ischemic stroke), valvular heart disease, and hemorrhagic stroke.
C. The risk of these diseases is increased by aging, lifestyle, environmental, and genetic factors (discussed below).
D. Atherothrombotic Cardiovascular Diseases
   1. The atherothrombotic cardiovascular diseases share a common pathophysiology, atherothrombosis, which involves the inter-related processes of **arteriosclerosis**, **atherosclerosis**, and **thrombosis**.
      a. Arteriosclerosis is a loss of elasticity of the arteries, which is characterized by thickening and hardening of artery walls.
      b. Atherosclerosis is a process whereby fatty material is deposited along the walls of arteries. This fatty material thickens, hardens, and may eventually block the artery. Atherosclerosis is just one of several types of arteriosclerosis.
      c. Thrombosis is a blood clot that forms in a blood vessel or heart chamber and remains there. A thrombus that travels from where it was formed to another location in the body is called an embolus (e.g., pulmonary embolism).
   2. Understanding of the development and progression of atherosclerosis (atherogenesis) is incomplete.
   3. Endothelial injury resulting in endothelial dysfunction and a subsequent inflammatory response is known to play a critical role in arteriosclerosis and atherosclerosis.
   4. Atherogenesis
      a. Figure 4-1 depicts the normal coronary artery wall.

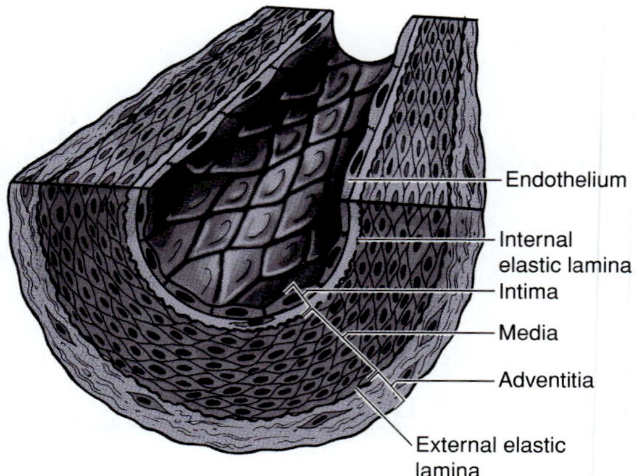

FIGURE 4-1. The normal coronary artery wall. The lumen is the inside cavity or channel where blood flows. The endothelium is a single layer of cells that form a tight barrier between blood and the arterial wall. It resists thrombosis, promotes vasodilatation, and inhibits smooth muscle cells from migration and proliferation into the intima. Damage to the endothelium increases the susceptibility of the artery to atherosclerosis. The intima is a very thin, innermost layer of the artery wall. Composed of predominantly connective tissue with some smooth muscle cells, it is where atherosclerotic lesions are formed. The thickest, middle layer of the artery wall, the media, is composed of predominantly smooth muscle cells. It is responsible for vasoconstriction or vasodilatation of the artery, and it can contribute to the atherosclerotic process through migration and proliferation of smooth muscle cells to the intima. The adventitia is the outermost layer of the artery wall. It provides the media and intima with oxygen and nutrients, and is not believed to have a significant role in the development of atherosclerosis. (From Ross R, Glomset J. The pathogenesis of atherosclerosis. *N Engl J Med* 295:369, 1976, with permission.)

      b. Atherosclerosis involves arterial injury and inflammation.
         1) Arterial injury (Figure 4-2)
            a) Chronic, excessive injury to endothelial cells initiating the process of atherogenesis can result from multiple causes including the following:
               (i) Tobacco smoke and other chemical irritants from tobacco.
               (ii) **Low-density lipoprotein cholesterol** (LDL-C).
               (iii) **Hypertension.**
               (iv) Glycated substances resulting from **hyperglycemia** and diabetes mellitus (DM).
               (v) Elevated plasma **homocysteine**.
               (vi) Infectious agents (e.g., *Chlamydia pneumoniae*, herpes viruses).
            b) Arterial (or endothelial) injury and insult results in endothelial dysfunction that alters the homeostasis around the vessel wall.
               (i) The end result can be ongoing, progressive atherosclerotic

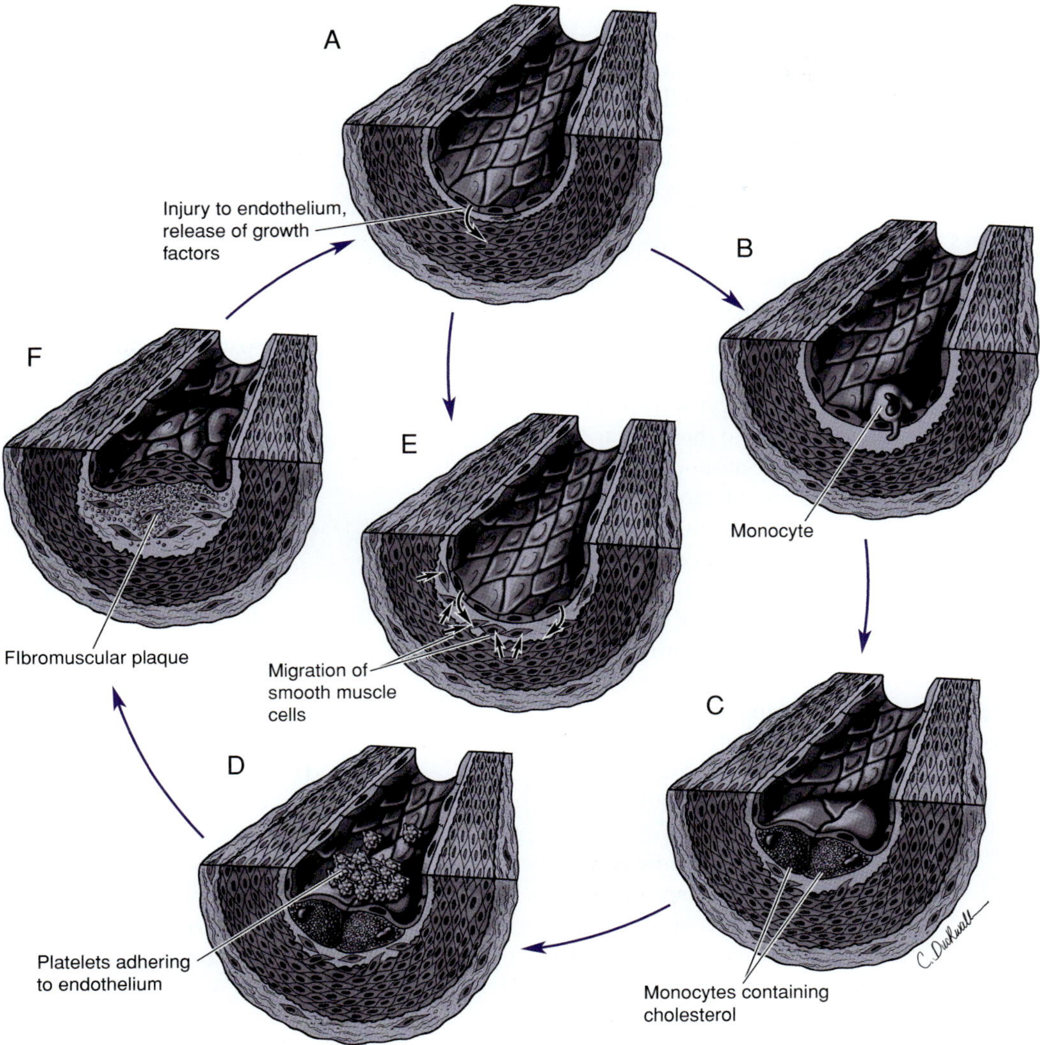

FIGURE 4-2. The atherosclerotic process-response to injury. A. Injury to endothelium with release of growth factors (*small arrow*). B. Monocytes attach to endothelium. C. Monocytes migrate to the intima, take up cholesterol, and form fatty streaks. D. Platelets adhere to the endothelium and release growth factors. F. The result is a fibromuscular plaque. An alternative pathway is shown with *arrows* from A to E to F, with growth factor-mediated migration of smooth muscle cells from the media to the intima (E). (From Ross R. The pathogenesis of atherosclerosis—an update. *N Engl J Med* 314:496, 1986, with permission.)

changes in the vessel and multiple lesion development.

c) Endothelial dysfunction caused by arterial wall injury results in an inflammatory response.
   (i) Increased adhesiveness.
      (a) Platelets adhere to the damaged endothelium (platelet aggregation), form small blood clots on the vessel wall (mural thrombi), and release growth factors and vasoconstrictor substances, such as thromboxane A_2.
      (b) Endothelial cells lose selective permeability, enabling cells and molecules to pass into the subendothelial space.
      (c) Endothelial cells lose antithrombotic properties, resulting in increased risk of clot formation and thrombus.
   (ii) Increased permeability to lipoproteins and other substances in the blood.
      (a) Endothelial cells secrete platelet-derived growth

factor, resulting in movement of smooth muscle cells into the intima.

(b) Endothelial cells attract other cells toward the intima that are involved in the development of atherosclerosis.
   i. Excess, oxidized low-density lipoprotein (LDL) particles accumulate in the arterial wall. They attract monocytes and other cells to the intima.
   ii. The monocytes mature into macrophages in the intima and promote mitosis and proliferation of these cells.
   iii. The release of additional growth factors and vasoactive substances continues.
   iv. Monocytes promote the uptake up more lipids, particularly LDL.
   v. These cells and connective tissue move from the media to the intima, producing fatty streaks or lesions. As they ingest more fatty substances, the fatty streak progresses to a fat-filled lesion.
   vi. As the process continues, smooth muscle cells accumulate in the intima and form a fibrous plaque.

(c) Early remodeling is the outward growth of the vessel to maintain lumen size in response to the enlarging plaque.

(d) As the plaque enlarges, the vessel lumen becomes occluded, obstructing blood flow. Other complications may include thrombus formation with occlusion, peripheral emboli, and weakening of the vessel wall.

(iii) Impaired **vasodilation**, increased **vasospasm**
   (a) Reduced secretion of vasodilating substances (e.g., endothelium-derived relaxing factor nitric oxide [EDRF-NO]) leads to abnormal vasoreactivity (increased vasoconstriction, decreased vasodilation, or both).

2) Atherosclerosis does not necessarily occur or progress in a stable, linear manner.
   a) Some lesions develop slowly and are relatively stable for long periods of time.
   b) Other lesions progress very quickly owing to frequent plaque rupture, thrombi formation, and intima changes.
   c) Partial regression of fatty, soft lesions is possible with aggressive multifactorial risk reduction. Modest results have been observed.
   d) Endothelial dysfunction can be reversed.
      (i) Many lifestyle behaviors relate specifically to either dysfunction or improved function (e.g. exercise, dietary fat content, appropriate management of stress-related events, maintaining optimal blood pressure, blood lipids and blood glucose).

E. **Acute Coronary Syndrome** (ACS)
   1. ACS is an umbrella term describing a group of clinical symptoms compatible with acute myocardial ischemia, including unstable angina pectoris and myocardial infarction (MI), and sudden cardiac death.
   2. ACS requires prompt cardiac care.

F. **Myocardial Ischemia**
   1. Insufficient blood flow to the heart muscle (myocardium) that occurs when myocardial oxygen demand exceeds the oxygen supply.
   2. Myocardial ischemia occurs when a coronary artery is partially or completely obstructed because of atherosclerosis, coronary thrombosis or coronary artery spasm.
   3. May be symptomatic (angina pectoris) or asymptomatic (silent myocardial ischemia).

G. **Angina Pectoris**
   1. Transient pain or discomfort in the chest (or adjacent areas) caused by myocardial ischemia.

a. Discomfort most commonly located in the areas of the chest, neck, cheeks or jaw, shoulder, upper back, or arms.
b. Most often described as constricting, squeezing, burning, or a heavy feeling.

2. Classic (typical) angina is initiated by factors such as exercise or stress, excitement, cold or hot weather; food intake, especially large meals or heavy, high fat meals; and it is relieved by rest or nitroglycerin.
3. Vasospastic (variant or Prinzmetal's) angina usually occurs at rest without any apparent precipitating event, such as exercise or stress. The cause of vasospastic angina is coronary artery vasospasm, often the result of abnormal endothelial function (reactivity).
4. The pain or discomfort is relieved by rest or nitrate medications within a short period of time (usually <15 minutes).

H. Unstable Angina Pectoris

1. Chest pain of new onset, or angina pectoris that lasts for a longer duration, at increased frequency; at a lower level of exertion than usual; or which occurs at rest.

I. Acute Myocardial Infarction (MI)

1. Prolonged myocardial ischemia (>60 minutes) that results in death **(necrosis)** of an area of the myocardium.
2. About 90% of MI result from formation of an acute thrombus in an atherosclerotic coronary artery.

V. PLAQUE RUPTURE—A MAJOR CAUSE OF CORONARY THROMBI

A. Endothelial dysfunction contributes to vasoconstriction of the coronary artery through reduced vasodilator substances, as well as a characteristic, abnormal vasoreactivity inherent in the dysfunctioning endothelium.

1. The healing process following an MI involves remodeling.
   a. Remodeling results in fibrous tissue residing among the necrosed myocardial tissue.
   b. The area of necrosis may increase secondary to residual ischemia following an acute MI, or may decrease because of collateral circulation.
2. Possible complications of MI include:
   a. Extension of the zone of ischemia to surrounding tissue, thus widening the necrosis.
   b. **Ventricular Aneurysm**
      1) Necrotic muscle fibers of the heart degenerate and remodel the ventricular wall, and may cause a thinning of the myocardial wall.
      2) During systole, these nonfunctional muscle fibers do not contract, but rather bulge outward (aneurysm).
      3) The presence of an aneurysm increases the risk of thrombus, ventricular arrhythmias, and heart failure.
   b. Ventricular Rupture
      1) Involves a mechanism similar to ventricular aneurysm, but the ventricular wall ruptures.
      2) Rupture of the ventricular free wall is often fatal.
         a) May be associated with cardiac tamponade or a large area of infarction in the ventricular free wall.
      3) Rupture of the ventricular septal wall is less often fatal and may be associated with chronic congestive heart failure (CHF).
   c. Papillary necrosis and rupture
      1) This necrosis and rupture of the papillary muscle(s) affects valvular function and results in severe mitral regurgitation, which can lead to heart failure or pulmonary edema.
   d. Left ventricular dysfunction
      1) Left ventricular dilation can be caused by weakening of the left ventricle owing to necrotic myocardium.
      2) It is often associated with chronic CHF.

B. Sudden Cardiac Death

1. Sudden, abrupt loss of heart function in a person with or without diagnosed CHD.
2. Death occurs immediately or shortly after symptoms appear (within 24 hours).
3. About half of all deaths from CHD are sudden and unexpected, regardless of the underlying disease.

C. Chronic Heart Failure **(congestive heart failure [CHF])**

1. A heart disease where there is an impairment in the ability of the ventricle to eject or to fill with blood.
2. Most commonly caused by CHD or other cardiovascular diseases, primarily affecting the elderly.
3. Impairment of heart function during systole or diastole.
   a. Some patients have either predominantly systolic or diastolic dysfunction, whereas others have both conditions concurrently.
   b. Systolic Dysfunction
      1) Diagnosed by a below-normal left ventricular ejection fraction.
      2) Coronary artery disease is the most common cause (ischemic left ventricular dysfunction).

3) Other causes may be identifiable, such as hypertension or valvular heart disease, or idiopathic (i.e., **idiopathic dilated cardiomyopathy**).

c. Diastolic Dysfunction

1) Impaired ventricular filling.
2) Diastolic dysfunction can result from restrictive cardiomyopathy, CHD, hypertrophic cardiomyopathy, infiltrative cardiomyopathies, or other unidentifiable conditions.
3) Signs and symptoms of heart failure include dyspnea, fatigue, exercise intolerance, and fluid retention, which can result in pulmonary or peripheral edema.
4) The natural history of CHF is progressive, although the rate of progression is highly variable.
   a) Three main stages of progression:
      (i) Ventricular dysfunction without definite symptoms (asymptomatic left ventricular dysfunction).
      (ii) Minimally symptomatic stage.
      (iii) Congestive symptoms of fluid overload.
5) The progression of CHF is directly related to the process of remodeling of the heart.
   a) The cardiac chambers enlarge and the walls of the ventricles hypertrophy.
      (i) This causes an increase in end-diastolic volume and preserves cardiac output.
   b) With continued remodeling, cardiac size becomes too great, resulting in:
      (i) Deterioration in cardiac output.
      (ii) Worsening symptoms.
6) The severity of CHF is classified as follows:
   a) Stage A: Patients at high risk for developing CHF, but who have no structural disorder of the heart.
   b) Stage B: Patients with structural heart disease, but no symptoms of CHF.
   c) Stage C: Patients with past or current symptoms of CHF with underlying structural heart disease.
   d) Stage D: Patients with end-stage disease requiring specialized treatment, such as mechanical circulatory support, continuous inotropic infusions, cardiac transplantation, or hospice care.

d. Once symptoms of congestion develop, median survival is only 2 to 3 years.

1) Sudden cardiac death is responsible for approximately 40% of deaths in CHF.

D. **Cardiomyopathy**

1. A heart disease characterized by a weakening of the myocardium that usually results in inadequate pumping function of the heart
2. May be caused by viral infections, MI, alcoholism, long-term, severe high blood pressure, or unknown causes
3. The three main types of cardiomyopathy are dilated, hypertrophic, and restrictive.
   a. Dilated cardiomyopathy involves enlargement of the heart muscle and is the most common type of cardiomyopathy.
   b. Restrictive cardiomyopathy is a group of disorders where there is abnormal filling of the heart chambers because of stiffness of the heart and the inability to relax normally during diastole.
   c. Hypertrophic cardiomyopathy is the thickening of the muscles that make up the heart.

D. Valvular Heart Disease

1. Disorders involving the valves of the heart (aortic, pulmonary, mitral, tricuspid)
2. Causes include degenerative heart disease, endocarditis (inflammation of the inner lining of the heart, often from infectious causes), CHD, rheumatic heart disease, connective tissue diseases (e.g., rheumatoid arthritis, ankylosing spondylitis), and iatrogenic (medical treatment) causes, such as radiation and pharmacologic therapies.
3. Two major classifications are stenotic and regurgitant valvular heart disease.
   a. Valvular stenosis is a condition characterized by the inability of a heart valve to open completely.
      1) Blood is pumped through a reduced passageway resulting in reduced blood flow.
   b. Valvular regurgitation is a condition characterized by the inability of a heart valve to close completely.
      1) This leads to regurgitation (blood leaking back through the valve when it should be closed).

E. Congenital Heart Defects

1. Congenital heart defects is a broad term that refers to diseases of the heart that were present at birth.
2. Congenital defects can include patent ductus arteriosus (mixing of blood between right ventricle and pulmonary artery), obstruction defects (e.g., aortic stenosis, pulmonary stenosis, and coarctation of the aorta), septal defects (e.g., atrial septal

defect [ASD], ventricular septal defect [VSD]), cyanotic defects (e.g., Tetralogy of Fallot, transposition of the great arteries), hypoplastic left-sided heart syndrome (underdevelopment of the left side of the heart).

3. Adults may have congenital heart diseases that may or may not have been repaired in childhood.

F. Peripheral Arterial Disease (**PAD**)
   1. Arteriosclerosis of the peripheral blood vessels (arteries that supply the legs and feet).
      a. May result in ischemia of the muscle supplied by the artery.
      b. Symptoms include claudication (pain in the thighs, calves, or feet on exertion or at rest), numbness, and cold legs or feet.
   2. Diagnosis is usually made using the supine resting and postexercise ankle brachial blood pressure index (ABI), segmental pressure measurements, pulse volume recordings, Doppler and duplex ultrasound. MRI, CT scans, and angiography may also be used.
   3. Severity can be classified by the Fontane Classification or by use of ABI.
      a. Fontane Classification
         1) Asymptomatic.
         2) Intermittent claudication.
         3) Distance to pain onset >200 m.
         4) Distance to pain onset <200 m.
         5) Pain at rest.
         6) Gangrene, tissue loss.

G. Stroke
   1. Stroke is an acute vascular event that is a leading cause of death and disability.
   2. Two types of stroke:
      a. Ischemic Stroke
         1) Decreased blood flow to a portion of the brain (ischemia) resulting in cell death.
         2) More common and potentially treatable with thrombolytic agents (<270 minutes on onset).
      b. Intracranial Hemorrhagic Stroke
         1) Sudden rupture of an artery in the brain, leading to compression of the brain structures.
         2) Caused by bleeding in the brain.
         3) Two types:
            a) Subarachnoid Hemorrhage
               (i) Sudden rupture of an artery in the brain, leading to blood filling the space surrounding the brain.
               (ii) Nontraumatic leakage or rupture of the Circle of Willis.
               (iii) May occur from an arteriovenous malformation.
               (iv) Symptoms include sudden onset of severe headache, neck stiffness, and loss of consciousness.
            b) Cerebral hemorrhage.
            c) Intracerebral hemorrhage most common in patients with hypertension.
            d) Caused by rupture of lenticulostriate artery (branch of middle cerebral artery).
      c. Stroke symptoms
         1) Sudden weakness of the face, arm, or leg, usually on one side of the body.
         2) May also include sudden numbness of the face, arm, or leg; sudden confusion, trouble speaking, or trouble understanding speech; sudden trouble seeing in one or both eyes; sudden trouble walking, dizziness, loss of balance or coordination; or sudden severe headache with no known cause.
      d. Diagnosis
         1) Symptoms evaluated using the National Institutes of Health (NIH) Stroke Scale.
         2) CT scan, MRI, Doppler (carotid, transcranial), cerebral arteriogram.
      e. Risk increased in presence of CVD risk factors, previous transient ischemic attack (TIA) or stroke, and previous MI.

VI. SIGNS AND SYMPTOMS OF CARDIOPULMONARY AND METABOLIC DISEASE

A. DEFINITION OF SIGN AND SYMPTOM

1. A sign is an objective symptom of a disease. This is something that the clinician observes or discovers on examination.
   a. Example: swelling of the ankles (edema).
2. A symptom is a subjective symptom of a disease. This is something the person (patient) experiences.
   a. Example: chest pain.
3. Major signs and symptoms of cardiovascular, pulmonary, and metabolic diseases are listed below (see also *GETP* Figure 2.3).
   a. Pain, discomfort (or other anginal equivalent) in the chest, neck, jaw, arms, or other areas, which may be caused by ischemia.
   b. Shortness of breath at rest or with mild exertion.
   c. Dizziness or syncope.
   d. **Orthopnea** or paroxysmal nocturnal dyspnea.

1) Orthopnea dyspnea: difficulty in breathing while lying down; inability to breathe easily unless sitting upright.
2) **Paroxysmal Nocturnal Dyspnea** (PND): waking at night short of breath.

d. Ankle edema (swelling).
e. Palpitations (the sensation of skipped heart beats) or tachycardia (rapid heartbeat).
f. Intermittent claudication (pain in the leg, typically calf or buttocks, particularly with exertion and relieved by rest).
g. Known heart murmur.
h. Unusual fatigue or shortness of breath with usual activities.

VII. RISK FACTORS FOR CARDIOVASCULAR DISEASE

A. PRIMARY RISK FACTORS—NONMODIFIABLE

1. Advancing age

a. Risk increases steeply with advancing age in men and women because of atherosclerosis accumulation.
b. About 50% of MIs occur in persons over age 65, 45% in those age 45 to 65, and 5% in those under age 45.

2. Gender

a. One-third of all adult men and women have some form of CVD.
b. The risk of CVD increases for both genders with advancing age.
c. Before age 75 years, the rate of CVD events is higher in men compared with women.
   1) The gender gap in a CVD event narrows with advancing age.
   2) A postmenopausal woman has two to three times the risk of CHD than a premenopausal woman of the same age.
d. The lifetime risk of developing CHD after age 40 years is 49% for men and 32% for women.
e. Woman have a higher mortality rate associated with MI and the prevalence of angina pectoris, CHF, sudden death, and stroke compared with men.

3. Family History

a. Children and siblings of a person with CAD are more likely to develop it themselves.
b. A positive family history carries excess risk even when accounting for modifiable risk factors.
   1) Risk increases with the number of relatives affected and at younger ages of onset.

B. PRIMARY RISK FACTORS—MODIFIABLE

1. Tobacco Smoking

a. Smokers are at roughly two and a half times greater risk for CAD than nonsmokers, although individual risk varies with extent of exposure (lifetime dosage).
b. The risk of heart disease decreases 50% within 1-year of smoking cessation and approaches that of a lifetime nonsmoker within 15 years.
c. Smoking has both acute (e.g., increased myocardial oxygen demand) and chronic effects (e.g., endothelial damage) on the myocardium and coronary vessels.
d. Smoking negatively influences other coronary artery disease risk factors (e.g., lowers high-density lipoproteins [HDLs]).

2. Dyslipidemia

a. There is a positive correlation between total cholesterol (TC) and LDL levels, the amount of fat, saturated fat, and cholesterol in the diet, and CAD mortality and morbidity.
b. TC, LDLs, and TGs contribute to the atherosclerotic process, whereas high-density lipoproteins (HDLs) are cardioprotective.
c. The National Cholesterol Education Program Adult Treatment Panel III (ATPIII) provides recommendations for the detection, evaluation, and treatment of high blood cholesterol in adults.
d. The aggressiveness of lipid management is determined by the absolute risk of developing CAD (e.g., MI, CAD death) over the next 10 years.
e. The primary target for management is LDL, especially in those with established CAD.

C. HYPERTENSION

1. Hypertension is classified according to the blood pressure classifications of the 2003 Seventh Report of the Joint Committee on Prevention, Detection, Evaluation, and Treatment of High Blood Pressure (JNC7) (See *GETP*, Table 3.1).
2. Recommendations for treatment are also available in the JNC7.
3. As blood pressure increases, so does the risk of cardiovascular disease.
   a. This holds true across all blood pressure ranges, including individuals classified as normal or prehypertensive.

   b. Hypertension has both acute (e.g., increased myocardial oxygen demand) and chronic effects (e.g., endothelial and renal dysfunction) on the myocardium.
4. Treatment of hypertension does not remove all of the cardiovascular risk associated with elevated blood pressure.

D. SEDENTARY LIFESTYLE

1. A sedentary lifestyle carries a risk for CVD similar to that of hypertension, dyslipidemia, and cigarette smoking.
2. A sedentary lifestyle can influence other CVD risk factors (e.g., increased blood pressure, decreased HDL cholesterol, decreased sensitivity to insulin resulting in elevated blood glucose levels, and increased overweight/obesity).
3. Persons who are physically inactive following a MI have significantly higher mortality rates than active individuals.

E. OVERWEIGHT/OBESITY

1. Overweight/obesity has a strong positive relationship with other risk factors for CAD, such as hypertension, dyslipidemia, and type 2 DM.
2. The risk for CVD is greater in persons with central (android or upper body) obesity than in those with peripheral (gynoid or lower body) obesity.
3. Waist circumference and waist-to-hip ratio (WHR) provide an index of central obesity.
4. Health risk increases with increasing waist circumference and WHR.
   a. Standards for risk vary with gender.
5. Classification of overweight and can also be based on body mass index (BMI).
   a. Overweight is defined as a BMI between 25 and 29.9 kg/m^2 and a person is considered obese at a BMI >30 kg/m^2.
6. Body fat is measured by use of skinfolds, bioelectrical impedance, hydrostatic weighing, air displacement measurements, and dual energy x-ray absorptiometry.
   a. Body fat status is defined by gender, age, and race or ethnicity.

F. DIABETES MELLITUS

1. Persons with diabetes mellitus (DM) are two to eight times more likely to develop CVD than persons of similar age, gender, and ethnicity without DM.
2. Asymptomatic (silent) myocardial ischemia is common in patients with DM.
3. Renal disease is a common complication of DM, which further increases the CVD risk.
4. Diabetes is highly prevalent, and about one-third of all cases of DM are undiagnosed and untreated.
5. A person with diabetes is considered as having CVD for purposes of CVD risk assessment and risk reduction.
6. Aggressive risk factor modification is recommended to reduce the CVD risk in patients with DM.

G. METABOLIC SYNDROME

1. The metabolic syndrome is a constellation of CVD risk factors that are of metabolic origin which appear to promote atherosclerotic CVD.
2. The metabolic risk factors include dyslipidemia (elevated TGs and apolipoprotein B, small LDL particles, and low HDL cholesterol concentrations), elevated blood pressure, elevated plasma glucose, a prothrombotic state, and a proinflammatory state.
3. It is not known if the metabolic syndrome results from one cause or multiple causes.
4. The most important underlying risk factors are abdominal obesity and insulin resistance. Aging, physical inactivity, hormonal imbalance, and genetic and ethnic factors are also associated with increased risk of metabolic syndrome.
5. The presence of metabolic syndrome doubles the risk of CVD and increases the risk of developing diabetes mellitus fivefold.
6. For purposes of CVD risk assessment and treatment, the metabolic syndrome is considered a CVD equivalent, so the person is considered as having CVD.
7. Criteria for the diagnosis of metabolic syndrome include the presence of at least three of the following five factors.
   a. Elevated waist circumference (≥102 cm [40 inches] in men; ≥88 cm [35 inches] in women).
      1) In Asian Americans, a lower cutpoint is appropriate. (≥90 cm [35 inches] in men; ≥80 cm [31 inches] in women).
   b. Elevated TGs (≥150 mg/dL [1.7 mmol/L]) or drug treatment for elevated TGs.
   c. Reduced HDL cholesterol (<40 mg/dL [1.03 mmol/L] in men; <50 mg/dL [1.3 mmol/L] in women; or drug treatment for low HDL).
   d. Elevated blood pressure (systolic blood pressure ≥130 mm Hg; diastolic blood pressure ≥85 mm Hg or drug treatment for hypertension).
   e. Elevated fasting glucose (≥100 mg/dL [5.6 mmol/L]) or drug treatment for elevated glucose.

H. EMERGING RISK FACTORS

1. Emerging (also termed nontraditional or novel risk factors) are factors that are associated with an increased risk of CVD, but whose causal link has not been proved with certainty.
2. These include factors such as poor oral health, dietary trans fat, homocysteine, lipoprotein (a), adhesion molecules, cytokines, fibrinogen, high sensitive C-Reactive protein, infectious agents, and subclinical atherosclerosis (coronary artery calcification, carotid artery plaque identified with ultrasound, endothelial dysfunction).
3. Routine screening for these factors is not recommended, but may be indicated for persons having certain characteristics (see statements by the American Heart Association for more details on these recommendations).

VIII. DIAGNOSIS OF CORONARY ARTERY DISEASE

A. ELECTROCARDIOGRAPHY (ECG)

1. A noninvasive, diagnostic test that records cardiac electrical currents by placing electrodes on the surface of the body. (See Chapter 12 for an extensive discussion of Electrocardiography.)
2. Can be administered at rest or during stress ("Stress Test") induced by exercise (exercise tolerance test [ETT]) or pharmacologic agents (e.g., dipyridamole, adenosine, dobutamine).
   a. May be combined with radionuclide imaging.
   b. Used to assess rhythm and conduction disturbances, chamber enlargement, ischemia, MI, and ventricular function.
      1) Various changes and combinations of ST segment abnormalities, presence of significant Q waves, and absence of R waves point to acute, recent, or old MI.
         a) ST segment depression suggests subendocardial ischemia.
         b) ST segment elevation suggests acute ischemia.
3. Certain cardiac conditions, illnesses, and medications may make interpretation of resting or exercise ECG difficult. More sensitive and specific tests (e.g., radionuclide imaging, echocardiography, positron emission tomography [PET], coronary angiography) may be needed to confirm or rule out ischemia (see Chapter 6, pg. 124 for definitions of sensitivity and specificity in exercise testing).

B. DIAGNOSTIC IMAGING

1. Radionuclide Scintigraphy (Perfusion Imaging)
   a. These tests assess the extent and location of both transient (ischemic) and fixed (necrotic) myocardial perfusion defects.
      1) The test may take place over several hours on 1 or 2 days.
   b. A radioisotope or a combination of radioisotopes such as thallium-201, technetium-99m, or technetium-99 sestamibi ("Cardiolite") is injected intravenously (IV) at rest and during or shortly after exercise or pharmacologic stress (dipyridamole [Persantine], dobutamine, or adenosine).
      1) These agents are taken up by the myocardium in proportion to the cardiac blood flow, so that areas with inadequate perfusion caused by myocardial ischemia or MI can be detected.
   c. Images are taken using planar, single-photon emission computed tomography (SPECT), or PET scans.
      1) In a normal heart, full perfusion is revealed in both scans.
      2) In an ischemic heart, unequal perfusion (a defect or cold spot) is present on the stress imaging, but not on the resting scan (i.e., the defect is "reversible").
      3) In a necrotic heart, unequal perfusion is shown in areas where scarring has occurred on both the resting and stress images (i.e., the defect is "fixed").
   d. The sensitivity and specificity for each type of scan are as follows:
      1) Planar: sensitivity 83%, specificity 88%.
      2) SPECT: sensitivity 89%, specificity 76%.
      3) PET: sensitivity 78%–100%, specificity 87%–97%.
2. Radionuclide ventriculography (RVG)
   a. Commonly called a multiple gated acquisition (MUGA) scan.
   b. Used to assess heart wall motion abnormalities, ejection fraction, systolic and diastolic function, and cardiac output.
   c. A bolus (first-pass technique) of radioisotope (such as technetium) is ejected in a central vein under resting conditions.
   d. The test can also be administered with exercise or pharmacologic stress (commonly done to assess complications of acute MI).
      1) The real-time exercise scans are recorded and compared with resting scans to evaluate changes in heart function under stressful conditions owing to areas of ischemia and MI.

3. **Echocardiography**
   a. Used to assess heart wall motion abnormalities, structural abnormalities, valvular function, systolic and diastolic function, ejection fraction, and cardiac output by use of ultrasound waves (echocardiogram).
      1) Most commonly involves the use of planar ultrasound, duplex ultrasound, and Doppler ultrasound.
   b. Resting and/or stress induced by exercise or dobutamine ("stress echocardiogram") images may be obtained.
      1) The real-time stress echocardiogram is recorded and compared with resting scans to evaluate changes in heart function under stressful conditions owing to areas of ischemia and MI.
   c. Radioactive isotopes may also be used (contrast echocardiogram).

C. CORONARY ANGIOGRAPHY

1. Considered to be the "gold standard" diagnostic technique for CHD.
2. The technique requires the placement of a catheter through an incision in the groin or arm area.
3. The catheter is then guided through the femoral or brachial artery through the coronary artery system.
4. A contrast medium or dye (radiopaque) with a vasodilator effect is injected during x-ray fluoroscopy, which allows for its visualization while flowing through the coronary tree.
5. Areas of narrowing can then be identified, located with respect to the coronary artery anatomy, and quantified for the level of stenosis within a given artery.
6. Often used in combination with ventriculography to assess heart wall motion abnormalities, cardiac ejection fraction, systolic and diastolic function, and cardiac output.

D. CORONARY CALCIUM ASSESSMENT

1. Two available technologies used to assess coronary artery calcium.
   a. Electron beam computed tomography (EBCT).
   b. Spiral tomography (CT).
2. The patient is prescanned to determine the length of the scanning field (i.e., the length of the heart).
3. Electrodes are placed on chest to allow imaging to be gated, or coordinated with the cardiac cycle.
   a. The scan takes approximately 30 seconds and requires a breath hold to minimize thoracic movement.
4. During this time 20–30 "slices" of the heart are scanned during the diastolic phase of the cardiac cycle.
   a. The scanned slices are reviewed to visualize the major coronary arteries.
5. Techniques based on the deposition of calcium in coronary atheromas show as whitened areas.
   a. The whitened areas can be quantified (i.e., scored) based on their intensity (i.e., Hounsfield unit). The greater the score, the greater the amount of calcium.
      1) Calcium detected in the coronary arteries is indicative of CHD.
      2) This technique cannot provide an assessment of the degree of stenosis in the arteries.
   b. These methods are currently not recommended routinely for the diagnosis or screening of coronary artery disease (CAD).
      1) May be useful in identifying preclinical CHD disease (before myocardial ischemia or infarction).
      2) The argument is that once the preclinical disease is found, the treatment of risk factors should be no different that if the coronary calcium score was not known.

IX. TREATMENT OF CORONARY ARTERY DISEASE

A. RISK FACTOR MODIFICATION

1. Aggressive control of modifiable risk factors may reverse, slow, or halt the progression of atherosclerosis.
   a. Resulting in a reduction of ischemia, angina, recurrent cardiac events, and revascularization.

B. PHARMACOLOGIC (DRUG) THERAPY

1. Platelet Inhibitors

   a. Platelet-inhibiting agents, such as aspirin, warfarin (Coumadin), or clopidogrel (Plavix), have been shown to significantly reduce cardiovascular events (mortality and morbidity) in persons with or at high risk for acute CVD events, including following revascularization procedures (percutaneous coronary interventions [PCI] and coronary artery bypass grafting [CABG].

2. Anti-ischemic Agents

   a. **β Adrenergic Blockers**
      1) Reduce ischemia by lowering myocardial oxygen demand for any given workload.

2) Lower blood pressure and control ventricular arrhythmias.
3) Reduce first-year mortality rate in patients after an MI by 20%–35%.

b. **Calcium Channel Antagonists**

1) They reduce ischemia at any given workload by altering the major determinants of myocardial oxygen supply and demand. Some calcium channel blockers reduce resting and exercise heart rate. All calcium channel blockers reduce resting and exercise blood pressure.
2) Have not been shown to reduce post-MI mortality.

C. NITRATES

1. Reduce ischemia by reducing myocardial oxygen demand with a small, concomitant increase in oxygen supply.
2. Both short- and long-acting forms are used to treat typical and variant angina.
3. Have not been shown to reduce post-MI mortality.

D. OTHER AGENTS

1. Angiotensin-converting Enzyme Inhibitors

a. Reduce myocardial oxygen demand by reducing systemic vascular resistance and, thus, may increase exercise tolerance in those with left ventricular dysfunction.
b. Vasodilatation of the systemic vasculature reduces resting and exercise blood pressure.

2. Aldosterone Antagonists

a. Spironolactone has been shown to improve survival in patients with CHF.
b. Blunts SA and AV node conduction, which results in a lower ventricular response (chronotropic effect) in those with atrial fibrillation or tachycardia.
c. Used in treatment of CHF.

3. Digitalis

a. Enhances contractility (positive inotropic) of myocardium resulting in increased stroke volume.
b. Blunts SA and AV node conduction, which results in a lower ventricular response (chronotropic effect) in those with atrial fibrillation or tachycardia.
c. Used in treatment of CHF.

4. Diuretics

a. Reduces blood pressure by increasing the renal excretion of sodium, potassium, and other ions, which results in a loss of water as urine.
b. Used when a mild reduction in blood pressure is warranted.
c. Slight effect on resting and exercise blood pressure; no effect on resting or exercise heart rate.
d. May increase exercise tolerance in those with CHF.

5. Lipid-lowering Therapy

a. The goal is to reduce the availability of lipids to the injured endothelium.
b. Lowering LDL and TC has been shown to be effective in decreasing progression and increasing regression of atherosclerosis.
c. Various classifications of lipid-lowering drugs work through different mechanisms:

1) Bile acid sequestrants, such as cholestyramine (Questran), colestipol (Colestid), and colesevelam (WelChol), lower LDL, but tend to elevate TGs. They work by binding bile acids and reducing recirculation through the liver.
2) Niacin (Nicobid) lowers LDL by inhibiting secretion of lipoproteins from the liver; it has no influence on TGs; it increases HDL.
3) The statin drugs, such as lovastatin (Mevacor), pravastatin (Pravachol), and simvastatin (Zocor), and atorvastatin (Lipitor) and rosuvastatin (Crestor) are also effective for lowering LDL and TC.
   a) They are less effective with decreasing TGs and elevating HDL, although the newer statins are more effective at raising HDLs than older statins.
   b) These compounds are also called 3-hydroxy-3-methyglutaryl coenzyme A (HMG-CoA) reductase inhibitors and work by affecting a primary metabolic pathway in the production of cholesterol, as well as by increasing the number of LDL receptors in the liver and, perhaps, directly reducing circulating LDL particles.
4) Fibric acid drugs, such as gemfibrozil (Lopid) and fenofibrate (Tricor), are effective for lowering elevated TG levels with a moderate reduction in LDL and elevation of HDL. They work by promoting lipolysis of very low-density lipoprotein (VLDL) TGs.

X. REVASCULARIZATION PROCEDURES

A. PERCUTANEOUS TRANSLUMINAL CORONARY ANGIOPLASTY (PTCA)

1. In PTCA, a catheter with a deflated balloon is inserted into the narrowed portion of the coronary artery.
2. The balloon is inflated and plaque is "flattened" inside the walls of the artery, resulting in an increased inner diameter of the artery.
3. The balloon is then deflated and the catheter removed. Most of these procedures now also involve the placement of a coronary artery stent (see below).
4. PTCA can be used in acute MI to interrupt an active infarction.
5. PTCA was typically reserved for younger patients, those with single-vessel disease, and those with stenosis distal to the occluded artery, but is now common in individuals at higher risk.
6. Restenosis with PTCA alone occurs within 6 months in approximately 30%–50% of patients. PTCA alone carries a greater risk of restenosis than either PTCA-stent or CABG surgery.

B. PTCA WITH CORONARY ARTERY STENT

1. A coronary artery stent is a mesh tube that acts as a "scaffold" to hold the walls of the artery open after PTCA, thereby improving blood flow and relieving the symptoms of CAD.
2. The stent is mounted on a balloon catheter that is inserted into the artery, inflated or expanded at the blockage site, and permanently implanted in the artery.
3. Stents are typically used in conjunction with PTCA in interventional therapy for CAD or MI.
4. Restenosis occurs within 6 months in up to about 10%–15% of patients.
5. The lower rate of restenosis of PTCA-stent has made the use of PTCA alone rare.
6. Newer drug-eluting stents (DES), stents that are coated with time release immunosuppressant (sirolimus) or chemotherapeutic (paclitaxel) agents, have been shown to have very low rates of restenosis (perhaps as low as 3%–4%).

C. ATHERECTOMY

1. Similar procedure as for PTCA.
2. A rotational atherectomy uses a high-speed rotating shaver to grind the plaque.
3. A transluminal extraction atherectomy cuts and vacuums away the plaque.
4. Can be used in conjunction with PTCA-stent.
5. Similar long-term outcomes as with PTCA.

D. LASER ANGIOPLASTY

1. Similar procedure as for PTCA.
2. End of catheter emits pulses of photons (laser beam) that vaporizes plaque.
3. Useful when PTCA catheter cannot be passed through an artery or if calcification is present.
4. May be used in conjunction with PTCA-stent.
5. Similar long-term outcomes as with PTCA.

E. CORONARY ARTERY BYPASS GRAFT SURGERY (CABGS)

1. In CABGS, a right or left mammary internal artery (RIMA or LIMA), saphenous vein (SVG), or other large vein is removed and attached to the base of the aorta and at other points below the stenosis of a coronary artery caused by plaque.
2. CABGS is indicated for patients with extensive multivessel disease who are unresponsive to pharmacologic treatment, have failed PTCA-stents, or other higher risk CAD patients.
3. Arterial and LIMA grafts are superior to SVG grafts in terms of patency (90% for arterial grafts versus less than 50% for venous grafts at 10 years).

XI. RISK STRATIFICATION

A. DEFINITION

1. Risk stratification consists of placing an individual in a risk group for untoward events based on sets of known risk factors.
2. Purpose
   a. The purpose of risk stratification is to provide:
      1) Guidance on the need for a medical examination and exercise test before participation in a moderate-to-vigorous exercise program.
      2) Guidance for monitoring and supervision during exercise testing and training.
      3) Assistance in making recommendations for occupational, recreational, or daily activity participation and any necessary restrictions.
      4) Assistance in making therapeutic recommendations for CVD treatment and risk factor reduction.
   b. Goal
      1) Increase the safety of exercise training in adult fitness and exercise-based cardiac rehabilitation programs.
      2) Increase efficacy of secondary prevention in exercise-based cardiac rehabilitation programs.

c. Criteria
   1) The criteria for an initial risk stratification are published by ACSM (*GETP* Figure 2.3) and is discussed in Chapter 6.
   2) Quantification of CVD risk in persons without CVD can be made using the Framingham Risk Equations (see *GETP* Chapter 5).
   3) Cardiac patients may be further stratified for risk of untoward events during exercise and for progression of disease using criteria published by the American Heart Association and the American Association of Cardiovascular and Pulmonary Rehabilitation (AACVPR) (see *GETP* Boxes 2.2 and 2.3).

XII. EFFECTS OF EXERCISE ON CARDIOPULMONARY AND OTHER DISORDERS

A. PULMONARY DISEASE

1. Exercise can improve musculoskeletal and psychosocial factors that typically limit exercise in persons with pulmonary disease.
2. Because pulmonary disease is commonly associated with CAD and CAD risk factors, exercise training can reduce the risk of CAD in persons with pulmonary disease.

XIII. CORONARY ARTERY DISEASE

A. Exercise has been shown to help reduce mortality and morbidity in persons with CAD.
B. The mechanisms responsible for a reduction in CVD events are varied, and include:
   1. The effects of exercise on other risk factors.
   2. Reduction in myocardial oxygen demand at rest and at submaximal workloads (resulting in an increased ischemic and angina threshold).
   3. Reduction in platelet aggregation.
   4. Improved endothelial-mediated vasomotor tone.

XIV. OBESITY

A. An increase in caloric expenditure through exercise, combined with a reduction in caloric intake, results in a caloric deficit.
B. Over time, a caloric deficit results in reduction of overall body fat and a likely reduction in central fat deposits.
C. Decreased body fat, especially reduced central obesity can reduce risk factors for CAD, including dyslipidemia, type 2 DM, and hypertension.
D. Exercising to induce a caloric deficit can preserve lean body mass. Dieting alone to produce a caloric deficit usually results in a loss of lean body mass.
E. A combination of exercise and diet is best for initial and long-term weight loss and maintenance of target weight.
F. The ACSM Position Stand On Appropriate Intervention Strategies For Weight Loss And Prevention Of Weight Regain For Adults recommends strategies to be incorporated into weight loss interventions.

XV. DYSLIPIDEMIA

A. Exercise has the beneficial effect of lowering TGs and raising HDLs.
   1. Exercise increases the activity of lipoprotein lipase (LPL), which frees VLDL and TG.
      a. TG levels are then decreased when they are utilized in metabolism by skeletal muscles during exercise.
   2. In addition, VLDL remnants serve as precursors to HDLs, which are cardioprotective.
   3. Exercise moderates the postprandial lipemia that ensues after a high-fat or moderately high-fat meal.
   4. To induce these beneficial changes, the volume (duration and frequency) of aerobic activity is more important than the intensity of activity.
B. Exercise can indirectly lower TC and LDLs.
   1. Lowering TC and LDLs is related more to caloric restriction, a reduction of dietary fat, saturated fat and cholesterol, and body fat reduction than to exercise training alone.
   2. However, because exercise training can result in body fat reduction, it can have an indirect effect on TC and LDL levels.

XVI. DIABETES MELLITUS (DM)

A. Exercise can improve insulin sensitivity and glucose metabolism in people with type 1 DM.
B. In people with type 2 DM, exercise can enhance fat loss, resulting in improved insulin sensitivity and glucose metabolism.
C. Exercise can favorably alter other risk factors typically associated with DM, including dyslipidemia and hypertension, and thus decrease the overall risk of CAD.
D. Aggressive pharmacologic therapy and behavior modification, which includes exercise training to reduce hyperglycemia, can lower the risk of microvascular complications (e.g., retinopathy, nephropathy, automatic neuropathy); recent studies also suggest a lower incidence of cardiovascular diseases (e.g., nonfatal MI and stroke).

XVII. HYPERTENSION

A. An average reduction of about 5–7 mm Hg in both systolic and diastolic blood pressure has been observed in patients with hypertension after an acute bout of exercise and as a result of chronic cardiorespiratory endurance and resistance exercise training.
B. Blood pressure remains decreased for up to 22 hours following an acute bout of exercise.
C. Exercise can reduce total peripheral resistance (TPR), and thus reduce blood pressure.
   1. Mechanisms for the change in TPR are probably related to changes in both sympathetic nervous system and vascular responsiveness through effects on endothelial function, vasoactive substances, and vascular remodeling.
   2. Exercise can reduce blood pressure through effecting weight loss and reducing risk factors for metabolic syndrome, which can affect vascular function.
   3. Further recommendations can be found in the ACSM Position Stand on Exercise and Hypertension.

XVIII. PERIPHERAL ARTERY DISEASE

A. Exercise training is effective in increasing walking distance and the onset of symptoms of intermittent claudication.
B. Exercise training can improve oxygen extraction from skeletal muscle. Increased oxygen extraction improves the relationship between oxygen supply and oxygen demand.
C. Exercise may improve the mechanical efficiency of walking, which, together with changes in the oxygen supply:demand ratio, improves the ability to walk longer or at higher intensities.
D. Maintenance of exercise training reduces the ill effects of deconditioning and risk factors associated with peripheral artery disease (e.g., hypertension, insulin resistance).
E. Physical activity is important as part of a comprehensive program of CVD risk reduction.

XIX. OSTEOPOROSIS

A. Exercise reduces the deleterious effects of deconditioning and the risk factors for osteoporosis associated with physical inactivity.
B. Exercise may help delay or halt the age-related decline in bone mass.
C. Resistance training may be more beneficial than aerobic training; weight-bearing exercise may be more effective at increasing bone mass than non–weight-bearing exercise.
D. Adaptations in bone are site specific to the limbs exercised.
E. Exercise training may also reduce the risk of falls by increasing muscle strength, posture, and balance.
F. Further information is available in the ACSM Position Stand on Physical Activity and Bone Health.

XX. ENVIRONMENTAL RISK FACTORS AND EXERCISE

A. HEAT

1. High ambient temperature and high relative humidity increase the risk of heat-related disorders, such as heat cramps, heat syncope, dehydration, heat exhaustion, and heat stroke.
2. Persons with hypertension or diabetes, obese individuals, unfit persons, pregnant women, children, the elderly, and individuals taking certain medications or alcohol may have particular difficulty adapting to high ambient temperature and high humidity, and thus are at increased risk for heat-related disorders.
   a. High ambient temperature and high humidity can produce increased heart rate response at submaximal workloads, and decreased oxygen consumption at maximal workloads.
   b. The wet bulb globe temperature is an index of environmental heat stress that is derived from measures of ambient temperature, relative humidity, and radiant heat. It provides guidance for exercise prescription to minimize the risk of developing heat-related illnesses.
   c. General guidelines for safe exercising in high ambient temperatures and humidity are listed in *GETP* pages 194–198.

B. COLD

1. Cold exposure results in vasoconstriction with resulting blood pressure elevation.
2. The elevation in blood pressure increases the oxygen demand on the heart. This lowers the angina threshold in patients who are susceptible to angina, and may provoke resting angina (variant or Prinzmetal's angina).
3. Breathing large volumes of cold, dry air can provoke exercise-induced asthma, general dehydration, and dryness or burning of the mouth and throat.
4. Use the wind chill equivalent, not the actual temperature, when gauging the risk of hypothermia and frostbite.

C. ALTITUDE

1. The primary consideration in exercise prescription at high altitude is to lower the exercise

intensity (absolute workload), for the following reasons:

   a. Acute exposure to high altitudes causes an increase in pulmonary ventilation, heart rate, and cardiac output at submaximal workloads.
   b. After acclimatization to high altitudes, persons generally experience a continued increase in pulmonary ventilation and heart rate response at submaximal workloads, but reduced cardiac output, stroke volume, and heart rate at maximal exercise.
   c. Even after exposure and training, there is approximately a 10% reduction in maximal oxygen consumption per 1,000 m of altitude above 1,500 m. These changes may lower the angina threshold.

2. Individuals with pulmonary hypertension, CHF, unstable angina, recent MI, or severe anemia may be at greater risk for traveling or exercising at high altitudes.

XXI. CARBON MONOXIDE

A. Prolonged exposure to carbon monoxide can reduce maximal oxygen consumption.
B. Individuals with CAD may experience lower thresholds for myocardial ischemia and angina, and are susceptible to arrhythmias induced by carbon monoxide exposure.
C. Guidelines for exercise prescription include avoiding carbon monoxide exposure, and decreasing the intensity and duration of exercise during periods, or in areas, of high ambient carbon monoxide levels (e.g., heavy motor vehicle traffic).

XXII. INFLUENCE OF DRUGS ON EXERCISE

A. Classes of drugs and a summary of their effects on resting and exercise electrocardiogram, heart rate, blood pressure, symptomatology, and exercise capacity are listed in *GETP* Table A.2.

Review Test

DIRECTIONS: Carefully read all questions and select the BEST single answer.

1. Which term is used to describe angina pectoris that occurs at rest without a precipitating event?
   A) Silent.
   B) Stable.
   C) Variant.
   D) Typical.

2. What term is used to refer to a group of pulmonary disorders characterized by limitations in airflow that are not fully reversible?
   A) Bronchitis.
   B) Asthma.
   C) Emphysema.
   D) Chronic obstructive pulmonary disease.

3. The primary effects of chronic exercise training on blood lipids include
   A) Decreased triglycerides and increased high-density lipoproteins.
   B) Decreased total cholesterol and low-density lipoproteins.
   C) Decreased high-density lipoprotein and increased low-density lipoproteins.
   D) Decreased total cholesterol and increased high-density lipoproteins.

4. Which physiologic responses would be expected to occur under conditions of high ambient temperature?
   A) Increased maximal oxygen uptake.
   B) Decreased heart rate at rest.
   C) Increased heart rate at submaximal workload.
   D) Decreased maximal heart rate.

5. Which of the following statements is true concerning the pathophysiology of coronary artery disease?
   A) Injury to the artery wall begins in the media.
   B) Platelets and thrombi form in the adventitia.
   C) The endothelium takes up lipids, especially low-density lipoproteins.
   D) Atherosclerotic lesions are formed in the intima.

6. A cardiac patient is taking a β-blocker medication. During an exercise test, you would expect
   A) ST segment depression because β-blockers depress the ST segment on the resting ECG.
   B) An increase in the anginal threshold compared with a test without the medication.
   C) No change in heart rate or blood pressure compared with a test without the medication.
   D) A slight decrease or no effect on blood pressure compared with a test without the medication.

7. The loss of elasticity (or "hardening") of the arteries is known as
   A) Atherosclerosis.
   B) Arteriosclerosis.
   C) Atheroma.
   D) Adventitia.

8. A transient deficiency of blood flow to the myocardium resulting from an imbalance between oxygen demand and oxygen supply is known as
   A) Infarction.
   B) Angina.
   C) Ischemia.
   D) Thrombosis.

9. Which of the following drugs is used during acute MI to dissolve blood clots, restore blood flow, and limit myocardial necrosis?
   A) β-blockers.
   B) Thrombolytic agent's therapy.
   C) Sestamibi.
   D) Coronary artery bypass graft surgery.

10. All of the following are suggestive of cardiovascular and pulmonary disease except
    A) A sharp, jabbing pain in the side when running.
    B) Dyspnea during strenuous exertion.
    C) Syncope during moderate-intensity exercise training.
    D) Substernal burning that occurs during exertion and dissipates with rest.

11. Modifiable primary risk factors for coronary artery disease include
    A) Hypertension, dyslipidemia, advancing age, and tobacco smoking.
    B) Homocysteine, lipoprotein (a), C-reactive protein, and gender.
    C) Obesity, diabetes mellitus, tobacco smoking, and sedentary lifestyle.
    D) Tobacco smoking, dyslipidemia, hypertension, and homocysteine.

12. What is the current state of knowledge on progression or regression of atherosclerosis in human coronary arteries?
    A) Regression of atherosclerosis has been observed in clinical studies.

B) Regression of atherosclerosis has yet to be observed in clinical studies.
C) Progression of atherosclerosis begins at puberty.
D) There is no difference in the rate of progression or regression between those who undergo usual medical care and those who aggressively control risk factors.

13. What is the correct term and definition to describe a potential complication that may occur after an acute myocardial infarction (MI)?
A) Expansion—another MI.
B) Aneurysm—bulging of the ventricular wall.
C) Extension—left ventricular dilation.
D) Rupture—coronary artery breaks open.

14. The goal of risk stratification is to
A) Determine prognosis.
B) Assess disease severity.
C) Confirm diagnosis.
D) Increase the safety of exercise participation.

15. A classic sign of subendocardial ischemia is
A) Angina.
B) ST segment depression.
C) ST segment elevation.
D) A pathologic Q wave.

16. Which of the following statements concerning the surgical treatment of coronary artery disease is true?
A) A coronary artery stent carries a lower rate of revascularization than does percutaneous transluminal coronary angioplasty.
B) Atherectomy is a prerequisite requirement for percutaneous transluminal coronary angioplasty.
C) Venous grafts are significantly superior to arterial grafts in terms of patency.
D) Long-term outcome of laser angioplasty is unknown and, thus, rarely used.

17. A possible mechanism by which chronic exercise training may reduce resting blood pressure in a person with hypertension is
A) An increase in plasma renin.
B) A higher cardiac output.
C) A reduced heart rate.
D) A lower stroke volume.

18. The relationship between heart rate (HR) and oxygen consumption in pulmonary cases is
A) Nonlinear.
B) Linear.
C) Exponential.
D) No relationship.

19. A sedentary lifestyle
A) Has a risk similar to that of hypertension, high cholesterol, and cigarette smoking.
B) Increases high-density lipoprotein (HDL) cholesterol.
C) Increases the sensitivity to insulin.
D) Has little influence on mortality rates after an MI.

20. Body fat appears to be most dangerous when
A) Weight for height exceeds 20% above recommended.
B) Body fat exceeds 25% for males and 30% for females.
C) Central (android) obesity is present.
D) Body mass index exceeds 25 kg/m^2.

21. All of the following are possible causes of restrictive lung disease except
A) Scoliosis.
B) Obesity.
C) Muscular dystrophy.
D) Cigarette smoke.

22. Which answer below best describes the condition of asthma?
A) Narrowing of the bronchial airways.
B) Alveolar destruction.
C) Ventilatory dead space.
D) Respiratory muscular atrophy.

23. The criteria for the diagnosis of metabolic syndrome includes the following
A) Elevated total cholesterol, obesity, diabetes, and physical inactivity.
B) Central obesity, elevated low-density lipoprotein cholesterol, diabetes, and physical inactivity.
C) Low high-density lipoprotein cholesterol, cigarette smoking, hypertension, and physical inactivity.
D) Central obesity, elevated triglycerides and low high-density lipoprotein cholesterol, hypertension, and insulin resistance.

24. All of the following risk factors for coronary artery disease can be modified by a regular and appropriate exercise training program except
A) Advancing age.
B) Diabetes mellitus.
C) Hypertension.
D) High-density lipoprotein cholesterol.

25. Emerging risk factors for coronary artery disease include
A) Advancing age, family history, and male gender.
B) Impaired fasting glucose, obesity, and hypertension.
C) Lipoprotein (a), advancing age, and male gender.
D) Homocysteine, lipoprotein (a), and fibrinogen.

ANSWERS AND EXPLANATIONS

1–C. Variant, or Prinzmetal's, angina is a form of unstable angina that occurs without provocation at rest owing to coronary vasospasm. Typical, or classic, angina is usually provoked by physical activity or other stressor and is relieved by rest or nitroglycerin. Stable angina is a form of typical angina that is predictable in onset, severity, and means of relief. Silent angina is not a medical term used to describe chest pain, because pain cannot be silent.

2–D. Bronchitis and emphysema are all forms of chronic obstructive pulmonary disease (COPD). Asthma is a separate category of pulmonary disease.

3–A. Chronic exercise training has its greatest benefit on lowering triglycerides (TGs) and increasing high-density lipoproteins (HDL). Changes in total cholesterol or low-density lipoprotein (LDL) cholesterol are influenced more by dietary habits and body weight than by exercise training.

4–C. Compared with a cool and dry environment, a higher metabolic cost exists at submaximal workloads when exercising in the heat and humidity. Thus, the exercise prescription should be altered by lowering the work intensity. Evaporation of sweat cools the skin; therefore, wiping away sweat would decrease evaporative cooling and heat loss. Heat loss by convection, such as that which occurs when a breeze is created by running, can be beneficial but not unless the workload of activity is reduced. It is necessary to exercise in the heat and humidity to become acclimated to the environment; it will not occur by being sedentary.

5–D. Atherosclerotic lesions are formed in the intima. Injury to the artery wall does not begin in the media but rather in the endothelial layer with subsequent platelet and clot formation. Monocytes adhere to the endothelium, move to the intima, and take up cholesterol. The adventitia, the outermost layer of the artery wall, is not involved in the development of atherosclerosis.

6–B. β-blockers increase the angina threshold by reducing myocardial oxygen demand at rest and during exercise. This occurs through a reduction in chronotropic (heart rate) and inotropic (strength of contraction) responses. Blood pressure is also reduced at rest and during exercise by a reduction in cardiac output (reduced chronotropic and inotropic response) and a reduction in total peripheral resistance. β-blockers do not produce ST segment changes on the resting ECG.

7–B. Arteriosclerosis, also called "hardening" of the arteries, is a loss of arterial elasticity and is associated with aging. Atherosclerosis is a form of arteriosclerosis characterized by an accumulation of obstructive lesions within the arterial wall. The adventitia, the outermost layer of the artery wall, provides the media and intima with oxygen and other nutrients.

8–C. Myocardial ischemia occurs when the oxygen supply does not meet oxygen demand resulting from decreased blood flow to the myocardium. This is usually owing to atherosclerotic lesions reducing blood flow or coronary artery spasm, both of which are the result of atherosclerosis. This process often leads to angina (symptoms) or myocardial infarction caused by a thrombosis.

9–B. Administration of streptokinase or t-PA (recombinant tissue plasminogen activator) within the first 1–2 hours after an MI may dissolve the clot causing the injury. This type of therapy, called thrombolytic therapy, is designed to restore blood flow and limit myocardial necrosis.

10–B. Dyspnea (shortness of breath) commonly occurs during strenuous exertion in healthy, well-trained persons and during moderate exertion in healthy, untrained persons. It should be regarded as abnormal, however, when it occurs at a level of exertion that is not expected to evoke this symptom in a given individual. Underlying cardiac arrhythmias can cause palpitations, even at rest. Syncope is loss of consciousness and is abnormal at rest or during any level of exertion. The location (substernal), character (burning), and provoking factor (exertion that dissipates with rest) of substernal burning are features of classic ischemia.

11–C. The primary modifiable risk factors for CAD are tobacco smoking, dyslipidemia, hypertension, sedentary lifestyle, obesity, and DM. The primary nonmodifiable risk factors for CAD are advance age, male gender, and family history. Emerging risk factors for CAD are numerous and include, for example, homocysteine, fibrinogen tissue plasminogen activator, lipoprotein (a), and C-reactive protein.

12–A. Clinical studies of cardiac patients have shown that long-term aggressive control of CAD risk factors can reduce or halt the rate of disease progression and may actually result in regression of atherosclerotic plaque. Individuals who aggressively attack, reduce, and control risk factors are more likely to see favorable results than individuals who undergo usual medical care. The process of atherosclerosis begins at birth.

13–B. A ventricular aneurysm is a bulging of the ventricular wall. Expansion is dilation of the left ventricle while extension is another MI. Rupture is an aneurysm that breaks open in the ventricular wall not the coronary artery.

14–D. The goal of risk stratification is to increase the safety of exercise training in adult fitness and exercise-based cardiac rehabilitation programs. Initial risk stratification tables are available from the American College of Sports Medicine. Cardiac patients may be further stratified using tables available from the American Heart Association, and American Association of Cardiovascular and Pulmonary Rehabilitation. Although risk stratification is based on the likelihood of experiencing an untoward cardiac event, it does not attempt to diagnose disease, predict prognosis, or determine disease severity. Different nomograms and tables are available for such information.

15–B. A classic sign of MI ischemia is ST segment alteration. ST segment depression suggests subendocardial ischemia, whereas ST segment elevation indicates transmural ischemia or acute MI. Pathologic Q waves point to transmural MI. Angina is a classic symptom, not a sign, of ischemia.

16–A. Restenosis occurs within 6 months in approximately 30%–50% of patients who have had a PTCA, whereas a stent has about a 25% failure rate and the drug-eluting stent having a restenosis rate in the low single digits. Atherectomy can be used along with PTCA and is useful when the PTCA catheter cannot pass through the artery, but atherectomy is not a prerequisite for PTCA. Internal mammary artery grafts are preferred over saphenous venous grafts because of superior patency (90% versus <50% at 10 years). About 25%–50% of patients will experience a restenosis within 6 months of laser angioplasty.

17–C. Blood pressure is the product of cardiac output and total peripheral resistance. A benefit of exercise training is a reduction in cardiac output and total peripheral resistance at any given workload, including rest. A lower cardiac output is probably owing to a reduction in heart rate as a result of an increased stroke volume and arteriovenous oxygen difference. Plasma renin is a catalyst for vasoconstriction. It is reduced, not increased, with exercise training.

18–B. Patients with pulmonary disease and apparently healthy individuals have a linear increase in heart rate to oxygen consumption. With pulmonary disease, the patient will be limited by some mechanism that ultimately results in inefficient pulmonary gas exchange. An attempt to correct for this factor will be shown by a high ventilation per unit of oxygen consumed ($\dot{V}E/\dot{V}O_2$), a high percentage of pulmonary ventilation to maximal voluntary ventilation ($\dot{V}E$/MVV), and a high respiratory rate.

19–A. The risk ratios of hypertension (2.1), high cholesterol (2.4), cigarette smoking (2.5), and physical inactivity (1.9) are similar. A sedentary lifestyle is associated with low HDL cholesterol and sensitivity to insulin (higher plasma glucose values). Studies have shown that, after an MI, a regular exercise training program can significantly reduce mortality rates in these patients as compared with those who are less active after an MI.

20–C. The distribution of body fat, rather than the overall quantity of fat, appears to be the most important predictor of the health risks associated with obesity. Individuals with abdominal fat (central obesity or android) are especially at increased risk for a variety of cardiovascular conditions than individuals with similar body fat levels but with more of their fat on the extremities. A waist-to-hip, or waist alone circumference can be used to assess risk of central obesity. Weight for height tables, body composition assessment, and body mass index provide indices of total excess weight or total fat weight, but do not provide a distribution of body fat.

21–D. Restrictive lung disease can be caused by a variety of factors that compromise the ability of the lungs and rib cage to expand outward and upward including, for example, scoliosis, muscular dystrophy, and obesity. Cigarette smoke is risk factor for chronic obstructive lung disease, a condition characterized by inflammation of the airways and impaired gas exchange.

22–A. Asthma is a narrowing or vasoconstriction of the bronchial airways that is initiated by some trigger such as, for example, dust or cigarette smoke. Destruction of the alveoli and impaired ventilation (dead space) is the pathophysiology of emphysema. When the muscles of respiration are comprised (e.g., muscular dystrophy), then restrictive lung disease can occur.

23–D. The metabolic syndrome is a cluster of lipid and nonlipid risk factors of metabolic origin. Excess body fat, particularly abdominal obesity, raised blood pressure, insulin resistance (with or without glucose intolerance), and dyslipidemia (elevated TG, and low HDL cholesterol) comprise this deadly quartet. The metabolic syndrome enhances the risk for heart disease exponentially.

24–A. A modifiable risk factor is one that be influenced by either surgical, pharmacologic, or behavioral intervention. Scientific studies have shown that a regular and appropriate exercise program can reduce the risk of developing DM, hypertension, and unfavorable HDL levels or it can be used as an adjunct treatment.

25–D. Primary risk factors are those that have shown a consistent causal link over time and have been proved with much certainty (e.g., advancing age, obesity, hypertension). Emerging risk factors are those that have been shown to be related to an increased risk, but their link has not been causal or consistent in nature. Although such factors (e.g., homocysteine, lipoprotein (a), fibrinogen) show promise as independent causes of CAD, additional studies are warranted to assess their complete significance to CAD.

Human Behavior and Psychosocial Assessment

CHAPTER 5

I. PSYCHOLOGICAL THEORIES: THE FOUNDATION FOR BEHAVIORAL CHANGE

A. PSYCHOLOGICAL THEORY

1. A **psychological theory** is a set of assumptions that account for the relationships between certain variables and the particular behavior of interest.
2. **Explanatory theories** have been developed to help explain certain behaviors.
3. Other theories have been developed to **guide interventions**, such as trying to create a change in personal behavior (e.g., increasing physical activity, eating healthier, quitting smoking).

B. PSYCHOLOGICAL THEORIES USED IN THE HEALTH AND FITNESS SETTING

1. Psychological theories provide the foundation for effective use of the strategies and techniques of **counseling and motivational skill-building for exercise adoption and maintenance.**
2. Psychological theories provide **a conceptual framework** for assessments, development of programs or interventions, application of cognitive-behavioral principles, and evaluation of program effectiveness.
3. **Program interventions** should be designed to:
   a. Build the skills of participants.
   b. Correct misunderstandings.
   c. Clarify relationships.
   d. Negotiate and solve problems.
   e. Establish a supportive relationship.
   f. Provide a target date for follow-up.
4. **Cognitive-behavioral principles** are the **methods used within programs** to improve motivational skills as suggested by the assessment. For example, **setting several small, short-term goals** to attain a long-term goal is likely to increase self-efficacy (self-confidence), as the person successfully reaches each short-term goal on the way to attaining the long-term goal.

C. LIMITATIONS OF PSYCHOLOGICAL THEORIES

1. Most psychological theories have been developed to explain the behaviors of individuals or small groups. They **cannot always explain the behavior of larger groups** (e.g., communities, groups of individuals with the same medical condition).
2. Psychological theories **may leave out important elements that may influence behavior** (e.g., sociocultural elements, age, gender).

II. THEORIES USED TO ENCOURAGE EXERCISE ADOPTION AND MAINTENANCE AND TO IMPROVE ADHERENCE

A. LEARNING THEORIES

Learning theories propose that an overall **complex behavior arises from many small, simple behaviors.** These theories propose that it is possible to **shape** the desired behavior by **reinforcing "partial behaviors"** and **modifying cues** in the environment.

1. **Reinforcement is the positive or negative consequence for performing or not performing a behavior.**
2. **Reinforcement can be simple**, such as saying "Good job!" to participants who have performed an exercise correctly or achieved an exercise goal. **Reinforcement can be complex**, such as earning points to earn incentives (e.g., T-shirts for exercising 3 days or more a week for a period of 1 month). **Positive consequences motivate behavior.** The two types of rewards that motivate individuals to change their behavior are called **intrinsic rewards** and **extrinsic** or **external rewards.**
   a. **Intrinsic rewards** are the benefits gained because of the rewarding nature of the activity. For example, an intrinsic reward would be feeling good about being able to perform an activity or skill, such as finally being able to

run 1 mile or to increase the speed of walking 1 mile.
   b. **Extrinsic** or **external rewards** are the positive outcomes received from others. This can include encouragement and praise or material reinforcements (e.g., T- shirts, water bottles, squeeze balls).
3. **External or internal stimuli (cues) can signal behaviors.** For example, many traditional, gym-based programs have participants keep their gym clothes packed **(behavioral cue)** to remind them that they are ready to go to the gym.
   a. Behaviors can be **habitual**, such as coming home from work, turning on the television, and sitting down for the remainder of the evening.
   b. Behaviors can be **cued from the engineered environment.** For example, the easy accessibility of elevators compared with stairways, which discourages stair climbing.
   c. **Internal cues** (e.g., fatigue, boredom) can make a person feel "too tired" to exercise.
4. The techniques of modifying cues and providing reinforcement seem to be **more effective for helping people to adopt a behavior than for maintaining a behavior.**
5. For people who are not ready to start an exercise program or who need help maintaining an exercise program, **additional tools or strategies for change are required.**

B. THE HEALTH BELIEF MODEL

1. The **Health Belief Model** assumes that people will engage in a given behavior (e.g., exercise) when:
   a. **They perceive threat of disease.**
   b. They believe they are susceptible to disease.
   c. They believe the threat is severe.
2. Taking action depends on whether **the benefits outweigh the barriers.**
3. The concept of **self-efficacy** (self-confidence) is a major component of this model.
4. This model also incorporates **cues to action** as being critical to adopting and maintaining a given behavior.

C. THE TRANSTHEORETICAL MODEL OF HEALTH BEHAVIOR CHANGE (STAGES OF CHANGE OR MOTIVATIONAL READINESS)

The **Transtheoretical Model (TTM) of health behavior** provides an awareness and understanding of choices and behaviors related to personal balance and health (or lack thereof) by considering the perceived costs and benefits within. **This model incorporates constructs from other theories,** including intention to change and processes (or strategies) of change.

1. The basic concepts of the **TTM** are:
   a. **People progress through five stages of change at varying rates.**
   b. In the process of change, **people move back and forth along the stage continuum.**
   c. People use different **cognitive and behavioral** processes or strategies.
   d. For **decisional balance**, people look at the **pros and cons of a given health behavior or choice** by performing a "cost-benefit analysis" designed to assist in considering change, understanding what is keeping them from change (payoffs), and providing them an incentive for change.
2. **The five stages of change or motivational readiness** applied to physical activity are:
   a. **Stage 1: Precontemplation**
      No physical activity or exercise is occurring, and the person has **no intention to start** within the next 6 months.
   b. **Stage 2: Contemplation**
      No physical activity or exercise is occurring, but the person has the **intention to start** within the next 6 months.
   c. **Stage 3: Preparation**
      Participation in some physical activity or exercise is occurring, but not at levels that meet the **Centers for Disease Control and Prevention/American College of Sports Medicine (CDC/ACSM) recommendations** and **current ACSM guidelines** for exercise prescription.
   d. **Stage 4: Action**
      The person is engaged in **physical activity or exercise that meets CDC/ACSM recommendations** for physical activity and **current ACSM guidelines,** but the person has not maintained this program for 6 months or longer.
   e. **Stage 5: Maintenance**
      Exercise or activity that meets current CDC/ACSM guidelines has been occurring **for 6 months or longer.**
3. Other key components of the **TTM** are the **processes of behavioral change.**
   a. **Processes** are various behavioral or cognitive **skills or strategies** that are applied during the different stages of change.

b. The model has numerous applications, depending on the stage of readiness.
c. In general, cognitive processes are the most efficient strategies for early stages, and behavioral processes are the most efficient strategies for later stages.
    1) The five cognitive processes include:
        a) Consciousness raising (increasing knowledge).
        b) Dramatic relief (warning of risks).
        c) Environmental reevaluation (caring about consequences to oneself and to others).
        d) Self-reevaluation (comprehending benefits).
        e) Social liberation (increasing healthy opportunities).
    2) The five behavioral processes include:
        a) Counter-conditioning (substituting alternatives).
        b) Helping relationships (enlisting social support).
        c) Reinforcement management (rewarding yourself).
        d) Self-liberation (committing yourself).
        e) Stimulus control (reminding yourself).

D. THE RELAPSE PREVENTION MODEL

1. The Relapse Prevention Model incorporates the identification of high-risk situations and the development of plans for coping with high-risk situations.
2. An important element of this model is to learn how to restructure thinking to distinguish between a lapse and a relapse and to develop flexibility in the approach for attaining exercise and physical activity goals. For example, exercise routines tend to get disrupted during the holiday seasons, but reminder phone calls from a friend may encourage continued participation.

E. THE THEORY OF REASONED ACTION (AND ITS LATER EXTENSION, THE THEORY OF PLANNED BEHAVIOR)

1. The Theory of Reasoned Action postulates that intention is the most important determinant of behavior.
2. In turn, attitudes and subjective norms influence intention.
    a. Attitudes are determined by positive and negative beliefs about the outcome or the process of performing the behavior.
    b. Subjective norms are influenced by perceptions about what others think or believe (normative beliefs).
    c. The Theory of Planned Behavior extends the Theory of Reasoned Action by incorporating perceived behavioral control, which is determined by perceived power and control beliefs.

F. SOCIAL COGNITIVE THEORY

1. The Social Cognitive Theory is one of the most widely used and comprehensive theories of behavioral change.
2. This dynamic model involves three major interacting influences: behavioral, personal, and environmental (*Figure 5-1*).
3. This theory contains several different concepts or constructs that are implicated in the adoption and maintenance of healthy behaviors that are used for increasing and maintaining physical activity or exercise.
    a. Observational learning implies that people can learn by watching others model a behavior and by perceiving the rewards that another person receives for engaging in that behavior. This is sometimes called vicarious reward.
    b. Behavioral capability means that the person has both the knowledge and the skill to perform the behavior.
    c. Outcome expectations and outcome expectancies are the anticipated benefits from engaging in the behavior.
        1) Outcome expectations are what the person anticipates the outcome will be for performing the behavior.
        2) Outcome expectancies are the values of that outcome.
    d. Self-efficacy is the confidence about performing a specific behavior. This construct has been one of the strongest predictors for adopting a program of regular exercise in many populations and in many settings.
    e. Self-control of performance refers to self-regulatory skills when directed toward a

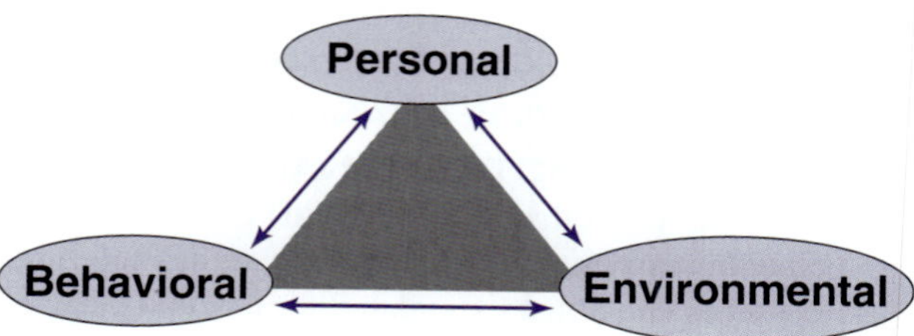

FIGURE 5-1. The Social Cognitive Theory takes into account reciprocal relationships between the personal, behavioral, and environmental factors.

specific goal. This includes the concepts of self-monitoring and goal setting.

f. Management of emotional arousal is the ability to deal with emotions appropriately by:
   1) Cognitive restructuring, as in thinking about the problem in a more constructive manner.
   2) Stress management techniques, as in controlling symptoms of emotional distress.
   3) Learning methods of effective problem solving.

g. Reinforcement is derived from operant learning theories, which state that a behavior is controlled by the consequences of the behavior and that the behavior will increase if positive reinforcement is applied or a negative reinforcement is removed. Social Cognitive Theory involves three types of reinforcement:
   1) Direct reinforcement, as described in operant conditioning.
   2) Vicarious reinforcement, as described in observational learning.
   3) Self-reinforcement, as would be applied in a self-control technique.

III. APPLYING CONCEPTS FROM THEORIES TO THE EXERCISE SETTING

A. ASSESSING THE PARTICIPANT AND DEVELOPING STRATEGIES TO INCREASE EXERCISE ADHERENCE

Various assessments can be used to determine behavioral needs as well as strategies to encourage initiation, adherence, and return to participation if an individual has experienced a relapse.

1. Assessing benefits and barriers entails using a decisional balance sheet.
   a. All of the perceptions about exercise programs, both negative (e.g., lack of time, too painful, too hard) and positive (e.g., makes you feel more energetic, helps you to lose weight, strengthens muscles), are written on a sheet of paper.
   b. Helping individuals see the benefits of exercising can increase the likelihood of continued participation in an exercise program.
   c. Using problem-solving techniques to remove exercise barriers, one by one, can help the participant learn how to find time and enjoyment with exercise and decrease the reasons for not being able to maintain a regular exercise program.
   d. As a participant finds more reasons to become active and reduces the number of reasons for inactivity, the decisional balance tips in the positive direction and improves adherence.
2. Assessing self-efficacy (i.e., self-confidence) means determining the degree to which individuals believe that they can perform the desired behavior.
   a. Self-efficacy can be assessed by use of a written questionnaire. Using a 1-to-5 or a 1-to-10 Likert scale, individuals rank how confident they are that they can exercise when it is raining or snowing, when they feel that they do not have the time, when they are tired, and so forth.
   b. Four ways to improve self-efficacy include the following:
      1) Listing Performance Accomplishments
         Example: The participant sets a goal of walking 1 mile continuously within a month by gradually increasing the weekly walking distance. The exercise professional assists by helping to set realistic, specific, short- and long-term goals.
      2) Observing Through Vicarious Experience
         Example: The participant observes the behavior of individuals who have made positive contributions to their health. They may say to themselves: "These people are like me—if they can do it, then I probably can."
      3) Using Verbal Persuasion
         Example: The exercise professional helps the participant to see how he or she might be able to understand the feasibility of a goal and how to best accomplish that particular goal. Unrealistic expectations are discouraged and continuous reinforcement and feedback are provided.
      4) Understanding Physiologic States
         Example: The exercise professional helps the participant to recognize and monitor the number of positive feelings that come from exercise. This is accomplished through reinforcing self-monitoring techniques, such as keeping an

exercise log or counting steps using a mechanical step-counter.

3. Techniques from learning theories, such as **shaping, reinforcement and antecedent control**, have been used to increase adoption and maintenance of exercise.
   a. **Shaping** involves setting a series of intermediate goals that lead to a long-term goal. Shaping is especially appropriate when:
      1) Applied to **increasing frequency, intensity, duration, or types** of activities.
      2) Initiating exercise programs in which the **long-term goals may be too difficult for a novice**.
   b. **Reinforcement** should be scheduled to occur both during and after exercise to offset any possible immediate negative consequences (e.g., feeling hot, sweaty, or out of breath). Reinforcement can take several forms:
      1) **Verbal encouragement**.
      2) **Material incentives** (based on **specific contingency contracts**).
      3) **"Natural" reinforcements** (e.g., stress relief, self-praise).
   c. **Antecedent control** uses techniques that prompt the initiation of behavior. Such prompts include:
      1) Using telephone reminders.
      2) Packing a gym bag for the next day before going to bed.
      3) Scheduling time for exercise in one's daily schedule.
      4) Scheduling "pop-up" reminders on the computer.
4. **Cognitive restructuring techniques** involve changing thought processes about a particular situation. These are particularly important for **adoption and maintenance of an activity**, as well as for **relapse prevention**.
   a. **Relapse prevention strategies** include helping the participant to **identify high-risk situations** that may lead to a lapse. **Plans are developed before a lapse occurs.** Then, if the lapse does occur, a plan is in place and a relapse is less likely.
   b. Another goal is the **elimination of "all-or-none" thinking.** Participants who have a momentary lapse in a regular exercise routine often label themselves as a failure, subsequently leading to elimination of the exercise routine altogether. By eliminating "all-or-none" perceptions, the relapse is labeled correctly as a slight disruption with encouragement to resume the regular exercise routine.

B. UNDERSTANDING CONFIDENCE LEVEL, PERCEIVED BENEFITS, AND EXERCISE BARRIERS

1. This provides a focus for the exercise professional to **set realistic goals and gradually shape and increase** exercise behavior.
2. As participants progress in a program, it is important for them to continue **to set goals and to plan for possible lapses.**

C. USING THE STAGES OF CHANGE MODEL TO INCREASE ADHERENCE

(See also the previous discussion of the Transtheoretical Model or TTM)

1. Precontemplation

Discussing benefits, learning from previous attempts, and understanding the change process may assist during this stage. For example, many people decide to become regular exercisers and then have difficulty in maintaining a regular exercise program.

a. Participants in this stage **may not be aware of the risks** associated with being sedentary, or they **may have become discouraged** by previous attempts to stay active and develop feelings of failure. Multiple attempts may be required to succeed.
b. The exercise professional should not assume that a participant in the precontemplation stage is ready for an exercise program.
c. **Counseling should center on achievable goals** with which success is relatively certain (e.g., a 10-minute walk during the work week). This may not be the desired or long-term outcome, but by using a gradual process of shaping, the exercise behavior can become more frequent and of longer duration.

2. Contemplation

Contemplators believe that the reasons for being inactive (e.g., "I am too tired" or "Exercise takes too much time") outweigh the benefits of initiating an exercise program. Useful approaches in this stage include:

a. **Discussing the benefits of exercise** and **helping the participant to problem-solve** to eliminate barriers. These techniques should increase the participant's confidence level and self-efficacy.

b. **Encouraging the individual to set specific short-term goals** (e.g., exercise for 20 minutes on specific days).

3. **Preparation**

Irregular exercise behavior is the hallmark of people in this stage.

a. **Further barrier reductions and continued building of self-efficacy** are important.
b. **Monitoring gains** and **rewarding the achievement of goals** are two methods for increasing confidence.
c. **Shaping by reinforcing small steps** toward an action is also important. Gradually increasing the time for, intensity of, and adherence to, exercise will assist in achieving the recommended levels of an exercise behavior.

4. **Action**

People in the action stage are at the **greatest risk of relapse.**

a. Instruction on **avoiding injury, exercise boredom, and exercise burnout** is important to those who have recently started an exercise program.
b. **Social support** (e.g., asking how it is going, what problems have arisen) and **praise** are the most important contributors to maintained activity.
c. **Planning for high-risk relapse situations** (e.g., vacations, sickness, bad weather, and increased demands on time) is important. The exercise professional can emphasize that a short lapse in activity can be a learning opportunity and not a failure. Planning can help to develop coping strategies and eliminate the "all-or-none" thinking that is sometimes typical of people who miss several exercise sessions and feel that they need to give up.

5. **Maintenance**

After 6 months of regular activity, participants are considered to be in the maintenance stage of exercise adoption.

a. In this stage, some coping strategies have been developed, but **risk for dropping out still remains present.**
b. **Scheduling check-in appointments** can help the maintainer to stay motivated.
c. **Continued feedback** is important. If a maintainer is absent for several sessions, a **prompt such as a telephone call or letter noting the absence** can help to re-establish maintenance.
d. **Planning for high-risk situations** (e.g., alternate activities, plans to begin exercise after a lapse, finding someone to exercise with, lowering initial exercise goals after a lapse) is also important.
e. It also helps to **revisit the benefits** and **reassess the goals** of physical activity.
f. **Boredom** can be minimized by including a variety of activities (e.g., performing rowing exercise followed by walking and cycling and ending with resistive training).

IV. UNDERSTANDING VARIABLES THAT INFLUENCE ACTIVITY LEVELS

A. DEMOGRAPHIC VARIABLES

1. Women tend to participate in less vigorous activity than men. Thus, many women may respond better to programs that incorporate low- to moderate-intensity activity.
2. Older age is associated with lower levels of physical activity, especially vigorous activity. Older individuals may respond better to programs that incorporate low-intensity activity.

B. COGNITIVE AND EXPERIENTIAL VARIABLES

1. **Previous experiences** with physical activity can influence the initiation of an exercise program.
2. An individual's **perception of his or her current health status** can affect current physical activity levels.
3. **Perceived enjoyment of physical activity** can affect adoption of and adherence to an exercise program.
4. **Access to exercise facilities** and **convenience of the exercise program** can also affect adoption of and adherence to such a program.

C. ENVIRONMENTAL AND PROGRAM FACTORS

1. Environmental and program factors are very important for the adoption and continued maintenance of an exercise program. These factors include:
   a. **Social support** from family, peers, and coworkers.
   b. **Weather** that is either too hot or too cold.
   c. **Increased flexibility or adaptability** of the exercise program (e.g., adding lifestyle components, home exercise, location, intensity, frequency).
   d. **Reminders** in the environment to exercise.
   e. **Neighborhood factors** (e.g., available sidewalks, stray animals, crime, streetlights).

V. EFFECTIVE COUNSELING TIPS

A. USING A THREE-FUNCTION MODEL OF PARTICIPANT-CENTERED EDUCATION AND COUNSELING

1. During information gathering, any or all of the following areas should be assessed for participants:
   a. Current level of knowledge.
   b. Attitudinal beliefs, intentions, and readiness to change.
   c. Previous experiences with exercise or physical activity skills.
   d. Behavioral skills.
   e. Available social support.
2. In developing a helping relationship, it is important to understand the process and to establish support.
   a. An effective process is interactive, assesses information central to the issues, asks questions of the participant, instructs, and takes into account a willingness to negotiate. Effective listening skills are essential in developing a helping relationship.
   b. Exhibiting feelings of acceptance develops a supportive relationship. If the exercise professional is judgmental, participants may not share information regarding their exercise behavior or lifestyle.
   c. It is also important to establish a supportive relationship. To do this, the exercise professional should:
      1) Exhibit empathy by restating expressed emotion (e.g., "This seems frustrating to you" or "I know how it feels to feel pain in your heels").
      2) Legitimize concerns (e.g., "I can understand why you might be concerned with travel out of town" or "I see why you might be worried about hurting your knees").
      3) Respect one's abilities and positive efforts (e.g., "You've worked hard to get this far" or "You have done so well after just a few weeks of exercise").
      4) Support by providing reinforcement and follow-up (e.g., "I'll be available to help you get on track and stay on track" or "Feel free to call me with any questions that may arise").
      5) Partner with the individual by stating your willingness to work together (e.g., "You won't be alone—I will be there to help you").
      6) Pay attention to nonverbal communication (e.g., eye contact, body posture, vocal quality).
3. Participant education and counseling is a multifactorial process that can involve various situations and issues. To counsel effectively about readiness to change, it is necessary to understand that waning motivation to exercise is universal. Effective counseling can assist a person who is experiencing a lapse (short break) to prevent it from turning into a relapse (longer period of inactivity) or a collapse (no plans for returning to exercise).
   a. During each counseling session, the five As should be used:
      1) Address the agenda (e.g., "I'd like to talk to you about . . . ").
      2) Assess (e.g., "What do you know about . . . ?" "How do you feel?" "What are you considering . . . ?").
      3) Advise (e.g., "I'd like you to perform. . . ").
      4) Assist (e.g., "How would you like for me to help you?" "What problems do you foresee?").
      5) Arrange follow-up (e.g., "We will set up a time for you to let me know how you did . . . ").
   b. Most sedentary people are not motivated to initiate exercise programs. If exercise is initiated, they are likely to stop within 3–6 months.
   c. Participants in the earlier stages benefit most from cognitive strategies (e.g., listening to lectures and reading books without the expectation of actually engaging in exercise). Those in the later stages depend more on behavioral techniques (e.g., reminders to exercise and developing social support to help them establish and maintain a regular exercise habit).

B. RECOGNIZING AND ACKNOWLEDGING INDIVIDUAL DIFFERENCES

1. Many ways exist to achieve a regular exercise or physical activity routine.
2. The Surgeon General's report on physical activity and health states that moderate-intensity lifestyle activity (e.g., brisk walking, gardening) performed for a total of 30–60 minutes at least five times a week produces important health benefits.
3. Some participants may feel more comfortable using this type of home-based approach rather than going to a health/fitness facility where

others might notice their appearance and skill level.

4. Some participants may not perceive that they can achieve 30 minutes continuously, and they may not be aware that activity benefits can be achieved by accumulating shorter bouts of exercise.
5. **Intermittent-activity prescriptions counteract the "all-or-none" thinking** (e.g., "I can't exercise for an hour so I might just as well not exercise at all") that leads to relapse.

C. DEALING WITH DIFFICULT PATIENTS

Despite best efforts, some patients are difficult to work with. Issues related to interaction with the exercise professional must be resolved before exercise goals can be achieved.

1. The **dissatisfied participant** is never pleased regardless of all efforts to please.
   a. The exercise professional must work hard at all times to remind the participant that **the professional's goal is to assist in achieving exercise adherence**.
   b. If dissatisfaction remains after developing all possible options, **state the options, acknowledge that they may not be ideal, and ask the participant for his or her preferred option.**
2. The **needy participant** wants more support than can be given. Often, a primary goal of needy individuals is simply to gain attention. The exercise professional should:
   a. **Establish specific expectations** of what is possible.
   b. **Remain focused** on the exercise or physical activity issues and the participant's behavioral skills.
   c. Remind the participant that the goal is health education and exercise adherence.
   d. Refer the participant for additional help (e.g., professional counseling from a psychologist or physician), if necessary.
3. The **hostile participant** may try to elicit hostility. When faced with such an individual, it is important to **maintain professionalism.**
   a. **Acknowledge** the participant's anger.
   b. Try to **determine whether you should address the underlying issue** or ask the participant what would make him or her feel less angry.
   c. If chronic hostility occurs, a **different exercise leader** may help to ameliorate the situation.
   d. If chronic hostility remains, the program director or health/fitness facility administrator should be consulted and the participant may be asked to leave.
4. The **shy participant** is usually pleasant but not talkative. Try asking probing and **open-ended questions** instead of those that just require yes or no answers.
5. The **chronic complainer** has a negative outlook on life and may have legitimate medical concerns (e.g., chronic joint or back problems) that cause pain during exercise. This individual may undermine efforts to create a socially supportive atmosphere. A chronic complainer may be asked to modify his or her behavior or to exit the program in favor of a more conducive exercise environment (e.g., one-on-one home exercise therapy with a personal trainer).
6. The **underexerter** does not work hard enough during exercise sessions to benefit from their prescribed rehabilitation. Sedentary individuals typically go through a period of adjustment during which time they must learn to tolerate increased levels of discomfort from exercise. To help the underexerter, the exercise professional should:
   a. Provide gentle but steady encouragement.
   b. Pair the underexerter with a peer who is at a more advanced stage in the exercise program.
   c. Work with the participant closely one-on-one, showing that person that a mild increase in exercise workload is tolerable and will not be hurtful.
7. **Overexerters** or **noncompliers** consistently work too hard during exercise sessions, potentially putting themselves at risk of **orthopedic** or **cardiopulmonary** complications. Overexerters may benefit from:
   a. Instruction on how to pace themselves to avoid counterproductive excessive effort.
   b. Information on the dangers of exercise overexertion for their particular medical condition.
   c. Being paired with a former overexerter who has modified his or her rehabilitation approach.
8. The class **disrupter** or **comedian** feels the need for extreme attention from the exercise professional or the class members. This need for attention may be channeled into a productive leadership role within the group (e.g., taking attendance). Any disrupter or comedian who is intimidating to others (either physically or verbally) or distracts from the program's goals should be dealt with directly by the exercise professional

or program director and may be asked to leave the program if the situation remains unresolved.

VI. PROBLEMS EXCEEDING YOUR LEVEL OF EXPERTISE

A. WHEN TO REFER PARTICIPANTS FOR FURTHER INTERVENTIONS

Referrals to other resources may be required when participants have **health problems** that may limit the types of exercises that can be performed. Participants identified as having significant psychosocial disturbances should always be referred to the appropriate mental health professional (e.g., **clinical social worker, psychologist, psychiatric nurse, psychiatrist,** or **chaplain**) before starting an exercise program.

1. Participants with **existing health problems** or **perceived health limitations** should be referred to their primary care physician for further evaluation or reassurance.
2. Participants with **psychological issues** (e.g., poor coping abilities, difficulty managing stress, depression, anxiety, chronic complaints of being overwhelmed) should be referred to a mental health professional or physician for further evaluation.
3. **Symptoms of depression or anxiety** (*Table 5-1*) are very serious. Participants with these symptoms should be referred to a physician or mental health professional as soon as possible.
4. **Anxiousness prior to a fitness assessment** may be accompanied by a high heart rate and rapid, shallow breathing. **Techniques for reducing pretest anxiety** include:
    a. Having the person sit quietly and perform **deep-breathing exercises.**
    b. **Giving thorough explanations,** and **allowing practice** with unfamiliar equipment.
    c. **Scheduling an additional practice session** on equipment to increase the participant's familiarity with staff, equipment, and setting.
5. Individuals dealing with **life crises** may experience emotional difficulties that affect their exercise behavior. Examples of life crises include marital difficulty, divorce, unemployment, and financial problems. These individuals should be referred to a mental health professional, as needed.
6. **Persons with substance abuse or eating disorders** should be referred to a physician or mental health professional.

TABLE 5-1. SYMPTOMS OF DEPRESSION AND ANXIETY

SYMPTOMS OF DEPRESSION	SYMPTOMS OF ANXIETY
■ Feeling sad or "down in the dumps" for >2 weeks. ■ Frequent crying or tearfulness ■ Having frequent discomforts or pains ■ Depressed or irritable mood most days of the week ■ Loss of interest or pleasure in activities (e.g., hobbies, work, sex, or being with friends) ■ A sudden change in weight (e.g., weight loss without dieting, gaining more >5% of body weight in 1 month) or a change in appetite ■ Inability to sleep or sleeping too much nearly every day (also early morning awakening) ■ Frequent feelings of worthlessness or inappropriate guilt ■ Difficulty in concentrating or making decisions ■ Frequent thoughts of death or suicide ■ Withdrawal from family and society	■ Having panic attacks (sudden episodes of fear and physiological arousal that occur for no apparent reason) ■ Rapid heart rate ■ Sweaty palms ■ Increased nervousness associated with going into crowded places (e.g., the mall or a gym) ■ Feeling "keyed up" or "on edge" most of the time ■ Unable to "calm down" or relax ■ Always fidgety or needing to move a body part ■ Rapid speech patterns

7. **When making referrals, the exercise professional should be acquainted with the physician or mental health professional and should follow up with the participant after the referral.**

B. PSYCHOLOGICAL DISTRESS

1. Signs of **significant psychosocial disturbance** may include any of the following:
    a. The inability for the participant to carry out routine activities of daily living (ADL).
    b. A significant disruption of normal lifestyle patterns in the participant or significant others.
    c. The inability to work at a normal occupational level.
    d. Any symptoms of depression.
    e. Acknowledgement by the patient, family member, or support person of psychosocial dysfunction and a reduction in their social support network.
    f. Excessively high or low scores with psychometric testing, depending on the survey used.
    g. Distorted perceptions of reality.

VII. MEASURING HEALTH AND BEHAVIOR CHANGE

A. PSYCHOSOCIAL ASSESSMENT

1. The psychosocial assessment is performed to establish baseline measures of behavioral or psychological constructs and to help assess change.
2. Psychosocial assessments help in understanding in what areas assistance might be required for the participant (e.g., building confidence, improving self-efficacy, lessening feelings of depression).
3. Psychosocial assessments lead to focusing on intervention strategies (e.g., setting and achieving realistic fitness goals to build confidence).
4. The psychosocial assessment component, including interviewing and scoring strategies employed by the exercise professional, is vital to the success of a cardiac or pulmonary rehabilitation program and in the health and fitness setting.
5. The psychosocial assessment survey is given to the participant by the exercise professional to be completed either at home (ideally without the help of a spouse or family member) or in the fitness setting.
6. After the survey is returned, the exercise professional may score the survey, either with hand-scoring or with a computer software program designed for that survey.
7. Once scored, the survey results are compared with normative data and the results are discussed with the participant. The scores may also be entered into a group database or registry for group analyses and benchmarking.
8. In some instances, the mental health professional of a cardiac or pulmonary rehabilitation program or health/fitness facility may score the survey and discuss the results with the participant.
9. Psychosocial assessment surveys are limited by the survey length and the scoring complexity.
10. Many programs now prefer simple, quick, effective, and easily scored surveys with easily understood language for the participant.

B. EVALUATION OF PSYCHOSOCIAL ASSESSMENT TOOLS

1. It is important that the psychosocial assessment tool selected for use in the program be adequately tested for validity, reliability, and feasibility.
2. The three types of validity measures are:
   a. Face validity, which indicates that the measure on the psychosocial assessment tool appears to measure what it is intended to measure.
   b. Content validity, which indicates that the measure captures the meaningful aspects of patient care.
   c. Construct validity, which indicates that the measure correlates well with other measures of the same aspects of patient care.
3. Test reliability indicates that the measure is likely to be reproducible across organizations and delivery settings. If the psychosocial assessment survey is given to a cohort of participants (e.g., those with congestive heart failure), similar results should be found in other groups of patients with congestive heart failure.
4. Test feasibility indicates that the data required for a particular measure are likely to be obtained with reasonable effort, at a reasonable cost, and within the period allowed for data collection.

C. HEALTH-RELATED QUALITY OF LIFE

1. Health-related quality of life (QOL) measurement is the primary focus of many psychosocial assessment tools. One definition of health-related QOL is the value assigned to duration of life as modified by impairments, functional states, perceptions, and social opportunities that are influenced by disease, injury, treatment or policy. A person's assessment of satisfaction with life involves two subjective considerations: how important a given domain is for that person, and how satisfied that person is with that domain. An individual can be dissatisfied with a domain that he or she considers to be of relatively little importance and, thus, continue to maintain a satisfactory overall QOL. Dissatisfaction with a domain of great importance to an individual, however, would clearly contribute to a lower QOL.
2. Before selecting an instrument for measuring health-related QOL, the purpose and objectives for the survey must be established, including those listed below:
   a. To evaluate changes (large or small) in a participant or group of participants over time related to an intervention, disease progression, or other agent of change.
   b. To judge the level of a participant or group of participant's QOL over time at specified intervals for determination of positive or negative change.
   c. As a basis for cost-utility analysis for economic evaluation of healthcare services.
   d. As a means to present QOL summary outcome data to program staff, supervisors, administrators, physicians, and healthcare providers.

D. GENERIC QOL SURVEYS

1. Generic QOL surveys are those given to all program participants, regardless of health or disease state. Generic QOL surveys are beneficial in that they:
   a. Apply to a heterogeneous population, regardless of existing conditions.
   b. Allow crosspopulation comparisons (i.e., comparisons with participants with varying health conditions).
   c. Address multiple issues related to limitations in health status (i.e., comorbid conditions, age).
   d. Are useful in cost-utility analysis for economic evaluation of health services.
2. Generic QOL surveys are limited in that they:
   a. Include items that are not relevant to all populations.
   b. Are less responsive to disease-specific issues.
   c. Require large numbers of respondents for accurate comparisons across populations.
3. Examples of Generic QOL surveys include the following:
   a. Nottingham Health Profile.
   b. DUKE Health Profile.
   c. Medical Outcomes Study Short Form (SF-36).
   d. Quality of Life Systemic Inventory.
   e. Sickness Impact Profile.

E. DISEASE-SPECIFIC (TARGETED) QOL SURVEYS

1. Disease-specific or targeted QOL surveys focus on participants with a particular disease state (e.g., cardiac, pulmonary, renal). These surveys are beneficial in that they:
   a. Are responsive to a specific population with the same disease or condition.
   b. Focus on relevant, problematic areas for a given population.
   c. Address issues related to clinical manifestations of a disorder.
   d. Measure small changes in specific conditions.
   e. Allow comparisons of a small cohort of respondents with the same disease.
2. Disease-specific QOL surveys are limited in that they:
   a. Are not sensitive to the combined effects of conditions when a comorbid condition exists.
   b. Do not allow comparisons between populations.
   c. Are not as well accepted by hospital administrators and payers as some generic QOL surveys.
   d. Are not sufficiently comprehensive to be used for economic evaluations.
3. Examples of cardiac-specific QOL surveys include the following:
   a. Minnesota Living with Heart Failure Questionnaire.
   b. Ferrans and Powers Quality of Life Index (QLI)—Cardiac Version.
   c. Seattle Angina Questionnaire.
   d. Quality of Life After Myocardial Infarction.
   e. Kansas City Cardiomyopathy Questionnaire.
4. Examples of pulmonary-specific QOL surveys include the following:
   a. Chronic Respiratory Disease Questionnaire (CRQ).
   b. Ferrans and Powers Quality of Life Index (QLI)—Pulmonary Version.
   c. St. George's Respiratory Questionnaire (SGRQ).
   d. Living with Asthma Questionnaire.
   e. Pulmonary Functional Status Scale (PFSS).

F. MEASUREMENT OF DEPRESSION, HOSTILITY, AND ANXIETY

1. Many psychosocial assessment surveys are specifically designed to measure levels of depression, hostility, and anxiety.
2. Recent research has identified depression as an independent risk factor for myocardial infarction and mortality and a major contributor to other adverse health states.
3. Psychological distress is an important predictor of hospitalization costs following a cardiac or pulmonary event.
4. Surveys that are used to assess depression, hostility, and anxiety include the following:
   a. Beck Depression Inventory II (BDI-II).
   b. Cook Medley Hostility Scale.
   c. Herridge Cardiopulmonary Questionnaire (HCQ).
   d. Cardiac Depression Scale (CDS).
   e. Center for Epidemiological Studies—Depression Mode Scale (CES-D).
   f. Jenkins Activity Survey (JAS).

G. DETERMINING DEGREES OF CHANGE IN PSYCHOSOCIAL STATUS

Many ways exist to determine if a score on a particular psychosocial assessment tool indicates a significant change in behavior or degree of psychosocial status. Degrees of change may be determined by assessing statistical significance, the minimal clinically significant change, or by comparisons with standardized normative values (e.g., ACSM, Cooper Institute, YMCA norms).

1. A **statistically significant change** is determined through comparisons of scores through mathematical analyses based on the population size and the sample characteristics.
2. The **minimal clinically significant change** in QOL or a specific behavior may be more practical for the exercise professional. This is defined as the smallest change in a given domain that a participant perceives as a beneficial or adverse response, or a change that would require a change in patient management.
3. The **minimal clinically significant change** may be estimated from theoretical arguments or statistical considerations, such as the standard error of the mean or test/retest reliability measurements. **Example**: the minimal clinically significant change on the **SF-36** survey is **5 points**, whereas on the **Ferrans and Powers Quality of Life Index—Pulmonary Version** the change is **2 points**.
4. Assessing the **minimal clinically significant change** allows the exercise professional to provide a more comprehensive explanation of a psychosocial survey score increase or decrease to a program participant, indicating a true change in behavior or psychosocial status.
5. Comparisons with **standardized normative values** by age (e.g., YMCA norms for sit-and-reach distance, Cooper Institute norms for level of fitness based on graded exercise test results of thousands of subjects, ACSM classification of overweight and obesity based on body fat percentage) can be extremely helpful for the exercise professional when discussing psychosocial assessment results with the participant. In this fashion, the participant gains insight into "yardstick" comparisons with people of the same age or disease classification with survey scores.

Review Test

DIRECTIONS: Carefully read all questions, and select the BEST single answer.

1. The cognitive theory of behavioral change includes all of the following concepts EXCEPT
   A) Dramatic relief (warning of risks).
   B) Reinforcement management (rewarding yourself).
   C) Helping relationships (enlisting social support).
   D) Counter-conditioning (substituting alternatives).

2. In which stage of motivational readiness is a person who is an irregular exerciser?
   A) Precontemplation.
   B) Contemplation.
   C) Preparation.
   D) Action.

3. Which of the following is an example of increasing self-efficacy by setting several short-term goals to attain a long-term goal?
   A) An application of cognitive-behavioral principles.
   B) Shaping.
   C) A component of antecedent control.
   D) An explanatory theory.

4. Which of the following is **not** considered a component for assessing the feasibility of a psychosocial measure?
   A) The data required for the measure are obtained with reasonable effort.
   B) The data required for the measure are obtained at reasonable cost.
   C) The data required for the measure are obtained from studies that report a significance level (P-value) of >0.05.
   D) The data required for the measure are obtained within the period allowed for data collection.

5. The minimal clinically significant change in a psychosocial assessment survey score:
   A) Is less practical than looking at the statistical significance of a psychosocial assessment survey score.
   B) Helps the exercise professional to give better "yardstick" comparisons to the participant when compared with other individuals who have taken the test.
   C) Can only be determined through statistical analyses performed by the exercise professional for a given psychosocial survey
   D) Is the highest degree of change score indicating a psychosocial improvement or decline.

6. In the Social Cognitive Theory, which three major dynamic interacting influences are postulated as determining behavioral change?
   A) Stage of readiness, processes of change, and confidence.
   B) Reinforcement, commitment, and social support.
   C) High-risk situations, social support, and perceived control.
   D) Personal, behavioral, and environmental.

7. Face validity in psychosocial research
   A) Is reproducible across organizations and delivery settings.
   B) Appears to measure what it is intended to measure.
   C) Captures the most meaningful aspects of patient care.
   D) Correlates well with other measures of the same aspect of healthcare.

8. An individual would **not** increase self-efficacy by
   A) Performance accomplishments.
   B) Vicarious experience.
   C) Using a decisional balance sheet.
   D) Verbal persuasion.

9. Which of the following stages define people having the greatest risk of relapse?
   A) Precontemplation.
   B) Contemplation.
   C) Preparation.
   D) Action.

10. Which of the following strategies can help a person to maintain his or her physical activity?
    A) Schedule check-in appointments.
    B) Reduce barriers to exercise.
    C) Increase the benefits of physical activity.
    D) All of the above.

11. Referrals to other sources, such as a mental health professional or physician, may be required if someone ___________
    A) Is noncompliant with a prescribed level of exercise.
    B) Is very shy and nontalkative.
    C) Has an eating disorder.
    D) None of the above.

12. Establishing specific expectations of what you are willing to do as a counselor and staying focused on exercise and physical activity issues and behavioral skills related to exercise are strategies for handling which type of participant?
    A) Dissatisfied participant.

B) Needy participant.
C) Hostile participant.
D) Shy participant.

13. Encouraging moderate-intensity activity and the accumulation of activity throughout the day are examples of
A) Allowing individuality in exercise choices.
B) Using the stages of change.
C) Relapse prevention counseling.
D) "All-or-none" thinking.

14. Which of the following is **not** considered a significant indicator of psychosocial distress?
A) The inability to carry out basic activities of daily living.
B) Driving consistently 20–30 mph over the speed limit.
C) A very high score on a psychosocial assessment survey, such as the Beck Depression Inventory-II.
D) Acknowledgement of a patient being depressed by a patient's spouse, partner, or friend.

15. Which of the following is an error that a healthcare provider may make?
A) Assume that most individuals are ready to change their behavior.
B) Encourage the accumulation of moderate-intensity activity throughout the day.
C) Legitimize a patient's concerns.
D) Use the five A's strategy for counseling.

16. The concept of shaping refers to ______________________
A) Using self-monitoring techniques (e.g., exercise logs).
B) Using visual prompts (e.g., packing a gym bag the night before) as reminders to exercise.
C) The process for establishing self-efficacy.
D) Setting intermediate goals that lead to a long-term goal.

17. Verbal encouragement, material incentives, self-praise, and use of specific contingency contracts are examples of
A) Shaping.
B) Reinforcement.
C) Antecedent control.
D) Setting goals.

18. The Health Belief Model assumes that people will engage in a given behavior, such as increasing their level of daily activity, when
A) There is a perceived threat of disease.
B) There is the belief of susceptibility to disease.
C) The risk of disease is nonthreatening to the individual.
D) Only A and B of the above.
E) None of the above.

19. The Transtheoretical Model of Health Behavior assumes that individuals
A) Move through the stages of behavioral change at a steady pace.
B) Only progress forward through the stages.
C) Move back and forth along the stage continuum.
D) Tend to use behavioral processes during the earlier stages of change.

20. If an individual is in the action stage, he or she
A) Has been physically active on a regular basis for <6 months.
B) Participates in some exercise, but does so irregularly.
C) Intends to start exercising in the next 6 months.
D) Has been physically active on a regular basis for >6 months.

21. Which of the following is not a cardiac-specific quality-of-life questionnaire?
A) Ferrans and Powers Quality of Life Index (QLI)—Cardiac Version.
B) Minnesota Living with Heart Failure Questionnaire.
C) Cook Medley Hostility Scale.
D) Seattle Angina Questionnaire.

22. The five A's of counseling are:
A) Address, Assess, Advise, Assist, and Arrange follow-up.
B) Address, Assess, Advise, Assist, and Act.
C) Address, Assess, Act, Assist, and Arrange follow-up.
D) Act, Assess, Advise, Assist, and Arrange follow-up.

23. Which of the following techniques would assist the anxious patient before an exercise test?
A) Ask the person to sit quietly in a chair for a few minutes.
B) Thoroughly explain the exercise test.
C) Familiarize the person with the exercise equipment by brief practice.
D) All of the above.

24. Which of the following is **not** a symptom of depression?
A) Irritability.
B) A change in sleeping patterns.
C) Hearing voices or unusual sounds.
D) Having frequent bouts of crying.

25. Which of the following are symptoms of anxiety?
A) Panic attacks.
B) Increased nervousness.
C) Feelings of being "on edge."
D) All of the above.

ANSWERS AND EXPLANATIONS

1–A. The cognitive theory of behavioral change includes counter-conditioning (e.g., substituting alternatives, such as taking a 20-minute walk instead of eating a donut), reinforcement management (e.g., rewarding yourself for a given behavior, such as watching your favorite television show for exercising a full 60 minutes), and helping relationships (e.g., having a running partner). Dramatic relief (warning of risks) is a cognitive process component of the TTM.

2–C. The stages of motivational readiness describe five categories of readiness to change or maintain behavior. As applied to physical activity or exercise, they are precontemplation (stage 1: no physical activity or exercise, and no intention to start within the next 6 months); contemplation (stage 2: no physical activity or exercise, but an intention to start within the next 6 months); preparation (stage 3: participation in some physical activity or exercise, but not at levels meeting current and standard guidelines); action (stage 4: physical activity or exercise that meets standard guidelines for physical activity, but for <6 months); and maintenance (stage 5: exercise or activity for 6 months or longer).

3–A. Applications of cognitive-behavioral principles are the methods used within programs to improve motivational skills as suggested by the assessment. For example, setting several small short-term goals to attain a long-term goal is likely to increase self-efficacy as the person successfully reaches each short-term goal on the way to attaining the long-term goal.

4–C. Assessing the feasibility of a psychosocial measure involves obtaining the data required with reasonable effort, at a reasonable cost, and within the period allowed for data collection. For the exercise professional, the psychosocial data required can be obtained from sources such as the participant's record or state or national registries.

5–B. The minimal clinically significant change in QOL or a specific behavior is the smallest change in a given domain that a participant perceives as a beneficial or adverse response, or a change that would require a change in patient management. Using this measure is often more practical than looking solely at statistical significance or normative values. Not all psychosocial surveys have been evaluated for minimal clinically significant change, but this number is increasing over time.

6–D. The Social Cognitive Theory is one of the most widely used and comprehensive theories of behavioral change. This theory is a dynamic model that asserts three major interacting influences: behavioral, personal, and environmental. The Social Cognitive Theory contains a number of different concepts of constructs that are implicated in the adoption and maintenance of healthy behavior and that are used for increasing and maintaining physical activity or exercise. They include observation learning, behavioral capability, outcome expectations, self-efficacy, self-control of performance, management of emotional arousal, and reinforcement.

7–B. Face validity evaluates the ability of the psychosocial assessment tool or test item to measure what it is intended to measure. If a survey is designed to measure the level of depression in a group of individuals with pulmonary disease, it needs to be validated with a large number of individuals with pulmonary disease to assess if it is truly measuring this particular psychological component in this population of patients.

8–C. Self-efficacy (self-confidence) is the degree to which individuals believe they can perform the desired behavior. It is possible to increase self-efficacy in four ways: performance accomplishments (e.g., setting a goal of walking 1 mile in a month by gradually increasing the weekly distance); vicarious experience (e.g., "This person is like me; if she can do it, then I probably can"); verbal persuasion (e.g., helping the person to see how he or she might understand the feasibility of a goal and a way to accomplish it); and physiologic states (e.g., getting the person to recognize and monitor the number of positive feelings that come from exercise). A decisional balance sheet would be used to assess the benefits and barriers of a given behavior.

9–D. People in the action stage are at the greatest risk of relapse. Instruction about avoiding injury, exercise boredom, and burnout is important for those who have recently begun an exercise program. Providing social support and praise are the most important contributors to maintained activity. Planning for high-risk, relapse situations (e.g., vacations, sickness, bad weather, increased demands on time) is also important. The exercise professional can emphasize that a short lapse in activity can be a learning opportunity and is not failure. Planning can help to develop coping strategies and to eliminate the "all-or-none" thinking sometimes typical of people who have missed several exercise sessions and think they need to give it up.

10–D. Many ways exist to help an individual maintain an exercise program. Such methods include scheduling exercise appointments, reducing barriers to exercise, providing incentives and rewards, and understanding all the benefits of exercise.

11–C. Referrals to other resources may be required when participants have health problems that may limit the types of exercise that can be performed. Existing health problems or perceived health limitations may be referred to a primary care physician for further evaluation and reassurance. Participants with psychological issues (e.g., eating disorders, poor coping, difficulty managing stress, depression, anxiety, chronic complaints of being overwhelmed) should be referred to a mental health professional for professional counseling or to their personal physician for evaluation.

12–B. Despite the best efforts, working with some individuals are difficult. Issues related to interaction with the exercise professional must be resolved before exercise goals can be achieved. The needy person wants more support than can be given. It is important, then, to establish specific expectations of what is possible and to remain focused on the exercise or physical activity issues and behavioral skills related to those issues. Often, a primary goal of the needy individual is to gain attention. It is important to remember that the exercise professional is not a trained counselor and, in some cases, it may be appropriate to refer that person for additional help.

13–A. Recognizing and acknowledging individual differences is an important component of effective counseling. A regular exercise or physical activity routine can be achieved in many ways. Many participants may not perceive that they can achieve 30 minutes of continuous physical activity, and they may not be aware that activity benefits can be achieved through the accumulation of shorter bouts of exercise. Intermittent-activity prescriptions counteract the "all-or-none" type of thinking that often leads to relapse.

14–B. Psychosocial dysfunction is characterized by the patient's inability to carry out the basic activities of daily living such as bathing, dressing, or eating. The patient may also exhibit very high (or low) scores on various psychosocial assessment questionnaires. One of the best indicators that the patient is suffering psychologically is testimony from the patient's spouse, family member, or friend indicating a significant change in that person's daily behavior. These changes could include excessive sleeping, frequent crying, or complaints of feelings of hopelessness.

15–A. Participants progress through various stages of change at varying rates and, in the process of changing, they move back and forth along the stage continuum. Different cognitive and behavioral processes or strategies are used during each stage. Discussing the benefits of physical activity and learning from previous attempts may assist those in the precontemplation stage. This group may not be aware of the risks associated with being sedentary, or they may have become discouraged by previous attempts to stay active and have feelings of failure. Multiple attempts may be required to succeed. The exercise professional should not assume that the participant in the precontemplation stage is ready for an exercise program.

16–D. Shaping is setting a series of intermediate goals that lead to a long-term goal. This is especially appropriate when applied to increasing frequency, intensity, duration, or types of activities. When initiating exercise programs in which the long-term goals may be too difficult for a novice, this strategy is particularly appropriate.

17–B. Reinforcement should be scheduled to occur both during and after exercise to offset any possible immediate negative consequences. Reinforcement can take the form of verbal encouragement, material incentives (based on contingency contracts), and natural reinforcements (e.g., stress relief, self-praise).

18–D. The Health Belief Model assumes that people will engage in a given behavior, such as increasing daily levels of activity, when there is a perceived threat of disease, a belief that they are susceptible to disease, and that the threat is severe. The individual will take action depending on whether the benefits of the activity outweigh the barriers. Self-efficacy (self-confidence) also plays a major role of the Health Belief Model.

19–C. The Transtheoretical Model of Change (Stages of Change or Motivational Readiness) incorporates constructs from other theories, including intention to change and processes (or strategies) of change. The basic concepts of this model are that people progress through five stages of change at varying rates and that, in the process of changing, they also move back and forth along the stage continuum. The model also holds that people use different cognitive and behavioral processes or strategies.

20–A. Stages of motivational readiness describe five categories of readiness to change or maintain behavior. As applied to physical activity or exercise, they are precontemplation (stage 1), contemplation (stage 2), preparation (stage 3), action (stage 4), and maintenance (stage 5). The action stage is when the person is engaged in physical activity or exercise that meets the current ACSM recommendations for physical activity, but has not maintained this program for 6 months or more.

21–C. The Ferrans and Powers Quality of Life Index (QLI)—Cardiac Version, Minnesota Living with Heart Failure Questionnaire, and Seattle Angina Questionnaire all are disease-specific assessment tools that have been thoroughly tested for validity and reliability in persons with cardiovascular disease. The Cook Medley Hostility Scale is a generic instrument designed to assess hostility levels in the general population.

22–A. Participant education and counseling is a multifactorial process that may involve a variety of situations and issues. For example, to counsel effectively about readiness to change, it is necessary to understand that waning motivation to exercise is universal. Effective counseling can assist a person who is experiencing a lapse (e.g., short break) to prevent it from turning into a relapse or collapse. During each counseling session, the five A's (address the agenda, assess, advise, assist, arrange follow-up) should be used.

23–D. Anxiousness before a fitness assessment may be accompanied by a high heart rate and rapid, shallow breathing. This may be alleviated by having the person sit quietly and use deep-breathing exercises. Thorough explanations and practice on unfamiliar equipment can also reduce anxiety before exercise testing. Scheduling an additional practice session on equipment to increase familiarity with staff, equipment, and setting may assist those unable to reduce pretest anxiety.

24–C. Symptoms of depression are serious and those who are experiencing these symptoms should be referred to a physician or professional counselor. Symptoms of depression include feeling sad or "down in the dumps" for more than a few weeks, tearfulness, withdrawal from social activities, excessive guilt, rapid weight loss or gain, feelings of fatigue, changing sleep patterns (e.g., early morning awakening), vague pains or discomfort, or expressions of wanting to die, including suicide attempts.

25–D. Symptoms of anxiety include panic attacks (sudden episodes of fear and physiologic arousal that occur for no apparent reason), increased nervousness associated with going into crowded places (e.g., the mall, a gym), or feeling "keyed up" or "on edge."

CHAPTER 6

Health Appraisal and Fitness Testing

I. PRETEST CONSIDERATIONS

A. HEALTH APPRAISAL

Essential information is required before exercise testing to identify any necessary modifications of test protocols, risk factors for contraindications to testing, or the need for referral to a physician.

1. Purpose

a. **Safety**
Provides health and fitness professionals with information that can lead to **identification of individuals for whom exercise requires limitations or modifications or is contraindicated.**

b. **Risk Factor Identification**
Many medical conditions increase the health risk associated with physical activity or exercise testing.
Health screening allows the health/fitness professional to **determine who may participate** and **who should be referred to a physician** before participation in exercise testing or physical activity.

c. **Exercise Prescription and Programming**
Information gathered allows the health/fitness professional to **develop specific exercise programs appropriate to the individual needs** and goals of the individual.

2. Health History

a. **Present History**
1) Known disease or symptoms of disease.
2) Activity level.
3) Dietary behaviors (including caffeine and alcohol intake).
4) Smoking and tobacco use.
5) Medication use (including recreational drugs), drug allergies.

b. **Past History**
1) Cardiorespiratory problems.
2) Orthopedic problems.
3) Recent illnesses or hospitalizations.
4) Exercise history.
5) Work history.

c. **Family History**
1) Onset of heart disease in first-degree relative before age 55 (men) or 65 (women).
2) Other significant disorders, including diabetes, hyperlipidemia, stroke, and sudden death in first-degree relatives.

d. **Health Screening Questionnaire**
1) A preparticipation health screening tool, such as the **Physical Activity Readiness Questionnaire (PAR-Q)**, should be completed before exercise testing (*Figure 6-1*).
2) The American Heart Association/American College of Sport Medicine (AHA/ACSM) Health Fitness Facility Preparticipation Screening Questionnaire could be used for individuals beginning a physical activity program in a health and fitness setting.
3) To solicit reliable information, the questionnaire should be completed in a **quiet, private area.**
4) **Review the responses** with the patient to confirm the accuracy of the information and to determine the health risk status.

3. Physical Assessment and Laboratory Tests

a. **Resting Heart Rate**
1) After the patient has been sitting quietly for 5 minutes, palpate the pulse at the radial or carotid artery for 30 seconds; normal resting heart rate (HR) is 60–100 beats per minute (bpm).
2) Peripheral pulses should be measured as well, as a screening tool for peripheral circulatory problems. Note strength of pulse (radial, pedal). Also look for signs of peripheral edema (i.e., pitting of tissue at the ankles).

b. **Resting Blood Pressure**
1) Because blood pressure (BP) can fluctuate, accurate BP assessment should

Physical Activity Readiness Questionnaire - PAR-Q (revised 1994)

PAR - Q & YOU

(A Questionnaire for People Aged 15 to 69)

Regular physical activity is fun and healthy, and increasingly more people are starting to become more active every day. Being more active is very safe for most people. However, some people should check with their doctor before they start becoming much more physically active.

If you are planning to become much more physically active than you are now, start by answering the seven questions in the box below. If you are between the ages of 15 and 69, the PAR-Q will tell you if you should check with your doctor before you start. If you are over 69 years of age, and you are not used to being very active, check with your doctor.

Common sense is your best guide when you answ... these questions. Please read the questions carefully and answer each one honestly: check YES ...

... heart condition and that you should only do physical activity

... physical activity?

... when you were not doing physical activity?

☐ ☐ 4. Do you lose your balance because of dizziness or do you ever lose consciousness?

☐ ☐ 5. Do you have a bone or joint problem that could be made worse by a change in your physical activity?

☐ ☐ 6. Is your doctor currently prescribing drugs (for example, water pills) for your blood pressure or heart condition?

☐ ☐ 7. Do you know of any other reason why you should not do physical activity?

If you answered

YES to one or more questions

Talk with your doctor by phone or in person BEFORE you start becoming much more physically active or BEFORE you have a fitness appraisal. Tell your doctor about the PAR-Q and which questions you answered YES.

- You may be able to do any activity you want—as long as you start slowly and build up gradually. Or, you may need to restrict your activities to those which are safe for you. Talk with your doctor about the kinds of activities you wish to participate in and follow his/her advice.
- Find out which community programs are safe and helpful for you.

NO to all questions

If you answered NO honestly to all PAR-Q questions, you can be reasonably sure that you can:

- start becoming much more physically active—begin slowly and build up gradually. This is the safest and easiest way to go.
- take part in a fitness appraisal—this is an excellent way to determine your basic fitness so that you can plan the best way for you to live actively.

DELAY BECOMING MUCH MORE ACTIVE:

- if you are not feeling well because of a temporary illness such as a cold or a fever—wait until you feel better: or
- if you are or may be pregnant—talk to your doctor before you start becoming more active.

Please note: if your health changes so that you then answer YES to any of the above questions, tell your fitness or health professional. Ask whether you should change your physical activity plan.

Informed Use of the PAR-Q: The Canadian Society for Exercise Physiology, Health Canada, and their agents assume no liability for persons who undertake physical activity, and if in doubt after completing this quesionnaire, consult your doctor prior to physical activity.

You are encouraged to copy the PAR-Q but only if you use the entire form

NOTE: if the PAR-Q is being given to a person before he or she participates in physical activity program or a fitness appraisal, this section may be used for legal or administrative purposes.

I have read, understood and completed this questionnaire. Any questions I had were answered to my full satisfaction.

NAME ______________________

SIGNATURE ______________________ DATE ______________________

SIGNATURE OF PARENT ______________________ WITNESS ______________________
or GUARDIAN (for participants under the age of majority)

© Canadian Society for Exercise Physiology
Société canadienne de physiologie de l'exercice

Supported by: Health Canada Santé Canada

FIGURE 6-1. PAR-Q form. (Reprinted from the 1994 revised version of the *Physical Activity Readiness Questionnaire* [PAR-Q and YOU]. The PAR-Q and YOU is a copyrighted, pre-exercise screen owned by the Canadian Society for Exercise Physiology.)

be based on two or more measurements and findings are compared with published standards.

2) Blood pressure should be measured with the patient in both the supine and standing positions to screen for **postural hypotension**. Measure the pressure immediate after the patient stands.

c. **Lung Capacity**

Lung capacity is tested by assessing airway patency and airflow volume and rate.

1) **Forced Vital Capacity (FVC)**
   a) This is the volume of air expired following a maximal inspiration.
   b) FVC assesses the degree of restrictive pulmonary disease.
2) **Forced Expiratory Capacity at 1 Second (FEV_1)**
   a) This is the proportion of the FVC expired in 1 second.
   b) FEV_1 assesses the degree of airway obstruction.
3) **Maximal Voluntary Ventilation (MVV)**
   a) This is the maximal volume of airflow per minute possible.
   b) MVV represents the mechanical limit of pulmonary function.

d. **Blood Tests**

Various blood tests may shed light on the patient's current health status and may help guide exercise programming. Typically, blood samples are drawn following an overnight fast; values are expressed in either milligram per deciliter (mg/dL) or millimole per liter (mmol/L).

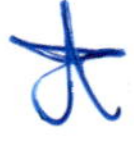

1) **Total Cholesterol (TC)**
This is the measure of the total amount of cholesterol in the blood. It includes all cholesterol fractions.

2) **Low-Density Lipoprotein (LDL)**
   a) An LDL is a cholesterol-carrying protein that tends to deposit cholesterol on arterial walls, greatly accelerating atherosclerosis.
   b) LDLs are also thought to act as free radicals and to cause damage to cell walls. **High levels increase risk.**

3) **High-density lipoprotein (HDL)**
An HDL is a cholesterol-carrying protein that tends to remove cholesterol from the blood.
   a) HDLs are also thought to remove cholesterol from cell walls, possibly reversing the progression of atherosclerosis. **High levels are desirable.**

4) **TC:HDL Ratio**
   a) **This ratio is a useful index of dyslipidemia.**
   b) **May be significant (>4.3) even if both TC and HDL are within normal limits.**

5) **Fasting Glucose**
   a) This is a measure of blood glucose level without the influence of a meal.
   b) **High levels are indicative of impaired glucose tolerance.**

6) Other Blood Tests
   a) Homocysteine: in adults, elevated levels ($>15\ \mu mol \cdot L^{-1}$) are linked to increase coronary artery disease (CAD) risk, stroke, thromboemboli, and peripheral artery disease.
   b) C-reactive protein (CPR) is a marker for inflammation, and can contribute information to predict coronary events. CPR can be lowered with aspirin and statin therapy.

B. CONTRAINDICATIONS AND RISK STRATIFICATION

1. Contraindications to Exercise Testing

Some persons have risk factors that outweigh the potential benefits derived from exercise testing (*Table 6-1*).

a. **Absolute contraindications** apply to individuals for whom exercise testing should not be performed until the situation or condition has stabilized.

TABLE 6-1. CONTRAINDICATIONS TO EXERCISE TESTING

Absolute
- A recent significant change in the resting ECG suggesting significant ischemia, recent myocardial infarction (within 2 days), or other acute cardiac event
- Unstable angina
- Uncontrolled cardiac dysrhythmias causing symptoms or hemodynamic compromise
- Symptomatic severe aortic stenosis
- Uncontrolled symptomatic heart failure
- Acute pulmonary embolus or pulmonary infarction
- Acute myocarditis or pericarditis
- Suspected or known dissecting aneurysm
- Acute systemic infection, accompanied by fever, body aches, or swollen lymph glands

Relative[a]
- Left main coronary stenosis
- Moderate stenotic valvular heart disease
- Electrolyte abnormalities (e.g., hypokalemia, hypomagnesemia)
- Severe arterial hypertension (i.e., systolic BP of >200 mm Hg and/or a diastolic BP of >110 mm Hg) at rest
- Tachydysrhythmia or bradydysrhythmia
- Hypertrophic cardiomyopathy and other forms of outflow tract obstruction
- Neuromuscular, musculoskeletal, or rheumatoid disorders that are exacerbated by exercise
- High-degree atrioventricular block
- Ventricular aneurysm
- Uncontrolled metabolic disease (e.g., diabetes, thyrotoxicosis, or myxedema)
- Chronic infectious disease (e.g., mononucleosis, hepatitis, AIDS)
- Mental or physical impairment leading to inability to exercise adequately

[a] Relative contraindications can be superseded if benefits outweigh risks of exercise. In some instances, these individuals can exercise with caution or use low-level endpoints, especially if they are asymptomatic at rest.
(Modified from Gibbons RA, Balady GJ, Beasely JW et al. ACC/AHA guidelines for exercise testing. *J Am Coll Cardiol* 30:260–315, 1997.)

b. **Relative contraindications** apply to those who might be tested if the potential benefit from exercise testing outweighs the relative risk of testing.

2. Risk Stratification

a. Patients initially can be classified into three risk strata: low risk, moderate risk, and high risk (*Table 6-2*).

Low risk: individuals who do not have signs or symptoms, or are diagnosed with, cardiovascular, pulmonary, or metabolic disease, and have no more than one cardiovascular disease (CVD) risk factor.

Moderate risk: individuals who do not have signs or symptoms, or are diagnosed with, cardiovascular, pulmonary, or metabolic disease, but have two or more CVD factors.

TABLE 6-2. CORONARY ARTERY DISEASE RISK FACTOR THRESHOLDS FOR USE WITH ACSM RISK STRATIFICATION

RISK FACTORS	DEFINING CRITERIA
Positive	
Family history	Myocardial infarction, coronary revascularization, or sudden death before 55 years of age in father or other male first-degree relative (i.e., brother or son), or before 65 years of age in mother or other female first-degree relative (i.e., sister or daughter).
Cigarette smoking	Current cigarette smoker or those who quit within the previous 6 months.
Hypertension	Systolic blood pressure of ≥140 mm Hg or diastolic ≥90 mm Hg, confirmed by measurements on at least two separate occasions, or on antihypertensive medication.
Hypercholesterolemia	Total serum cholesterol of >200 mg/dL (5.2 mmol/L) or high-density lipoprotein cholesterol of <35 mg/dL (0.9 mmol/L), or on lipid-lowering medication. If low-density lipoprotein cholesterol is available, use >130 mg/dL (3.4 mmol/L) rather than total cholesterol of >200 mg/dL.
Impaired fasting glucose	Fasting blood glucose of ≥110 mg/dL (6.1 mmol/L) confirmed by measurements on at least 2 separate occasions (7).
Obesity[a]	Body Mass Index of ≥30 kg · m^{-2} (8), or waist girth of >100 cm (9).
Sedentary lifestyle	Persons not participating in a regular exercise program or meeting the minimal physical activity recommendations[†] from the U.S. Surgeon General's report (10).
Negative	
High serum HDL cholesterol[b]	>60 mg/dL (1.6 mmol/L).

[a] Professional opinions vary regarding the most appropriate markers and thresholds for obesity; therefore, exercise professionals should use clinical judgment when evaluating this risk factor.
[b] Accumulating 30 minutes or more of moderate physical activity on most days of the week. It is common to sum risk factors in making clinical judgments. If high-density lipoprotein (HDL) cholesterol is high, subtract one risk factor from the sum of positive risk factors because high HDL decreases coronary artery disease (CAD) risk.
(Adapted from Expert Panel on Detection, Evaluation, and Treatment of High Blood Cholesterol in Adults. Summary of the second report of the National Cholesterol Education Program (NCEP) expert panel on detection, evaluation, and treatment of high blood cholesterol in adults (Adult Treatment Panel II). *JAMA* 1993;269:3015–3023.)
[1] Equation from Brozek J, Grande F, Anderson J, Keys A. Densitometric analysis of body composition: Revision of some quantitative assumptions. *Ann NY Acad Sci* 1963;110:113–140, 1963.
[2] Equation from Siri WE. Body composition from fluid spaces and density. *Univ Calif Donner Lab Med Phys Rep,* March 1956. Published with permission from University of California-Berkeley.

High risk: individuals who have one or more signs or symptoms, or are diagnosed with, cardiovascular, pulmonary, or metabolic disease.

b. Following identification of an individual's risk status, the exercise leader or health or fitness specialist should make an informed decision whether the individual should be tested or permitted to exercise, according to the guidelines provided in Figure 2-4 in the *Guidelines for Exercise Testing and Prescription,* 8th edition.

c. Pretest likelihood: determine the individual's likelihood of having disease based on the information obtained before the exercise test. This is an important step in determining the type of exercise test (functional, diagnostic) best suited to the individual.

C. INFORMED CONSENT

1. Purpose

a. Ethical Considerations
   1) A well-designed consent form provides the patient with sufficient information to enable an **informed decision** about participation.
   2) It **details the expectations** of the patient so that full knowledgeable participation is possible.

b. Legal Concerns
   Although not a legal document, the use of a well-designed consent form provides written documentation that the person was made aware of the procedures, limitations, **risks** and discomforts, as well as the **benefits** of exercise.

2. Limitations of Informed Consent

a. **Does not provide legal immunity** to a facility or individual in the event of injury.
b. **Does provide evidence** that the patient was made aware of the **purposes, procedures, and risks** associated with the test or exercise program.
c. Negligence, improper test administration, inadequate personnel qualifications, and insufficient safety procedures are **expressly not covered** by informed consent.
d. **Legal counsel** should be sought during the development of the document.

3. Content

a. **Purpose.**
b. **Procedures** explained in lay terminology.
c. Potential **risks** and **discomforts.**
d. Expected **benefits.**
   1) To the participant.
   2) To society.
e. **Responsibilities** of the participant.
f. Provision of an **opportunity to ask questions** and have them answered.

g. Confidentiality of results.
h. Right of participant to refuse or withdraw from any aspect of the procedures.
i. Signatures.
   1) Participant.
   2) Test supervisor or administrator.
   3) Guardian for those younger than 18 years of age.
   4) Witness(es).
j. Dates of Signatures.

4. Administration

a. The consent form should be presented to the patient in a private, quiet setting.
b. The order of activities associated with the completion of the document should be as follows:
   1) Private, quiet reading of the document.
   2) Private, verbal explanation of the contents of the document with a verbally expressed opportunity to ask questions for which answers are provided.
   3) Signing and dating the document.
   4) Presentation of a copy of the signed document to the participant, for his or her keeping.

D. PATIENT PREPARATION

1. Patient teaching includes a description of the test and specific and general instructions, such as:
   a. Avoid eating, smoking, and consuming alcohol or caffeine within 3 hours before testing.
   b. Avoid exercise or other strenuous physical activity on the day of the test.
   c. Get adequate sleep the night before the test.
   d. Wear comfortable, loose-fitting clothing.
2. Preparing for electrocardiographic (ECG) monitoring involves abrading the patient's skin with a rough pad or sandpaper to remove dead skin cells, followed by cleansing with alcohol and scrubbing with gauze, and then applying the ECG electrodes using the anatomic landmarks described in Chapter 1 (Figure 1-14).

II. FITNESS TESTING: GENERAL CONSIDERATIONS

A. PURPOSE

1. Education

A well-planned and implemented battery of fitness assessment provides information to current and potential exercisers about the various aspects of health-related fitness. The results of fitness assessment provide a patient with information useful in making possible lifestyle decisions.

2. Exercise Prescription

Data collected via appropriate fitness assessments assist the instructor in developing safe, effective programs of exercise based on the individual's current fitness status.

3. Progress Evaluation

Baseline and follow-up testing provides evidence of progression toward fitness goals.

4. Motivation

Fitness assessment provides information needed to develop reasonable, attainable goals. Progress toward, or attainment of, a goal is strong motivation for continued participation in an exercise program.

5. Risk Stratification

Results of fitness assessment, when used in tangent with diagnostic equipment, can sometimes detect the presence of signs of heart disease, which may influence both the exercise prescription and subsequent assessment.

B. RISKS ASSOCIATED WITH EXERCISE TESTING

1. Peak or Symptom Limited Testing

a. The risk of death during or immediately after an exercise test is 1/10,0000.
b. The risk of acute myocardial infarction during or immediately after an exercise test is 1/2,500.
c. The risk of a complication requiring hospitalization is 1/500.

2. Submaximal Exercise Testing

The submaximal cycle ergometer test recommended by the ACSM has resulted in no reported deaths, myocardial infarctions, or morbid events when care has been taken to ensure careful patient screening and compliance with appropriate pretest instructions, and appropriate supervision during the test.

C. SAFETY

To maximize safety during the assessment, each of the following items should be assessed:

1. Site.

a. Emergency Plans.
   1) Written, posted emergency plans.
   2) Posted emergency numbers.
   3) Regularly scheduled practices of responses to emergency situations,

including a minimum of one announced and one unannounced drill.

b. Room Layout
The equipment and floor space should be arranged to allow safe and fast exit from the facility in an emergency.

2. **Equipment**

a. Maintenance
Develop a written document that includes procedures for all daily, weekly, and monthly activities associated with maintaining each piece of equipment.

b. Positioning
The equipment used for testing should be positioned to ensure maximal visual supervision of the patient.

c. Cleanliness
Develop a written document that includes procedures for all daily, weekly, and monthly activities associated with cleaning each piece of equipment.

3. **Personnel**

a. Certifications
Personnel should have the appropriate and current certification(s) to carry out their responsibilities effectively and safely (e.g., CPR, American College of Sports Medicine Health/Fitness Specialist [ACSM H/FS]).

b. Training
The personnel should be trained, updated, and standardized for inter and intratester reliability periodically.

D. TEST ORDER

When a battery of fitness assessments is administered to a patient in a single session, the following order of tests is recommended:

1. **Resting Measurements**
Measurements such as HR, BP, blood analysis.

2. **Body Composition**
Some methods of assessing body composition are sensitive to the hydration status. Because some tests of cardiorespiratory or muscular fitness may have an acute effect on hydration, it is inappropriate to conduct such assessments before the body composition assessment.

3. **Cardiorespiratory Fitness**
Assessments of cardiorespiratory fitness often use heart rate as a predictive measurement. Assessing muscular fitness or flexibility can produce an increase in HR. The cardiorespiratory assessment must therefore be conducted before any other assessment that may affect HR.

4. **Muscular Fitness**

a. When assessing both muscular and cardiorespiratory fitness the same day, muscular fitness should be assessed after cardiorespiratory fitness.

b. Strenuous assessments of cardiorespiratory fitness should be followed by an appropriate recovery period before tests of muscular fitness are attempted.

5. **Flexibility**
Flexibility is most appropriately assessed after the person has warmed up well and has been given time to stretch.

E. TEST TERMINATION

Clearly written instructions and regular practice will help to ensure that an assessment is conducted in a manner that is both safe and provides valid, useful information.

1. **Criteria for Stopping A Test**

a. Attainment of Desired Performance
The fitness professional must be familiar with the testing procedures to ensure recognition of the desired endpoint of the assessment. This may be a predetermined HR endpoint, specific respiratory exchange ratio (RER) as measured by gas analysis, or a perceptual endpoint (e.g., rating of perceived exertion [RPE]).

b. Patient or Equipment Complications

1) Signs and symptoms consistent with guidelines for test cessation (see Box 5-2 from *ACSM's Guidelines for Exercise Testing and Prescription,* 8th ed).
2) Abnormal exercise responses (dyspnea, angina, ECG signs of ischemia, drop in blood pressure).
3) Equipment failure.
4) Patient asks to stop.

2. **Procedures**

a. In non–life-threatening situations, an active cool-down should be completed.

b. In life-threatening situations, the test should be terminated, the patient should be removed from the testing equipment, and the site's emergency plan should be put into operation.

F. INTERPRETATION OF RESULTS

1. **Data Reduction**

a. Equations used to predict a fitness score should be appropriate to both the tests conducted and the patient.

b. Comparison to published norms will assist in data interpretation.

2. Normative Data

a. Selection

The norms against which results are compared should meet the following criteria:

1) Appropriate to the test administered.
2) Appropriate to the age, gender, and history of the patient.

b. Standard Error of the Estimate

1) The standard error of the estimate is an indication of the error of the estimate compared with the actual measurement of the variable.
2) Knowledge of the standard error of the estimate associated with a test is critical to the appropriate interpretation of the results.
3) Reports to patients should clearly indicate the error associated with the testing.

3. Repeated Assessment

a. Methods

Follow-up assessment of any fitness component should **use the same test**, including procedures and protocols, as that used during the original assessment. It is therefore essential to keep precise records of all assessments.

b. Timing

Repeat testing should be conducted only **after sufficient time for alteration in the fitness component is assessed**. The fitness professional should therefore be aware of the time course needed for physiologic adaptations.

c. Pre- and Postdifferences

Care should be taken when interpreting small changes in fitness scores from time point to time point. Often, such changes are within the error of estimate of the procedures used.

G. BODY COMPOSITION ASSESSMENT

Body composition assessment measures the **relative proportions of fat versus fat-free (lean) tissue** in the body. This is commonly reported as **percent body fat**, thus identifying the proportion of the total body mass composed of fat. **Fat-free mass** is then determined as the **balance of the total body mass.**

1. Hydrostatic (Underwater) Weighing

a. Principle

This method is based on **Archimedes' principle** that a body immersed in water is buoyed by a counterforce equal to the weight of the water displaced. Because bone and muscle are more dense than water and fat is less dense than water, a person with more fat-free body mass weighs more in water than a person of the same weight with a greater percentage of body fat.

b. Procedure

1) The patient is suspended from a scale in water, submerges under the water surface, and exhales as much air as possible, holding his or her breath for 5 seconds while weight is recorded.
2) **Body density is then determined** through the following formula:

$$\textit{Body Density} = \frac{\textit{Weight in air} - \textit{Weight in Water}}{\textit{Density of water} - \textit{Residual Volume}}$$

3) **Residual volume** (RV), the remaining volume of air in the lungs after forced exhalation is either estimated based on age, gender, and forced vital capacity or measured directly (e.g. helium dilution method).
4) Equations are then used to **convert body density into body fat percentage**; the two most common equations are:

$$\%\ fat = (457/\textit{Body Density}) - 414.2$$

$$\%\ fat = (495/\textit{Body Density}) - 450$$

c. Measurement Error

1) Inaccurate measurement or estimation of lung residual volume.
2) The great variability in bone density among individuals.
3) Error is approximately 2%–3% when procedures are performed correctly.

2. Skinfold Measurements

a. Principle

1) This technique assumes a relationship between subcutaneous fat and overall body fat, a predictable pattern of body fat distribution for men and for women, and a given fat-free density.
2) **Age** is accounted for because of changes in body fat distribution with age. With aging, more fat is stored internally, thus altering the meaning of a given skinfold measure.
3) **Body fat equations** are specific to age, gender, and ethnicity (*Table 6-3*).

b. Procedure

1) The **measurement technique** involves using the thumb and index finger to grasp a fold of skin 1 cm above the site being measured (*Table 6-4*), placing the

TABLE 6-3. SKINFOLD PREDICTION EQUATIONS

ETHNICITY	GENDER	AGE	EQUATION
1 Black	Males	18–61	Db (g/cc) = 1.1120 − 0.00043499 (Σ7SKF chest, abdomen, thigh, triceps, subscapular, suprailiac, midaxillary) + 0.00000055 $(\Sigma 7SKF)^2$ − 0.00028826 (age).
2 Black	Females	18–55	Db (g/cc) = 1.0970 − 0.00046971 (Σ7SKF chest, abdomen, thigh, triceps, subscapular, suprailiac, midaxillary) + 0.00000056 $(\Sigma 7SKF)^2$ − 0.00012828 (age).
3 White	Males	18–61	Db (g/cc) = 1.109380 − 0.0008267 (Σ3SKF chest, abdomen, thigh) + 0.0000016 $(\Sigma 3SKF)^2$ − 0.0002574 (age).
4 White	Females	18–55	Db (g/cc) = 1.0994921 − 0.0009929 (Σ3SKF triceps, suprailiac, thigh) + 0.0000023 $(\Sigma 3SKF)^2$ − 0.0001392 (age).
5 Hispanic	Females	20–40	Db (g/cc) = 1.0970 − 0.00046971 (Σ3SKF chest, abdomen, thigh, triceps, subscapular, suprailiac, midaxillary) + 0.00000056 $(\Sigma 7SKF)^2$ − 0.00012828 (age).
6 Black and white	Males	≤18	%BF = 0.735 (Σ2SKF triceps, calf) + 1.0.
7 Black and white	Males (SKF >35 mm)	≤18	%BF = 0.735 (Σ2SKF triceps, subscapular) + 1.6.
8 Black and white	Males (SKF >35 mm)	≤18	%BF = 0.783 (Σ2SKF triceps, subscapular) − 0,008 $(\Sigma 2SKF)^2$+1*.
9 Black and white	Females	≤18	%BF = 0.610 (Σ2SKF triceps, calf) + 5.1.
10 Black and white	Females (SKF >35 mm)	≤18	%BF = 0.546 (Σ2SKF triceps, subscapular) + 9.7.
11 Black and white	Females (SKF >35 mm)	≤18	%BF = 1.33 (Σ2SKF triceps, subscapular) − 0.013 $(\Sigma 2SKF)^2$ − 2.5.

(Adapted from Heyward VH, Stolarcyzk LM: Applied Body Composition Assessment. Champaign, IL, Human Kinetics, 1996, pp 173–185.)

* = intercept substitutions based on maturation and ethnicity for boys:

Age	Black	White
Prepubescent	−3.2	−1.7
Pubescent	−5.2	−3.4
Postpubescent	−6.8	−5.5

caliper jaws perpendicular to the fold, and recording the measurement on the caliper.

2) Hold the fold as the jaws compress, take the measure after 1–2 seconds.

3) Rotate measures from one site to the next. Record two measurements at each site; if these vary by more than 1 cm, then a third measurement is taken and the two closest measurements are averaged.

c. Measurement Error

1) Inaccurate calipers.
2) Poor technique.
3) The patient does not fit norms for standard equations (e.g., odd body fat distribution, deformation).
4) Improper site identification.
5) Error is approximately 4% when performed correctly and the optimal equation is used.

3. Anthropometry

a. Theoretical Basis

1) Measurements of height, weight, and girths provide information about the relative distribution of body mass compared with "standard" distributions.
2) The addition of anthropometric measurements to skinfold measurements may be used to predict body fatness.

b. Procedures

Height and weight should be measured, and appropriate sites for the anthropometric measures are required.

c. Measurement Error

1) Inaccurate stance for assessing height.
2) Unfamiliarity with the use of balance scales.
3) Incorrect location of circumference site.
4) Incorrect placement of the tape measure around the body segment to be measured.
5) Inappropriate tension in the use of the tape measure.
6) Approximately 3%–8% error.

4. Body Mass Index (BMI)

a. This basic weight-for-height ratio can be quickly determined using a standard nomogram. The results are compared with a standard table to classify obesity according to BMI value (*Table 6-5*).

b. BMI is commonly used in large population studies. It has been found to correlate with incidence of certain chronic diseases, such as hyperlipidemia.

c. **BMI should not be used to assess an individual's body fat** during a fitness assessment, because it does not take into account fat-free density and skeletal mass.

TABLE 6-4. STANDARDIZED DESCRIPTION OF SKINFOLD SITES AND PROCEDURES

Skinfold Site	
Abdominal	Vertical fold; 2 cm to the right side of the umbilicus
Triceps	Vertical fold; on the posterior midline of the upper arm, halfway between the acromion and olecranon processes, with the arm held freely to the side of the body
Biceps	Vertical fold; on the anterior aspect of the arm over the belly of the biceps muscle, 1 cm above the level used to mark the triceps site
	Chest/pectoral Diagonal fold; one-half the distance between the anterior axillary line and the nipple (men) or one-third of the distance between the anterior axillary line and the nipple (women)
Medial calf	Vertical fold; at the maximal circumference of the calf on the midline of its medial border
Midaxillary	Vertical fold; on the midaxillary line at the level of the xiphoid process of the sternum. (An alternate method is a horizontal fold taken at the level of the xiphoid or sternal border in the midaxillary line.)
Subscapular	Diagonal fold (at a 45° angle); 1 to 2 cm below the inferior angle of the scapula
Suprailiac	Diagonal fold; in line with the natural angle of the iliac crest taken in the anterior axillary line immediately superior to the iliac crest
Thigh	Vertical fold; on the anterior midline of the thigh, midway between the proximal border of the patella and the inguinal crease (hip)

Procedures

- All measurements should be made on the right side of the body
- Caliper should be placed 1 cm away from the thumb and finger, perpendicular to the skinfold, and halfway between the crest and the base of the fold
- Pinch should be maintained while reading the caliper
- Wait 1 to 2 seconds (and not longer) before reading caliper
- Take duplicate measures at each site and retest if duplicate measurements are not within 1 to 2 mm
- Rotate through measurement sites or allow time for skin to regain normal texture and thickness

(From *ACSM's Guidelines for Exercise Testing and Prescription,* 8th ed. Philadelphia: Lippincott Williams & Wilkins, 2010, p 67.)

TABLE 6-5. CLASSIFICATION OF OBESITY ACCORDING TO BODY MASS INDEX (BMI) VALUES

	BMI (kg · m^{-2})
Underweight	<18.5
Normal	18.5–24.9
Overweight	25.0–29.9
Obesity, class	
I	30.0–34.9
II	35.0–39.9
III	≥ 40

(Modified from *ACSM's Guidelines for Exercise Testing and Prescription,* 8th ed. Baltimore: Williams & Wilkins, Table 4.1, p. 63.)

TABLE 6-6. WAIST-TO-HIP CIRCUMFERENCE RATIO (WHR) STANDARDS FOR MEN AND WOMEN

	DISEASE RISK RELATED TO OBESITY			
AGE	LOW	MODERATE	HIGH	VERY HIGH
Men				
20–29	<0.83	0.83–0.88	0.89–0.94	>0.94
30–39	<0.84	0.84–0.91	0.92–0.96	>0.96
40–49	<0.88	0.88–0.95	0.96–1.00	>1.00
50–59	<0.90	0.90–0.96	0.97–1.02	>1.02
60–69	<0.91	0.91–0.98	0.99–1.03	>1.03
Women				
20–29	<0.71	0.71–0.77	0.78–0.82	>0.82
30–39	<0.72	0.72–0.78	0.79–0.84	>0.84
40–49	<0.73	0.73–0.79	0.80–0.87	>0.87
50–59	<0.74	0.74–0.81	0.82–0.88	>0.88
60–69	<0.76	0.76–0.83	0.84–0.90	>0.90

(With permission from Heyward VH, Stolarcyzk LM: *Applied Body Composition Assessment.* Champaign, IL: Human Kinetics, 1996, p 82.)

5. **Waist-to-Hip Ratio (WHR)**
   A simple index of upper versus lower body fat distribution, WHR is a predictor of disease risk related to fat distribution. Waist circumference and hip circumference are measured; then, WHR is calculated using a standard nomogram and compared with available standards (*Table 6-6*).

6. **Bioelectrical Impedance Analysis (BIA)**
   a. This quick, noninvasive method of measuring fat and fat-free body mass is relatively inexpensive and does not require a highly skilled technician.
   b. In the most common form of BIA, four electrodes are placed on the individual's skin (typically two on the right hand and two on the right foot), and a high-frequency, low-level excitation current is sent through the body.
   c. Because electrical conductivity varies based on the fat content of tissue (fat-free tissue is a good conductor, whereas fat is not), the measured resistance to current flow reflects body composition.
   d. Measurement Error
      1) Inappropriate skin preparation.
      2) Inaccurate electrode placement.
      3) Lack of adherence to pretest diet or exercise recommendations.
      4) Use of inappropriate prediction equation.
      5) Inadequate hydration.
      6) Body temperature.
      7) Approximately 4%–7% error when performed correctly.

7. **Near-Infrared Interactance**
   a. This technique, based on principles of light absorption and reflection, uses near-infrared spectroscopy to measure body composition.
      1) A fiberoptic probe is placed on a body site (e.g., biceps), and the infrared beam penetrates the skin.
      2) The measurement of reflected light is related to subcutaneous fat.
      3) Approximately 4%–7% error when performed correctly.

8. **Dual-Energy X-ray Absorptiometry**
   a. In this technique, an emitter passes photons at two different energies (one deep, one shallow) through body tissue, and a scanner analyzes the energy that passes through the tissue.
   b. A computer calculates fat, bone, and muscle tissue based on pixel strength.

H. CARDIORESPIRATORY FITNESS

1. **Assessment Purpose**
   a. To measure variables, such as HR, BP, and oxygen uptake ($\dot{V}O_2$) during exercise, to evaluate the body's ability to absorb, distribute, and utilize oxygen, and to help screen for CAD.
   b. To collect baseline and follow-up information for charting a patient's fitness program progress to help motivate an individual by establishing and meeting reasonable fitness goals.

2. **Basic Skills Needed to Assess Cardiorespiratory Fitness**
   a. **Heart Rate Determination**
      1) **Palpation**
         a) Heart rate can be determined by counting the number of pulses in a given period of time (10–30 seconds).
         b) The most common sites at which the pulse can be palpated include:
            (i) The radial artery.
            (ii) The carotid artery.
      2) **Auscultation**
         a) A stethoscope can be placed over the left aspect of the midsternum, or just under the pectoralis major.
         b) The HR can be counted as the number of heart beats in a given period of time (10–30 seconds).
      3) **Electronic Monitoring**
         a) Radio frequency transmitters.
            (i) A chest strap with embedded electrodes is fastened around the chest just under the pectoral muscles.
            (ii) The electrodes sense the electrical current associated with the electrical activity of the heart to measure HR.
         b) Pulsatile blood flow monitors.
            (i) Sensors affixed to the ear lobe or finger sense the pulsing of blood.
            (ii) Some devices are currently not effective in monitoring exercise heart rate.
   b. **Blood Pressure Measurement**
      The most standard BP measuring equipment includes a **sphygmomanometer** and a **stethoscope**.
      1) **Sphygmomanometer**, with three important components:
         a) A cloth cuff placed around the upper arm. Encased in the cuff is a bladder made of rubber or similar material.
         b) A diaphragmatic bulb and valve used to increase or decrease the pressure in the cuff.
         c) A mercury column or preferably aneroid (air pressure) manometer, used to indicate the pressure in the cuff.
      2) **Stethoscope**, with two important components:
         a) A diaphragm to focus sound waves.
         b) Earpieces to direct the sound waves.
   c. **Rating of Perceived Exertion (RPE) Determination**
      1) Provides the exercise professional with an indication of a subjective assessment of the relative intensity of the exercise.
      2) Correlates well with such physiologic measures as percent of maximal heart rate and percent $\dot{V}O_2$max. Currently, there are two widely used scales for assessing RPE:
         a) Original scale.
            (i) Ratings are 6–20.
            (i) The scale was developed largely on the basis of the linear response of $\dot{V}O_2$max and heart rate to changing exercise intensity.
         b) Revised scale.
            (i) Ratings are 0–10.
            (ii) The revised scale is based on the $\dot{V}O_2$max and heart rate responses to exercise, but also

to lactate accumulation and ventilation during exercise.

3. **Timing of Measurements During Assessments**
During most graded exercise tests, the following measurements are taken at the times indicated:
   a. **Heart Rate**
      1) During a 2-minute stage: every minute.
      2) During a 3-minute stage: at minutes 2 and 3, and additionally at every subsequent minute until steady state is achieved.
   b. **Blood Pressure**
   Measured once during each stage, toward the end of the stage.
   c. **Rating of Perceived Exertion (RPE)**
   Assessed once during each stage, toward the end of the stage.
   d. **Sequence of Measurements**
   For most graded exercise tests (with 3-minute stages), it is practical to take the measurements according to the following schedule:
      1) Minute 2:00–HR.
      2) Minute 2:15–RPE.
      3) Minute 2:30–BP.
      4) Minute 3:00–HR.

4. **Equipment Calibration**
Accuracy of instrumentation is essential for valid assessments of cardiorespiratory endurance as well as for all other areas of health-related fitness. All equipment should be calibrated at regular intervals. A regular schedule for equipment calibration should be established for all testing equipment.
   a. **Cycle Ergometer**
   Work rate is determined by **resistance** and **distance flywheel traveled per revolution** multiplied **revolutions per minute.**
      1) **Resistance**
         a) On most mechanically braked ergometers, calibration requires identification of the attachment of the resistance pendulum to the resistance belt.
         b) The zero mark on the resistance indicator is checked and adjusted as required.
         c) A known weight is hung from the point at which the resistance belt is attached to the pendulum.
         d) The resistance should be checked at each resistance that might be used during testing.
         e) Any discrepancies in the resistance markings are noted on a new scale fastened over the original resistance markings.
      2) **Distance Per Revolution**
      The distance the flywheel travels per revolution of the pedal must be accurately determined by measuring the circumference of the flywheel, then determining the number of flywheel revolutions per pedal revolution.
      3) **Revolutions Pedaled Per Minute (rpm)**
      Because the work rate on a cycle ergometer is expressed in kg · m/min, it is necessary to check the accuracy of the device used to determine rpm.
      A mechanical or electronic metronome may be checked for accuracy using an accurate clock or stopwatch.
   b. **Treadmill Calibration**
      1) **Speed**
      Calibrating the speed of a motorized treadmill requires knowledge of both the length of the treadmill belt and the number of revolutions of the belt per minute.
         a) The length of the belt can be measured using a long cloth tape or a rolling measuring device.
         b) The treadmill rpm is determined by marking a fixed point on the belt, and a corresponding point on the treadmill frame or other fixed object and measuring the time needed for a fixed number of revolutions (e.g., 20 for slower speeds, 50 for higher speeds).
      2) **Grade**
         a) The treadmill grade is expressed as the relationship of rise to run. The run is the distance between two fixed points on the floor or other flat surface. The rise is the difference between two perpendicular distances measured from the belt surface to the floor.
         b) Treadmill grade is determined by dividing the rise by the run, and expressing the result as a percent.

5. **Protocol Selection**
Test selection is influenced by the purpose and goals of the exercise test and also by characteristics of the person being tested.
   a. Maximal Testing.
      1) A maximal exercise test can be most effective in detecting CAD and

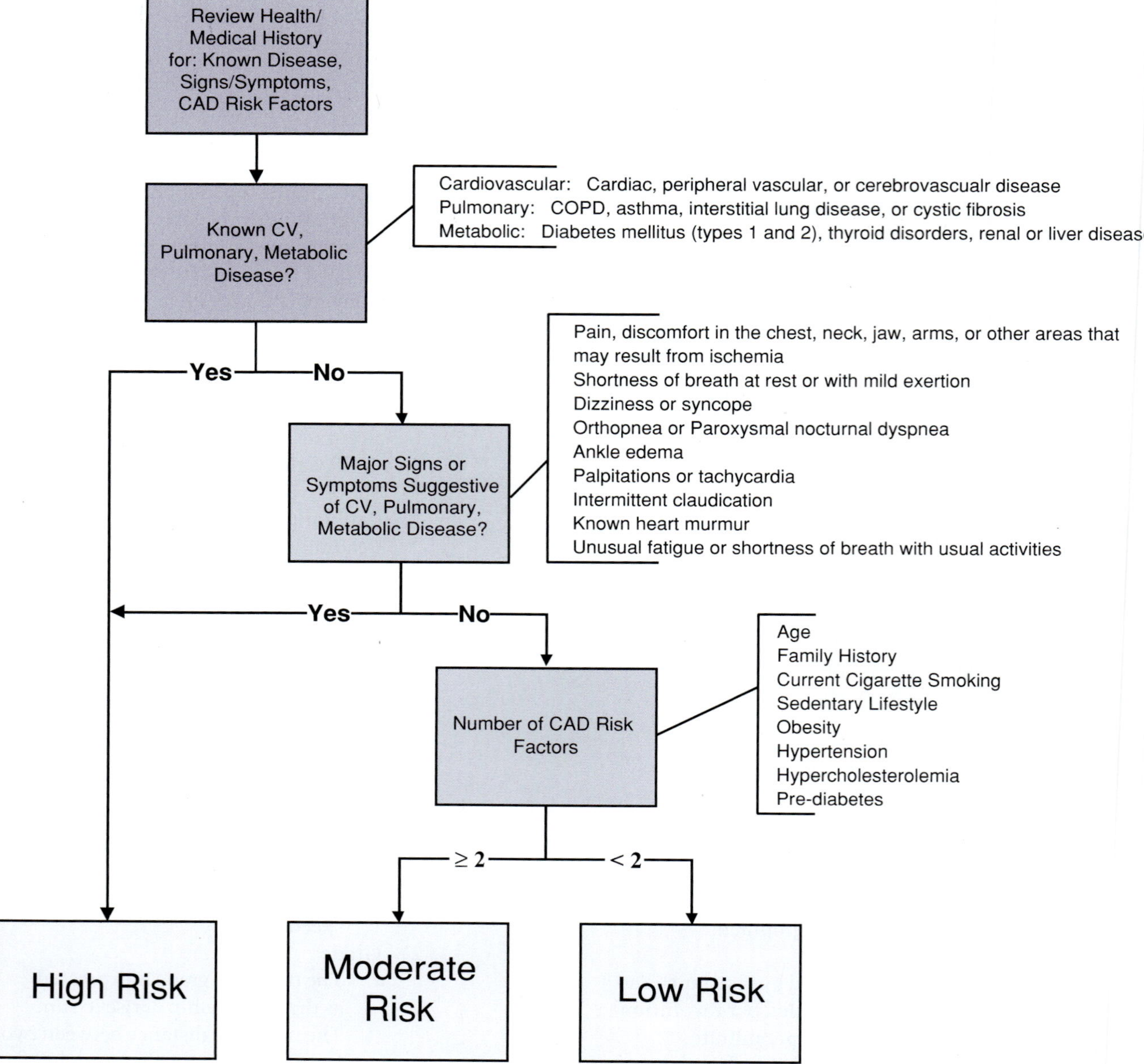

FIGURE 6-2. Risk Stratification.

accurately measuring $\dot{V}O_2$max (using on-line measurements of expired gases or estimated using prediction equations).

2) The choice of maximal testing should be based on the reason for the exercise test (e.g., CAD screening or functional capacity measurement).
3) Maximal testing is expensive, and guidelines for testing various populations and age groups should be followed (*Figures 6-2 and 6-3*).

b. **Submaximal Testing**

1) Submaximal exercise tests are used extensively to assess fitness, evaluate changes in fitness following a training program, and provide an estimate of $\dot{V}O_2$max used to establish an initial training program.
2) Submaximal testing estimates $\dot{V}O_2$max based on the assumed linear relationship between HR and $\dot{V}O_2$max. Heart rate is measured at multiple workloads during the test, and $\dot{V}O_2$max at an

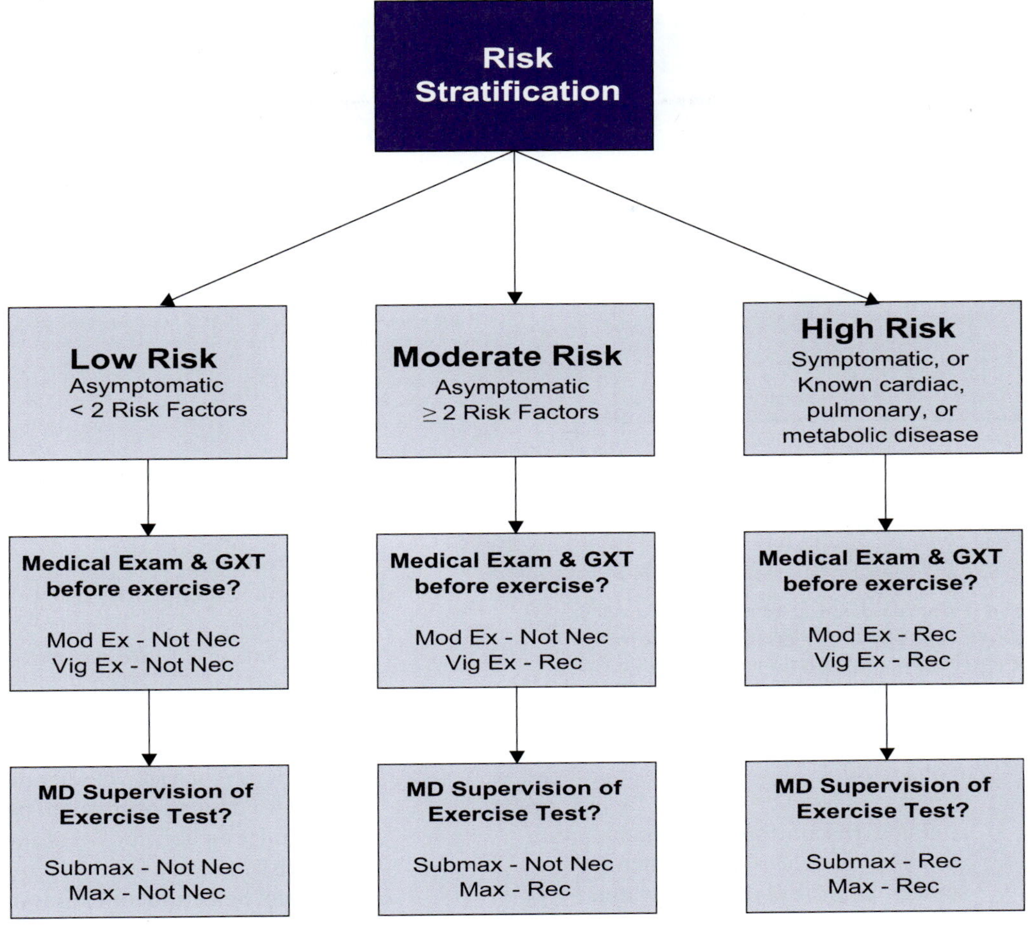

Mod Ex: Moderate intensity exercise; 40-60% of VO_2max; 3-6 METs; "an intensity well within the individual's capacity, one which can be comfortably sustained for a prolonged period of time (~45 minutes)"

Vig Ex: Vigorous intensity exercise; > 60% of VO_2max; > 6 METs; "exercise intense enough to represent a substantial cardiorespiratory challenge"

Not Nec: Not Necessary; reflects the notion that a medical examination, exercise test, and physician supervision of exercise testing would not be essential in the preparticipation screening, however, they should not be viewed as inappropriate

Rec: Recommended; when MD supervision of exercise testing is "Recommended," the MD should be in close proximity and readily available should there be an emergent need

FIGURE 6-3. Exercise testing and testing supervision recommendation based on risk stratification.

estimated maximal HR is calculated (*Figure 6-4*).

3) **Submaximal testing is based on several assumptions:**
   a) Measurements are made while the patient is at steady state.
   b) There is a linear relationship between HR and $\dot{V}O_2max$.
   c) Maximal HR is similar for all individuals in a given age group.
   d) Mechanical efficiency is the same for all patients.

c. **Discontinuous and Continuous Protocols**
   1) In a **discontinuous test protocol**, the test is momentarily stopped, measurements are obtained, and the test is then

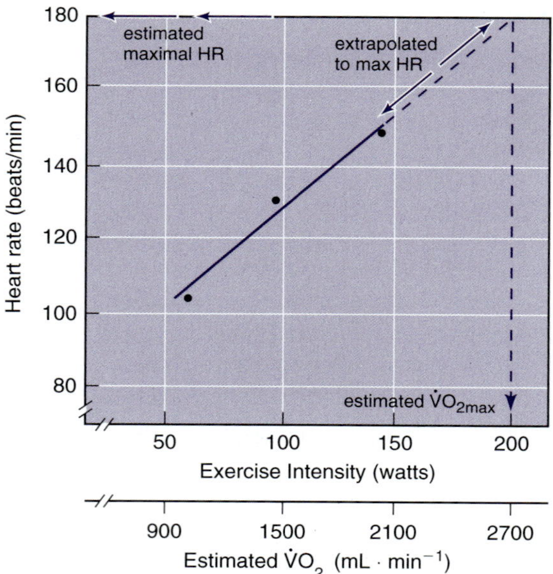

FIGURE 6-4. Heart rate obtained from at least two (more are preferable) submaximal exercise intensities may be extrapolated to the age-predicted maximal heart rate. A vertical line to the intensity scale estimates maximal exercise intensity from which an estimated $\dot{V}O_2$max can be calculated. (Redrawn with permission from *ACSM's Guidelines for Exercise Testing and Prescription*, 8th ed. Baltimore: Lippincott Williams & Wilkins; 2010, p. 79.)

resumed. Discontinuous protocols are usually used only in special circumstances, because of the lengthy time required for such a test. Examples include:

a) Individuals being tested using arm ergometry, stopping for BP measurement.

b) Persons with claudication who develop leg pain and need rest periods.

TABLE 6-7. FIELD FITNESS TESTING FOR CHILDREN[a]

FITNESS/HEALTH COMPONENT	FIELD TEST
Aerobic capacity	1-mile walk/run
Muscular strength and endurance	Curl-ups
	Pull-ups/push-ups
Flexibility	Sit-reach/V-sit reach
Agility	Shuttle run
Body composition	Body mass index/skinfolds

[a] For detailed descriptions of specific test items, see the following publications: *Fitnessgram: The Test Administration Manual.* Dallas, Institute for Aerobics Research, 1994; and President's Council on Physical Fitness and Sports: *The Presidential Physical Fitness Award Program.* Washington, DC, 1997.

(From *ACSM's Guidelines for Exercise Testing and Prescription,* 6th ed. Philadelphia: Lippincott Williams & Wilkins, 2000, p 218.)

2) A **continuous test protocol**, the most common form, involves multiple stages of increasing work intensity with no stoppages.

d. **Protocol Selection for Overweight Patients**

1) During weight-bearing exercise, a patient's absolute oxygen costs are directly proportional to his or her body mass.

2) In some cases, weight-supported exercise, such as cycle ergometry, is preferred for an overweight person to minimize orthopedic stress and reduce the risk of injury.

e. **Protocol Selection for Children**

1) **Physical fitness testing** is common in school-based physical education programs to evaluate skill-related fitness and, most importantly, health-related fitness (*Tables 6-7 and 6-8*).

2) **Clinical exercise testing** is also performed to screen for preexisting cardiorespiratory disease in children.

TABLE 6-8. PROTOCOLS SUITABLE FOR GRADED EXERCISE TESTING OF CHILDREN

MODIFIED BALKE TREADMILL PROTOCOL

SUBJECT	SPEED (mph)	INITIAL GRADE (%)	INCREMENT (%)	STAGE DURATION (min)
Poorly fit	3.00	6	2	2
Sedentary	3.25	6	2	2
Active	5.00	0	2.5	2
Athlete	5.25	0	2.5	2

THE McMASTER CYCLE TEST

HEIGHT (cm)	INITIAL LOAD (W)	INCREMENTS (W)	STEP DURATION (min)
<120	12.5	12.5	2
120–139.9	12.5	25	2
140–159.9	25	25	2
≥160	25	50 (boys)	2
	25 (girls)		

(Adapted from Skinner J. *Exercise Testing and Exercise Prescription for Special Cases,* 2nd ed. Philadelphia: Lea & Febiger, 1993.)

3) **Challenges** involved in testing children include the difficulty in assessing changes in physical fitness as a result of training or maturation.
4) **Contraindicated** in children include:
   a) Acute inflammatory disease.
   b) Myocardial infarction.
   c) Pulmonary disease.
   d) Renal disease.
   e) Hepatitis.
   f) Uncontrolled congestive heart failure.
   g) Severe systemic hypertension.
   h) Use of any medication that affects the cardiovascular response to exercise.

f. **Protocol Selection for the Elderly**
1) Exercise testing in the elderly must take into account **age-related changes** in cardiovascular and other physiological variables, including:
   a) Maximal heart rate.
   b) Maximal cardiac output.
   c) Maximal oxygen uptake.
   d) Resting and exercise blood pressure.
   e) Residual volume.
   f) Vital capacity.
   g) Reaction time.
   h) Muscular strength.
   i) Bone mass.
   j) Flexibility.
   k) Glucose tolerance.
   l) Body fat percentage.
2) Other factors to consider include the great **variations in physiologic status** in elderly person because of differing levels of activity and the presence of underlying disease.
3) Modifications to standard test protocols may be needed for severely deconditioned patients or those with physical limitations.
4) Given the longer adaptation time to a workload in the elderly compared with younger adults, a **prolonged warm-up phase is recommended.**

g. **Protocol Selection for Patients with Cardiorespiratory Disorders**
1) Exercise testing may help differentiate exercise-induced breathlessness from dyspnea caused by cardiorespiratory disease.
2) Oxygen uptake, ventilation, and oxygen saturation should be measured during exercise testing, because desaturation is possible during exercise.
3) Test protocol selection should be individualized, because each person will respond differently; protocols should be adjusted to achieve a test duration of 8–12 minutes.

6. Modes of Exercise Testing

a. **Field Tests**

These tests can be administered with minimal equipment and in patients with varying conditions.

1) **Cooper 12-minute test:** The subject must cover the greatest distance possible during the 12-minute test period. $\dot{V}O_2max$ is estimated based on the distance covered.
2) **1.5-mile test:** The subject must cover 1.5 miles as rapidly as possible. $\dot{V}O_2max$ is estimated based on this time.
3) **Rockport One-Mile Fitness Walking Test:** This submaximal test requires the subject to walk 1 mile as fast as possible, with HR measured for 15 seconds immediately posttest. $\dot{V}O_2max$ is predicted based on gender, time, and HR.
4) **Six-minute walk test:** This test requires a 100 ft (30 m) indoor hallway. Subjects are asked to walk as far as they can during the 6 minutes. Distance is marked off every 3 m. A chair is available if the subject needs to stop to rest during the test.
5) **Limitations:** Although these tests are easy to administer, they have certain limitations:
   a) An individual's motivation may influence test performance and thus the accuracy of the test.
   b) Persons unaccustomed to the test may pace themselves inappropriately, which can affect results.
   c) Because the patient is not monitored (i.e., HR, BP, symptoms), individuals at risk or older patients should not be tested using this method, unless monitoring equipment and personnel is nearby (i.e., during the 6-minute walk test).

b. **Nuclear and Radionuclide Imaging**

In these exercise tests, radioactive substances are injected into the bloodstream to visualize aspects of the circulatory system more closely; this technique helps increase test sensitivity and specificity.

1) **Perfusion Imaging**
   a) During the last minute of a standard stress test, thallium-201 is injected into the bloodstream. Thallium-201 enters myocardial cells in proportion to the amount of blood flow to those cells, and emits energy detectable with a scintillation counter.
   b) Images of the myocardium can be constructed immediately following a stress test and 4–24 hours later. Areas with little or no perfusion immediately following a test indicate areas of ischemia; any "cold spots" remaining 4–24 hours later indicate necrotic tissue.
   c) Areas of reversible ischemia will reperfuse and cold spots will disappear in later testing.
   d) **Single-photon emission computed tomography (SPECT)** enhances sensitivity and also allows for multidimensional viewing.
2) **Ventriculography**
   To visualize the resting and exercise cardiac function related to cardiac output, ejection fraction, and wall motion, a test such as a **multiple gated acquisition study (MUGA)** is performed.
   a) Technetium 99m (TC 99) is injected into the bloodstream, where it attaches to red blood cells.
   b) Areas where the blood pools, such as the ventricles, are visualized by the technetium emissions.
   c) Changes in ejection fraction or wall motion abnormalities may be indicative of a failing heart or compromised blood flow through the coronary circulation.

c. **Exercise Echocardiography**
   This technique uses ECG monitoring to identify the cardiac cycle, along with high-frequency sound waves to evaluate cardiac wall motion and pump function. Measurements can be made during or immediately after stationary cycle ergometry.

d. **Pharmacologic Testing**
   1) In some instances, an individual is not able to complete an exercise stress test owing to muscular limitations, neurologic disability, peripheral vascular disease, or other conditions that prevent that person from achieving a sufficient work intensity to provide an accurate cardiovascular assessment.
   2) **Two common tests** are used that do not involve exercise, but rather use drug-induced changes in cardiovascular work.
      a) **Dipyridamole (Persantine) Perfusion Imaging**
         (i) Infusion of dipyridamole causes vasodilation of normal coronary arteries, with little effect on narrowed arteries. Reduced flow to diseased arteries ("cardiac steal" reveals itself via ischemic signs or symptoms).
         (ii) Dipyridamole is often used in conjunction with a nuclear imaging agent (e.g., thallium) and a nuclear imaging technique (e.g., thallium scanning, SPECT).
         (iii) Arteries are visualized before and after drug administration and the findings are compared.
      b) **Dobutamine Testing**
         (i) Dobutamine infusion elevates heart rate and increases myocardial oxygen demand.
         (ii) When used in concert with echocardiography, dobutamine testing can elicit heart wall motion abnormalities.

e. Holter ECG Monitoring
   1) This test is used to track ECG abnormalities during the course of a day.
   2) Generally, a single-lead ECG is connected to a battery pack and a recorder.
   3) ECG monitoring is done continuously for up to 24 hours and recorded. The patient records his or her activities during the day, as well as any symptoms experienced during these activities.
   4) ECG tracings are reviewed and compared with the patient's activity log to identify precipitating events for ECG abnormalities.

I. MUSCULAR FITNESS

1. Muscular Strength Assessment

a. **Purposes**
   1) To determine maximal strength to create a prudent strength training program.

2) To monitor progress and revise the strength training program.
3) To determine physical strength for performing standardized work tasks (i.e., pre-employment screenings).

b. **Resistance Training Methods**
1) In **isotonic (free-weight) training**, the weight is held constant through the range of motion (ROM); speed can vary with the person's movement.
2) In **isokinetic training**, the speed of movement is kept constant through the ROM; force can vary with the person's movement.
3) In **variable-resistance training**, the weight is altered using mechanical assistance to compensate for changes in the muscle's ability to generate force owing to changes in the lever system.
4) In **isometric (static) training**, the joint angle remains constant while force is exerted.

c. **Strength-Testing Devices**
1) **Cable tensiometer:** This device measures static strength by measuring force exerted while pulling on a steel cable. Various limbs can be tested, and by varying the length of the cables the different joint angles can be assessed.
   a) **Advantages:** It can assess strength for almost all major muscle groups, and results are reliable.
   b) **Disadvantage:** Strength is assessed statically, so results may not apply to dynamic movements in demonstrating strength.
2) **Dynamometer**
   This is a more portable static strength-testing device that generally tests leg, back, and forearm strength.
   a) **Advantages:** Portable, less cumbersome than cable tensiometers, and numerous persons can be tested quickly.
   b) **Disadvantages:** Only a limited number of muscle groups can be tested and reliability is questionable.
3) **Strain Gauge**
   a) Thin electroconductive material is placed over machined metal parts and connected to an electrical source. As force is exerted, the gauge is bent or deformed, altering its electrical conductivity; measurement of the change in conductivity reflects the amount of force generated.
   b) For example, a strain gauge is installed on the crank arm of a cycle ergometer pedal; as the cyclist pushes on the crank (pedals), the arm bends, changing the strain gauge's conductivity and allowing measurement of force.

d. **One-Repetition Maximum (1-RM) Testing**
1) Assesses the maximal amount of weight that can be lifted one time for a given exercise.
2) Begins with a weight that the person can lift easily. Following a successful lift, the patient rests for 2–3 minutes, 5–10 pounds of weight are added, and the patient lifts again.
3) Generally, four to six trials are needed to determine the 1-RM.
4) Advantages.
   a) It is easy to administer, and multiple muscle groups can be tested.
   b) The same equipment used for testing can often be used for training.
   c) It also provides a measure of dynamic strength, which is most applicable to real-world settings.
5) Disadvantages.
   a) In unconditioned individuals, posttest muscle soreness is likely.
   b) Strength is limited by the weakest point in the ROM.
   c) The tester needs to take into account the skill involved with each lift, and ensure that the person being tested can safely and effectively perform the lifts.
6) Submaximal Tests to Estimate Strength
   a) Submaximal lifts to fatigue are commonly used to estimate the 1-RM.
   b) The weight used for the submaximal assessment must be carefully selected so that the person performs from 2–14 repetitions before fatigue.

e. **Equipment**
Common equipment includes:
1) Free weights, such as barbells and dumbbells, which require the lifter to determine the planes of movement.
2) Variable-resistance machines, for which the plane and range of movement are limited by the machine and the

resistance is increased by adding additional plates of weight to the stack lifted.
3) Isokinetic machines, which limit movement to a constant velocity.
4) Isometric equipment (e.g., handgrip dynamometers), which measure strength at a constant joint angle.

f. Safety
To reduce the risk of injury during assessments of muscular strength, the following items should be addressed:
1) One or more properly trained spotters should assist the lifter.
2) Proper form should be demonstrated by the exercise professional and required of the lifter.
3) The lifter should be coached to breathe during both concentric (exhale) and eccentric (inhale) movements. This will help reduce BP changes as a result of Valsalva maneuvers.
4) Adequate rest should be provided between lifting attempts.

g. Special Considerations
1) Muscle force varies over joint ROM because of changes in joint angle; therefore, dynamic muscle strength testing (1-RM) is not useful for establishing strength throughout the ROM.
2) Acceleration and inertia can both influence the performance of a dynamic strength test; thus dynamic strength testing should be standardized with regard to velocity.
3) Body position must be stabilized to isolate the muscle group being tested.

2. Muscular Endurance Assessment

These techniques assess an individual's ability to exert a submaximal force repeatedly.

a. Static Endurance
1) A submaximal force is held for as long as possible; time is measured as an index of endurance performance.
2) The same devices used to assess static strength can be used. In addition, measuring the drop-in force with time will give an index of fatigue or muscular endurance.

b. Dynamic Endurance
1) Maximal repetitions completed at a set percentage of 1-RM or body weight, taking into account the size of the muscle mass being assessed (e.g., chest endurance, 50% 1-RM or 60% of body weight; biceps endurance, 50% 1-RM or 15% of body weight).
2) **Isokinetic endurance** measures the number of repetitions completed above 50% of maximal torque.
3) **Calisthenic tests** include sit-ups, push-ups, and pull-ups. The number of repetitions is assessed with the individual lifting his or her own body weight.
4) Persons who are not physically fit may be able to complete only a few repetitions; thus, these tests may be more useful for assessing strength than for assessing endurance.

3. Flexibility Assessment

a. Definition
1) The **functional range of motion about a joint**.
2) Flexibility is specific to each joint, and therefore can vary from one joint to another.
3) The functional ROM refers to **the ability to move the joint without incurring pain** or a limit to performance.

b. Rationale for Assessment
1) Inadequate flexibility is associated with decreased performance of activities of independent living and decreased ability to engage in specific physical movements.
2) Flexibility can decrease quickly with chronic disuse or can improve significantly with appropriate exercise intervention.

c. Procedure
1) Depending on the joint, **flexion, extension, rotation, abduction, adduction, supination, pronation, or deviation can be assessed** (*Table 6-9* and *Figure 6-5*).
2) An individual should **warm up** before flexibility testing by lightly exercising the joint to be tested; this promotes a more accurate measure of flexibility and reduces the risk of injury.
3) Measurements are taken with the limb starting in an anatomically neutral position to improve reliability.
4) **Repeated measurements** of flexibility are essential to ensure accurate assessment of ROM.

d. Measurement Devices
1) Portable and cost-effective, **goniometers** consist of two arms that

TABLE 6-9. RANGE OF MOTION OF THE MAJOR JOINTS

JOINT	MOTION	AVERAGE RANGES (degrees)
Spinal		
Cervical	Flexion	0–60
	Extension	0–75
	Lateral flexion	0–45
	Rotation	0–80
Thoracic	Flexion	0–50
	Rotation	0–30
Lumbar	Flexion	0–60
	Extension	0–25
	Lateral flexion	0–25
Upper Extremity		
Shoulder	Flexion	0–180
	Extension	0–50
	Abduction	0–180
	Adduction	0–50
	Internal rotation	0–90
	External rotation	0–90
Elbow	Flexion	0–140
Forearm	Supination	0–80
	Pronation	0–80
Wrist	Flexion	0–60
	Extension	0–60
	Ulnar deviation	0–30
	Radial deviation	0–20
Thumb	Abduction	0–60
	Flexion	
	Carpal-metacarpal	0–15
	Metacarpal-phalangeal	0–50
	Inter-phalangeal	0–80
	Extension	
	Carpal-metacarpal	0–20
	Metacarpal-phalangeal	0–5
	Interphalangeal	0–20
Fingers	Flexion	
	Metacarpal-phalangeal	0–90
	Proximal Interphalangeal	0–100
	Distal Interphalangeal	0–80
	Extension	
	Metacarpal-phalangeal	0–45
Lower Extremity		
Hip	Flexion	0–100
	Extension	0–30
	Abduction	0–40
	Adduction	0–20
	Internal rotation	0–40
	External rotation	0–50
Knee	Flexion	0–150
Ankle	Dorsiflexion	0–20
	Plantarflexion	0–40
Subtalar	Inversion	0–30
	Eversion	0–20

(From *ACSM's Resource Manual for Guidelines for Exercise Testing and Prescription*, 3rd ed. Baltimore: Williams & Wilkins, 1998, p 369.)

intersect at a disc that can measure 360° of movement. One arm is held on the stationary portion of the limb, while the other moves with the portion of the joint that moves.

2) **Inclinometers and fleximeters** are either handheld or attached to a limb, head, or trunk to measure ROM. These devices, which have a high measurement reliability, are excellent to use when use of a goniometer is not feasible.
3) **Tape measures** can accurately measure lateral trunk flexion and lumbar flexion as well as changes in ROM in the carpometacarpal and interphalangeal joints.

III. CLINICAL EXERCISE TESTING

A. INDICATIONS

1. Predischarge Exercise Testing Following Myocardial Infarction
   a. This is done to determine minimal standards of functional capacity, to **evaluate the client's ability to perform activities of daily living (ADL).**
   b. Testing is also conducted to evaluate the effectiveness of medications and the patient's hemodynamic response to exercise.
   c. This testing can reassure the patient (and family members) of the patient's capacity for physical work.
2. Postdischarge Exercise Testing Following Myocardial Infarction or Cardiac Surgery
   a. Testing can demonstrate the **degree of improvement since discharge**; maximal testing is usually conducted 3–6 weeks after the event.
   b. Results are used to design an exercise program, identify signs or symptoms, and to aid decisions on medication adjustments.
3. Diagnostic Testing and Determination of Disease Severity and Prognosis
   a. Maximal testing with measures of HR, BP, and ECG is the most cost-effective screening tool for detecting signs and symptoms of heart disease.
   b. Individuals diagnosed with heart disease are also tested to determine the presence and extent of myocardial ischemia, and to provide information on prognosis.
   c. Disease severity can be inferred from the shape or slope of the ST depression (upsloping, flat, or down-sloping), as well as the magnitude of depression.
   d. In addition, left ventricular function can be evaluated through measurements of maximal metabolic equivalent (MET) capacity as well as maximal systolic BP achieved.

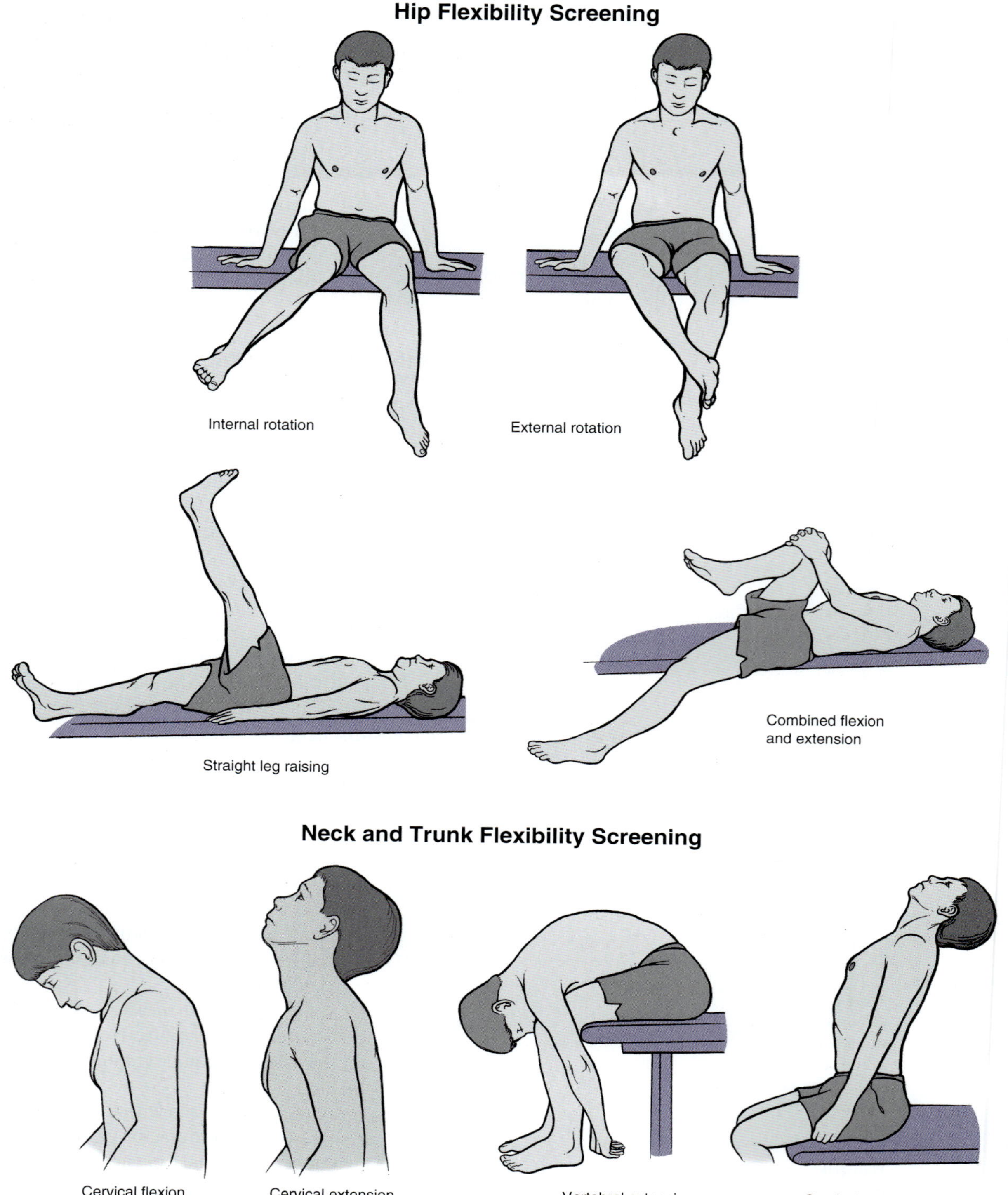

FIGURE 6-5. Top: Hip flexibility screening. Internal rotation involves flexing the hip and knee and moving the leg as far to the side as possible by rolling the thigh. External rotation involves moving the leg as far as possible past the midline by rolling the thigh outward. Straight leg raising consists of keeping the contralateral lower extremity in full extension while lifting the other extremity without bending the knee. Note limited hamstring flexibility. In the combined test of hip flexion and extension, one bent hip and knee are brought as close to the chest as possible, while allowing the other limb to drop over the edge of the table into extension (Thomas Test for hip extension). Bottom: Neck and trunk flexibility screening. In cervical flexion, the chin should touch the chest. Cervical extension involves bending the head as far as possible posteriorly. In vertebral flexion, with the hips and knees bent, the trunk should touch the anterior thighs. Vertebral extension involves backward movement of the trunk as far posterior as possible without hip extension. (Reprinted with permission from *ACSM's Resource Manual for Guidelines for Exercise Testing and Prescription*, 6th ed. Baltimore: Lippincott Williams & Wilkins, 2010.)

4. Functional Capacity Testing
Testing is useful in determining appropriate levels of activity and aerobic fitness, and providing feedback related to fitness improvements as part of a training program.

B. EXERCISE TEST MODALITIES AND PROTOCOLS

1. Treadmill
In this common test modality, the patient walks or runs at a predetermined pace on a treadmill whose grade can be adjusted. By raising the grade of the treadmill, the tester increases stress on this person. ECG and BP readings evaluate the effects of this stress.
   a. In the **Bruce protocol**, work rate is increased in 3-MET increments in 3-minute stages by gradually increasing both the grade and speed of the treadmill. Although this protocol is widely used, it may not be appropriate for less-fit individuals.
   b. For those who can complete only a submaximal protocol, the **modified Bruce protocol** may be used. This involves gradually increasing the grade while maintaining a constant low speed (1.7 mph).
   c. A variation of the Bruce protocol is the **ramp protocol**, which uses both grade and speed increases, but at a slower pace than in the Bruce protocol, to increase work rate.
   d. Other treadmill protocols include the **Balke-Ware**, **Naughton** (both most appropriate for those who are less fit), and **Ellestad** (appropriate for individuals who are fit).

2. Cycle Ergometer
   a. Cycle ergometry has several advantages over the treadmill:
      1) It keeps the upper body stable, ensuring more accurate ECG and BP measurements.
      2) It supports the individual's body weight, making it more appropriate for those with poor balance.
      3) It allows work rate to be set more precisely.
   b. Protocols can be easily individualized; most use stage durations of 2–5 minutes and work rate increments of 15–50 watts.

C. MEASUREMENTS

1. **Heart rate and blood pressure** are measured repeatedly before, during, and after the exercise test (*Table 6-10*), see also Box 4.4 in GETP 8th ed., p. 81.
2. Ideally, three **ECG leads** are monitored, one each from the lateral, inferior, and anterior views. One of those leads should be V_5 to pick up most ST segment changes.

TABLE 6-10. SEQUENCE OF MEASURES FOR HEART RATE, BLOOD PRESSURE, RATING OF PERCEIVED EXERTION (RPE), AND ELECTROCARDIOGRAM (ECG) DURING EXERCISE TESTING

Pretest	
(1)	12-lead ECG in supine and exercise postures
(2)	Blood pressure measurements in the supine position and exercise posture
Exercise[a]	
(1)	12-lead ECG recorded during last 15 seconds of every stage and at peak exercise (3-lead ECG observed/recorded every minute on monitor)
(2)	Blood pressure measurements should be obtained during the last minute of each stage[b]
(3)	Rating scales: RPE at the end of each stage, other scales if applicable
Posttest	
(1)	12-lead ECG immediately after exercise, then every 1–2 minutes for at least 5 minutes to allow any exercise-induced changes to return to baseline
(2)	[a]Blood pressure measurements should be obtained immediately after exercise, then every 1–2 minutes until stabilized near baseline level
(3)	Symptomatic ratings should be obtained using appropriate scales as long as symptoms persist after exercise

[a] In addition, these referenced variables should be assessed and recorded whenever adverse symptoms or abnormal ECG changes occur.
[b] Note: An unchanged or decreasing systolic blood pressure with increasing workloads should be retaken (i.e., verified immediately).
(From *ACSM's Guidelines for Exercise Testing and Prescription*, 6th ed. Philadelphia: Lippincott Williams & Wilkins, 2000, p 102.)

3. Monitoring for any **clinical signs** (e.g., changes in gait, skin color, or responsiveness) that may develop during the test helps identify test termination criteria and enhances patient safety.
4. The patient's subjective report of **rating of perceived exertion (RPE)** reflects his or her perception of work effort during testing.
   a. RPE can help determine the test endpoint, as well as information to be used in a future exercise prescription.
   b. The patient is instructed to report his or her perception of effort during the last minute of each work stage, generally using a scale of 1–10 or 6–20.
5. **Perceptual scales** (e.g., 1–4, with 1 representing minimal discomfort and 4 severe discomfort), allow an individual to express his or her degree of perceived angina or dyspnea during testing; this can be done nonverbally with hand signals (*Figure 6-6*).

D. INDICATIONS FOR TERMINATING AN EXERCISE TEST are classified as **absolute or relative** (*Table 6-11*.)

E. POSTEXERCISE PERIOD

1. **Active recovery**, involving walking or riding the cycle ergometer with a light load for 3–6 minutes, helps maintain venous return and prevents

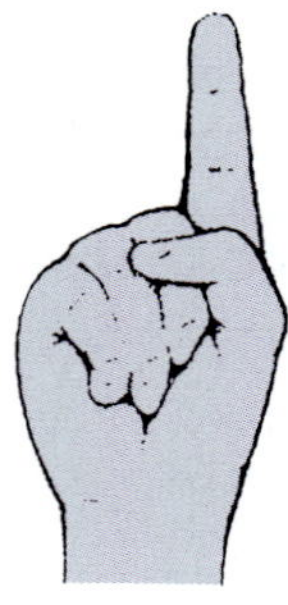
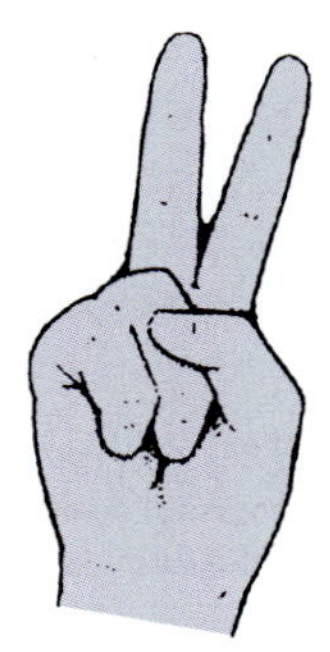
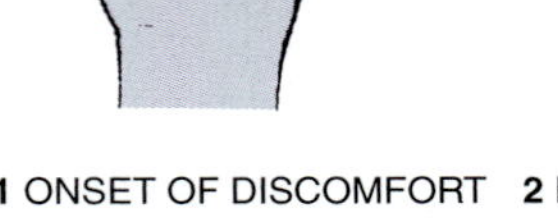

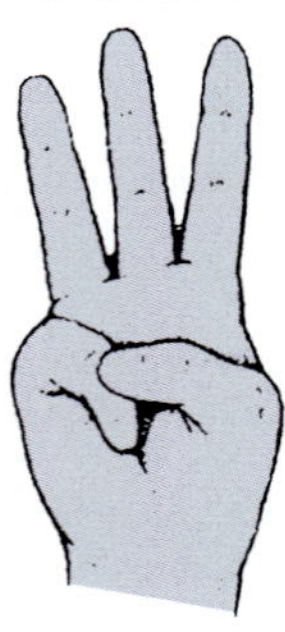
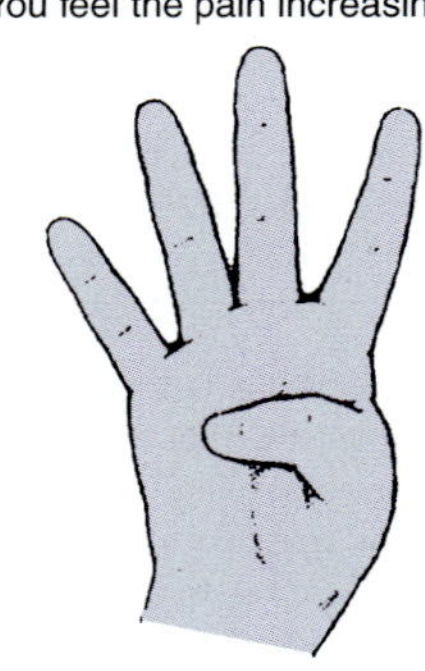
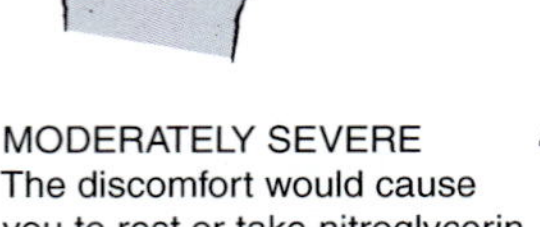

FIGURE 6-6. Nonverbal rating scale for exertional chest discomfort. The scale is particularly useful with gas exchange techniques. A rating of 3 is the appropriate endpoint. (Reprinted with permission from *ACSM's Resource Manual for Guidelines for Exercise Testing and Prescription*, 6th ed. Baltimore: Lippincott Williams & Wilkins, 2010.)

TABLE 6-11. INDICATIONS FOR TERMINATING EXERCISE TESTING

Absolute Indications
Drop in systolic blood pressure of ≥10 mm Hg from baseline blood pressure despite an increase in workload, when accompanied by other evidence of ischemia
Moderate to severe angina
Increasing nervous system symptoms (e.g., ataxia, dizziness, or near syncope)
Signs of poor perfusion (cyanosis or pallor)
Technical difficulties monitoring the electrocardiogram (ECG) or systolic blood pressure
Subject's desire to stop
Sustained ventricular tachycardia
ST elevation (≥10 mm) in leads without diagnostic Q-waves (other than V_1 or aVR)
Relative Indications
Drop in systolic blood pressure of ≥10 mm Hg from baseline blood pressure despite an increase in workload, in the absence of other evidence of ischemia
ST or QRS changes such as excessive ST depression (>2 mm horizontal or downsloping ST-segment depression) or marked axis shift
Arrhythmias other than sustained ventricular tachycardia, including multifocal premature ventricular contractions (PVCs), triplets of PVCs, supraventricular tachycardia, heart block, or bradyarrhythmias
Fatigue, shortness of breath, wheezing, leg cramps, or claudication
Development of bundle-branch block or intraventricular conduction delay that cannot be distinguished from ventricular tachycardia
Increasing chest pain
Hypertensive response[a]

[a] Systolic blood pressure >250 mm Hg or a diastolic blood pressure of >115 mm Hg. (Reprinted with permission from Gibbons RA, Balady GJ, Beasely JW et al. ACC/AHA guidelines for exercise testing. *J Am Coll Cardiol* 1997;30:260–315.)

blood pooling, hypotensive response, and compromised cardiac output.

2. Heart rate, ECG, and BP are monitored throughout active recovery, after which the patient is instructed to lie supine until ST changes have returned to baseline and HR falls below 100 bpm.

F. INTERPRETATION OF RESULTS
1. The value of a stress test depends on proper test performance, careful monitoring, and understanding the sensitivity and specificity of the test to make informed decisions regarding further testing or exercise prescription.
2. **Prognostic implications** are based on sensitivity and specificity.
   a. **Sensitivity** refers to the percentage of cases in which exercise testing accurately identifies the presence of CAD.
      1) **Current sensitivity** for detecting CAD using the exercise stress test **is about 70%.**
      2) **Sensitivity is enhanced by the following factors:**
         a) The patient exercises to near-maximal levels of exertion.
         b) Multiple-lead ECG is used.
         c) Other criteria besides ECG are assessed (e.g., BP response, symptoms).
      3) A **false-negative** stress test finding indicates a normal, or negative stress test (i.e., no signs of CAD) in individuals who actually have CAD (*Table 6-12*).
   b. **Specificity** refers to the percentage of cases in which the exercise test accurately rules out CAD.
      1) Using standard criteria for detecting CAD, the exercise stress test has about an 84% specificity (84% of healthy people tested show no signs or symptoms of CAD).
      2) A **false-positive** stress test finding indicates CAD in individuals who actually do not have CAD (*Table 6-13*).

TABLE 6-12. FACTORS THAT LOWER SENSITIVITY (FALSE-NEGATIVE FINDINGS)

- Failure to reach an ischemic threshold
- Monitoring an insufficient number of leads to detect electrocardiographic (ECG) changes
- Failure to recognize non-ECG signs and symptoms that may be associated with underlying cardiovascular disease (CVD) (e.g., exertional hypotension)
- Angiographically significant CVD compensated by collateral circulation
- Musculoskeletal limitations to exercise preceding cardiac abnormalities
- Technical or observer error

(From *ACSM's Resource GTEP*, 8th ed. Baltimore: Williams & Wilkins.)

IV. ASSESSING FITNESS IN OTHER POPULATIONS

A. CHILDREN

1. Purpose

a. Assessment of health status.

b. Comparison with criterion-referenced standards.

c. Determination of change resulting from exercise programs.

2. Considerations

a. In performing laboratory assessments of cardiovascular function, a **treadmill is preferable to a cycle ergometer.**

b. Inexperience, local muscle fatigue, inability to maintain cadence, and the short attention span of children make it difficult for many children to complete a cycle ergometer test.

c. Closure of the epiphyseal plates is not complete until after puberty. Therefore, it is **not recommended that children perform maximal tests for muscular strength.**

3. Modifications

a. **Treadmill Tests**

Keep speed constant, adjusting only the grade.

b. **Cycle Ergometer Tests**

Adjustments to the ergometer, including modifications to the handlebars, seat post, and pedal crank arms, are often required to fit the smaller anatomy.

4. Protocols

Recommended field tests for assessing health-related physical fitness in children include 1-mile or 1/2-mile run or walk, BMI, pull-ups, sit-ups, push-ups, and sit-and-reach test. (Refer to pages 187–189, in *ACSM's Guidelines for Exercise Testing and Prescription*, 8th edition.)

B. OLDER ADULTS

1. Purpose

Fitness testing is conducted in older adults for the same reasons as in younger adults, including exercise prescription, evaluation of progress, motivation, and education.

2. General Considerations

a. Adults of any specified age will vary widely in their physiologic response to exercise testing.

b. Deconditioning and disease often accompany aging. These factors must be taken into account in selecting appropriate fitness test protocols.

c. Adaptation to a specific workload is often prolonged in older adults. Therefore, a prolonged warm-up, followed by small increments in workload, is recommended.

3. Modifications

Test stages in graded exercise tests should be prolonged, lasting at least 3 minutes to allow the participant to reach steady state.

4. Protocols

a. Choose protocols that account for musculoskeletal and aerobic impairments.

b. Most protocols have 1–2 MET increments, with stages lasting 2–5 minutes.

c. **A variety of exercise test protocols may be found on Figure 5.3** *ACSM's Guidelines for Exercise Testing and Prescription*, 8th edition.

TABLE 6-13. CAUSES OF ABNORMAL ST-CHANGES IN THE ABSENCE OF OBSTRUCTIVE CORONARY ARTERY DISEASE

- Resting repolarization abnormalities (e.g., left bundle-branch block)
- Cardiac hypertrophy
- Accelerated conduction defects (e.g., Wolff-Parkinson-White syndrome)
- Digitalis
- Nonischemic cardiomyopathy
- Hypokalemia
- Vasoregulatory abnormalities
- Mitral valve prolapse
- Pericardial disorders
- Technical or observer error
- Coronary spasm in the absence of significant coronary artery disease
- Anemia
- Female gender

(From Box 6.4 of *ACSM's Guidelines for Exercise Testing and Prescription*, 8th ed. Baltimore: Williams & Wilkins, 2010.)

Review Test

DIRECTIONS: Carefully read all questions and select the BEST single answer.

1. A patient's health screening should be administered before:
   A) Any contact with that person.
   B) Any physical activity by the patient.
   C) Fitness assessment or programming.
   D) The initial "walk-through" showing of a facility.

2. A well-designed consent document developed in consultation with a qualified legal professional provides your facility with:
   A) Documentation of good-faith effort to educate those using the facility.
   B) Legal documentation of a person's understanding of assessment procedures.
   C) Legal immunity against lawsuits.
   D) No legal benefit.

3. Relative contraindications for exercise testing are conditions for which:
   A) A physician should be present during the testing procedures.
   B) Exercise testing should not be performed until the condition improves.
   C) Exercise testing will not provide accurate assessment of health-related fitness.
   D) Professional judgment about the risks and benefits of testing should determine whether to conduct an assessment.

4. A male client is 42 years old. His father died of a heart attack at age 62. He has a consistent resting blood pressure (measured over 6 weeks) of 132/86 mm Hg, and a total serum cholesterol of 5.4 mmol/L. Based on his coronary artery disease risk stratification, which of the following activities is appropriate?
   A) Maximal assessment of cardiorespiratory fitness without a physician supervising.
   B) Submaximal assessment of cardiorespiratory fitness without a physician supervising.
   C) Vigorous exercise without a prior medical assessment.
   D) Vigorous exercise without a prior physician-supervised exercise test.

5. During calibration of a treadmill, the belt length was found to be 5.5 m. It took 1 minute, 40 seconds for the belt to travel 20 revolutions. What is the treadmill speed?
   A) 4 m/min.
   B) 66 m/min.
   C) 79 m/min.
   D) 110 m/min.

6. Which of the following would most appropriately assess a previously sedentary 40-year-old woman's muscular strength?
   A) Using a 30-lb (18-kg) barbell to perform biceps curls to fatigue.
   B) Holding a handgrip dynamometer at 15 lb (7 kg) to fatigue.
   C) Performing modified curl-ups to fatigue.
   D) Using a 5-lb (2.2-kg) dumbbell to perform multiple sets of biceps curls to fatigue.

7. Flexibility is a measure of the:
   A) Disease-free range of motion about a joint.
   B) Effort-free range of motion about a joint.
   C) Habitually used range of motion about a joint.
   D) Pain-free range of motion about a joint.

8. Which of the following is a **FALSE** statement regarding an informed consent?
   A) The informed consent is not a legal document.
   B) The informed consent does not provide legal immunity to a facility or individual in the event of injury to an individual.
   C) Negligence, improper test administration, inadequate personnel qualifications, and insufficient safety procedures are all items that are expressly covered by the informed consent.
   D) The consent form does not relieve the facility or individual of the responsibility to do everything possible to ensure the safety of the individual.

9. An individual must be given specific instructions for the days preceding a fitness assessment. Which of the following is **NOT** a necessary instruction to a patient for a fitness assessment?
   A) Avoid liquids for 12 hours before the test.
   B) Do not drink alcohol, use tobacco products, or drink caffeine at least 3 hours before the test.
   C) Avoid strenuous exercise or physical activity on the day of the test.
   D) Get adequate sleep the night before the assessment.

10. Hydrodensitometry (hydrostatic weighing, underwater weighing) has several sources of error. Which of the following is **NOT** a common source of error when using this technique to determine body composition?
    A) Measurement of vital capacity of the lungs.

B) Interindividual variability in the amount of air in the gastrointestinal tract.
C) Interindividual variability in the density of individual lean tissue compartment.
D) Measurement of residual volume.

11. The definition of cardiorespiratory fitness is:
A) The maximal force that a muscle or muscle group can generate in a single effort.
B) The coordinated capacity of the heart, blood vessels, respiratory system, and tissue metabolic systems to take in, deliver, and use oxygen.
C) The ability to sustain a held maximal force or to continue repeated submaximal contractions.
D) The functional range of motion about a joint.

12. Adults age physiologically at individual rates. Therefore, adults of any specified age will vary widely in their physiologic responses to exercise testing. Special consideration should be given to the older adult when giving a fitness test because:
A) Age is often accompanied by deconditioning and disease.
B) Age predisposes the older adult to clinical depression and neurologic diseases.
C) The older adult cannot be physically stressed beyond 75% of age-adjusted maximum.
D) The older adult is not as motivated to exercise as a younger person.

13. Which of the following statements about underwater weighing is true?
A) It can divide the body into bone, muscle, and fat components.
B) It is a test that assumes standard densities for bone, muscle, and fat.
C) It will divide the body into visceral and subcutaneous fat components.
D) It is a direct method of body composition assessment.

ANSWERS AND EXPLANATIONS

1–B. A person should not be allowed to engage in any physical activity, including fitness assessment, at your facility before his or her health risk status has been determined. Informational meetings or "walk-throughs" of the facility that do not incorporate physical activity do not require health screening.

2–A. An appropriately prepared consent form is a written document that provides evidence that you made a good-faith effort to inform the individual of the procedures, risks, and benefits of the activities in which he or she would participate. The document does not provide legal immunity against lawsuits.

3–D. Identification of risk conditions for exercise testing includes familiarization with those conditions that may increase risk but that may not necessarily preclude fitness assessment. Such conditions are called "relative" contraindications. Conditions that do preclude testing until they have stabilized are "absolute" contraindications.

4–B. The patient has only one risk factor, hypercholesterolemia, with total serum cholesterol >5.2 mmol/L. He is, however, classified as "older" for exercise purposes because he is older than 40 years of age. Consequently, it is recommended that he should have medical clearance and an exercise test before engaging in vigorous exercise and that a physician should supervise any maximal assessment of cardiorespiratory fitness.

5–B. The belt length is 5.5 m. Twenty revolutions equals 110 m total distance (20 revolutions × 5.5 m/ revolution). This distance was traveled in 100 seconds (60 + 40), resulting in a speed of 1.1 m/sec (110 m/100 sec). Converting this to meters/min (1 min = 60 sec) results in a treadmill speed of 66 m/min.

6–A. Muscular strength is most appropriately assessed via either a determination of 1-RM, or through lifting a submaximal weight that an individual can lift at most 2–14 times. A weight of 30 lb (18 kg) for a previously sedentary middle-aged woman is probably an adequate weight to allow 2 to 14 repetitions. The held handgrip exercise, the modified curl-ups, and the 5-lb dumbbell exercise meet the criteria for muscular endurance assessments.

7–D. Range of motion may be limited by pain. This decreases the function of the joint. Therefore, flexibility is limited by painful actions. Disease status and effort can affect the range of motion. The range of motion habitually used is not necessarily an indication of the complete range of motion through which an individual can move.

8–C. Negligence, improper test administration, inadequate personnel qualifications, and insufficient safety procedures are all items that are expressly NOT covered by the informed consent. The informed consent is also not a legal document; it does not provide legal immunity to a facility or individual in the event of injury to a person and it does not relieve the facility or individual of the responsibility to do everything possible to ensure the safety of an individual.

9–A. The person should wear appropriate, comfortable, loose-fitting clothing, be adequately hydrated, avoid alcohol, tobacco, caffeine, and food for at least 3 hours before the test; avoid strenuous exercise or physical activity on the day of the test; and get adequate sleep the night before the test.

10–A. It is the measurement of residual volume of air in the lungs and not the vital capacity of the lungs that is a source of error. Residual volume is difficult to measure directly and is often estimated using vital capacity.

11–B. The maximal force that a muscle or muscle group can generate in a single effort is the definition of muscular strength. The ability to sustain a held maximal force or to continue repeated submaximal contractions is the definition of muscular endurance. The functional range of motion about a joint is the definition of flexibility. The coordinated capacity of the heart, blood vessels, respiratory system, and tissue metabolic systems to take in, deliver, and use oxygen is the definition of cardiorespiratory fitness.

12–A. Fitness testing is conducted in older adults for the same reasons as in younger adults, including exercise prescription, evaluation of progress, motivation, and education. Age is often accompanied by deconditioning and disease and these factors must be taken into consideration when selecting appropriate fitness test protocols. In addition, adaptation to a specific workload is often prolonged in older adults (a prolonged warm-up, followed by small increments in workload are recommended). Test stages in graded exercise tests should be prolonged, lasting at least 3 minutes, to allow the participant to reach a steady state. An appropriate test protocol should be selected to accommodate these special needs.

13–B. Underwater weighing is based on the concept that the human body can be divided into a fat component and fat-free component. Fat is expressed relative to body weight (this includes all fat). This is an indirect method of measurement, because fat is not actually separated by dissection.

Clinical Exercise Study Questions

DIRECTIONS: Carefully read all questions and select the BEST single answer.

1. A patient with a functional capacity of 7 METs, an ejection fraction of 37%, and 1 mm ST depression on exertion
   A) Should not exercise until his or her ejection fraction is > 50%.
   B) Is considered a low risk.
   C) Is considered a moderate risk.
   D) Is considered a high risk.

2. The most accurate screening method for signs and symptoms of coronary artery disease is a:
   A) Maximal exercise test with a 12-lead ECG.
   B) Submaximal exercise test with a 12-lead ECG.
   C) Discontinuous protocol, stopping at 85% of maximal heart rate.
   D) Continuous protocol, stopping at 85% of maximal heart rate.

3. What is the best test to help determine ejection fraction at rest and during exercise?
   A) Angiogram.
   B) Thallium stress test.
   C) Single-proton emission computer tomography test.
   D) Multiple gated acquisition (blood pool imagery) study.

4. A "cold spot" that is detected in the inferior portion of the left ventricle during a stress test and resolves 3 hours later most likely indicates:
   A) An old inferior myocardial infarction.
   B) A myocardial infarction that is healing.
   C) Reversible myocardial ischemia.
   D) The need for multiple bypass surgery.

5. What is the best test of cardiovascular function for individuals who are obese, have claudication in their legs, and have limited mobility owing to neurologic damage from uncontrolled diabetes?
   A) Dipyridamole or dobutamine testing and assessment of cardiovascular variables.
   B) Discontinuous treadmill exercise test.
   C) Resting echocardiogram.
   D) Continuous submaximal cycle ergometer test.

6. Although 12-lead testing is the optimal ECG configuration, if only one lead can be used, which one should it be?
   A) Lead II.
   B) Lead AV_L.
   C) Lead V_5.
   D) Lead V_1.

7. Which of the following is an indication for terminating an exercise test?
   A) The patient requests test termination.
   B) The respiratory exchange rate exceeds 0.95.
   C) The maximal heart rate exceeds 200 bpm.
   D) The rating of perceived exertion exceeds 17 on the standard scale.

8. Given the sensitivity of the exercise ECG, stress testing conducted on 100 cardiac rehabilitation patients with documented coronary artery disease (CAD) would be expected to produce what results?
   A) All 100 clients would show ECG indicators of CAD.
   B) About 50 clients would show ECG indicators of CAD.
   C) About 30 clients would show ECG indicators of CAD.
   D) About 70 clients would show ECG indicators of CAD.

9. What action should you take for a 55-year-old person who has three risk factors for heart disease and complains of fatigue on exertion?
   A) Conduct a submaximal stress test without the presence of a physician.
   B) Conduct a maximal diagnostic stress test in the presence of a physician.
   C) Use a questionnaire to evaluate activity and not conduct a test.
   D) Start the person exercising slowly and test after 6 weeks.

10. For a patient taking a β-blocker who has lowered resting blood pressure and heart rate, which of the following statements is true?
    A) A submaximal test will provide the best estimate of that person's fitness.
    B) A submaximal test may underestimate that person's fitness.
    C) A submaximal test may overestimate that person's fitness.
    D) The patient should be tested only when not taking the medication.

11. Two individuals have the same body weight, gender, ethnic background, and skinfold measurement results. One is 25-years of age; the other, 45 years of

age. Given this scenario, which of the following statements is accurate?

A) They both have the same percentage of body fat.
B) The 25-year-old is fatter.
C) The 45-year-old is fatter.
D) Who is fatter cannot be determined from the information given.

12. Lead V_1 is located at the

A) Fifth intercostal space, left sternal border.
B) Midclavicular line, fourth intercostal space.
C) Fourth intercostal space, right sternal border.
D) Midclavicular line, lateral to the xiphoid process.

13. Following termination of a stress test, a 12-lead ECG is:

A) Monitored immediately, then every 1–2 minutes until exercise-induced changes are at baseline.
B) Monitored immediately, then at 2 and 5 minutes after the test.
C) Monitored immediately only.
D) Monitored and recorded only if any signs or symptoms arise during recovery.

14. For a patient who has a contraindication for exercise testing but could benefit greatly from the information gained through testing, which of the following statements is true?

A) The contraindication is considered a relative contraindication.
B) The contraindication is considered an absolute contraindication.
C) The patient should not be tested until the contraindication is resolved.
D) A submaximal test is the only test that the patient should complete.

ANSWERS AND EXPLANATIONS

1–C. Moderate risk individuals have signs or symptoms that suggest possible cardiopulmonary or metabolic disease or two or more risk factors. Other moderate risk criteria include functional capacity < 6–8 METs 3 weeks after a clinical event; shock or congestive heart failure during a recent myocardial infarction (MI); moderate left ventricular dysfunction (ejection fraction 31%–49%); exercise-induced ST-segment depression of 1–2 mm; and reversible ischemic defects.

2–A. A maximal stress test requires the heart to work at its peak capacity. If heart disease is present, then signs or symptoms should be detected. A submaximal test may not stress the heart sufficiently to allow detection of ischemia.

3–D. A multiple gated acquisition (MUGA) study may be performed to assess resting and exercise cardiac function related to cardiac output, ejection fraction, and wall motion. In this test, technetium 99m is injected into the blood stream, where it attaches to red blood cells. Areas where the blood pools, such as the ventricles, are visualized by the technetium emissions.

4–C. During a standard stress test, a patient is connected to an intravenous line. During the last minute of exercise, thallium-201 is injected into the blood stream. Thallium enters myocardial cells in proportion to the amount of blood flow to those cells, and emits energy detectable with a scintillation counter. Images of the myocardium can be constructed immediately following a stress test and 4–24 hours later. Areas with little or no perfusion immediately following a test indicate areas of ischemia. Persistence of these "cold spots" for 4–24 hours later indicates necrotic tissue. Areas of reversible ischemia will reperfuse, and cold spots will disappear in later testing.

5–A. In some instances, individuals are not able to complete a stress test because of muscular limitations, neurologic disability, peripheral vascular disease, or other conditions that prevent them from achieving a sufficient work intensity to provide an accurate cardiovascular assessment.

6–C. During the test, three leads should be monitored, one each from the lateral, inferior, and anterior views. Research has shown that one of these leads should be V_5, as it will pick up most ST-segment changes.

7–A. Criteria are classified as absolute or relative indications. These criteria are based both on measured physiologic responses and on symptoms displayed by the patient. However, under any test condition, if the individual being tested requests that the test be stopped, then it must be stopped.

8–D. Sensitivity refers to the percentage of cases in which exercise testing accurately identifies the presence of coronary artery disease (CAD). Although the exercise ECG is not completely sensitive to detecting CAD, it is the most cost-effective first-line screening tool. Current sensitivity for detecting CAD using the exercise stress test is about 70%.

9–B. A maximal exercise test can be most effective in detecting CAD as well as allowing the technician to measure maximal oxygen uptake ($\dot{V}O_2max$). Therefore, when screening for CAD, a maximal diagnostic stress test (ECG, physician supervision) is recommended.

10–C. Submaximal testing estimates $\dot{V}O_2max$ based on the assumed linear relationship between heart rate and $\dot{V}O_2max$. Heart rate is measured at multiple workloads during the test, and $\dot{V}O_2max$ at an estimated maximal heart rate is calculated. Submaximal testing is based on several assumptions:

- Measurements are done while the client is at steady state.
- The relationship between heart rate and $\dot{V}O_2max$ is linear.
- Maximal heart rate is similar for any given age.
- A β-blocker will change the reliability of the assumption, showing a lower heart rate for a given workload, thus predicting a higher achievable workload (and thus $\dot{V}O_2max$).

11–C. Age is accounted for in skinfold equations because of the changes in body fat distribution with age. With aging, more fat is stored internally, altering the meaning of a given skinfold measure. Thus, the same skinfold for an older man indicates a higher relative body fat than a younger man of equivalent size and sum of skinfold.

12–C. The position for lead V_1 is located by palpating along the intercostal spaces to the fourth space; the electrode is placed along the right sternal border.

13–A. The 12-lead ECG should be recorded immediately after exercise, then every 1–2 minutes for 5 minutes or until exercise-induced ECG changes are at baseline.

14–A. *Relative contraindications* include patients who might be tested if the potential benefit from exercise testing outweighs the relative risk. *Absolute contraindications* refer to individuals for whom exercise testing should not be performed until the situation or condition has stabilized.

Safety, Injury Prevention, and Emergency Care

CHAPTER 7

I. GENERAL CONSIDERATIONS

A. All forms of exercise, from clinical testing to supervised exercise and from cardiac rehabilitation to general fitness programs, entail some risk (*Table 7-1*).

B. Every clinical exercise physiologist, exercise specialist, health/fitness specialist, and personal trainer must understand the risks associated with exercise testing and training, be able to implement preventive measures, and know how to respond in case of injury or medical emergency.

C. Every clinical testing and exercise program must have an **emergency response system** to respond to injuries and medical emergencies.

D. Every health/fitness testing and exercise program must **have and practice** an emergency plan to respond to injuries and medical emergencies, conduct and document mock drills, and update the emergency plan as appropriate for potential injuries and medical emergencies that may occur in a health/fitness setting.

II. RISK OF PARTICIPATION IN EXERCISE

A. PHYSICAL DEMANDS

At higher intensities, the potential exists for either **injury** or an **emergency situation** that requires an appropriate and timely response.

B. BENEFITS SHOULD OUTWEIGH RISKS

The exercise professional must create as safe an environment as possible by:

1. **Understanding the risks.**
2. Being able to **implement preventive** measures.
3. Having **knowledge regarding the appropriate care of injuries.**
4. **Creating, practicing, and implementing emergency plans** in the event of a medical emergency.

C. POTENTIAL SOURCES OF RISK

1. Exercise Equipment

Exercise equipment can **malfunction**, not be properly calibrated properly, be **used incorrectly**, or be in **disrepair** or **poor condition.**

2. Environment

The exercise environment must be **clean** and properly **maintained.**

3. Staff

Staff must be **qualified (e.g., have proper certification), trained**, act in a **responsible and safe** manner, and **design safe exercise programs based on risk stratification, medical history, and exercise testing data if available.**

4. Medical History

The exercise professional must **know the patient's medical history, medication use (including prescription and over-the-counter [OTC] drugs), and restrictions.**

5. Individual Factors

a. **Age.**
b. **Extent of exercise or athletic experience.**
c. **Medical history.**
d. **Lack of experience and familiarity** with equipment.
e. **Lack of knowledge** about proper principles of exercise.
f. Poor body alignment or poor execution of an exercise.

D. PREVENTION STRATEGIES FOR STAFF AND CLIENTS

1. Think about safety.
2. Exercise intelligently.
3. Purchase good equipment and supplies.
4. Perform routine maintenance check of equipment.
5. Use proper technique.
6. Follow the rules.
7. Train staff on a regular basis; frequency and amount of training will depend on staff credentials and knowledge, clientele, and employee turnover.
8. Offer members a general orientation to the facility, including proper use of exercise equipment.
9. In a group exercise setting, staff should understand the following:
   a. Exercise space for each person (e.g., size of the room, number of participants).

TABLE 7-1. POSSIBLE MEDICAL COMPLICATIONS OF EXERCISE

Cardiovascular Complications
- Cardiac arrest
- Ischemia
  - Angina
  - Myocardial infarction
- Arrhythmias
  - Supraventricular tachycardia
  - Atrial fibrillation
  - Ventricular tachycardia
  - Ventricular fibrillation
  - Bradyarrhythmias
  - Bundle branch blocks
  - Atrioventricular nodal blocks
- Congestive heart failure
- Hypertension
- Hypotension
- Aneurysm rupture
- Underlying medical conditions predisposing to increased complications
  - Hypertrophic cardiomyopathy
  - Coronary artery anomalies
  - Idiopathic left ventricular hypertrophy
  - Marfan syndrome
  - Aortic stenosis
  - Right ventricular dysplasia
  - Congenital heart defects
  - Myocarditis
  - Pericarditis
  - Amyloidosis
  - Sarcoidosis
  - Long QT syndrome
  - Sickle-cell trait

Metabolic Complications
- Volume depletion
- Dehydration
- Rhabdomyolysis
- Renal failure
- Electrolyte disturbances

Thermal Complications
- Hyperthermia
  - Heat rash
  - Heat cramps
  - Heat syncope
  - Heat exhaustion
  - Heat stroke
- Hypothermia
- Frostbite

Pulmonary Complications
- Exercise-induced asthma
- Bronchospasm
- Pulmonary embolism
- Pulmonary edema
- Pneumothorax
- Exercise-induced anaphylaxis
- Exacerbation of underlying pulmonary disease

Gastrointestinal Complications
- Vomiting
- Cramps
- Diarrhea

Endocrine Complications
- Amenorrhea
- Complications in those with diabetes
  - Hypoglycemia
  - Hyperglycemia
  - Retinal hemorrhage
- Osteoporosis

Neurologic Complications
- Dizziness
- Syncope (fainting)
- Cerebral vascular accident (stroke)
- Insomnia

Musculoskeletal Complications
- Mechanical injuries
- Back injuries
- Stress fractures
- Carpal tunnel syndrome
- Joint pain or injury
- Muscle cramps or spasms
- Tendonitis
- Exacerbation of musculoskeletal diseases

Overuse Complications
- Overuse syndromes
- Overtraining
- Overexercising
- Shin splints
- Plantar fasciitis

Traumatic Injuries
- Bruises
- Strains and sprains
- Muscle and tendon tears and ruptures
- Fractures
- Contusions and lacerations
- Bleeding
- Crush injuries
- Blunt trauma
- Internal organ injury
  - Splenic rupture
  - Myocardial contusion
- Drowning
- Head injuries
- Eye injuries
- Death

(From *ACSM's Resource Manual for Guidelines for Exercise Testing and Prescription*, 6th ed. Baltimore, Lippincott Williams & Wilkins, 2010.)

b. Temperature and humidity of the space.
c. Fitness level and special needs of participants.
d. Proper flooring to match group activity.
e. Appropriate warm-up, cool-down, exercise progression, and sequencing.

III. SAFETY IN THE FACILITY

A. AREAS OF SAFETY

1. Specific Areas of Safety

a. Building design.
b. Physical plant.
c. Fixtures.
d. Furniture.
e. Equipment.
f. Program design.
g. Staff training.

2. Americans with Disabilities Act (ADA)

a. The ADA lists specific standards that enhance safety and access for both **disabled and nondisabled** exercisers.
b. The ADA is especially important for fitness facilities because of the **variety of individuals that may participate** in exercise programs.

3. ACSM Health/Fitness Facility Standards and Guidelines *(Third Edition, 2007)* for Signage in Health/Fitness Facilities

a. Facilities must post appropriate caution, danger, and warning signage where conditions warrant.
b. Facilities must post appropriate emergency and safety signage pertaining to fire and related emergency situations, as required by federal, state, and local codes.
c. Facilities must post all required ADA and Occupational Safety and Health Administration (OSHA) signage.
d. All signage must conform to American National Standards Institute (ANSI) standards.

B. CREATION OF A SAFE ENVIRONMENT

1. This is a primary responsibility in all fitness facilities.
2. Managers and staff must **meet a standard of care for safety** in developing and operating facilities and equipment by **looking beyond obvious safety parameters**.
3. **Environmental factors** (e.g., temperature, humidity, ventilation, altitude, pollution) must be monitored and controlled, because physiologic

response to exercise performance and health can be affected by these conditions.

a. **High temperature** can lead to dehydration, dizziness, syncope, heat exhaustion, and even heat stroke.
    1) Strategies to alleviate heat stress include:
        a) Wear light colored clothing made of materials that allows for heat loss and sweat evaporation.
        b) Reschedule exercise for a cooler time of day or indoors.
        c) Reduce intensity and add rest breaks.
b. **Low temperature** can lead to dehydration caused by considerable loss of water from respiratory passages, reduced coordination, chills, hypothermia, and potentially frostbite.
    1) Wear layers of clothing to reduce heat loss in cold temperatures.
    2) Refer to Wind Chill Index tables for guidelines for time required for frostbite to occur in exposed skin. (For the complete table, please refer to Figure 8.2 in *ACSM's Guidelines for Exercise Testing and Prescription*, 8th ed., p. 200.)
c. **High humidity** reduces the evaporative loss of sweat, which can reduce the body's ability to control core temperature and can lead to heat illness.
    1) Refer to Wet-Bulb Globe temperature (WBGT) and National Institute for Occupational Safety and Health (NIOSH) tables for guidelines for safe exercise duration.
d. Exposure to **high altitude** can lead to headaches, nausea, and altitude sickness.
    1) Ascend slowly to reduce risk of altitude sickness. Sleeping at a lower altitude at night may also reduce the symptoms.
    2) Eat a high-carbohydrate diet to reduce symptoms of acute mountain sickness.
    3) Avoid exercise until symptoms resolve.
e. In addition to affecting performance negatively, **pollution** can lead to wheezing, coughing, and irritation of the eyes, nose, and mouth.
    1) Choose a time of day (specific to the season) when pollution levels are lowest.
    2) Moderate intensity and duration are key to limit exposure to pollutants.
    3) Check local meteorologic authorities for specific information on air quality.

C. EQUIPMENT

1. Includes pieces used for **testing cardiovascular, strength**, and **flexibility**, and **rehabilitation, pool, locker room, and emergency equipment.**
2. **Criteria for equipment selection include:**
    a. Proper anatomic position.
    b. Ability to adjust to different body sizes.
    c. Quality of design and materials.
    d. Durability.
    e. Repair history.
    f. Cost.
    g. Size of equipment relative to space availability.
    h. Equipment can be used for multi- or single-purpose exercises.
3. **Test the equipment** before purchase, and follow the manufacturer's instructions for installation.
4. **Inspect the equipment** regularly for cleanliness, disrepair, and proper functioning to allow early recognition of problems.
5. **Other safety considerations include:**
    a. All **electrical plugs** should be secured and grounded.
    b. Treadmills should have easily accessible **emergency cutoff switches.**
    c. **Safety instructions should be mounted** on all equipment.
    d. Machines should **restrict joint movements beyond the normal range of motion.**

D. FURNITURE AND FIXTURES

1. **Locker room and reception furniture** are used frequently and should be selected for **ergonomics, durability, ability to disinfect and clean, and safety.**
2. **Inspection, routine maintenance, and cleaning** are equally important with furniture.
3. Lighting should be bright enough to see signage and records clearly and prevent falls, and it should create a positive, motivating atmosphere while meeting with federal, state, and local building code standards.

E. SURFACES

1. Proper surfaces must be provided to **prevent slips and falls.**
2. Surface selection **should meet minimal standards** for the activity being carried out and should **comply with the ADA** requirements or standards.
3. Maintenance includes:
    a. Proper cleaning and disinfecting.
    b. Removal of oil and dust.
    c. Inspection for cracks, holes, exposed seams, and warping.

F. SUPPLIES AND SMALL EQUIPMENT

1. This category of equipment includes heart rate (HR) monitors, blood pressure (BP) units, stopwatches, headphones, skinfold calipers, metronomes, exercise gloves, and so forth.
2. Equipment **must be in proper working order and calibrated.**
3. Devices that do not function correctly may provide incorrect information and precipitate an unsafe situation.

G. ROUTINE AND REQUIRED MAINTENANCE AND REPAIRS

1. Help to ensure that equipment; furniture; heating, ventilation, and air conditioning; lights; and so on **function safely** and according to specifications.
2. **Increase the life of the equipment.**
3. **Reduce the risk of a mechanical problem.**
4. A **routine maintenance schedule** for exercise equipment should be in place.
   a. Service contracts may provide suggested equipment maintenance schedule.
   b. Routine maintenance should be documented.
5. A procedure for reporting problems and a repair process that reduces downtime should include **documentation of the problem, repair history, and resolution of the problem** (*Figure 7-1*).

H. MAINTENANCE AND HOUSEKEEPING

1. Contribute to safety by presenting a clean environment.
2. Help to maintain proper equipment functioning.
3. Slippery surfaces, dirty equipment and furniture, poorly maintained ventilation, and equipment in disrepair **increase the risk of accidents.**
4. Equipment and fixtures must be **regularly cleaned and disinfected.**
   a. **Written standards** must outline clearly the procedure for routine cleaning and maintenance.
   b. Solutions and materials must be **safe** for the skin and **hypoallergenic.**
   c. The professional staff should have a role in the cleaning and maintenance of exercise equipment. **Knowledge of procedures and chemical safety** is critical.
      1) Material Safety Data Sheets (MSDS) should be kept on file for all chemicals used in the facility.
      2) Cleaning solutions and chemicals must be stored properly.

IV. WEIGHT ROOM SAFETY

A. WEIGHTS

The use of weights—either machine or free weights (e.g., dumbbells, barbells)—increases the risk of injury because of the **amount of weight used, improper alignment, improper technique, fatigue, and improper behavior.**

B. METHODS TO INCREASE SAFETY

1. **Spotting:** A second person assists in the initial lift, correcting the lifter's technique and lifting the weight to safety if the lifter is unable to handle the weight.
2. **Buddy system:** Exercise with a partner who can offer encouragement and motivation, knowledge of correct technique, and assistance if a problem develops.
3. **Speed of movement:** Movements should be controlled with a slow, smooth pace (~3 seconds concentric, ~3 seconds eccentric).
4. **Range of motion (ROM):** ROM should be controlled such that weights are not repetitively banged against one another and are carefully returned to their start position at the end of each set.
5. **Replacing weights:** A safe environment requires returning weights to their proper place after exercise.
6. **Placement of equipment:** Adequate space between machines, free weight equipment, and weight benches is important for safety.
7. **Equipment inspection and routine maintenance.**

V. TESTING AND EVALUATION AREA

This area must be safely organized and similarly prepared for emergencies. Equipment should include:

A. Sphygmomanometer, stethoscope, mask, mouth guard, and gloves for cardiopulmonary resuscitation (CPR), first-aid kit, and automated external defibrillator (AED).
B. Telephone to activate the public emergency medical system (EMS).
   1. Should have **posted, written procedures to activate the EMS** (e.g., 911).
   2. Should include the following instructions:
      a. **Identify** yourself, your location, specific point of entry, and the phone number.
      b. **Provide** a clear and succinct **explanation** of the problem (e.g. life-threatening versus non–life-threatening emergency) and type (e.g., musculoskeletal versus cardiac).

Fitness Equipment Repair Chart

Date	Equipment	Serial No.	Problem	Date repaired	Order No.	Cost

FIGURE 7-1. An example of a repair log for fitness equipment. (From *ACSM's Resource Manual for Guidelines for Exercise Testing and Prescription,* 4th ed. Philadelphia, Lippincott Williams & Wilkins, 2001, p 646.)

c. Obtain medical history, medications, and emergency contact information from facility files (if known) for EMS technicians.
d. Provide vital signs and state of consciousness.
e. Explain the treatment actions taken and their results.

C. Back board and neck board
A total body back board and neck board are not required in the testing area, but they should be immediately accessible.

D. Emergency equipment
1. Emergency equipment must be:
   a. Clearly marked.
   b. Readily accessible at all times.
   c. Calibrated and maintained regularly with documentation of such actions.
2. Necessary emergency equipment includes:
   a. Telephones with the numbers of the EMS or 911, physicians, cardiac code team (clinical setting), police, fire, and building security (if applicable).
   b. First-aid kits.
   c. First-responder bloodborne pathogen kits (infection control kit).
   d. Latex gloves.
   e. Blood pressure kit with stethoscope.
   f. CPR masks or mouthpieces.
   g. Resuscitation bags (clinical setting).
   h. Oxygen (clinical setting).
   i. Back board for performing CPR.
   j. Splints.
   k. Defibrillator (clinical facility) or automatic external defibrillator (AED) (fitness facility).
   l. Crash cart with emergency medications and supplies (e.g., epinephrine, dextrose, blood glucose meter) in the clinical setting.
3. Staff should know how to use and routinely practice (at least quarterly) the use of emergency equipment. Training and drills should be documented, reviewed with the Medical Director, and revised as appropriate.

VI. SAFETY DURING EXERCISE TESTING AND TRAINING

A. PARTICIPANT/PATIENT SAFETY

1. Monitoring for Signs of Fatigue and Distress
During exercise testing, the clinical exercise specialist monitors the patient's HR and rhythm (on an electrocardiogram [ECG]), BP, rating of perceived exertion (RPE), respiration, and other parameters for signs of fatigue or distress.
   a. Manifestations of cardiac or pulmonary distress necessitate stopping the test immediately and, possibly, initiating the emergency response system.
   b. Less severe manifestations (e.g., lightheadedness, muscular fatigue, intermittent premature ventricular contractions, mild wheezing) may not necessitate immediate test termination.
2. Indications for stopping an exercise session include those listed in Chapter 6, Table 6-11), as well as the following:
   a. Signs of confusion or inability to concentrate.
   b. Dizziness.
   c. Convulsions.
   d. Physical injury.
   e. Nausea.
   f. Physical or verbal manifestations of severe fatigue.
   g. The patient requests to stop.

B. STAFF SAFETY

Fitness and healthcare professionals must have an appropriate level of professional education, work experience, or certification to prescribe, instruct, monitor, or supervise physical activity programs. (For recommended competency criteria for program supervisors, instructors, counselors, and personal trainers, please refer to Table 6-11 in *ACSM's Health/Fitness Facility Standards and Guidelines*, 3rd ed.).

1. Fitness and clinical exercise staff must demonstrate professional competence with all programs and use of exercise or testing areas. Staff competency must be documented.
2. Safety of the exercise staff can be maximized by following federal OSHA standards.
   a. Wash hands thoroughly before working with a patient.
   b. Wear gloves, goggles, and other protective clothing (when necessary) when any possibility of exposure to bloodborne pathogens exists.
   c. Keep cords out of the path of both staff and patients to eliminate the possibility of trips or falls.
   d. Keep long hair and loose clothing from catching on equipment.

VII. MEDICATIONS AND SAFETY

Various medications can affect a patient's response to exercise testing or training. (For a full review, please refer to Tables 5-2 and 5-3 in *ACSM's Health/Fitness Facility Standards and Guidelines*, 3rd ed.)

Appendix A in ACSM's Guidelines for Exercise Testing and Prescription, 8th edition.

VIII. SAFETY PLANS

A. Clearly outline procedures for maintaining a safe environment and reducing the risk of accidents. Plans should include regional conditions such as tornados, hurricanes, bomb threats, where such conditions may occur more frequently.

B. Appropriate safety plans include:
   1. Fire
      a. Procedures for evacuation and contacting authorities.
      b. Regular inspection of fire extinguishers.
      c. Procedures for the use of fire extinguishers, signage, and documentation of staff training.
   2. Power Failure
      a. Procedures that reduce the risk of power outages and electrical malfunction.
      b. Procedures for evacuation and contacting the authorities.
      c. Routine drills should be conducted to document the functionality of back-up power and lighting in the event of an emergency to ensure participant safety in both the health/fitness and clinical settings.
   3. Flood
      a. Procedures to reduce the risk of flooding in areas such as the pool, shower, and whirlpool.
      b. Procedures for clean-up and salvage.
   4. Earthquake
      a. Procedures for evacuation and contacting authorities.
      b. Procedures for safety of equipment and persons in the facility.
   5. Tornado
      a. Procedures for evacuation and contacting authorities.
      b. Procedures for safety of equipment and persons in the facility.
   6. Bomb Threat
      a. Procedures for staff handling calls of a bomb threat (e.g., getting information about the caller, questions to ask, checking for background noise).
      b. Procedures for evacuation and contacting authorities.
   7. Bloodborne Pathogens and Hazardous Waste
      a. OSHA has specific standards that must be posted and closely adhered to when applicable.
      b. All staff must be familiar with and trained in these procedures. Training must be documented.
      c. Proper disposal of "contaminated" items can be obtained from your local health department.
      d. Biohazard bags should be readily available.
   8. Staff Certification in First Aid, CPR, AED, and ACLS
   9. Posted Information
      a. Clearly visible signs should be posted for evacuation routes, fire extinguishers, first-aid kits, CPR mouth shields, location of AED, and for activating the EMS (911) or code team.
      b. Emergency procedures should be posted adjacent to all phones to assist in enacting the emergency plan.

IX. PROPER DOCUMENTATION

Events should be recorded. This includes written policies and procedures, rules, patient and client rights, as well as the benefits and risks of exercise programs. Such documents offer important protection against liability and negligence for both facilities and professional staff. Liability insurance and legal assistance is recommended as well, because laws differ from state to state. Also, the individual staff members, as well as the facility, may be subject to legal action.

A. PARTICIPANT AGREEMENTS

1. Participant agreements define the risks and rewards of an exercise program, exact type of exercise program, and who shares the risk and responsibility for the participant's exercise. It combines a waiver, informed consent, an assumption of risk agreement, and other protective language into one stand-alone document (*Figure 7-2*).
2. An attorney should assist in creating these forms.

B. INFORMED CONSENT

Informed consent provides detailed explanation of the test or exercise program, including:

1. Potential benefits and risks.
2. Purpose of the test or exercise program.
3. Participant responsibilities.
4. Opportunity for the participant to ask questions.

C. WAIVERS

1. Waivers allow the participant to release the exercise professional or facility from liability for any acts of negligence.

SAMPLE

PARTICIPANT'S RELEASE AND AGREEMENT

I, the undersigned, hereby agree to participate in an exercise class and/or program ("Program") offered by the XYZ Health Club. I understand that there are inherent risks in participating in a program of strenuous exercise. I warrant and represent that I am in acceptable health and that I may participate in the Program. I agree that I have been honest in my statements regarding my health and medical history and if there are any medical or health conditions or problems, I further agree to obtain a physician's clearance before participating in the Program. If restrictions exist, I will inform XYZ Health Club at the time and allow XYZ Health Club staff to contact my physician for additional information.

I agree that XYZ Health Club shall not be liable or responsible for any injuries to me or illnesses resulting from my participation in the Program and I expressly release and discharge XYZ Health Club and it employees, agents, and assigns, from all claims, actions or judgements which I or my heirs, executors, administrators or assigns may have or claim to have against XYZ Health Club, and/or its employees, agents or assigns for all injuries, illnesses or other damage which may occur in connection with my participtation in the Program. This release shall be binding upon my heirs, executors, administrators, and assigns.

I have read this release and agreement and I understand all of its terms. I execute it voluntarily and with full knowledge of its significance.

Signature: ______________________ Date: ______________

Print name: ______________________

Witness: ______________________ Date: ______________

FIGURE 7-2. A sample of a participant's release and agreement.

2. Waivers may offer a form of **protection** for both the **instructor** and the **facility**.

D. INCIDENT REPORTS

1. Incident reports are a record of an incident, accident, or event that involves **unusual circumstances**, such as a participant not following club policies or rules, or some other **unusual incident, injury, or medical emergency**.
2. These reports should include:
   a. **Detailed documentation** of the entire incident without speculative or opinionated information.
   b. Names and contact information of **involved participants and witnesses**.
   c. All **actions by staff** to resolve the problem or emergency situation.
   d. Any **follow-up action** required or taken.

X. EMERGENCY MANAGEMENT

Safe and effective management of an emergency situation will ensure the best care and protection for participants, staff, and facility. All plans must be specific and tailored to individual program needs and local standards. (For a sample plan for nonemergency and emergency situations, please refer to Appendix B, Tables B-1 through B-4 in *ACSM's Guidelines for Exercise Testing and Prescription*, 8th ed.)

A. EMERGENCY PLAN

1. **An emergency plan is mandatory** in all testing and exercise areas.
2. **The emergency plan must specify** the following:
   a. The specific responsibilities of each staff member.
   b. The methods to activate the emergency procedures.
   c. The required equipment.
   d. Predetermined contacts for emergency response and specific information to forward to appropriate medical personnel.
   e. A map of emergency exits, emergency equipment locations, phones, fire alarms, and fire extinguishers.
   f. Step-by-step actions to take for each common medical emergency (both life-threatening and non–life-threatening),

nonmedical emergency (e.g., flood, power outage, fire), and disaster (natural or man-made).

3. All emergency incidents must be documented with dates, times, actions, people involved, and outcomes.
4. The plan should be practiced, and staff attendance should be documented with both announced and unannounced drills, at a minimum, on a quarterly basis.

B. STAFF ROLE

The professional staff role during an emergency should include:

1. Control of the situation by implementing the emergency plan and taking charge.
2. Maintain order and calm, especially regarding the victim, and also the crowd.
3. Activate the EMS, if necessary.
4. Assure that proper documentation, follow-up, and review of the event occur.

C. STAFF TRAINING

All staff, including nonclinical staff, should be trained in the emergency plan and training should be documented.

1. Staff training includes in-services, safety plans, and emergency procedures.
2. In-services with physicians, nurses, and paramedics are especially recommended.
3. Review and update emergency plans, as necessary, including regularly scheduled drills.
4. Exercise staff should have training in the proper use of emergency equipment.
5. CPR and AED and first aid certification should be current in all staff. Basic life support is mandatory, and advanced cardiac life support is recommended for clinical staff.
6. Staff should be fully trained to recognize:
   a. Absolute and relative contraindications to exercise.
   b. Absolute and relative reasons for terminating an exercise test or exercise session.
7. A physician should be present or nearby in every clinical exercise test setting to assist with or manage emergencies.

XI. GENERAL EMERGENCY RESPONSE GUIDELINES

A. CONTACTS

1. Activating the EMS

a. This may entail calling a paramedic or ambulance group or an emergency medical team within the facility.

b. Information to communicate includes:
   1) Patient's location, including cross streets, and the telephone number.
   2) Patient's status, including vital signs.
   3) Symptoms and actions that led to the emergency.
   4) Actions of the exercise staff in caring for the patient after the onset of symptoms.

2. Communicating with a Physician or Other Appropriate Medical Professional

a. Report the signs and symptoms associated with the emergency, as well as the patient's status before the start of the test.
b. State the patient's current vital signs and symptoms.
c. Ask for recommendations.

3. Contacting the Patient's Family Physician

The patient's family physician should be contacted, particularly if a physician is not present at the facility.

a. Indicate to the family physician that a medical emergency has occurred with one of his or her patients.
b. Be prepared to report the symptoms associated with the emergency as well as the patient's status before the start of the test.
c. Present vital signs, current symptoms, and actions being taken (e.g., patient transported to the nearest emergency room).
d. Ask for recommendations.

4. Contacting the Patient's Family or Emergency Medical Contact

a. Explain the situation in whatever detail needed.
b. Indicate if the patient has been transported to a hospital or emergency department and how the family can find that location.
c. Give the family your name and contact information and assist the family in any other way possible.

B. INITIAL ACTIONS

1. Initial monitoring during a medical emergency should include:
   a. HR through palpation or ECG.
   b. Heart rhythm through ECG.
   c. BP.
   d. Respiration.
   e. Oxygen saturation if monitor available.
   f. Physical signs of complications, including:
      1) Loss of balance.
      2) Convulsion or seizure.

3) Shivering.
4) Cold, clammy skin.
5) Verbal and nonverbal expression of pain and description of location, type, and intensity of pain.

g. Blood glucose level in patients with diabetes.

2. First aid procedures should be initiated as indicated (*Table 7-2*).
3. After the patient is stabilized, he or she should be transported to a facility (e.g., hospital, medical center, physician's office) or department (e.g., emergency room) for appropriate treatment.

C. FOLLOW-UP ACTIONS

After an emergency incident, follow-up with the patient serves several purposes.

1. It clarifies the patient's current medical status, aiding in understanding the causes of the emergency.
2. It provides more information regarding the consequences of the staff's actions to help determine whether the response to the emergency was effective.
3. It allows the staff to finalize the incident report, with a final analysis of the patient's status (which may not be known until days after the incident).

D. DOCUMENTATION

1. Careful documentation of an emergency event provides important information for the safety of the patient, management of the program, and protection of the staff and facility.
2. Information should include:
   a. Time line of events.
   b. Names and contact information of all people involved, including witnesses.
   c. Actions taken by the staff to resolve the emergency situation.
   d. All communications with medical personnel, family, and other staff.
   e. Follow-up actions.

XII. INJURY PREVENTION

A. PREPARTICIPATION SCREENING

Preparticipation screening may uncover medical and physical risks to exercise. Standards for preactivity screening:

1. All facilities offering exercise equipment or other exercise programs and activities or services must offer a general preactivity cardiovascular screening to all new members and prospective users.
2. All specific preactivity screening tools must be interpreted by qualified staff and the results of the screening must be documented.
3. If a facility becomes aware that an individual has a known cardiovascular, metabolic, or pulmonary disease, that person must be advised to consult with a qualified healthcare provider before beginning a physical activity program.

   (For a complete list, please refer to Table 2-1 in *ACSM's Health/Fitness Facility Standards and Guidelines*, 3rd ed.)

B. IMPROVED FITNESS

1. Musculoskeletal fitness may reduce the risk of injury.
2. Physiologic fitness may help to prevent many chronic medical conditions.
3. All four components of fitness are important and should be a part of all fitness programs.
   a. Conditioning should be well balanced among cardiovascular, flexibility, strength, and endurance as well as throughout the muscle groups and major joints.
   b. The progression of exercise training should be gradual.
   c. Flexibility is an important component of fitness and may contribute to injury prevention.
   d. Warm-up and cool-down
      1) Prepares the body for exercise and safely returns the body to a resting state.
      2) May prevent complications (e.g., musculoskeletal injury, cardiac crisis, dizziness) that can result from immediate changes in exercise intensity.
   e. Rest
      1) Is an important part of conditioning.
      2) Can facilitate recovery from the stress of exercise.
      3) Can reduce the risk of injury.
      4) Includes rest between exercises and exercise sessions as well as that prescribed for acute injury.

C. PROPER INSTRUCTION

Proper instruction assists in decreasing injury risk and avoiding emergency situations.

D. EXERCISE CLOTHING AND EQUIPMENT

1. Gloves, helmets, protective glasses, and so on are important to safety during certain modes of exercise.
2. Clothing should fit properly and be layered to maintain warmth (in cold environments) or be appropriate for hot or humid environments.
3. Shoes must be appropriate for the exercise or sport.

TABLE 7-2. BASIC FIRST AID GUIDELINES FOR CARDIOPULMONARY AND METABOLIC CONDITIONS

CONDITION	FIRST AID PROCEDURES
Angina (pain, pressure or tingling in the chest, neck, jaw, arm, and/or back)	If individual develops new symptomatic chest pain: Stop activity; rest or sit in recumbent position. Check pulse and BP (and cardiac rhythm if appropriate). Activate EMS or evaluate by a physician. If unresponsive, check breathing and pulse; begin CPR if necessary. If patient suffers from chronic stable angina: Stop exercise and rest; give medication (if appropriate) and consult primary physician.
Bradycardia	Stop activity, assess vital signs, secure airway, ensure defibrillator is available. Activate EMS system.
Tachycardia	Stop activity, assess vital signs, secure airway, ensure defibrillator is available. Activate EMS system.
Cardiac Arrest	Assess responsiveness. If unresponsive activate EMS and get AED. Check ABCs. If no pulse and no breathing, perform CPR until defibrillator is attached. Operate AED to analyze and attempt defibrillation, if indicated (follow equipment manufacturer instructions). After one shock or after any "no shock indicated": Perform 2 minutes of CPR beginning with compressions.
Fainting (syncope)	Leave the victim lying down; elevate legs, if no injury is suspected. Maintain an open airway; turn victim on his or her side if vomiting occurs. Loosen any tight clothing. Take BP and pulse if possible. Seek medical attention, because this is a potentially life-threatening situation and the cause of fainting must be determined.
Hypoglycemia (symptoms include diaphoresis, pallor, tremor, tachycardia, palpitation, visual disturbances, mental confusion, weakness, light-headedness, fatigue, headache, memory loss, seizure, and coma)	Stop activity and check blood glucose levels. May become life-threatening; seek medical attention to treat cause. Give oral glucose solutions (e.g., Kool-Aid with sugar, nondiet soft drinks, juice); if patient is able to ingest solids, gelatin sweetened with sugar, candy, or fruit may be given.
Hyperglycemia (symptoms include dehydration, hypotension, reflex tachycardia, osmotic diuresis, impaired consciousness, nausea, vomiting, abdominal pain, hyperventilation, acetone odor on breath)	Stop activity and check blood glucose levels. Administer fluids if conscious; turn head to side if vomiting. May be life-threatening if it leads to diabetic ketoacidosis. Seek immediate medical attention. Rehydrate with intravenous normal saline. Correct electrolyte loss (K^+). Assist in administering insulin.
Dyspnea, labored breathing	Stop activity; maintain open airway. Help administer bronchodilator, if prescribed. Try pursed-lip breathing. If signs and symptoms persist, activate EMS.
Tachypnea	Stop activity; maintain open airway. If signs and symptoms persist, activate EMS.
Hyperventilation	Have the individual slow the rate of respiration and concentrate on breathing in through the nose and exhaling through the mouth; inhaling and exhaling through one nostril; or breathing slowly into a paper bag.
Asthma or bronchospasm	Preventative: Patient should avoid known irritants, and cold, dry, or polluted air. Stop activity; maintain open airway. Give bronchodilators via nebulizer if prescribed for patient. Give oxygen by nasal cannula if available. If signs and symptoms persist, activate EMS.
Hypotension/shock	Stop activity and remove patient from exercise area, if possible. Position in a supine position. Activate EMS. Elevate legs unless fracture, head, neck, or back injury is suspected. Maintain an open airway and normal body temperature. Monitor vital signs (pulse, blood pressure). Call for immediate advanced life support measures, because this is a life-threatening emergency that requires intensive monitoring of vital signs and administration of intravenous fluids and drugs to maintain adequate tissue perfusion during evaluation to determine the cause (e.g., hypovolemia, cardiogenic shock, sepsis).

ABC, airway, breathing, circulation; AED, automated external defibrillator; BP, blood pressure; EMS, emergency medical services.

TABLE 7-3. GENERAL INJURY CLASSIFICATIONS

INJURY	MAJOR SIGNS AND SYMPTOMS
Muscle	
Acute	
Contusions	Soft-tissue hemorrhage, hematoma, ecchymosis, movement restriction
Strains	Movement pain, local tenderness, loss of strength or ROM
Tendon injuries	Loss of strength or ROM; palpable defect
Muscle cramps/spasms	Involuntary muscle contraction; muscle pain
Acute-onset muscle soreness	Muscle pain, fatigue; resolves when exercise has ceased
Delayed-onset muscle soreness	Muscle stiffness 24 to 48 hours after exercise; tenderness and pain.
Chronic	
Myositis/fasciitis	Local swelling and tenderness
Tendonitis	Gradual onset, diffuse or localized tenderness and swelling, pain, loss of strength
Tenosynovitis	Crepitus, diffuse swelling, pain
Bursitis	Swelling, pain, some loss of function
Joint	
Acute	
Sprains	Swelling, pain, joint instability, loss of function
Acute joint synovitis	Pain during motion, swelling, pain
Subluxation/dislocation	Loss of limb function, deformity, swelling, point tenderness
Chronic	
Osteochondrosis	Joint locking, swelling, pain, disability
Osteoarthritis	Pain, articular crepitus, stiffness, reduced ROM
Capsulitis/synovitis	Joint edema, reduced ROM, joint crepitus
Bone	
Periostitis	Pain over bone, especially under pressure
Acute fracture	Deformity, bone point tenderness, swelling and ecchymosis
Stress fracture	Vague pain that persists when attempting activity; point tenderness

ROM, range of motion.

E. HYDRATION

1. Hydration is not always appropriately driven by thirst.
2. Hydrate adequately before, during, and after exercise.
3. May need to adjust hydration, carbohydrate, and electrolyte intake based on environmental conditions and length of exercise session.

XIII. CONTRAINDICATIONS TO EXERCISE TESTING AND TRAINING

For certain individuals, the risks for complications during exercise testing and training outweigh the potential benefits.

A. Identifying an individual's contraindications to exercise testing and training (*Table 6-1*) involves:
   1. Reviewing the medical history.
   2. Assessing cardiac risk.
   3. Evaluating physical examination findings.
   4. Evaluating laboratory test results.

B. Persons with absolute contraindications should not undergo exercise testing or training until those conditions are stabilized and they are cleared by their physician.

C. A person with relative contraindications may undergo exercise testing and training only after careful analysis by a physician of his or her risk-to-benefit ratio.

D. In rare cases, clinical exercise testing may still be performed for a patient with contraindications to guide drug therapy.

XIV. MUSCULOSKELETAL INJURIES

The incidence of exercise-related injury varies, depending on the type of activity (weight-bearing versus non–weight-bearing), frequency, intensity, and duration of exercise. The risk of musculoskeletal injury increases for all levels of participation with increasing physical activity, intensity, and duration of training (*Table 7-3*).

A. RISK FACTORS

1. Extrinsic Factors

a. Excessive load.

b. Training errors.
   1) Poor technique.
   2) Excessive stress on joints.
   3) Spine not in a neutral position.

c. Adverse environmental conditions.

d. Faulty equipment, clothing, or footwear.

e. Overtraining (overuse) signs and symptoms.
   1) Decline in performance.

2) Chronic fatigue and muscle soreness.
3) Increased submaximal heart rate.
4) Sleep disturbances.
5) Overuse injuries.
6) Prolonged recovery from typical training sessions or events.

f. Exercise or playing surface.
g. Skill level.
h. Level of competition.

2. Intrinsic Factors

a. Fitness level.
b. Body composition.
c. Anatomic abnormalities or alignment.
d. Gender.
e. Age.
f. Previous injury.
g. Disease.
h. Restricted range of motion.
i. Muscle weakness and imbalance.
j. Joint or ligamentous laxity.

3. High-Risk Stretches

a. Standing toe touch.
b. Barré stretch.
c. Hurdler's stretch.
d. Full neck circles.
e. Knee hyperflexion.
f. Yoga plough.

B. BASIC PRINCIPLES OF PRE- AND POSTINJURY CARE FOR MUSCULOSKELETAL INJURIES

1. Objectives are to **decrease pain, reduce swelling, and prevent further injury and loss of function.**
2. Objectives usually can be met by:
   a. "RICES": Rest, Ice, Compression, Elevation, and Stabilization.
      1) **Rest** prevents further injury and ensures initiation of the healing process.
      2) **Ice** reduces swelling, bleeding, inflammation, and pain.
      3) **Compression** reduces swelling and bleeding.
      4) **Elevation** decreases blood flow, controls edema, and increases venous return.
      5) **Stabilization** reduces muscle spasm in the injured area by assisting in the relaxation of associated muscles.
   b. Heat
      1) Is used to relieve pain and muscle spasms and increase blood flow.
      2) Should not be applied during the acute inflammatory phase.
   c. Splints or Casts
      1) May be used to immobilize the area and improve healing.
      2) Immobilization is used primarily for fractures and severe sprains.
   d. Medications
      1) May be used to reduce swelling and inflammation.
      2) May be used to treat the pain associated with swelling.
   e. Care of Low Back Injury
      1) Neutral spine during exercise (pain-free).
      2) Aerobic exercise.
      3) Unloaded flexion and extension of spine (cat stretch).
      4) Single leg extension holds.
      5) Abdominal curl-ups.
      6) Horizontal isometric side support.
      7) Low weight, high repetitions to emphasize muscular endurance.
   f. Ergonomics
      Improper workplace ergonomics can place stress on various joints and muscles, which may contribute to postural imbalances. Some work station areas that can be addressed are:
      1) Seat height, depth; knee, hip, and feet position; and arm rest placement.
      2) Keyboard height and mouse placement.
      3) Computer monitor distance and height.
      4) Document placement.

XV. OTHER MEDICAL EMERGENCIES AND ASSOCIATED TREATMENT

Serious complications rarely occur during an exercise session. When complications do occur, however, the exercise staff must be prepared to take appropriate action (*Tables* 7-2 and 7-4).

A. HEAT EXHAUSTION AND HEAT STROKE

1. Move patient to a cool or shaded area.
2. Administer chilled fluids and electrolytes, if the patient is conscious.
3. Have the patient lie down.
4. Elevate the feet.
5. Remove excess clothing.
6. Cool with water (externally). Fan the patient.
7. Seek immediate medical attention.

B. FAINTING

1. Place the patient in the supine position, with the feet elevated above the head if no injury is suspected.
2. Maintain an open airway.
3. Administer fluids if conscious.
4. Loosen tight clothing.
5. Take BP and HR, if possible.

TABLE 7-4. FIRST AID GUIDELINES FOR COMMON INJURIES AND ENVIRONMENTAL EMERGENCIES

INJURY OR EMERGENCY	SIGNS AND SYMPTOMS	FIRST AID
Common Musculoskeletal and Skin Injuries		Calm and reassure the individual; monitor for signs of shock.
Closed skin wounds (blisters, corns)	Pain, swelling, infection	Clean with antiseptic soap; apply sterile dressing, antibiotic ointment.
Open skin wounds (lacerations, abrasions, incisions, puncture wounds)	Pain, redness, bleeding, swelling, headache, mild fever	Apply direct pressure to stop bleeding; clean with soap or sterile saline; apply sterile dressing to protect from contamination and infection; if bleeding continues, apply more pressure and dressings and elevate limb (if no fracture is suspected); refer to physician for stitches or tetanus shot. Remind individual to watch for signs of infection, keep the area clean and dry, and change dressing as needed.
Contusions (bruises)	Swelling, localized pain, loss of function if severe	RICES; apply padding for protection if necessary.
Strains[a]		
Grade I	Pain, localized tenderness, tightness	RICES.
Grade II	Loss of function, hemorrhage	RICES; refer for physician evaluation if victim has impaired function.
Grade III	Palpable defect	Immobilization; RICES; immediate referral to physician.
Sprains[a]		
Grade I	Pain, point tenderness, strength loss, edema	RICES.
Grade II	Hemorrhage, measurable laxity	RICES; physician evaluation.
Grade III	Palpable or observable defect	Immobilization; RICES; immediate referral to physician.
Fractures		
Stress	Pain, point tenderness	Physician evaluation; rest.
Simple	Swelling, disability, pain	Immobilize with splint; physician evaluation; radiography.
Compound	Bleeding, swelling, pain, disability	Immobilize; control bleeding; apply sterile dressing; immediate physician evaluation.
Environmental and Exercise Intolerance Conditions		
Dehydration	No early symptoms; fatigue; weakness; dry mouth; loss of work capacity; increased response time.	Drink water; fluid and salt replacement. Can occur in warm or cool conditions.
Hypothermia	Shivering, but may stop with extreme drops in core temperature; loss of coordination; muscle stiffness; fatigue or drowsiness; lethargy	Move to a warm area. Activate the EMS, and transport to hospital; remove wet clothing, and replace with dry, warm clothing, encourage drinking hot liquids.
Frost bite	Burning sensation at first; coldness; numbness; tingling. Skin color white or grayish, yellow to reddish violet to black.	Move to a warm area and remove wet clothing. Check ABCs; monitor vital signs; care for shock. Drink warm carbohydrate-containing fluids if conscious. External warming; treat as a burn (cover affected area with dry sterile dressings). **Do not rewarm frostbitten area if there is a danger of refreezing. Do NOT rub affected area.** Activate EMS or transport to the hospital.
Hyperthermia		
Heat cramps	Acute, painful, involuntary muscle spasms	Stop activity; rest in a cool environment; administer fluids; stretch or massage cramp.
Heat syncope	Weakness, fatigue, hypotension, pale skin, syncope	Move to cool area; place in a supine position with legs elevated; administer fluids if conscious; check blood pressure.
Heat exhaustion	Profuse sweating, cold and clammy skin, multiple muscle spasms, headache, nausea, loss of consciousness, dizziness, tachycardia, insecure gait, low blood pressure; body temperature normal to slightly increased.	Move to cool area; remove excess clothing and cool if body temperature is elevated; place supine, with feet elevated; administer fluids, monitor vitals and body temperature; refer for physician evaluation. **Activate EMS if rapid improvement is absent.**
Heat stroke	Hot and dry skin, but can be sweating; dyspnea; confusion; often unconscious. Can result in death.	**Activate the EMS, and transport to hospital immediately.** Remove clothing, dowse with cool water and fan; wrap in cool, wet sheets; administer fluids if conscious; cease cooling when core temperature reaches approximately 101°F.
Hyponatremia (relatively rare)	Disorientation, confusion, headache, vomiting, lethargy, swelling of hands and feet. Can result in death.	**Activate the EMS, and transport to hospital immediately.** Do not administer fluids unless instructed by a physician.

[a] Signs and symptoms for each grade include those for the grade below the one listed (i.e., signs and symptoms of grade II also include those of grade I, and signs and symptoms of grade III include those of grades I and II).

ABC, airway, breathing, circulation; CPR, cardiopulmonary resuscitation; EMS, emergency medical system; RICES: rest, ice, compression, elevation, stabilization.

(Parts of table modified from ACSM's *Resource Manual for Guidelines for Exercise Testing and Prescription, 2nd ed.* Baltimore, Lippincott Williams & Wilkins, 2006.)

6. Seek medical attention if the patient remains unconscious.
7. Check blood sugar if monitor is available and patient does not respond immediately, especially if diabetic.

C. SIMPLE AND COMPOUND FRACTURES

1. Immobilize and splint the extremity.
2. Seek immediate medical attention.

D. SEIZURE

1. Do not restrain the person during convulsions.
2. Attempt to ensure safety by seeing that the person does not injure herself or himself.
   a. Remove surrounding objects with which the patient may come into contact, resulting in injury.
   b. Place a cushion (towel or pad) under the head to avoid additional trauma.
3. Roll patient to side once seizure ends.
4. Seek medical attention.

E. BLEEDING

1. Follow precautions regarding bloodborne pathogens.
2. Using a sterile dressing, apply direct pressure over the site to stop the bleeding.
   a. Apply additional dressing and pressure if bleeding continues.
   b. Do not remove blood-soaked dressings.
3. Protect the wound from contamination.
4. Elevate the injured area if necessary to control bleeding.
5. Seek medical attention if stitches may be required.

F. SUDDEN CARDIAC ARREST

Incidence is 0.4 in 10,000 clinical exercise tests.

1. Signs and Symptoms

a. Loss of consciousness.
b. Rapid onset of fatigue.
c. Ventricular tachycardia with or without pulse or breathing.
d. Ventricular fibrillation.
e. Patient may have chest pain or other symptoms before cardiac arrest.

2. Response

a. **If the patient is breathing and has a pulse:**
   1) Call the EMS immediately and get AED.
   2) Place the individual in the recovery position (prone, with one knee and hip slightly flexed) with the head to one side to avoid airway obstruction. **Do not attempt this position with patients who have suspected cervical spine injury.**
   3) Stay with the person, and continue to monitor his or her vital signs.
b. **If the patient is suspected of not breathing or having a pulse:**
   1) Assess airway, breathing, and pulse.
   2) Call the EMS or code team and call for crash cart with defibrillator and AED.
   3) Perform CPR, as appropriate, depending on presence of breathing and a pulse until an AED is available.
   4) Defibrillate shockable rhythms, and continue CPR as needed.
   5) Assist the medical staff or EMS in caring for the patient.

G. MYOCARDIAL INFARCTION (MI)

An MI is ischemic myocardial necrosis resulting from an abrupt reduction in blood flow to the myocardium. Reduced blood flow often results from arterial plaque buildup that occludes the coronary arteries.

1. Signs and Symptoms

a. Visceral pain described as pressure or aching that radiates down the left arm, chest, back, or jaw (angina).
b. Gastrointestinal upset.
c. Dyspnea or shortness of breath.
d. Shock.
e. Ventricular fibrillation.
f. Bradycardia.
g. Cool, clammy skin.
h. Nausea and vomiting.

2. Response

a. Terminate exercise immediately, place in seated or supine position (whichever is most comfortable).
b. Start physician evaluation if in clinical setting or call EMS.
c. If chest pain is not relieved immediately, give a nitroglycerin and oxygen per ACLS protocol in clinical setting.
d. Monitor HR and BP.
e. Assist as needed with the administration of medications and equipment or supply setup.
f. Stay with the patient, and continue to monitor his or her vital signs.
g. Be prepared to begin CPR, or employ the AED or defibrillator if rhythm is shockable.

H. HYPERGLYCEMIA

Hyperglycemia is an abnormally high blood glucose level (>300 mg/dL) that can impair function and, if severe, can become an emergency situation (diabetic ketoacidosis).

1. **Signs and Symptoms**
   a. Confusion and weakness.
   b. Headache.
   c. Sweet, fruity breath odor.
   d. Thirst.
   e. Nausea and vomiting.
   f. Reflex tachycardia.
   g. Abdominal tenderness.
   h. Hyperventilation.

2. **Response**
   a. Call the EMS.
   b. Check blood glucose level.
   c. Rehydrate and correct electrolyte loss through fluid administration.
   d. Assist patient or physician or nurse in administering insulin.
   e. Turn the patient's head to one side if he or she is vomiting.

I. TRANSIENT ISCHEMIC ATTACK OR STROKE

Transient ischemic attacks (sudden, brief ischemic attacks) are caused by a lack of oxygen to the brain owing to a blockage in the carotid, neck or cerebral artery.

1. **Signs and Symptoms**
   a. Confusion.
   b. Pain in jaw or neck.
   c. Severe headache.
   d. loss of vision and voluntary movement.
   e. Loss of coordination.
   f. Facial drop.
   g. Slight paralysis of one side (hemiparesis).
   h. Difficulty speaking (aphasia).
   i. Burning or tingling sensation in extremities.
   j. Fatigue.

2. **Response**
   a. Stop exercise immediately.
   b. Have the person sit or lie down.
   c. Contact the physician or EMS.
   d. Monitor vitals, give oxygen if hypoxic (clinical setting).
   e. Establish time of onset of symptoms if possible.

J. INTERNAL CARDIAC DEFIBRILLATOR DISCHARGE

Internal cardiac defibrillators (ICD) are implanted devices that defibrillate life-threatening arrhythmias. If a device discharges, the patient should immediately stop exercise and be placed in a supine position and monitored for signs and symptoms.

1. **Signs and Symptoms**
   a. Severe, sudden chest pain.
   b. Dyspnea.
   c. Muscle contractions in the chest or abdomen associated with discharge.
   d. Loss of consciousness.
   e. Abnormal heart rhythm (ventricular tachycardia or fibrillation).
   f. Cardiac arrest if the defibrillator fails to discharge or convert the rhythm.

2. **Response**
   a. If the patient is stable (appropriate HR, BP, and heart rhythm) following device discharge, contact the physician for recommendations.
   b. If the patient is experiencing multiple discharges or is unstable, call the EMS or the physician immediately.
   c. Place the patient in the recovery position, with the head turned to one side.
   d. Stay with the patient, and monitor his or her vital signs.
   e. **If on assessment the patient is not breathing or does not have a palpable pulse:**
      1) Perform CPR. However, avoid pressure or contact within the area of defibrillator application. **Note:** It is not harmful to be touching a patient when an ICD discharges, but rescuers may feel a tingle when the ICD discharges.
      2) If an ICD fails, an AED or manual defibrillator should be used to convert pulseless ventricular tachycardia or ventricular fibrillation. Care should be taken to avoid placement of paddles over the ICD.

   Note: For a variety of reasons an ICD may discharge when it should not. However, the device must be analyzed by a physician or nurse to know whether or not the ICD is appropriately firing. Whenever an ICD discharges, it should be assumed that the patient has had a life-threatening arrhythmia.

K. SERIOUS ARRHYTHMIAS

1. Various arrhythmias can develop during exercise testing and training. Those considered to be serious and that require emergency attention include:
   a. **Ventricular fibrillation.**
   b. **Ventricular tachycardia.**
   c. **Atrial fibrillation** or atrial flutter.
   d. **Supraventricular tachycardia.**
   e. **Severe or symptomatic bradycardia.**

2. Response

The most severe arrhythmias (ventricular tachycardia, ventricular fibrillation) may be a result of an MI and require defibrillation to control.

a. Stop activity.
b. Maintain airway, check vital signs, give oxygen, and identify rhythm.
c. Check for signs of poor perfusion, activate EMS, physician, or code team if appropriate.
d. Be prepared to shock or start CPR if necessary.

L. HYPOGLYCEMIA

Actual blood glucose levels that elicit hypoglycemic symptoms are highly individualized. Generally, however, levels of <80 mg/dL or a rapid drop in glucose may be problematic. However, patients may have symptomatic hypoglycemia at higher blood sugar levels. (For a complete list, please refer to Table 9-2 in *ACSM's Guidelines for Exercise Testing and Prescription*, 8th ed.)

1. Signs and Symptoms

a. Tremors.
b. Tachycardia.
c. Diaphoresis.
d. Visual disturbances.
e. Confusion.
f. Headache.
g. Fatigue.
h. Light-headedness.
i. Convulsions or seizures.
j. Excessive hunger.

2. Response to a Hypoglycemic Emergency

a. If a glucose monitor is available, check blood sugar.
b. If blood sugar is low or no equipment is available to check glucose and patient is a diabetic, immediately give the patient an **oral glucose solution** (e.g., orange juice, nondiet soft drink, sugar packet or glucose gel tube or tablets) if conscious. If unconscious, use sugar granules or glucose gel.
c. Monitor the patient's signs and symptoms, and blood glucose.
d. If the patient is unable to ingest oral glucose, becomes unstable or unresponsive, or if blood sugars do not respond to oral glucose, contact EMS and the physician immediately.
e. Keep the patient comfortable and safe.

M. BRONCHOSPASM

Bronchospasm is an obstruction of the airway caused by spasm of airway smooth muscle, edema of airway mucosa, increased mucus secretion, or injury.

1. Signs and Symptoms

a. Dyspnea.
b. Hyperventilation.
c. Coughing.
d. Wheezing.
e. Chest tightness.
f. Dizziness.

2. Response

a. Stop activity.
b. Maintain an open airway.
c. Assist in administering a bronchodilator if prescribed by a physician. Try pursed lip breathing if no relief.
d. Help in administering oxygen if available.
e. Monitor vitals, including oxygen saturation.
f. Replace fluids and electrolytes.
g. Keep the patient calm to reduce his or her anxiety.
h. If signs and symptoms persist, activate EMS or physician.

N. HYPOTENSION AND SHOCK

When blood pressure becomes so low that perfusion is affected, the patient will become symptomatic. In most exercise settings, if treated promptly, hypotension will resolve quickly.

1. Signs and Symptoms

a. Chills.
b. Syncope or loss of consciousness.
c. Bradycardia.
d. Dizziness.
e. Confusion.

2. Response

a. Stop activity.
b. Have the patient lie supine with the feet elevated, if no injury is suspected.
c. Maintain an open airway and assess vitals.
d. Monitor vital signs, and maintain normal body temperature. If the patient is conscious, give oral fluids.
e. Activate EMS or alert physician if symptoms do not resolve quickly and BP does not improve. In patients with hypotension, the cause of the hypotension should be determined so it can be treated (e.g. dehydration, postexercise hypotension).

XVI. COMMON CATEGORY I MEDICATIONS ADMINISTERED IN MEDICAL EMERGENCIES

For a complete list of medications, please refer to Appendix A, Table A-1 in *ACSM's Guidelines for Exercise Testing and Prescription, 8th edition.*

A. **Epinephrine** is an endogenous catecholamine that optimizes blood flow to the heart and brain by increasing aortic diastolic pressure and preferentially shunting blood to the internal carotid artery (enhancing cerebral blood flow).
B. **Lidocaine or amiodarone** is an antiarrhythmic agent that decreases automaticity in the ventricular myocardium.
C. **Oxygen** ensures adequate arterial oxygen content and greatly enhances tissue oxygenation.
D. **Atropine** is a parasympathetic blocking agent used in the treatment of bradyarrhythmias.

Review Test

DIRECTIONS: Carefully read all questions, and select the BEST single answer.

1. The clinical exercise physiologist shares a responsibility to
   A) Implement measures to stop disease.
   B) Make patients look healthy.
   C) Implement preventive measures to reduce the risk of medical emergencies.
   D) Develop a plan to reduce the physical demands of exercise testing.

2. Which of the following is NOT considered to be a benefit of follow-up in an emergency situation?
   A) It provides information regarding the patient's current status, which may help to determine the cause of the emergency.
   B) It provides statistics that will help to justify the emergency response program.
   C) It allows the staff to finalize the incident report.
   D) It provides information to determine the consequences of the staff's actions.

3. Which of the following actions involving termination of exercise testing is correct?
   A) Immediately terminate the test if muscular fatigue occurs.
   B) Initiate the test termination process when cardiac complications occur.
   C) Initiate the test termination process when intermittent premature ventricular contractions are detected on ECG.
   D) Immediately terminate the test when intermittent premature ventricular contractions are detected on ECG without an active cool-down.

4. Safety procedures for clinical staff help protect them from
   A) Bloodborne pathogens.
   B) Theft.
   C) Violent patients.
   D) Work-related injuries.

5. The treatment modality RICES includes all of the following EXCEPT
   A) Covering.
   B) Ice.
   C) Stabilization.
   D) Rest.

6. Which of the following statements about emergency equipment is MOST important?
   A) Each piece of equipment should be painted a specific color for easy identification.
   B) Use of emergency equipment should be practiced routinely.
   C) Emergency equipment should include pencils, not pens.
   D) Emergency equipment should be kept clean at all times.

7. Identifying a patient's risk of complications is important. Which of the following is NOT considered to be a common aspect of the risk identification process?
   A) Laboratory results.
   B) Assessment of cardiac risk.
   C) Review of medical history.
   D) Assessment of work history.

8. Symptoms of hyperglycemia include all of the following EXCEPT
   A) Acetone odor on breath.
   B) Confusion.
   C) Bradycardia.
   D) Slurred speech.

9. Emergency procedures and safety include which of the following?
   A) Injury prevention.
   B) Basic principles for exercise training.
   C) Metabolic injuries.
   D) Emergency consequences.

10. Category 1 medications include all of the following EXCEPT
    A) Lidocaine.
    B) Oxygen.
    C) Xylocaine.
    D) Epinephrine.

11. The emergency response system (EMS) is:
    A) A combination of the ambulance and the emergency room.
    B) Critical for the staff to be able to respond adequately to an emergency.
    C) The protocol used to practice safety plans.
    D) Required by most health departments.

12. In developing an emergency plan, program administrators must take into account all of the following factors EXCEPT
    A) Type of flooring.
    B) Type of electrical wiring.
    C) Ventilation, temperature, and humidity.
    D) Types of exercise equipment.

13. Documentation in the context of emergency response commonly refers to
    A) Records of each exercise session.
    B) Records of attendance.
    C) Records of all emergency situations.
    D) Manuals for all emergency equipment.

14. A patient who exhibits tachycardia, diaphoresis, light-headedness, and visual disturbances may be experiencing
    A) Hypoglycemia.
    B) Congestive heart failure.
    C) Hyperglycemia.
    D) Hypotension.

15. Which of the following is NOT part of an emergency plan?
    A) The plan should list the schedule of each staff member so that they can all be accounted for during an emergency.
    B) The plan must be written.
    C) The plan should outline each specific action.
    D) The staff should be prepared and trained in the plan.

16. The physician's role in an emergency plan is
    A) Not important, because most facilities are hospital-based and the emergency room is nearby.
    B) Not significant, because a physician is not necessary when testing is conducted.
    C) Optional, depending on feasibility.
    D) Critical, because the physician must be available to handle emergency situations.

17. What is OSHA?
    A) A state agency that licenses medical facilities.
    B) A federal agency that sets standards for staff and patient safety.
    C) An agency that certifies a managed care organization.
    D) A state agency that inspects emergency protocols within medical facilities.

18. The preparation of professional staff should include training in
    A) Advanced basic life support and ENT.
    B) CPR and AED and basic life support.
    C) CPR and AED and EMS.
    D) Advanced cardiac life support and ENT.

19. Which of the following is NOT considered to be an absolute contraindication to exercise testing?
    A) Unstable angina.
    B) Psychosis.
    C) Suspected myocarditis.
    D) Moderate valvular heart disease.

20. Which of the following manifestations is NOT an indication for stopping an exercise test?
    A) Subject requests to stop.
    B) Diastolic BP >115 mm Hg.
    C) Intermittent premature ventricular contractions.
    D) Failure of testing equipment.

21. Serious complications during an exercise session
    A) Occur more often with women.
    B) Rarely occur.
    C) Occur at a rate of 1 in 3,000 hours of exercise.
    D) Occur more often during the late hours because of client fatigue.

22. The exercise staff's role when an injury or emergency occurs should be to:
    A) Control the situation by implementing the emergency plan and taking charge.
    B) Find someone to implement the emergency plan.
    C) Get everyone out of the facility to avoid chaos.
    D) Hope that an emergency contact is available to help with the situation.

23. In preventing injuries, hydration is very important, because
    A) It controls breathing and the Valsalva maneuver.
    B) It helps to regulate carbohydrate utilization during cardiovascular exercise.
    C) It helps to regulate body temperature and electrolyte balance.
    D) It helps to prevent blood pooling during the cool-down.

24. What US legislation is critical for operators of fitness facilities to understand and adhere to regarding safety?
    A) The Americans with Handicaps Act.
    B) The Civil Rights Act of 1966.
    C) The Health Portability Act of 1996.
    D) The Americans with Disabilities Act.

25. What is the most appropriate action in assisting a person having a seizure?
    A) Hold the person down so that he or she does not hurt himself or herself.
    B) Do not restrain the person, but be sure that he or she is in a safe area.
    C) Place a wedge in the person's mouth so that he or she does not swallow the tongue.
    D) Ignore the person, and allow the seizure to pass.

26. One of the **first** actions that an exercise professional should consider in preventing injury is to
    A) Teach the individual how to warm-up and cool-down.
    B) Instruct the person on safety procedures when using the facility.
    C) Conduct a preparticipation screening.

D) Instruct the individual on how to use the exercise equipment safely.

27. How should an exercise professional advise a person with regard to progression of the exercise program?
A) The progression should be gradual and slow.
B) The progression should be at specific increments based on a calendar schedule (e.g., add 10% every 2 weeks).
C) Be aggressive in increasing the program to increase fitness.
D) The program should progress only when the participant feels ready.

28. How can exercise equipment add to the risk of participation?
A) Because it is expensive.
B) Because it is hard to move.
C) Because it is used incorrectly.
D) Because of the time having to wait to use it.

29. Prevention strategies to reduce the risk of injury of staff and clients must include
A) Following the rules and policies.
B) Keeping the equipment clean.
C) Hiring good front-desk staff.
D) Developing clever, unique programs.

30. An equipment maintenance plan should include
A) A floor plan.
B) A participant advisory statement.
C) A document that records maintenance and repair history.
D) Temperature and humidity readings.

31. In cleaning the facility and equipment, of what must an operator be aware?
A) That signs are written clearly.
B) That surfaces are brightly colored.
C) That solutions and cleaning materials are safe for the skin and hypoallergenic.
D) That disinfectants smell pleasant.

32. Which of the following are symptoms of heat exhaustion?
A) Hypotension.
B) Hot dry skin.
C) Bradycardia and low body temperature.
D) Bronchospasms and hyperventilation.

33. RICES refers to
A) Relaxation, Ice, Compression, Energy, and Stabilization.
B) Relaxation, Incremental heat, Care for injury, Energy, and Standardization.
C) Rest, Ice, Common sense, Energy, and Standardization.
D) Rest, Ice, Compression, Elevation, and Stabilization.

34. Complaints of pain in the chest with associated pain radiating down the left arm may be signs of
A) Cardiac crisis.
B) Hypotension.
C) Seizure.
D) Heartburn.

35. Beyond the general safety parameters, such as keeping equipment in good repair, a facility must create a safe environment for any individual, especially
A) Guest participants.
B) Staff.
C) Healthcare providers.
D) Special populations.

36. Weight room safety should include
A) A phone.
B) Lifting gloves and back belts.
C) Male trainers to help with spotting.
D) Safe passageways and use of the buddy system.

37. Fire, bloodborne pathogens, and power outage should all be included in
A) Facility insurance.
B) Safety plans.
C) Maintenance plans.
D) Testing by the facility and staff.

38. The potential benefits and risks of an exercise test should be written in what document?
A) Description of services.
B) Safety plan.
C) Informed consent.
D) Exercise waivers.

39. Documentation offers important
A) Liability and negligence protection.
B) Liability and risk protection.
C) Safety and communication programs.
D) Billing and classification tools.

40. Emergency procedures should be
A) Given to all who join the facility.
B) Put away in a safe place.
C) Posted under each phone.
D) Posted above each fire extinguisher.

41. Which of the following is NOT a principle of low back care?
A) Abdominal curl-ups.
B) Unloaded flexion or extension of the spine.
C) Neutral spine during all exercises.
D) Controlled leg press or squat with light weights.

42. What is the exercise professional's primary responsibility in conducting an exercise test?
A) Maintaining a safe environment by not putting the person being tested in danger.
B) Making sure that the data collected are accurate.
C) Completing the test.
D) Encouragement and support.

43. What are some of the risks for musculoskeletal injury?
    A) Poor signage in the facility.
    B) Extrinsic factors: intensity, terrain, equipment.
    C) Intrinsic factors: frequency, attitude, gender.
    D) Membership type.

44. Chronic soreness and fatigue are symptoms of
    A) Hyperglycemia.
    B) Strain.
    C) Overuse injury.
    D) Hypoglycemia.

45. Exercise clothing
    A) Creates an important fashion statement.
    B) Should be bright so that you are easily seen in an aerobics class.
    C) Has only one rule: be comfortable.
    D) Must be safe and perform appropriately, like the exercise equipment.

ANSWERS AND EXPLANATIONS

1–C. The clinical exercise physiologist must understand the risks of exercise while realizing the benefits. If the benefits clearly outweigh the risks, preventive measures should be implemented to reduce that risk. The clinical exercise physiologist cannot eradicate or cure disease; he or she can only work to help prevent or reduce the symptoms of disease. The clinical exercise physiologist is concerned with the patient's health, not with the patient's appearance.

2–B. The follow-up is an important function following an incident. Justification of a program has no relevance when investigating an incident. The primary concern should be the health status of the patient and the cause of the emergency. The patient's present status is, indeed, part of the follow-up, because it will provide medical information that can help to determine the cause of injury. Also, information from the patient can help to piece together the specific actions of the incident. In addition, this follow-up information will help staff members to complete their report, because they may learn new and helpful information that should be included. The final report with the follow-up information will assist program administrators in determining the consequences of their actions.

3–C. Intermittent premature ventricular contractions (PVCs) are not a serious concern, so the tester can begin the test termination process instead of terminating the test immediately. Muscular fatigue and intermittent PVCs do not require immediate termination of the test; initiating the test termination process is appropriate. Cardiac complications are considered to be very serious and require immediate termination, not merely initiation of the test termination process.

4–A. Because of the importance of infection control, bloodborne pathogens must be a concern for all staff, and OSHA regulations help to protect both patients and staff. Theft and violent patients may be concerns but are not part of any emergency plan. The plan may include injuries in general but not work-related injuries specifically.

5–A. Covering is not part of RICES. Compression is the "C" component.

6–B. Routine practice in using emergency equipment is an important part of the emergency plan to ensure that staff members know how to use the equipment correctly in an emergency situation. Identification of equipment through tagging, not color, is important. Whether to use pens or pencils is irrelevant, and although equipment should be kept clean, this is not an essential part of emergency equipment protocol.

7–D. Work history is not a relevant part of the identification process. Work history most likely will not provide any meaningful information regarding the risk of medical emergencies. The review of medical history is very important and can identify significant cardiac risk factors. Assessment of laboratory results may indicate signs of potential cardiac or pulmonary risk, which could contraindicate exercise testing. Assessment of cardiac risk is critical to the determination of potential complications and clearly is part of the identification process.

8–C. Tachycardia, not bradycardia, is a possible sign of hyperglycemia. Elevated blood sugar overloads the endocrine system; confusion and slurred speech are common responses to this overload. Acetone or sweet odor of the breath is a common sign of hyperglycemia owing to the elevated levels of glucose in the system.

9–A. Injury prevention often is overlooked, but it is an important part of a facility's emergency procedures and safety program. All exercise professionals should understand how to avoid emergencies. Basic principles for exercise training are important for general day-to-day operations but not for emergency procedures.

10–C. Xylocaine, although similar to lidocaine, is not an antiarrhythmic agent, but lidocaine is. Thus, Xylocaine cannot help to stabilize the heart in a cardiac crisis. Oxygen often is overlooked as a drug, but it helps to keep tissues alive. Epinephrine optimizes blood flow to the heart and brain and is an important category 1 medication.

11–B. The emergency response system is designed to help the staff adequately handle emergencies. The ambulance and emergency room as well as the protocols used to practice safety procedures may be a part of an emergency response plan, but they are not part of the emergency response system. Health departments do not regulate emergency response systems.

12–D. Flooring and electrical wiring are important factors in the risk of accidents. Environmental factors can increase the risk of crises; for example, poor air quality, high temperatures, and high humidity can cause pulmonary difficulties and increase the risk of heat exhaustion.

13–C. Documentation of every aspect of an emergency situation is an important component of any emergency response system. Records of exercise sessions and attendance may be important for standard operations, but they are not important for emergency response. Equipment manuals should be on file, but are not considered to be documentation in this context.

14–A. Common signs and symptoms of hypoglycemia include tachycardia, diaphoresis, lightheadedness, and visual disturbances. Congestive heart failure and hypotension do not produce tachycardia. Hyperglycemia does not produce diaphoresis.

15–A. Accounting for staff in an emergency is not essential. Writing down the plan is essential so that the staff can read it as part of their training as well as have a document to refer to during an emergency. Delineating specific actions by each staff member in an emergency situation and training the staff in these actions obviously are integral parts of any emergency plan.

16–D. Communication with the physician is very important during a medical crisis, and exercise staff should have a ready means of communicating with a physician in the event of an emergency. A physician should be nearby, but not necessarily in the room, during any exercise test.

17–B. OSHA is a federal agency that sets safety standards for staff and patients. The National Committee for Quality Assurance (NCQA) is an accreditation agency that inspects and certifies MCOs.

18–B. CPR and AED and basic life support are important certifications in the care of medical emergencies. There is no advanced basic life support certification. Neither EMS nor ENT are appropriate emergency care training for exercise staff.

19–D. Individuals with moderate valvular heart disease are able to function under the stress of exercise, especially if they are under the care of a cardiac specialist and receive permission to undergo an exercise test. Unstable angina may lead to a significant cardiac crisis when exercise is introduced, so it is considered to be an absolute contraindication with exercise. Psychosis is a significant emotional distress and can lead to difficulties in completing the exercise test, so it is considered to be an absolute contraindication. Myocarditis is an absolute contraindication of exercise testing, because inflammation of the heart's muscular walls can cause severe cardiac complications with the increased stroke volume and HR associated with the stress of exercise.

20–C. Intermittent PVCs do not pose a danger to an exerciser, so the test should not be halted. The exercise specialist must be able to accurately measure workload, blood pressure, and HR response to exercise. Thus, an exercise test should always be stopped if any of the equipment fails to operate. In addition, the test should be terminated if the subject requests to stop. A rise in diastolic BP >115 mm Hg is an indication for stopping an exercise test.

21–B. Medical complications and injury can and do occur in an exercise setting. Serious complications rarely occur, however. No data suggest that women suffer more serious complications with exercise than men. Also, no data support the statements that serious complications occur late in the day and that serious complication occurs at a rate significantly lower than 1 in 3,000 hours of exercise. In truth, this rate is closer to 1 in 3,000,000 hours of exercise.

22–A. One of the exercise staff's responsibilities when an injury or emergency occurs is to control the situation by implementing the emergency plan and taking charge. Staff should make sure the proper actions are taken to ensure the safety and care of injured persons. One of those actions is to instruct the people around him or her to help implement the plan. It is inappropriate for the staff to sit back and let someone else implement the plan or hope that an emergency contact can take control of the situation. Controlling the situation and instructing those around the staff is the primary role, and getting people out of the facility may only happen under certain situations.

23–C. Hydration is one of the most important principles of exercise. Two of the effects of hydration are regulating body temperature and electrolyte balance. If either is out of balance because of dehydration (lack of appropriate hydration), it can lead to weakness, loss of work capacity, and heat exhaustion. Hydration does not affect breathing, carbohydrate utilization, or blood pooling.

24–D. The ADA protects individuals with any disability from discrimination of access. Fitness facilities must provide free and easy access to all disabled individuals throughout the facility. The Americans with Handicaps Act does not exist, and the Civil Rights Act was enacted in 1964, not in 1966. The Health Portability Act involves employees with health insurance and is not related to safety.

25–B. Most people having seizures display convulsing actions. With a convulsing seizure, the safest action is to not restrain the person and to let the convulsion pass. It is not safe to hold the person down or try to wedge anything into the victim's mouth. Make the area safe for the person by clearing any objects that he or she may contact.

26–C. Before starting a fitness program, it is important to understand an individual's medical history and risk of a crisis during exercise. A preparticipation screening can help to establish this understanding and prevent injury or crisis. Teaching the warm-up and cool-down procedures prevents injury, but it is not the first thing that you do. The same argument applies to teaching safety procedures and safe use of the equipment.

27–A. It is always safest to advise participants to progress in a fitness program gradually and slowly. This advice also increases the chance for program success and increased motivation. Using the calendar method does not take into account individual effects in adjusting to exercise. Participants may not be ready to progress when the calendar indicates that it is time to do so, just as they do not always know when to increase or may not be aggressive enough. Always taking an aggressive approach increases the risk of injury, because the increase may be too much too soon.

28–C. Using exercise equipment incorrectly can place excess stress on muscles and joints and increase the risk of injury, which adds to the risk of participation. The expense and ability to move exercise equipment have no bearing on the risk of participation. The time that one waits also does not add to the risk, unless an exerciser uses the equipment incorrectly.

29–A. One of the critical aspects in preventing injuries is to follow the rules and policies, which are made to prevent problems. Keeping the equipment clean and hiring good front-desk staff are important and can help to prevent problems, but they are not considered to be prevention strategies. Unique programs are designed to attract exercise participants, not to prevent risk.

30–C. The maintenance plan ensures that the exercise equipment is functioning properly and safely. Records that document maintenance and repairs are important in tracking when to maintain equipment and to make sure that repairs are conducted and completed. A floor plan is not necessary in a maintenance plan. Temperature and humidity readings should be included in a program plan (when necessary) but not a maintenance plan. A participant advisory statement does not exist.

31–C. When cleaning a facility, it is very important that the solutions used do not cause skin problems or allergic reactions. A safe facility must avoid these problems. Cleaning a facility usually does not involve signs or require particular colors of surfaces. A pleasant smell is nice to have, but this does not prevent problems or allergic reactions.

32–A. Heat exhaustion symptoms can vary and usually include low blood pressure, cold and clammy skin, multiple muscle spasms, headache, nausea, tachycardia, and normal to elevated body temperature. Hot, dry skin is a symptom of heat stroke.

33–D. RICES refers to Rest (let the injury heal without stress), Ice (reduces swelling and promotes healing), Compression (reduces swelling), Elevation (reduces swelling), and Stabilization (reduces muscle spasm by assisting in relaxation of associated muscles). Energy, incremental heat, standardization, and common sense do not decrease swelling, promote healing, reduce muscle spasm, or reduce the stress to the injury.

34–A. Symptoms of a cardiac crisis (e.g., heart failure, heart attack) include pain in the chest and pain radiating down the left arm. Hypertension, not hypotension, is a possible cause of a cardiac crisis. A seizure and heartburn are not associated with a cardiac crisis.

35–D. A safe environment is very important, and this fact is most important to many of the special populations that may have difficulty negotiating their way around a facility because of injury, disability, or age. Healthcare providers, staff, and guests are important, but in most cases, they do not require special attention regarding safety.

36–D. The weight room can be a dangerous place if safety is not a priority. Dumbbells, plates, and bars can fall or be thrown and cause injury. Safe passageways reduce the risk of an exercises getting hit by another person exercising. The buddy system helps with spotting and instruction, which reduces the risk of injury. A phone can cause distractions. Lifting gloves and belts may be helpful to individuals in easing the burden of lifting, but they are not critical for safety. Female trainers can be just as effective as male trainers in spotting.

37–B. Safety plans help to educate and guide staff in developing and maintaining a safe facility. The safety plan should include procedures for a fire, a power outage, and the exposure to bloodborne pathogens. Facility insurance addresses fire and, possibly, power outages, but it does not address bloodborne pathogens. Maintenance plans address the repair and maintenance of the equipment, but they do not address any of the three factors listed in the question. Testing by staff may involve bloodborne pathogens, but this has no involvement in fires or power outages.

38–C. Informed consent is a document that an individual reads, or that is read to him or her by a staff member, explaining the exercise test to be conducted in detail along with the potential benefits and risks, the purpose of the test, and the patient's responsibilities. The informed consent does not explain the services. The safety plan is designed to create a safe exercise environment and does not discuss potential benefits or risks. Exercise waivers are designed to release the exercise professional from negligence.

39–A. Documentation provides a record of events and a written description of the rules, rights, and risks of the program. These documents are designed to ensure the safety of both the exercisers and the staff. They also are designed to protect the facility and staff from liability or negligence issues, because they promote safety and reduce the risk of injury. Documentation does not protect against risk, but it provides tools to help reduce it. Program design or policies are written into documents, but they are not the programs. Documentation also may be tools for billing and classification, but it is not necessarily as important as computer software or the management of the data needed for both of these programs.

40–C. Emergency procedures should be easy to find so that the staff can act quickly to handle the emergency, not spend time looking for the procedures. The procedures should be placed by the phones, because they often are used in an emergency to dial 911 and to initiate emergency help. Emergency procedures should not be given to patients, because they should not be involved in enacting them. Only the staff should implement the emergency procedures. Placing the procedures in a safe place does not make them easy to find when they are needed. By the phones is a better place than by the fire extinguishers to put the emergency procedures, because unlike a fire extinguisher, a phone is used in almost all emergencies.

41–D. Leg press and squats with any type of weight adds compression to the spine, which can have significant adverse effects in the care of a low back injury. It is very important to increase flexibility and muscular strength without excessive load or compression. Abdominal curl-ups, unloaded flexion or extension of the spine (cat stretch), and maintaining a neutral spine during exercise are principles that do not place unnecessary load or compression on the spine and serve to increase both the flexibility and strength of supporting structures.

42–A. Safety is the most important responsibility for an exercise professional. An exercise professional must never endanger anyone. Accurate data are good to obtain, but this is secondary to safety. Completing the test and encouragement also are goals, but not the top priority, of the fitness specialist.

43–B. Included with the many risks for musculoskeletal injury are extrinsic or outside factors. If intensity is too high, the joints and muscles could be overstressed. Rough or uneven terrain can lead to falls. Poorly designed or maintained equipment can cause breakdowns or incorrect positioning, which in turn can cause injury. Signage usually does not lead to injury, and membership type is not a factor in musculoskeletal injury. Although intrinsic factors are included in the risks, frequency is not an intrinsic factor, so this answer is incorrect.

44–C. Chronic soreness, fatigue, sleep disturbances, and decline in performance are all symptoms of an overuse injury. Overtraining is another term used for this condition, which often occurs in individuals who are training for competition or who become obsessed with fitness training. Hyperglycemia and hypoglycemia are related to blood glucose levels and do not exhibit chronic soreness. A strain may show as a symptom; however, fatigue usually is not associated with this condition.

45–D. Exercise clothing is also exercise equipment and, as with the exercise machines that are used, it is critical that exercise clothing be safe and perform adequately. If not, then the risk of injury is increased. Fashion statements do not mean that the clothes are safe and perform appropriately. Bright clothing is not important in an aerobics class. Although comfort is important, safety and function are more important.

Exercise Programming

CHAPTER 8

I. INTRODUCTION

A. PURPOSE OF EXERCISE PROGRAMS
   1. Enhancement of physical **fitness for activities of daily life**, recreation, or competitive athletic endeavors.
   2. Primary or secondary **disease prevention**.
   3. Enjoyment, hobby, **stress management**, and psychological well-being.

B. CURRENT PHYSICAL ACTIVITY RECOMMENDATIONS
   1. Adults should engage in **moderate-intensity** physical activities for at least 30 minutes on 5 or more days of the week, according to the Centers for Disease Control and Prevention (CDC)/American College of Sports Medicine (ACSM). Moderate-intensity is any activity that burns 3.5–7 kcal/min such as leisurely bicycling, briskly walking, or push-mowing the lawn.
      –OR–
      Adults should engage in **vigorous-intensity** physical activity 3 or more days/week for 20 or more minutes per occasion, according to Healthy People 2010. Vigorous-intensity is any activity that burns >7 kcal/minute.
   2. Health benefits can be accrued with moderate amounts of physical activity (e.g., 30 minutes of walking, or 15 minutes of jogging); however, individuals may achieve even greater health benefits by increasing the time spent or intensity of those activities. In October of 2008, the Federal Government issued its first-ever Physical Activity Guidelines for Americans (PAGA). The science-based guidelines provide Americans aged 6 and older with recommendations for physical activity. Table 8-1 summarizes key points in the Federal Guidelines. The PAGA aligns closely with the ACSM and AHA jointly published guidelines.
   3. The 2005 Dietary Guidelines for Americans put out by the Department of Health and Human Services recommends that to reduce the risk of chronic disease, adults should engage in at least 30 minutes of moderate-intensity physical activity, above usual activity, at work or home on most days of the week. They recommend, however, that for adults to properly manage weight, they must engage in approximately 60 minutes of moderate-intensity activity most days; to sustain weight loss, adults should perform 60–90 minutes of moderate-intensity activity most days.
   4. In late 2008, an advisory committee (including several fellows of the ACSM) will make science-based recommendations that will be used to develop the first ever federal guidelines to focus on physical activity.
   5. Children and adolescents should participate in at least 60 minutes of moderate-intensity physical activity most days of the week, preferably daily (Dietary Guidelines for Americans). The CDC recommends that parents set a positive example by leading active lifestyles themselves, make physical activity fun for children, and limit the time children watch television or play video games to no more than 2 h/day.
   6. ACSM recommends that adults participate in **resistance training** 2–3 times per week, performing a minimum of 8–10 different exercises, 3–20 repetitions, and 1–3 sets that train all major muscle groups.
   7. ACSM's **flexibility training** guidelines recommend that stretching be preceded by a warm-up and be performed a minimum of 2–3 days per week, ideally 5–7 days per week, stretching to the point of tightness at the end of the range of motion but not to the point of pain, and holding each stretch for 15–30 seconds with 2–4 repetitions for each stretch. Flexibility training may include slow-sustained stretching, partner stretching, yoga, Pilates, or Tai chi. All major muscle groups should be stretched.

C. The ACSM recommends a target range of 150–400 kcal of energy expenditure per day.
   1. The lower end of this range (1,000 kcal/week) is associated with a significant health benefit. For some individuals with health problems or poor physical fitness, <1,000 kcal/wk may result in enhanced health (see GETP 8th, Chapter 7).
   2. Based on a dose-response relationship, individuals should be encouraged to move toward the upper end of the recommended range as their fitness improves.

TABLE 8-1. SUMMARY OF 2008 FEDERAL ACTIVITY GUIDELINES FOR AMERICANS

Children and Adolescents (aged 6–17)

- Children and adolescents should do 1 hour (60 minutes) or more of physical activity every day.
- Most of the 1 hour or more a day should be either moderate- or vigorous-intensity aerobic physical activity.
- As part of their daily physical activity, children and adolescents should do vigorous-intensity activity on at least 3 days per week. They also should do muscle-strengthening and bone-strengthening activity on at least 3 days per week

Adults (aged 18–64)

- Adults should do 2 hours and 30 minutes a week of moderate-intensity, or 1 hour and 15 minutes (75 minutes) a week of vigorous-intensity aerobic physical activity, or an equivalent combination of moderate- and vigorous-intensity aerobic physical activity. Aerobic activity should be performed in episodes of at least 10 minutes, preferably spread throughout the week.
- Additional health benefits are provided by increasing to 5 hours (300 minutes) a week of moderate-intensity aerobic physical activity, or 2 hours and 30 minutes a week of vigorous-intensity physical activity, or an equivalent combination of both.
- Adults should also do muscle-strengthening activities that involve all major muscle groups performed on 2 or more days per week.

Older Adults (aged 65 and older)

- Older adults should follow the adult guidelines. If this is not possible due to limiting chronic conditions, older adults should be as physically active as their abilities allow. They should avoid inactivity. Older adults should do exercises that maintain or improve balance if they are at risk of falling.

From: http://www.health.gov/paguidelines/

3. Weekly caloric expenditure in excess of **2,000 kcal/week** has been shown to be successful for short- and long-term weight control as well as for primary and secondary prevention of chronic disease.
4. Taking 10,000 steps per day has been shown to significantly reduce the risk for developing coronary heart disease. Using vertical displacement units (also known as step counters or pedometers) can be very beneficial in motivating individuals to become or increase physical activity.

D. Components of a comprehensive exercise program include:
   1. **Warm-up.**
   2. **Cardiovascular endurance (aerobic) exercise stimulus.**
   3. **Resistance exercise.**
   4. **Cool-down.**
   5. **Flexibility training.**

II. ESSENTIAL COMPONENTS OF AN EXERCISE PRESCRIPTION

A. Development of a systematic, individualized exercise prescription depends on the thoughtful, scientific integration of five essential components into a structured exercise program (*Table 8-2*):
   1. **Mode (type or kind of activity).**
   2. **Frequency (how often).**
   3. **Intensity (how hard).**
   4. **Duration (how long).**
   5. **Progression (how to change or advance the exercise prescription).**

B. These essential components are applied in an exercise program regardless of the participant's age, gender, health status, or fitness level.

C. Consideration of the **limitations**, **needs**, and **goals** of each individual will result in a more individualized, safer, and effective exercise program.

D. The following data obtained from a graded exercise test provide the basis for the exercise prescription:
   1. **Heart rate (HR).**
   2. **Blood pressure (BP).**
   3. **Rating of Perceived Exertion (RPE).**
   4. **Ventilatory values.**
   5. **Blood lactic acid values.**

III. CARDIOVASCULAR ENDURANCE EXERCISE

A. The ability to take in, deliver, and use oxygen is dependent on the function of the circulatory systems and cellular metabolic capacities.

B. The amount of expected improvement in cardiovascular endurance fitness is directly related to the frequency, intensity, duration, mode, and progression of exercise.

C. Maximal oxygen uptake ($\dot{V}O_{2max}$) **is genetically limited and may increase between 5% and 30% with training.** An obese individual could expect to increase his or her relative $\dot{V}O_{2max}$ more than a person who has already obtained an ideal body weight because $\dot{V}O_{2max}$ has an inverse relationship with body mass.

D. MODE

Mode is the type or kind of exercise.

   1. Cardiovascular endurance exercise is most effective when **large muscle groups** are engaged in **continuous, rhythmic** (aerobic) activity.
   2. Various activities such as walking, jogging, cycling, swimming, rowing, stair climbing, aerobic dance ("aerobics"), water exercise, in-line skating, snow-shoeing, cross-country skiing, or rolling your wheelchair may be incorporated to increase enjoyment and improve compliance.
   3. The potential for musculoskeletal injury increases when excessive weight-bearing activity is performed, although this same type of activity may enhance bone health.

TABLE 8-2. RECOMMENDED FITT FRAMEWORK FOR THE *F*REQUENCY, *I*NTENSITY AND *T*IME OF AEROBIC EXERCISE FOR APPARENTLY HEALTHY ADULTS[a]

HABITUAL PHYSICAL ACTIVITY/EXERCISE LEVEL	PHYSICAL FITNESS CLASSIFICATION[c]	FREQUENCY		INTENSITY[b]			TIME		
		kcal · wk^{1}	d · wk^{-1}	HRR/$\dot{V}O_2R$	% HR_{max}	PERCEPTION OF EFFORT[d]	TOTAL DURATION PER DAY (min)	TOTAL DAILY STEPS DURING EXERCISE[e]	WEEKLY DURATION (min)
Sedentary/no habitual activity/exercise/ extremely deconditioned	Poor	500–1,000	3–5	30%–45%	57%–67%	Light-moderate	20–30	3,000–3,500	60–150
Minimal physical activity/no exercise/ moderately-highly deconditioned	Poor-fair	1,000–1,500	3–5	40%–55%	64%–74%	Light-moderate	30–60	3,000–4,000	150–200
Sporadic physical activity/ no or suboptimal exercise/moderately to mildly deconditioned	Fair-average	1,500–2,000	3–5	55–70%	74%–84%	Moderate-hard	30–90	≥3,000–4,000	200–300
Habitual physical activity/ regular moderate to vigorous intensity exercise	Average-good	>2,000	3–5	65%–80%	80%–91%	Moderate-hard	30–90	≥3,000–4,000	200–300
High amounts of habitual activity/regular vigorous intensity exercise	>Good-excellent	>2,000	3–5	70%–85%	84%–94%	Somewhat hard-hard	30–90	≥3,000–4,000	200–300

kcal, kilocalories; $\dot{V}O_2R$, oxygen uptake reserve; HRR, heart rate reserve; $\%HR_{max}$, % age-predicted maximal heart rate.
[a] See Table 7-1 for exercise type (T) in *Guidelines for Exercise Testing and Prescription*, 8th edition.
[b] The various methods to quantify exercise intensity in this table may not necessarily be equivalent to each other.
[c] Fitness classification based on normative fitness data categorized by $\dot{V}O_{2max}$.
[d] Perception of effort using the ratings of perceived exertion (RPE) (11,32), OMNI (37,38,48), talk test (33) or feeling scale (17).
[e] Total steps based on step counts from a pedometer.
Note: These recommendations are consistent with the United States Department of Health & Human Services Physical Activity Guidelines for Americans, available at http://www.health.gov/PAGuidelines /pdf/paguide.pdf (October 7, 2008).

4. Comfortable, supportive walking or running shoes are important.
5. Selection of mode should be based on the desired outcomes, focusing on the exercises most likely to **sustain participation** (adherence and compliance) and enjoyment. Keep in mind that regularly using a variety of modes can be advantageous in both preventing repetitive use injuries and enhancing adherence.
6. **Stair Climbing**
   a. Necessary equipment is commonly found in fitness centers.
   b. An upright posture is important to avoid low back trauma.
   c. Weak quadriceps and gluteals may cause dependence on handrails for support, reducing the intensity of the exercise.
7. **Aerobics** is often performed in a group setting.
   a. Intensity is usually controlled by music and choreographed movement patterns.
   b. HR may not be an accurate indicator of intensity when arm movement is vigorously added to the routine.
   c. RPE is an appropriate indicator of intensity.
   d. **High-impact aerobics**
      1) Involve movement patterns in which both feet leave the floor simultaneously.
      2) May require significant energy expenditure.
      3) Increase the potential for musculoskeletal injury.
      4) Are appropriate for highly fit individuals and not advised for overweight individuals.
   e. **Low-impact aerobics**
      1) Involve movement patterns in which one foot remains in contact with the floor at all times.
      2) Produce low-impact forces and low incidence of musculoskeletal injury.
      3) Are appropriate for beginning exercisers and individuals who are moderately overweight provided that they are injury-free at the start.
      4) Can be increased in intensity by using greater horizontal displacement during movement.
   f. **Step aerobics**
      1) Involve choreographed movement patterns performed on and off bench steps varying in height from 4–12 inches.
      2) Have an energy cost that ranges from 6–11 metabolic equivalents (MET).
      3) Should be reduced in cadence for individuals who are less fit (functional capacity, <8 MET).
   g. **Water (aquatic) exercise**
      1) Allows the buoyancy properties of water to reduce the weight-bearing load, decreasing the incidence of musculoskeletal injury.
      2) May allow those with injuries to exercise during rehabilitation.
      3) May be altered in intensity by changing the speed of movement or the depth of the water or by using resistive devices (e.g., fins, hand paddles).
      4) Involves walking, jogging, and dance activity.
      5) Typically combines the benefits of the buoyancy and resistive properties of water, providing an aerobic stimulus as well as enhancing muscular strength and endurance.
      6) May benefit special population groups:
         a) Obese.
         b) Pregnant.
         c) Arthritic or those individuals with fibromyalgia.
         d) Elderly.
   h. **Cycling**
      1) A non–weight-bearing activity with a low incidence of musculoskeletal injury.
      2) A stationary cycle ergometer may be used if exercise testing and training workload must be quantified. Outdoor road cycling or mountain biking can provide individuals with a fun method to actively experience the outdoors, provided that they ride safely (i.e., wear bicycle helmets and observe rules of the road/trail).
      3) Some limiting factors to cycling are local muscle fatigue of the upper leg and expense of good equipment.

E. INTENSITY

Intensity is the relative (physiologic) difficulty of the exercise (i.e. how hard the exertion feels).

1. Intensity and duration interact and are inversely related.
   a. Improvements in aerobic fitness from low-intensity, longer duration exercise such as an easy run for 90 minutes, are similar to those with higher intensity interval training such as various quantities of intervals between 30 seconds and 4 minutes in duration.
   b. This becomes a consideration when developing an exercise prescription for individuals who prefer low-intensity over high-intensity exercise or the opposite.
2. Risk of orthopedic and other complications increases with higher intensity activity; however,

high-intensity interval training can be extremely time-efficient for those individuals who have less time available for physical activity.

3. Factors to consider when determining intensity for a particular individual include:
   a. Current level of fitness.
   b. Age and current cardiovascular risk factors.
   c. Medical conditions and medications that may influence exercise performance.
   d. Current or increased risk of orthopedic injury.
   e. Individual preference.
   f. Program objectives or performance goals.
4. Exercise intensities are recommended within the range of 55%–90% of maximum HR or 40%–85% of oxygen uptake reserve ($\dot{V}O_2R$) or HR reserve (HRR) (*Figure 8-1*).
   a. Lower intensities (40%–49% of HRR) elicit a favorable response in individuals with low fitness levels. For individuals with a $\dot{V}O_{2max}$ <40 mL · kg^{-1} · min^{-1}, a minimal intensity of 30% $\dot{V}O_2R$ can improve $\dot{V}O_{2max}$. An HRR of 20% or maximum HR of 50% may be sufficient for developing aerobic fitness in healthy adults who have a $\dot{V}O_2max$ <30 mL · kg^{-1} · min^{-1}.
   b. For most individuals, an intensity of **60%–80% of HRR** (via the **Karvonen Formula**, see Figure 8-1) or **77%–90% maximum HR** is reasonable for improvement of cardiovascular endurance fitness.
   c. Use of the actual maximum HR from a graded exercise test is preferable to estimating the maximum HR based on age.
   d. When exercising in a hot, humid, or air polluted environment, cardiac drift may occur in which HR elevates not because of the workload of the exercise but because of increased core temperature. An individual should exercise at a lower HR in such conditions to avoid health complications from the heat. Exercising at high altitudes can also elevate HR above normal levels because of the lower amount of oxygen available. Heart rates should be adjusted down in this setting as well.
5. The RPE can be used as an adjunct to the HR for regulating intensity.
   a. The ACSM recommends an intensity that will elicit an RPE within a range of 12–16 on the original 6–20 (Borg) scale.
   b. The RPE is considered to be a reliable indicator of exercise intensity; some learning is required on the part of the participant.
   c. The RPE is particularly useful when a participant is unable to monitor his or her pulse accurately or when the HR response to exercise is altered by medications.
   d. **The RPE should be individually determined on different exercise modes.**
6. An **MET** can also be used to regulate intensity. One MET is the caloric consumption of an individual while at complete rest. The unit is commonly used with aerobic exercise to estimate the intensity of the workout. A workout of 2–4 METs is considered light, whereas intensive running (8 min/mile, or 12 km/h) or climbing can yield workouts of 12 or more METs. METs are often used in cardiac rehabilitation exercise programs.
7. The HR-$\dot{V}O_2$ relationship can be plotted to determine the exercise intensity (*Figure 8-2*).
8. An abnormal response to a graded exercise test or individual exercise limitations must be considered when prescribing intensity.
   a. The ACSM recommends that exercise at intensities eliciting the following signs or symptoms should be avoided:
      1) Exercise-induced angina.
      2) Inappropriate BP changes.
      3) Musculoskeletal discomfort.
      4) Leg pain.
      5) Any sign or symptom that causes premature termination of the exercise test.
   b. The training HR is set at 10 bpm lower than the HR when signs or symptoms of intolerance are present (see above).

		220		220
Age		**-25**		**-25**
Max Heart Rate		**195**		**195**
Resting Heart Rate		**-75**		**-75**
Heart Rate Reserve		120		120
50-85%		**x .6**		**x .8**
		72		96
Resting Heart Rate		+75		+75
Target Heart Rate	**60% HRR=147**	**147**	**80% HRR=171**	**171**

FIGURE 8-1. Calculation of 50%–85% of the heart rate reserve (HRR) based on a 25-year-old individual with a resting heart rate of 75 bpm. (From Karvonen M, Kentala K, Mustala O: The effects of training on heart rate: A longitudinal study. *Annales Medicinae Experimentalis et Biological Fennial* 1957;35:307–315.)

F. DURATION

Duration is the time or length of an individual exercise session (how long the session is).

1. The ACSM recommends 20–60 minutes of continuous or intermittent aerobic activity.
2. Caloric expenditure and cardiovascular endurance conditioning goals may be achieved with exercise sessions of moderate duration (20–30 min).

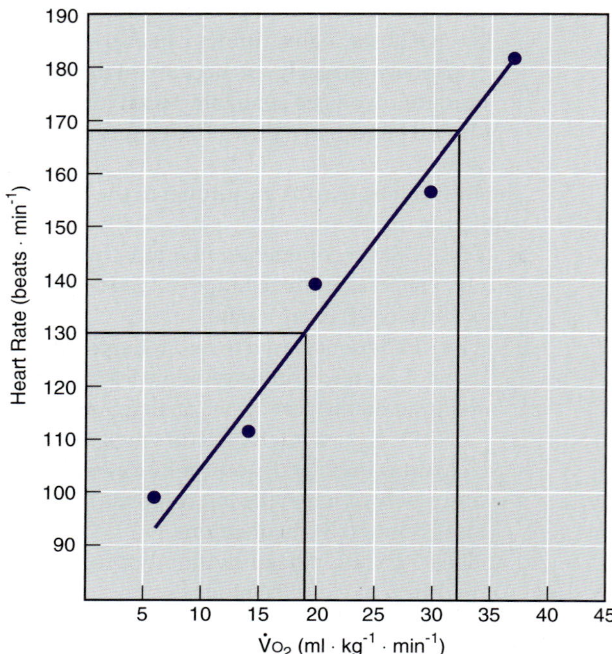

FIGURE 8-2. A line of best fit has been drawn through the data points on this plot of heart rate and oxygen consumption data observed during a hypothetical maximal exercise test in which maximal oxygen consumption ($\dot{V}O_{2max}$) was observed to be 38 mL · kg^{-1}· min^{-1} and maximal heart rate was 184 bpm. A target heart rate range was determined by finding the heart rates that correspond to 50% and 85% of $\dot{V}O_{2max}$. For this individual, 50% of $\dot{V}O_{2max}$ was approximately 19 mL · kg^{-1}· min^{-1}, and 85% of $\dot{V}O_{2max}$ was approximately 32 mL · kg^{-1}· min^{-1}. The corresponding target heart rates are approximately 130 and 168 bpm, respectively. (From *ACSM's Guidelines for Exercise Testing and Prescription*. 8th Ed. Baltimore: Lippincott Williams & Wilkins, 2010, Figure 7.1, p 159.)

3. High-intensity or short-duration exercise programs are associated with increased potential for injury.
4. Excessive duration is associated with decreased compliance.
5. Increases in exercise duration should be instituted as adaptation occurs without signs of intolerance.
6. Deconditioned individuals may benefit from multiple, short-duration exercise sessions (5–10 min) with frequent rest periods.
7. An inverse relationship exists between the intensity and duration of training.
8. Greater musculoskeletal and cardiovascular risk may occur with short-duration, high-intensity exercise compared with lower intensity, longer duration exercise.
9. Interval training programs using bouts of lower intensity exercise can be effective for improving cardiovascular endurance fitness.
   a. Intermittent exercise may allow for increased caloric expenditure and enhanced interest compared with continuous aerobic activity.
   b. Intermittent exercise may be particularly useful for beginning or deconditioned exercisers.
   c. Intermittent exercise programmed for health or fitness purposes should be aerobic in nature and not exceed an intensity of 85% of HRR.

G. FREQUENCY

Frequency is the number of exercise sessions per day and per week.

1. The ACSM recommends physical activity on most (preferably all) days of the week.
2. Frequency interacts with both intensity and duration.
3. Individual goals, preferences, limitations, and time constraints may affect frequency.
4. Frequency also is influenced by lifestyle and convenience.
5. Deconditioned people may benefit from lower intensity, shorter duration exercise performed at higher frequencies per day or per week.
6. An exercise frequency of more than 5 days per week generally is used for athletic performance enhancement or weight loss.

H. PROGRESSION

Progression is the systematic changes in exercise prescription (e.g., intensity, duration, frequency) necessary to increase fitness. Progression is not mutually exclusive to cardiorespiratory training. It is important for resistance training as well. Fitness professionals should be able to effectively teach progression of exercise to improve muscular fitness. Example: progressing a standing lunge to a walking lunge and then perhaps to a walking lunge with dumbbells.

1. The rate of progression depends on health or fitness status, age, goals, and compliance.
2. Improvement depends on systematic progression of frequency, intensity, or duration.
3. Increasing the frequency and duration of an activity before increasing the intensity is preferred.
4. **Adaptation**
   a. Occurs when an individual can adequately respond to the demands of a particular exercise stressor.
   b. Depends on health or fitness status and the relative mix of frequency, intensity, duration, and mode of exercise.
5. Most participants adapt more easily and comfortably to smaller increases in the intensity, duration, and frequency of exercise.
6. Few objective markers are available for short-term adaptation (1–3 weeks). Some indicators may be:
   a. Improvements in motor patterns.
   b. Lower RPE or exercising HR at the same workload.

c. Subjective evaluation through communication between the exercise professional and the individual.
7. The rate of adaptation is affected by compliance with the exercise program.
8. Increase the duration by 10%–20% per week until the relevant goal is attained.
9. Once the duration goal is attained, increase the intensity by 5%–10% every sixth training session.

I. STAGES OF CONDITIONING
1. **Initial**
a. Warm-up: 10–15 minutes.
b. Moderate intensity: 40%–60% of HRR.
c. Interval: 15 minutes, progressing to 30 minutes.
d. Frequency: 3–4 days per week.
2. **Improvement**
a. 50%–85% of HRR.
b. Progress duration by 10%–20% per week or as tolerated if longer.
c. Progress intensity by 5%–10% every 2 weeks until the relevant goal is attained.
d. Lasts approximately 4–8 months.
3. **Maintenance**
a. Goals have been attained.
b. Attainment of average fitness (50th percentile in all heath-related fitness parameters) is a reasonable goal.
c. Maintain fitness with a variety of activities.

J. WARM-UP
Warm-up involves low-intensity, large muscle group activity specific to the exercise to be performed.
1. Physiologic changes induced by appropriate warm-up exercises include:
a. Increased muscle temperature.
b. Increased muscle blood flow.
c. Increased ease of dissociation of oxygen from hemoglobin.
d. Increased muscle enzyme activity.
e. Increased elasticity of muscle and connective tissue.
f. Decreased muscle viscosity.
2. Benefits of specific warm-up routines include enhanced performance and, perhaps (inconsistently demonstrated in the literature), prevention of musculoskeletal and cardiovascular complications.
3. Five to 10 minutes should be allowed for the warm-up.
4. Stretching may be included after the large muscle activity.

K. COOL-DOWN
Cool-down is low- to moderate-intensity, large-muscle-group activity performed for approximately 5–10 minutes. Physiologic changes induced by appropriate cool-down exercises include:
1. Enhanced venous return.
2. Enhanced transport of metabolic byproducts away from skeletal muscle.
3. Gradual return of HR and BP to preexercise levels.
4. Skeletal muscle and connective tissue may be less viscous and more pliable after the exercise stimulus; therefore, the cool-down period may be an appropriate time to enhance flexibility through stretching.

L. CONTRAINDICATIONS TO EXERCISE
The ACSM specifies medical conditions that preclude safe participation in exercise testing and exercise programs. See Table 6-1 for a complete listing of these conditions.

M. TERMINATION OF AN EXERCISE SESSION
The ACSM specifies the conditions that require termination of a test or an exercise session. See Table 6-12 for a complete listing of these conditions.

IV. FLEXIBILITY

A. Refers to the range of motion (rom) or mobility of a joint.
B. Is necessary for optimal musculoskeletal health and physical activity.
C. Optimal musculoskeletal function requires that an adequate rom be maintained in all joints.
D. Activities that enhance or maintain musculoskeletal flexibility should be included in comprehensive preventive or rehabilitative exercise programs.
E. Although flexibility can improve acutely, scientific evidence regarding how long the effect may last is lacking. Ballistic (bouncing) stretching and proprioceptive neuromuscular facilitation are not recommended inclusions for most general exercise programs.

F. RISKS OF STRETCHING
1. Correct body alignment and joint position are critical for effectiveness and to minimize the risk of musculoskeletal injury.
2. Some common stretching exercises may be potentially harmful to the musculoskeletal system and, in the general population, should be avoided or modified (*Figure 8-3*).

V. MUSCULAR STRENGTH AND ENDURANCE

Muscular strength is the maximal amount of resistance that a muscle or a group of muscles can overcome. **Muscular endurance** is the ability of a muscle or a group of muscles to overcome a submaximal resistance several times consecutively.

A. INTRODUCTION
1. Maintenance or Improvement of Muscular Strength and Endurance.

CONTRAINDICTATED/HIGH-RISK EXERCISE		ALTERNATIVE EXERCISE
Straight Leg Full Sit-ups	Risk: Stress on lower back due to utilization of hip flexors with origin in the lumbar spine; exercise primarily targets hip flexors	Crunches
Double Leg Raises	Risk: Hyperextends low back due to utilization of hip flexors with origin in the lumbar spine	Single Leg Raises-Opposite Knee Flexed
Full Squats	Risk: Patellar tendon forces during deep knee bending are 7.6 times body weight (7), increasing the risk of chondromalacia meniscal tears; individuals with previous injury to ligamental structures and menisci are at increased risk for injury	Squats to 90 Degrees of Knee Flexion-Knee Over Ankle (90°)
Hurdler's Stretch	Risk: Knee flexion at end range of motion with rotational forces on hinge joint may stress the medial collateral ligament and menisci	Seated Hamstring Stretch
Plough	Risk: Loaded neck flexion can sprain cervical ligaments and increase pressure in cervical disks	Double Knee to Chest
Back Hyperextension	Risk: Hyperextension of the back	Back Extension to Normal Standing Lumbar Lordosis
Full neck rolls	Risk: Stretches cervical ligaments, increases cervical disc pressure and may impinge arterial flow, resulting in dizziness	Lateral Neck Stretches
Flexion with rotation	Risk: Flexion with rotation increases pressure on spinal disks	Supine Curl-ups with Flexion followed by Rotation
Standing toe touch	Risk: Increases pressure in lumbar disks and overstretches lumbar ligament	Standing Hamstring Stretch, Back Flat

FIGURE 8-3. Common high-risk exercises and recommendations for alternative exercises. (Adapted from *ACSM's Resource Manual for Guidelines for Exercise Testing and Prescription.* 3rd ed. Baltimore: Williams & Wilkins, 1998, p 644.)

a. Muscular strength and endurance are critical to the performance of activities of daily life.
b. Increased strength enables performance of normal physical activity with less physiologic strain and at reduced risk for musculoskeletal injury.
c. Improvements in muscular strength and endurance generally result from enhanced neuromuscular and metabolic function and, perhaps, increased size of individual muscle fibers.
d. The ability to realize substantial increases in muscle size is hormonally mediated and, probably, genetically limited.
e. **Resistance training should be included as an integral part of comprehensive preventive and rehabilitative exercise programs.**

2. Health benefits of resistance training include:
   a. Improved performance of activities of daily living with less physiologic stress.
   b. Maintenance of functional independence.
   c. Decreased risk of bone mineral loss.
   d. Maintenance of lean body mass.
   e. Decreased risk of low back pain.
3. **Intensity** usually is prescribed as the percentage of the maximal voluntary contraction.
   a. Volitional fatigue is the inability to move a resistance through an ROM with proper biomechanical form.
   b. The number of repetitions to volitional fatigue varies inversely with resistance.
   c. Exercise to volitional fatigue is safe, provided that good technique is maintained.
   d. Adaptation of the resistance training exercise prescription often is necessary in individuals with cardiovascular disease, hypertension, or those with complications associated with diabetes as well as other chronic disease conditions.
   e. A particular set of resistance training exercises should be terminated when the resistance cannot be moved through the full ROM during successive repetitions with good technique, including proper breathing.
   f. Relative exercise intensity should be similar for men and women.
   g. Resistance may be increased (by 2.5–5 pounds) when the desired number of repetitions can be completed with good technique.
   h. One exercise session per week has been shown to maintain strength for up to 3 months provided that intensity remains constant.
   i. The increase in resistance training intensity can be achieved by altering any one of the following variables while keeping the others constant.
      1) Number of repetitions.
      2) Decreasing speed of movement.
      3) Avoiding "locking out" a joint during multijoint exercises (e.g., bench press, leg press).
   j. Intensity should be reduced for people with cardiovascular or other chronic disease.
   k. The HR is not a valid indicator of resistance exercise intensity.

B. MODES OF EXERCISE FOR RESISTANCE TRAINING

1. Free weights require balance and some skill to perform exercises properly and safely, and they often require a partner for safety.
2. Machines (e.g., Nautilus, Universal, Keiser) also known as selectorized equipment may be safer than free-weight exercise for older or novice participants.
3. Rubber tubing, medicine balls, large therapy balls, bosu balls, air pillows, and so forth also may be used for core or resistance training.
4. Choice of resistance training mode should be based on safety, equipment availability, and individual preference.

C. EXERCISE PRESCRIPTION

1. Select a mode of exercise that is comfortable and provides full ROM.
2. Include 8–10 major muscle group exercises.
3. Program activity with attention to time efficiency, because exercise training programs lasting longer than 1 hour usually are associated with lower compliance.
4. The order of the exercises may be left to individual preference; however, arms should be exercised after the torso, if possible. Fatigue of the smaller arm muscles may limit the ability to adequately stress the larger torso muscles (triceps fatigue may limit bench press activity).
5. ACSM Recommendations.
   a. Healthy individuals should perform **one set** of each exercise **to volitional fatigue**.
   b. Choose a (limited) range of repetitions between 3 and 20 (e.g., 3–6, 8–12, 6–10).
   c. These exercises should be performed on two or three nonconsecutive days per week. Training 1 day per week will maintain strength for several weeks.
   d. Different exercises for a given muscle group may be performed every two or three training sessions.
   e. **Proper breathing** instruction for individuals who are unfamiliar with resistive training is necessary.
      1) Exhaling with the concentric (the lift or hard part) phase of the exercise and

inhaling with the eccentric (controlled lowering) phase of each repetition is recommended.

2) **The Valsalva maneuver** (a forced expiration against a closed airway; also known as holding your breath) **should be discouraged** during resistance exercise, because it may be accompanied by a significant increase in arterial BP.

f. Perform both the lifting and lowering phases of the exercise in a **controlled** manner at moderate to slow speeds (3-second concentric, 3-second eccentric) over the full ROM.

g. Maintain Proper Mechanics.
   1) Heavy resistance should not be performed with improper technique.
   2) If correct biomechanical form cannot be maintained, the resistance should be decreased.

h. Allow sufficient time for rest between exercises to perform the next exercise properly.

i. Training with a partner may be beneficial for safety and motivation.

D. TRAINING PRINCIPLES

1. **Specificity**
   Training effects resulting from an exercise program are specific to the exercise performed and to the muscles involved. For example, individuals wanting to strengthen their triceps would perform exercises such as triceps cable push-downs or two-handed overhead triceps extensions that target the triceps not a preacher curl that would work the biceps.
2. **Overload**
   This principle states that each workout should place a demand on the muscle or muscles that is greater than that in the previous workout session. Overload can be achieved by:
   a. Increasing the resistance or weight.
   b. Increasing repetitions.
   c. Increasing sets.
   d. Decreasing the rest period between sets or exercises.
3. **Progression**
   This principle is defined as an increase in workload to maintain overload.

VI. CONDITIONS REQUIRING MODIFICATION OF EXERCISE PROGRAMS

A. OSTEOPOROSIS

1. Increased risk of fractures of the wrists, hips, and lumbosacral regions.
2. Reductions in bone mass are most prevalent in sedentary individuals and progress at a more rapid rate following menopause.
3. Weight-bearing exercise is most effective in maintaining or increasing bone density, but such exercise may be harmful in those with advanced osteoporosis.
4. Resistance training.
   a. Include exercises that direct the load over the long axis of the bone (e.g., leg press, shoulder press).
   b. Frequency: two or three times per week.
   c. Repetitions: 8–10.
   d. Intensity: RPE of 13–15.
   e. Include functional exercises (e.g., balance).
   f. Include flexibility exercises 5–7 days/week.
   g. Spinal flexion may be contraindicated.
5. Aerobic Activity.
   a. Mode: aquatic, walking, cycling.
   b. Frequency: 3–5 days/week.
   c. Duration: 20–60 minutes, continuous or intermittent.
   d. Intensity: 40%–70% of HRR.
6. Special Considerations.
   a. Pain is a contraindication to exercise.
   b. Avoid high-impact or ballistic activity.
   c. Excessive trunk flexion and twisting activities increase compressive forces and may increase the risk of vertebral fracture.

B. HYPERTENSION

1. **Hypertension** is defined as a resting systolic BP $\geq$140 mm Hg and/or a resting diastolic BP $\geq$90 mm Hg.
2. Most hypertensive cases can be classified as primary (of unknown origin) and typically warrant multifactorial therapy, including some or all of the following:
   a. Pharmacologic management.
   b. Dietary management.
   c. Weight loss.
   d. Relaxation therapies.
3. Exercise is an effective tool in managing hypertension, with a reduction of 5–8 mm in both systolic and diastolic BP after daily exercise training.
4. If resting BP is $\geq$160/100 mm Hg, drug therapy is indicated either before or coincident with initiation of an exercise program.
5. Aerobic exercise.
   a. Cardiovascular endurance activities (e.g., walking, cycling, swimming) are appropriate.
   b. Frequency: 3–7 days/week.
   c. Duration: 30–60 minutes.
   d. Intensity: 40%–70% of HRR.

e. Multiple bouts of short-duration (10–15 minutes), low-intensity activity (e.g., walking) throughout the day may provide a viable option for control of BP.

6. Resistance exercise.
   a. Resistance exercise should be included for those with hypertension, but not as the primary form of activity.
   b. Isometric exercise, Valsalva maneuvers, and maximal effort should be specifically avoided.
   c. Terminate a set when the RPE is between 13 and 15.
   d. High-repetition, low-intensity (e.g., resistance) programs are usually recommended.
7. Special considerations.
   a. Exercise is contraindicated if preexercise systolic BP is >200 mm Hg or diastolic BP is >110 mm Hg.
   b. Terminate an exercise session if exercise systolic BP is >220 mm Hg or diastolic BP is >105.
   c. For those on vasodilator medications, prolong cool-down and avoid abrupt postural change.
   d. β-blockers attenuate the HR and necessitate use of the RPE.

C. DIABETES MELLITUS

1. A metabolic disorder characterized by hyperglycemia (fasting plasma glucose, >126 mg/dL).
2. Blood glucose levels that define diabetes according to the American Diabetes Association (ADA) in the 2004 Clinical Practice Guidelines are as follows:
   a. A fasting plasma glucose of <100 mg/dL (5.6 mmol/L) is normal.
   b. A fasting plasma glucose of 100–125 mg/dL (5.6–6.9 mmol/L) is impaired.
   c. A fasting plasma glucose of ≥126 mg/dL (7.0 mmol/L) indicates a provisional diagnosis of diabetes.
3. This condition is associated with increased risk for cardiovascular disease, renal failure, neuropathic disorders, and ophthalmic dysfunction, including blindness.
4. Benefits of exercise include:
   a. Improved insulin sensitivity.
   b. Increased glucose control.
   c. Decreased body fat (for type 2 diabetes).
   d. Improved lipid profile.
5. Classification.
   There are two major classifications of diabetes mellitus.
   a. Type 1 is caused by insulin deficiency and usually is an immune-mediated diabetes mellitus.
   b. Type 2 is caused by insulin resistance and generally is associated with obesity. Most cases of diabetes involve type 2.
   c. **The treatment goal for diabetes is glucose control**, which is accomplished through diet, medications. and exercise.
6. Complications.
   a. Can include autonomic neuropathy, peripheral neuropathy, claudication, hypertension, retinopathy, and nephropathy.
   b. Often necessitate modification of the exercise program.
7. Aerobic exercise.
   Exercise has an "insulinlike" effect on blood glucose through enhanced insulin-receptor sensitivity. Therefore, avoidance of hypoglycemia during or after exercise is important.
   a. Frequency: 3–7 days/week.
      1) Those with type 2 diabetes should strive to expend at least 1,000 kcal/week.
      2) Daily exercise may provide for better glycemic control.
   b. Intensity: 50%–80% of HRR.
   c. Duration: 20–60 minutes.
8. Resistance training.
   a. Lower intensity.
   b. Consider complications.
9. Special considerations.
   a. Monitor glucose pre- and postexercise, especially during the initial stages of an exercise program.
   b. Exercise is contraindicated if the fasting glucose level is >250 mg/dL with ketones or >300 mg/dL without ketones.
   c. Carbohydrate intake and insulin dosage should be adjusted before exercise (e.g., decrease insulin, increase carbohydrate intake).
   d. Avoid injecting insulin into exercising muscle; abdominal injection is recommended.
   e. Consume carbohydrates following late-evening exercise to avoid nocturnal hypoglycemia.
   f. Maintain adequate hydration.
   g. Clothing should allow proper thermoregulation so that any signs of hypoglycemia are not masked.

D. OBESITY

Obesity is an excess accumulation of body fat, particularly intra-abdominal fat, that is associated with increased health risks(e.g., hypertension, coronary artery disease, type 2 diabetes).

1. Currently, approximately 65% of Americans are estimated to be overweight (body mass index [BMI], >25 kg · m^{-2}), and more than 30% estimated to be obese (BMI, >30.0 kg · m^{-2}).

2. Fat loss is best attained through a combination of diet and aerobic exercise.
3. Even modest weight loss (5%–10%) is associated with clinically significant health improvements.
4. Prevention of further weight gain should be a priority.
5. The objective of exercise programs for the treatment of obesity should be to maximize caloric expenditure safely.
6. Generally, the rate of weight loss should be gradual, not exceeding 2–3 pounds (7,000–10,500 kcal) per week.
7. Objective Evidence of Obesity.
   a. BMI: $>30\ kg \cdot m^{-2}$.
   b. Waist circumference.
      1) Males: >102 cm.
      2) Females: >88 cm.
   c. Body fat.
      1) Men: >25%.
      2) Women: >32%.
      3) Variability in measurement often makes this value difficult to interpret and apply.
      4) Use this measure in conjunction with BMI and waist circumference.
8. Aerobic exercise.
   a. Mode.
      1) Walking is a generally accessible activity and should be within the tolerance limits of most obese persons.
      2) Cross-training with combinations of weight-bearing and non–weight-bearing activities may be effective.
      3) Non–weight-bearing activities (e.g., cycling, water exercises) should be included for persons with lower extremity orthopedic problems.
   b. Frequency: 5–7 days/week.
   c. Intensity: 40%–60% of HRR, progressing to 50%–75%.
   d. Duration: 45–60 minutes.
      1) Initial weekly training volume should be approximately 150 minutes/week, progressing to 200 to 300 minutes/week.
9. Resistance training is recommended as an adjunct to an aerobic exercise program, but it is not the primary means for caloric expenditure.
10. Special Considerations.
   a. Adequate thermoregulation often is a problem.
   b. Equipment modification may be necessary (e.g., wider seats on cycles and rowers).
   c. Behavior modification strategies should be included in the management of obesity.

E. PREGNANCY

1. Exercise is generally considered to be safe both during and after pregnancy if overheating is avoided, activities with a high risk of falling are avoided, high altitude training is avoided, and adequate fuel and oxygen are available for the mother and the fetus.
2. The American College of Obstetricians and Gynecologists (ACOG) has established contraindications to exercise during pregnancy (see http://www.acog.org).
3. Aerobic exercise.
   a. Frequency: 3–7 days/week.
   b. Intensity: RPE of 11–13.
   c. Duration: 30–40 minutes.
4. Resistance training.
   a. Decreased intensity.
   b. Avoid Valsalva maneuvers such as holding the breath. Breathe in on the easy part of the exercise and out on the exertional part.
5. Special considerations.
   a. Avoid exercise in the supine posture after the first trimester.
   b. Pregnancy requires an additional 300 kcal/day, so additional calories must be consumed to meet the needs of exercise and pregnancy.
   c. Avoid motionless standing during and in the short term after exercise, because it may exacerbate venous blood pooling.
   d. Avoid all risk of abdominal trauma.
   e. Facilitate thermoregulation.
      1) Consider temperature and humidity when planning and performing exercise.
      2) Wear proper clothing.
      3) Maintain adequate hydration.
      4) Avoid extreme intensity and duration of exercise.
   f. Consume between 30 and 50 g of carbohydrate before exercise.

F. CHILDREN AND ADOLESCENTS

1. Children ages 5–12 should:
   a. Frequency and duration: ≥60 minutes of age-appropriate physical activity on all or most days of the week.
   b. Activities that are intermittent in nature (active play) should be emphasized.
   c. Several bouts of physical activity lasting ≥15 minutes each day is ideal.
   d. It is important to use a wide variety of physical activities with children.
   e. Extended periods (≥2 hours) of inactivity are discouraged during daytime hours.

2. Resistance training for children:
   a. Avoid overly intense or maximal (one repetition maximum [1-RM]) resistance training.
   b. Training should be varied and appropriate to size, strength, and maturity.
   c. Repetitions: 8–15.
   d. Focus on participation and proper technique rather than resistance.
   e. If a prepubescent child cannot perform a minimum of eight repetitions in good form, the resistance is too heavy and should be reduced.

G. OLDER (ELDERLY) INDIVIDUALS

It is important to emphasize the activities of daily living (ADLs) in this population. ADLs refer to the basic tasks of everyday life, such as eating, bathing, dressing, toileting, and transferring. When people are unable to perform these activities, they need help to cope, either from other human beings or mechanical devices or both. Although persons of all ages may have problems performing the ADLs, prevalence rates are much higher for the elderly than for the nonelderly. Within the elderly population, ADL prevalence rates rise steeply with advancing age and are especially high for persons aged $\geq$85 years. Regular physical activity may help older individuals perform ADLs as well as maintain independence longer.

1. Cardiorespiratory fitness for older individuals:
   a. The exercise modes used for older individuals should be those that do not impose excessive orthopedic stress, such as walking, aquatic exercise, and stationary cycling.
   b. A group exercise setting can provide needed social reinforcement enhancing adherence.
   c. Intensity: Start at very low intensities and gradually build up. Initially increase duration rather than intensity.
   d. Many older individuals have a wide variety of medical conditions and are subsequently on several forms of medication.
2. Resistance training for older individuals.
   a. Exercise should be closely supervised.
   b. One set of 10–15 repetitions at a perceived exertion level of 12–13 should be used on 8–10 exercises that use all major muscle groups.
   c. Use machines (selectorized equipment) as opposed to free weights because balance is often an issue with older people.
   d. Allow ample time during transition between exercises.

H. ARTHRITIS

Two main forms of arthritis are osteoarthritis and rheumatoid arthritis. Exercise should be avoided during arthritic flare-ups. Morning exercise should be avoided if possible because of morning stiffness.

1. Cardiorespiratory training

a. Frequency: 3–5 times/week.
b. Intensity: 40% or 50%–85% HRR or $\dot{V}O_2R$, 55% or 65%–90% HRmax, 12–16 RPE.
c. Duration: 20–60 minutes, start initially in short bouts (10 minutes).
d. Mode: Walking, cycling, and especially aquatic exercises are preferred. Water exercise may reduce pain and stiffness and decrease reliance on nonsteroidal anti-inflammatory drugs. Functional activities should be performed daily. Cross-training should be incorporated if possible.

2. Resistance training

a. Frequency: 2–3 times/week.
b. Intensity: Volitional fatigue or stop two to three repetitions before volitional fatigue.
c. Duration: 1 set of 3–20 repetitions, 8–10 exercises include all major muscle groups. Circuit training can be valuable for arthritic individuals because it typically involves one set per exercise done at relatively low resistance levels often for a set time period on each exercise as opposed to a certain number of repetitions on each exercise.

3. Flexibility Training

a. Frequency: Minimal 2–3 days/week; ideally, 5–7 days/week, 1–2 times daily.
b. Intensity: Stretch to tightness at the end of the ROM but not to pain.
c. Duration: 15–30 seconds, repeat each stretch 2–4 times, static stretch all major muscle groups.

VII. DOCUMENTATION OF EXERCISE PROGRAMMING

It is extremely important for fitness professionals to record all exercise sessions of participants. The frequency, intensity, mode, duration, and progression for each exercise session should be clearly documented to note improvement as well as for legal liability.

Review Test

DIRECTIONS: Carefully read all questions and select the BEST answer.

1. Which of the following is NOT an appropriate treatment activity for inpatient rehabilitation of a patient on the second day after coronary artery bypass graft (CABG) surgery?
   A) Limit activities as tolerated to the development of self-care activities, ROM for extremities, and low-resistance activities.
   B) Limit upper body activities to biceps curls, horizontal arm adduction, and overhead press using 5-pound weights while sitting on the side of the bed.
   C) Progress all activities performed from supine to sitting to standing.
   D) Measure vital signs, symptoms, RPE, fatigue, and skin color and perform electrocardiography before, during, and after treatments to assess activity tolerance.

2. Which of the following situations indicates progression to independent and unsupervised exercise for a patient after CABG surgery in an outpatient program?
   A) The patient exhibits mild cardiac symptoms of angina, occurring intermittently during exercise and sometimes at home while reading.
   B) The patient has a functional capacity of >8 MET with hemodynamic responses appropriate to this level of exercise.
   C) The patient is noncompliant with smoking cessation and weight loss intervention programs.
   D) The patient is unable to palpate HR, deliver RPEs, or maintain steady workload intensity during activity.

3. Which of the following issues would you include in discharge education instructions for a patient with congestive heart failure to avoid potential emergency situations related to this condition at home?
   A) Record body weight daily, and report weight gains to a physician.
   B) Note signs and symptoms (e.g., dyspnea, intolerance to activities of daily living), and report them to a physician.
   C) Do not palpate the pulse during daily activities or periods of light-headedness, because an irregular pulse is normal and occurs at various times during the day.
   D) Both A and B.

4. Initial training sessions for an individual with severe chronic obstructive pulmonary disease (COPD) most likely would NOT include
   A) Continuous cycling activity at 70% of $\dot{V}O_2$ max for 30 minutes.
   B) Use of dyspnea scales, RPE scales, and pursed-lip breathing instruction.
   C) Intermittent bouts of activity on a variety of modalities (exercise followed by short rest).
   D) Encouraging the patient to achieve an intensity either at or above the anaerobic threshold.

5. Symptoms of claudication include
   A) Cramping, burning, and tightness in the calf muscle, usually triggered by activity and relieved with rest.
   B) Acute, sharp pain in the calf on palpation at rest.
   C) Crepitus in the knee during cycling.
   D) Pitting ankle edema at a rating of 3+.

6. Treatment for claudication during exercise includes all of the following EXCEPT
   A) Daily exercise sessions.
   B) Intensity of activity to maximal tolerable pain, with intermittent rest periods.
   C) Cardiorespiratory building activities that are non–weight-bearing if the plan is to work on longer duration and higher intensity to elicit a cardiorespiratory training effect.
   D) Stopping activity at the onset of claudication discomfort to avoid further vascular damage from ischemia.

7. During an exercise test, a patient exhibits angina symptoms and a 1-mm down-sloping ST-segment depression at a HR of 129 bpm. His peak exercise target HR should be set at
   A) 128 bpm.
   B) 109–119 bpm.
   C) 129 bpm.
   D) 125–128 bpm.

8. Special precautions for patients with hypertension include all of the following EXCEPT
   A) Avoiding muscle strengthening exercises that involve low resistance.
   B) Avoiding activities that involve the Valsalva maneuver.
   C) Monitoring for arrhythmias in a person taking diuretics.
   D) Avoiding exercise if resting systolic BP is >200 mm Hg or diastolic BP is >115 mm Hg.

9. According to the most recent National Institutes of Health's *Clinical Guidelines for the Identification, Evaluation, and Treatment of Overweight and Obesity in Adults*, recommendations for practical clinical assessment include
   A) Determining total body fat through the BMI to assess obesity.
   B) Determining the degree of abdominal fat and health risk through waist circumference.
   C) Using the waist-to-hip ratio as the only definition of obesity and lean muscle mass.
   D) Both A and B.

10. An individual with type 1 diabetes mellitus checks her fasting morning glucose level on her whole-blood glucose meter (fingerstick method), and the result is 253 mg/dL (14 mmol/L). A urine test is positive for ketones before her exercise session. What action should you take?
   A) Allow her to exercise as long as her glucose is not >300 mg/dL (17 mmol/L).
   B) Do not allow her to exercise this session and notify her physician of the findings.
   C) Give her an extra carbohydrate snack and wait 5 minutes before beginning exercise.
   D) Readjust her insulin regimen for the remainder of the day to compensate for the high morning glucose level.

11. A 62-year-old, obese factory worker complains of pain in his right shoulder on arm abduction; on evaluation, decreased ROM and strength are noted. You also notice that he is beginning to use accessory muscles to substitute movements and to compensate. These symptoms may indicate
   A) A referred pain from a herniated lumbar disk.
   B) Rotator cuff strain or impingement.
   C) Angina.
   D) Advanced stages of multiple sclerosis.

12. All of the following are special considerations when prescribing exercise for a person with arthritis EXCEPT
   A) The possible need to splint painful joints for protection.
   B) Periods of acute inflammation result in decreased pain and joint stiffness.
   C) The possibility of gait abnormalities as compensation for pain or stiffness.
   D) The need to avoid exercise of warm, swollen joints.

13. What common medication taken by patients with end-stage renal disease requires careful management for those undergoing hemodialysis?
   A) Antihypertensive medication.
   B) Lithium.
   C) Cholestyramine.
   D) Cromolyn sodium.

14. Which of the following is an appropriate exercise for persons with diabetes and loss of protective sensation in the extremities?
   A) Prolonged walking.
   B) Jogging.
   C) Step-class exercise.
   D) Swimming.

15. A person taking a calcium-channel blocker will likely exhibit which of the following responses during exercise?
   A) Hypertensive response.
   B) Increased ischemia.
   C) Improved anginal thresholds.
   D) Severe hypotension.

16. During the cool-down phase of an exercise session, participants should be encouraged to
   A) Rehydrate.
   B) Decrease the intensity of activity quickly to decrease cardiac afterload.
   C) Limit the cool-down period to 5 minutes.
   D) Increase the number of isometric activities.

17. Muscular endurance training is best accomplished by
   A) Performing four to six repetitions per set.
   B) Using high resistance.
   C) Incorporating high repetitions.
   D) Performing isometric exercises only.

18. Transitional care exercise and rehabilitation programs are NOT appropriate for
   A) Persons with functionally limiting chronic disease.
   B) Persons with comorbid disease states.
   C) Asymptomatic persons with a functional capacity of 10 MET.
   D) Persons at 1 week after CABG surgery.

19. Which of the following is TRUE regarding exercise programming with VVI-mode programmed pacemakers?
   A) Persons with VVI pacemakers may be chronotropically (HR) competent with exercise but require longer warm-up and gradual increase in intensity during the initial exercise portion of their session.
   B) Persons who are chronotropically competent are tachycardic at rest and should not exercise at low intensities.
   C) BP response is not a good marker of intensity effort in those with VVI pacemakers and need not be evaluated during an exercise session.
   D) Persons with VVI pacemakers must avoid exercise on the bicycle ergometer because of the

location of the ventricular lead wire and potential for displacement.

20. Controlling pool water temperature (83°F to 88°F), avoiding jarring and weight-bearing activities, and avoiding movement in swollen, inflamed joints are special considerations for exercise in
   A) Patients after atherectomy.
   B) Patients with angina.
   C) Patients with osteoporosis.
   D) Patients with arthritis.

21. Which of the following is a resistive lung disease?
   A) Asthma.
   B) Tuberculosis.
   C) Cystic fibrosis.
   D) Emphysema.

22. A specific benefit of regular exercise for patients with angina is
   A) Improved ischemic threshold at which angina symptoms occur.
   B) Increased myocardial oxygen demand at the same submaximal levels.
   C) Eradication of all symptoms.
   D) Elevation of BP.

23. Which of the following is NOT a benefit of increased flexibility?
   A) Increased muscle viscosity, allowing easier and smoother contractions.
   B) Reduced muscle tension and increased relaxation.
   C) Improved coordination by allowing greater ease of movement.
   D) Increased ROM.

24. Which of the following statements regarding warm-up is FALSE?
   A) Muscle blood flow is increased as a result of warm-up.
   B) A gradual increase in HR occurs as a result of warm-up.
   C) Peripheral vasoconstriction occurs as a result of warm-up.
   D) Between 5 and 10 minutes should be allotted for a warm-up period.

25. Which of the following statements regarding cool-down is FALSE?
   A) The emphasis should be large muscle activity performed at a low to moderate intensity.
   B) Increasing venous return should be a priority during cool-down.
   C) The potential for improving flexibility may be improved during cool-down as compared with warm-up.
   D) Between 1 and 2 minutes are recommended for an adequate cool-down.

26. All of the following are examples of aerobic exercise modalities EXCEPT
   A) Weight training.
   B) Walking.
   C) Bicycling.
   D) Stair climbing.

27. A target HR equivalent to 85% of HRR for a 25-year-old man with a resting HR of 75 bpm would be equal to
   A) 195 bpm.
   B) 166 bpm.
   C) 177 bpm.
   D) 102 bpm.

28. The appropriate exercise HR for an individual on β-blocking medication would generally be
   A) 75% of HRR.
   B) 30 bpm above the standing resting HR.
   C) 40% of HRR.
   D) $(220 - \text{age}) \times 0.85$.

29. The recommended cardiorespiratory exercise training goal for apparently healthy individuals should be
   A) 15 minutes, six times per week, at 90% of HRR.
   B) 30 minutes, three times per week, at 85% of HRR.
   C) 60 minutes, three times per week, at 85% of HRR.
   D) 30 minutes of weight training, three times per week, at 60% of HRR.

30. In an effort to improve flexibility, the ACSM recommends
   A) Proprioceptive neuromuscular facilitation.
   B) Ballistic stretching.
   C) The plough and hurdler's stretches.
   D) Static stretches held for 10–30 seconds/repetition.

31. An appropriate exercise for improving the strength of the low back muscles is
   A) Straight leg lifts.
   B) Parallel squats.
   C) Spinal extension exercises.
   D) Sit-ups with feet anchored.

32. Which of the following statements regarding exercise leadership is FALSE?
   A) The exercise leader should be sufficiently fit to exercise with any of his or her participants.
   B) Most people are not bored by exercise and can easily find time to participate in an exercise program.
   C) The exercise leader should adjust the exercise intensity based on individual differences in fitness.
   D) Periodic fitness assessment may provide evidence of improvement in fitness for some participants.

33. Which of the following statements regarding exercise for the elderly is FALSE?
   A) A decrease in maximal HR is responsible for reductions in the maximal oxygen consumption as persons age.
   B) A loss of fat-free mass is responsible for the decrease in muscular strength as persons age.
   C) The ACSM recommends a cardiorespiratory training intensity of 50%–70% of HRR for older adults.
   D) Resistance exercise training is not recommended for older adults.

34. Which of the following medications have been shown to be most effective in preventing or reversing exercise-induced asthma?
   A) β_2-agonists.
   B) β-blockers.
   C) Diuretics.
   D) Aspirin.

35. The exercise leader or health and fitness specialist should modify exercise sessions for participants with hypertension by
   A) Shortening the cool-down to <5 minutes.
   B) Eliminating resistance training completely.
   C) Prolonging the cool-down.
   D) Implementing high-intensity (>85% of HRR), short-duration intervals.

36. Osteoporosis is more prevalent in
   A) Women who have never been pregnant.
   B) Black women.
   C) Women who are involved in activities that place stress on the wrists, hips, or lumbosacral region.
   D) Postmenopausal women.

37. The goal for the obese exercise participant should be to
   A) Sweat as much as possible.
   B) Exercise at 85% of HRR.
   C) Perform resistance exercise three to five times per week.
   D) Expend 300–500 calories per exercise session.

38. Which of the following statements regarding exercise for persons with controlled cardiovascular disease is TRUE?
   A) Resistance exercise training is dangerous and should be avoided.
   B) A physician-supervised exercise test is not necessary to establish exercise intensity.
   C) Anginal pain is normal during exercise, and participants should be pushed through the pain.
   D) Exercise intensity should be set at a HR of 10 bpm less than the level at which signs or symptoms were evidenced during an exercise test.

39. All of the following factors are important to consider when determining exercise intensity EXCEPT
   A) An individual's level of fitness.
   B) The risk of cardiovascular or orthopedic injury.
   C) Any previous history participating in organized sports.
   D) Individual preference and exercise objectives.

40. When determining the intensity level, the RPE is a better indicator than percentage of maximal HR for all of the following groups EXCEPT
   A) Individuals on β-blockers.
   B) Aerobic classes that involve excessive arm movement.
   C) Individuals older than 65 years.
   D) Individuals involved in high-intensity exercise.

41. Using the original Borg scale, it is recommended that the exercise intensity elicit an RPE within the range of
   A) 8–12.
   B) 12–16.
   C) 14–18.
   D) 6–10.

42. The MINIMAL duration of exercise necessary to achieve improvements in health for deconditioned individuals is
   A) 20 minutes continuously.
   B) 30 minutes continuously.
   C) Multiple sessions of >10 minutes in duration throughout the day.
   D) Two sessions of 20 minutes throughout the day.

43. Which of the following is a method of strength and power training that involves an eccentric loading of muscles and tendons followed immediately by an explosive concentric contraction?
   A) Super sets.
   B) Split routines.
   C) Plyometrics.
   D) Periodization.

44. The safety of resistance exercise is dependent on all of the following EXCEPT
   A) Having a personal trainer.
   B) Proper breathing.
   C) Speed of movement.
   D) Body mechanics.

45. The recommended muscular strength and endurance training program for apparently healthy individuals should be
   A) One set of 8–12 repetitions, 8–10 separate exercises, 2 days/week.
   B) Two sets of 6–8 repetitions, 8–10 separate exercises, 2 days/week.
   C) One set of 8–12 repetitions, 8–10 separate exercises, 4–5 days/week.

D) Two sets of 6–8 repetitions, 8–10 separate exercises, 4 days/week, and alternating days for legs and upper body.

46. Which the following statements regarding intensity of resistance training is FALSE?
   A) The number of repetitions to volitional fatigue will vary inversely with resistance.
   B) It is necessary to determine the 1-RM to establish training intensity.
   C) Exercise to volitional fatigue is not dangerous from a musculoskeletal standpoint provided that good exercise form is maintained.
   D) Exercise intensity should be similar for male and female participants.

47. The recommended cardiorespiratory endurance exercise training program for older individuals should be
   A) 40%–60% of maximum HR, 20–30 minutes continuously, 3 days/week.
   B) 50%–70% of HRR, 20–30 minutes (multiple sessions of 5–10 min), 3 days/week.
   C) 40%–60% of maximal HR, 20–30 minutes (multiple sessions of 5–10 min), 3 days/week.
   D) 50%–70% of HRR, 20–30 minutes continuously, 3 days/week.

ANSWERS AND EXPLANATIONS

1–B. Strenuous and resistive upper body exercises and activity can cause injury to the sternum immediately after CABG surgery. Such exercises should be avoided until the sternum and chest incisions have healed.

2–B. Progression to a more independent self-managed program is encouraged for those who have a good functional capacity, exhibit appropriate hemodynamic and electrocardiographic responses to exercise and recovery, are asymptomatic, have stable resting HR and BP, manage risk factor intervention strategies safely and effectively, demonstrate knowledge of the disease process, and are compliant with their program.

3–D. Symptoms of worsening heart failure (e.g., leg edema, activity intolerance, dyspnea, orthopnea, paroxysmal dyspnea) must be explained to patients. A weight gain of 3–5 pounds since the last appointment should be reported. During symptoms of light-headedness or chest discomfort, palpating the pulse provides helpful information if the heartbeat suddenly becomes irregular during these episodes. Development of an arrhythmia should be reported to the physician.

4–A. A person with severe chronic obstructive pulmonary disease who is just beginning an exercise program would not be able to tolerate vigorously intense exercise for prolonged periods because of limitations, such as dyspnea, muscle weakness, and cardiovascular deconditioning, as a result of previous inactivity.

5–A. Sharp, palpable pain over an area typically indicates fasciitis or tendonitis. Crepitus in the knee indicates inflammation, arthritis, and other joint structural problems. Ankle edema indicates poor venous return in conditions such as right-sided heart failure and is not an indication of an atherosclerotic artery.

6–D. Patients with claudication are encouraged to exercise at an intensity that causes intense pain (grade III) or unbearable pain (grade IV). This is followed by a full-recovery rest period.

7–B. Peak exercise HR is set at 10–20 bpm below the ischemic level (which was symptomatic, downsloping ST-segment depression at 129 bpm).

8–A. Low-resistance muscle-strengthening exercises can be performed by those diagnosed with hypertension if they follow appropriate lifting techniques and avoid the Valsalva maneuver. In addition, hemodynamic parameters (HR and BP) and medications should be controlled.

9–D. The BMI can be used to classify overweight and obesity levels. In addition, waist circumference has been found to be a better marker of abdominal fat content than the waist-to-hip ratio.

10–B. Whole-blood glucose values generally are 10%–15% lower than plasma glucose levels. Those with type 1 diabetes should avoid exercise when ketones are present at a glucose level of >240 mg/dL (14 mmol/L) or if glucose levels >300 mg/dL (17 mmol/L) regardless of whether ketosis is present. Carbohydrate snacks are taken only when glucose levels are too low to help maintain proper glycemic control during exercise. Only a physician can prescribe changes in medication regimen.

11–B. The subdeltoid bursa, supraspinatus muscle, and nerves become impinged between the coracoid and acromion process with shoulder abduction. The resulting pain leads to decreased ROM, disuse, and muscle atrophy. Such impingement of the rotator cuff is common in assembly line workers performing repetitive overhead tasks.

12–B. During periods of acute arthritic inflammation, affected joints will be painful, stiff, hot, and swollen. These joints should not be exercised and may need to be protected to allow the person to perform other motor tasks.

13–A. The process of hemodialysis interacts with antihypertensive medications and lowers the drug level, causing a potentially severe hypertensive response. To avoid such a reaction, patients may skip their hypertension medication on dialysis days.

14–D. Prolonged walking, jogging, and step classes are high-impact or weight-bearing activities that can lead to sores, ulcers, or fractures in those with loss of sensation in the feet (peripheral neuropathy).

15–C. Patients with angina who are taking calcium-channel blockers will improve their exercise capacity response to exercise regimens.

16–A. A longer cool-down period of 10–15 minutes (or longer for certain disease states) and a gradual decrease in intensity will provide a smoother recovery period and avoid sudden adverse hemodynamic responses and associated symptoms.

17–C. Muscular endurance (the ability to sustain prolonged muscular contractions) is best accomplished by using lighter weights and performing more repetitions per set.

18–C. Transitional or home care rehabilitation can be provided through nursing homes, rehabilitation hospitals, or clinics to those needing supervised care for exercise or activities of daily living.

19–A. Chronotropically competent VVI patients often are bradycardic at rest but have good atrioventricular conduction. Gradual increases in activity are recommended to allow the sinus node time to respond. The BP should be monitored during exercise to help assess intensity levels.

20–D. Patients with arthritis should avoid exercising joints that are acutely inflamed and they will benefit from non–weight-bearing pool exercises in warm water. Patients with cardiac diagnoses are not limited to non–weight-bearing activities and do not have inflamed joints as a result of their disease. Individuals with osteoporosis benefit from exercise that decreases the rate of bone loss.

21–B. Obstructive lung diseases are "flow" obstructions, including asthma, cystic fibrosis, interstitial lung disease, chronic bronchitis, and emphysema. Restrictive lung diseases are those involving restricted lung capacity because of disease or damage of the lungs, including lupus, pulmonary edema, tuberculosis, and lung cancer.

22–A. The ischemic threshold is predictable in patients with stable angina. A benefit of regular exercise for patients with angina is an improved ischemic threshold at which angina symptoms occur. In addition, myocardial oxygen demand decreases, as do the BP and HR responses to submaximal exercise.

23–A. Increased flexibility provides numerous benefits, including reduced muscle tension, increased relaxation, increased ease of movement, improved coordination, increased ROM, improved body awareness, improved capability for circulation and air exchange, decreased muscle viscosity (causing contractions to be easier and smoother), and decreased soreness associated with other exercise activities.

24–C. Peripheral vasoconstriction would be a negative consequence of warm-up if it occurred. Appropriate warm-up activities promote increased muscle blood flow and increased oxygen delivery. This is accomplished through peripheral vasodilation. Typically, a 5- to 10-minute time frame will allow for a gradual increase in HR, an increase in body temperature, and a slight reduction in pH. These changes will facilitate increased oxygen consumption. Although more research is needed to determine the effects of warm-up on musculoskeletal injury rates, it seems that even from a psychological perspective, warm-up may prevent injury during exercise.

25–D. The primary purpose of cool-down is to increase venous return, and this is accomplished by low-intensity, large-muscle activity. This type of activity also aids the removal of lactic acid. Evidence of an effective cool-down is an HR of <100 bpm and a systolic BP within 10 mm Hg of preexercise levels. Between 5 and 10 minutes will allow these changes to occur and provide time for some attention to flexibility exercises. The potential for improving flexibility is increased when the body is warm and the muscles and connective tissue are more pliable, as is the case after (versus before) exercise.

26–A. Weight training is not considered to be an aerobic exercise. Although some increases in maximal oxygen consumption have been shown from circuit weight training, this is not considered to be a very effective means for improving cardiorespiratory fitness. Large-muscle group activity, performed in rhythmic fashion for a prolonged period, is the most efficient means of stressing the aerobic energy system.

27–C. Using 220 minus age (25) yields 195. Subtract 75 (resting HR) to yield the HRR (120). Multiply 120 by 0.85 (85%) to yield 102, and then add the resting HR (75) back in to yield 177 as the target HR.

28–A. β-blocking medications blunt the HR response at rest and during exercise, but the linear relationship between HR and oxygen consumption remains consistent with β-blocking medication. It is appropriate to program exercise at a percentage of HRR (75% is well within the correct range, but 40% HRR is not within guideline standards).

29–B. Although additional improvements in maximal oxygen consumption may be seen when exercise is performed at >85% of HRR or when duration >30 minutes and at frequencies greater than three times per week, these improvements are minimal and accompanied by increased risk of musculoskeletal injury.

30–D. The proprioceptive neuromuscular facilitation is impractical, because it requires a partner and potential for injury exists if the stretch is applied too vigorously. Ballistic stretching may induce soreness and actually impede the ability to stretch. The plough and hurdler's stretches are potentially harmful exercises that compromise the neck and knee, respectively. Isometric activity involves exerting force against an immovable object and is considered to be an inefficient form of muscle-strengthening exercise. Static stretches held for 10–30 seconds per repetition are effective and carry a low risk of injury.

31–C. Straight leg lifts are potentially harmful to the low back and actually stress the hip flexors and the abdominals. Squats primarily involve the gluteals and the quadriceps. The erector spinae are the prime movers for spinal extension. Spinal flexion requires the abdominals to contract while placing the low back muscles on a slight stretch. Sit-ups exercise the abdominal musculature and, if performed with the feet anchored or to a full ROM, will involve the hip flexors.

32–B. Unless creative program strategies are employed, most people become bored with exercise. The exercise leader may be able to increase exercise program compliance by offering variety in programming, providing adequate instruction and encouragement, keeping participants free of injury, and demonstrating progress through exercise testing. A comprehensive exercise program that can be completed in no more than 1 hour, three times per week, should be developed for all participants who are interested in health and fitness. The idea is to minimize the time commitment while providing for maximal response.

33–D. Resistance exercise training for older adults is highly recommended to slow the typical age-related loss of lean tissue. Additional benefits include increases in bone density and improved functional capacity. Attention should be given to the overall health status of the individual, and appropriate modifications should be made if cardiovascular, metabolic, or musculoskeletal problems are present.

34–A. β_2-agonists provide effective bronchodilation with relatively minimal side effect. β-lockers are prescribed for cardiovascular concerns, including hypertension. Diuretics also are used to treat hypertension and congestive heart failure. Aspirin is used to reduce pain and fever, but it provides no pulmonary effect. Theophylline has a slow onset of action and many associated side effects.

35–C. A prolonged cool-down of 5–10 minutes will enhance venous return and the hypotensive effects that are associated with many antihypertensive medications.

36–D. Osteoporosis is reduction in bone mass per unit of volume. Reduced bone mass is more prevalent in sedentary individuals and progresses at a more rapid rate in women following menopause. This condition increases the risk for fractures of the wrists, hips, and lumbosacral regions and is considered to be a significant source of debilitation in older adults.

37–D. The goal for weight loss would be to expend 300–500 kcal/exercise session in combination with a reduced caloric intake that would yield a total caloric deficit of no more than 1,000 kcal/day or 7,000 kcal/week. The recommended rate of weight loss should not exceed 1 or 2 pounds per week to ensure adequate nutrition and health. The emphasis in weight-loss exercise programs should be large muscle group, aerobic-type exercise at a level of intensity that will allow the greatest caloric expenditure for the time spent exercising, with attention also being given to musculoskeletal and cardiovascular safety.

38–D. According to the ACSM, individuals with known disease should have a clinical exercise test before exercise participation to determine safe levels of exercise for the participant. Exercise intensity should be set at 1 MET below the level where signs or symptoms are evidenced. An HR of 10 bpm less than the HR where signs or symptoms are evidenced also may be used. Whenever anginal pain is evidenced during exercise, the exercise should be terminated and appropriate medical attention sought.

39–C. The risk of orthopedic and, perhaps, cardiovascular complications may be increased with high-intensity activity. Factors to consider when determining the appropriate intensity include the individual's level of fitness, use of medications that may influence exercise performance, risk of cardiovascular or orthopedic injury, individual preference regarding exercise, and individual program objectives.

40–D. The RPE is particularly useful when participants are incapable of monitoring their pulse or when medications such as β-blockers alter the HR response to exercise. Excessive arm movements (e.g., in high-intensity exercise) make it difficult to feel and accurately count the pulse rate.

41–B. The RPE is particularly useful when participants are incapable of monitoring their pulse or when medications such as β-blockers alter the HR response to exercise. The ACSM recommends an exercise intensity that will elicit an RPE within a range of 12–16 on the original Borg scale.

42–C. The ACSM recommends 20–60 minutes of continuous aerobic activity. Typically, adequate caloric expenditure and cardiorespiratory conditioning goals may be met with exercise sessions of moderate duration (20–30 min). Individuals who are very deconditioned may benefit from multiple exercise sessions of short ($\leq$10 min) duration. Increases in duration may be instituted as evidence of adaptation without undue fatigue or injury occurs.

43–C. Plyometrics is a method of strength and power training that involves an eccentric loading of muscles and tendons followed immediately by an explosive concentric contraction. This stretch-shortening cycle may allow enhanced force generation during the concentric (shortening) phase.

44–A. The safety of resistance exercise is dependent on the proper execution of a given exercise. Spotting, proper breathing, movement speed, and body mechanics are all central to safe exercise performance.

45–A. The ACSM recommends that one set of 8–12 repetitions of exercise should be performed to volitional fatigue at least 2 days each week.

46–B. Intensity is defined as a percentage of a person's momentary ability to perform an activity (e.g., how difficult the exercise is, amount of effort during the exercise). It is the percentage of the maximal voluntary contraction in resistance exercise. It is not the percentage of 1-RM unless all other variables (e.g., individual exercise, movement speed, number of repetitions) are kept constant.

47–B. The health status of the individual should be carefully considered when establishing intensity. Generally, a conservative approach should initially be taken. The ACSM recommends an intensity of 50%–70% of HRR for older adults.

Nutrition and Weight Management

CHAPTER 9

I. WEIGHT-RELATED TERMS

A. OVERWEIGHT

The Centers for Disease Control and Prevention (CDC) defines **overweight** as body weight that is higher than what is considered healthy for a specific height.

B. OBESITY

Obesity refers to excess body fat based on some sort of quantitative assessment such as body composition or body mass index (BMI).

1. Body Composition Assessment

a. Evaluation of the body's fat to nonfat (lean) components.
   1) Lean components include muscle, bone, water, blood.
   2) Fat stores include subcutaneous, intraabdominal, and intramuscular fat.
   3) Estimating total lean mass = total body mass − fat mass.
   4) **Percent fat** (% fat) is the amount of total body weight that is fat only, based on body composition assessment. To estimate total fat mass: total body weight × percent body fat.

b. Established norms for age and gender.

c. Typically assessed by:
   1) **Skinfold** calipers.
   2) **Bioelectrical impedance.**
      (i) Handheld devices commonly used in health clubs.
      (ii) Home-use devices such as bathroom scales with special options.
      (iii) Laboratory devices using electrode placement on dorsum of hand and foot.
   3) **Hydrostatic (underwater) weighing.**
   4) **Dual-Energy X-ray Absorptiometry (DXA or DEXA).**
   5) **Air displacement plethysmography.**

d. Error associated with the assessment of body composition ranges from 1%–3% with hydrostatic weighing, DXA, and air displacement plethysmography.

e. Higher errors are found with skinfold and bioelectrical impedance measurements despite that these are the most common methods used in most fitness centers.
   1) Follow manufacturer instructions or established protocol for measurement.
   2) Accurate skinfolds depend on:
      i) Skill and experience of tester.
      ii) Equation used for prediction.
   3) Bioelectrical impedance accuracy affected by:
      i) Hydration.
      ii) Time of last exercise session.

2. Body Mass Index (BMI)

a. BMI is calculated as body weight in kilograms divided by body height in meters squared ($kg \cdot m^{-2}$).

b. Disease Risk Classification.

BODY MASS INDEX	CLASSIFICATION
$<18.5\ kg \cdot m^{-2}$	Underweight.
$18.5–24.9\ kg \cdot m^{-2}$	Normal.
$25.0–29.9\ kg \cdot m^{-2}$	Overweight
$30.0–39.9\ kg \cdot m^{-2}$	Class I Obesity
$35.0–39.9\ kg \cdot m^{-2}$	Class II Obesity
$40.0\ kg \cdot m^{-2}$	Class III Obesity

c. Cannot differentiate body composition; therefore, may not be best indicator for athletic populations who may have high BMI yet appropriate body composition levels.

d. Most commonly used to compare large data sets in research studies or to examine BMI over time.

C. ANOREXIA NERVOSA

1. A clinically diagnosed eating disorder exemplified by very thin physical appearance.
   a. Body weight at least 15% below the lowest value expected for height.
   b. BMI $\leq 17.5\ kg \cdot m^{-2}$.
2. Energy intake too low to maintain normal body weight.
3. Intense obsession with food and portions.

4. **Distorted self body image perception** (appearance very thin, but self-perception is overweight).
5. Intense fear of weight gain or becoming fat.
6. Other psychological issues such as low self-esteem, feelings of guilt, and self-disgust.
7. Health complications include osteoporosis, menstrual irregularities, electrolyte imbalances, cardiac arrhythmias, and loss of muscle mass.
8. Occurs mostly in females, but is also seen in males, especially those who participate in sports with appearance or weight requirements.
9. Whites more affected, but increasing incidence is seen in other races and ethnicities.
10. More prevalent in high school and college age groups, but incidence increasing in adult women in ages 25–40 years.
11. Although medical treatment is required, exercise professionals can play a supportive role by referring persons who are suspected of having eating disorders to physicians or mental healthcare providers.

D. BULIMIA NERVOSA

1. A clinically diagnosed eating disorder.
2. Body weight could be underweight, overweight, or normal weight.
3. Binging involves eating large amounts of food over a small period of time a minimum of twice per week for several months.
4. Health complications include gastrointestinal disturbances, wearing away of teeth enamel, pancreatitis, electrolyte imbalances, and esophageal rupture.
5. Purging Behaviors.
   a. Vomiting.
   b. Laxative abuse.
   c. Excessive exercise.
   d. Sauna suits.
   e. Diuretics.
6. Occurs mostly in females, but is also seen in males, especially those who participate in sports with aesthetic or weight requirements.
7. More common in whites, but increasing incidence in other races and ethnicities.
8. More prevalent in high school and college age groups, but incidence increasing in adult women in ages 25–40 years.
9. Although medical treatment is required, exercise professionals can play a supportive role by referring individuals who are suspected of having eating disorders to physicians or mental healthcare providers.

E. BODY COMPOSITION AND HEALTH

1. High Body Fat

High body fat is associated with risk of obesity-related diseases such as:

a. Diabetes.
b. Coronary artery disease.
c. Heart failure.
d. Stroke.
e. Certain cancers such as pancreatic, colon, possibly breast and prostate.
f. Sleep apnea.
g. Arthritis.
h. Hypertension (high blood pressure).

2. Low Body Fat

Low body fat may be advantageous for appearance or for participation in certain sports, but low body fat could occasionally be a symptom of disease, especially with a drastic or unintended weight loss. The participant should seek medical care to evaluate the possibilities of:

a. Eating disorders, such as anorexia or bulimia nervosa.
b. Digestive diseases and other diseases of nutrient absorption abnormalities.
c. Cancer.
d. Type 1 diabetes or other metabolic disorders.

II. BODY FAT DISTRIBUTION AND HEALTH

A. FAT DISTRIBUTION AND DISEASE

1. Body Fat Distribution Patterns

a. Where an individual predominantly stores his or her body fat has a role in risk of certain chronic diseases such as type 2 diabetes, coronary artery disease, high blood pressure (hypertension), and certain cancers.
   1) Central or **android pattern** (commonly known as "apple" shaped). This body fat is located mostly in the abdominal area versus hips and thighs and is more common in men but seen in women, more so after menopause. Another common term is "abdominal obesity."
   2) Peripheral or **gynoid pattern** ("pear" shaped). Body fat is located mostly in the hips and thighs versus waist and is more common in women, but occasionally seen in men.
   3) Body fat distribution:
      a) **Waist-to-hip ratio** (WHR) is the ratio of the waist circumference divided by the hip circumference.

Values of WHR >0.95 in men and >0.86 in women are associated with increased risk of type 2 diabetes, coronary artery disease, and hypertension.

b) **Waist circumference**, according to recent research, may be a more important measurement than WHR, because it may be a better estimate of abdominal obesity. Increased chronic disease risk appears with waist circumference values of >40 inches (102 cm) in men and >35 inches (88 cm) in women.

B. HEALTH RISKS ASSOCIATED WITH CENTRAL (ABDOMINAL) OBESITY

1. Abdominal obesity is more strongly correlated with certain metabolic risk factors than just overweight or obesity by BMI alone, such as insulin resistance, high blood pressure, elevated fasting blood glucose level, and dyslipidemia.
2. The term **metabolic syndrome** is used when several coronary artery disease risk factors occur at the same time in combination with abdominal obesity.
3. The risk factors linked with metabolic syndrome act to increase cardiovascular disease and diabetes morbidity and mortality in a synergistic way.
4. Management of metabolic syndrome includes lifestyle changes in diet and exercise, quitting smoking (if applicable), and likely the use of pharmacologic intervention.

III. MODIFYING BODY COMPOSITION

A. One pound of body fat contains stored energy in the amount of **3,500 kcal.** To lose 1 lb of body fat, an energy deficit of 3,500 kcal must be created. Theoretically, to lose 1 lb of body fat in 1 week, there must be an energy deficit of 500 kcal from the diet every day, a surplus energy expenditure of 500 kcal every day, or some combination of both to result in a 3,500 kcal difference in energy expenditure during the course of the week of body fat reduction.

B. Weight losses of >1–2 lb/week (0.5–1.0 kg) are not recommended and may result in decreased resting metabolic rate from loss of lean body mass.

C. There may be weight losses >2 lb in the initial weeks of a weight loss program, but this is often owing to normal weight fluctuations, measurement error, or water loss.

D. Aerobic activities should be emphasized to create an energy deficit.

E. Individual differences exist in rates of energy expenditure and with different aerobic activities, but a good estimation is 1 mile (0.6 km) of walking or jogging expends 100 kcal. Theoretically, for persons to lose a pound of body fat per week, they would have to expend 500 kcal every day, or walk or jog the equivalent of 5 miles (8 km) every day, without making changes to their regular diet.

F. Because most people expend <500 kcal/exercise session, it will take longer for them to create a sufficient energy deficit to lose 1 lb (0.5 kg).

G. There is elevated resting metabolic rate after exercise, and this additional energy expenditure may or may not have an effect on weight loss.

H. Preservation of lean body mass may affect both resting metabolic rate and weight management.

I. It is possible for patients to find a satisfactory program to produce a sufficient energy deficit from both diet and exercise to aim for a 1 lb. (0.5 kg) weight loss per week.

J. Research findings from weight management studies indicate that persons who maintain healthy eating habits and perform **regular exercise** demonstrate better outcomes for long-term weight management.

K. Assess stages of change using **Transtheoretical Model** and set goals appropriately (refer to Chapter 5, Section II.C.).

L. Utilize Social Cognitive Theory Concepts.

IV. INAPPROPRIATE METHODS FOR WEIGHT LOSS

Although many persons are often looking toward the latest big fad for weight loss, the only safe and effective methods involve eating healthy foods while consuming fewer total daily kilocalories, performing regular physical activity through aerobic exercise, and maintaining or increasing lean body mass by resistance training. Despite extensive knowledge of these principles by consumers, exercise professionals must educate exercise participants regarding fads and myths that are inappropriate for weight loss.

A. **Spot reduction**, exercising a particular body part, does not lead to weight or fat loss over that body part.

B. **Saunas, sweat suits, and body wraps** can lead to a rapid weight loss, owing to fluid loss, but are not recommended for weight loss because of many safety concerns such as risk of electrolyte imbalances from dehydration and heat exhaustion or heat stroke. These methods are ineffective for body fat loss because weight lost is from water, which is rapidly regained once normal hydration resumes.

C. **Vibrating belts** are passive movement devices that are used to "break down" fat. In reality, these are ineffective for weight loss because no such breakdown takes place and there is little or no actual energy expenditure by the person using these devices.

D. **Electrical stimulators** are inappropriate for weight loss because they rely on spot reduction and there is little or no actual energy expenditure by the user.

E. **Fad and starvation diets,** such as packaged foods, food combinations, or supplements; and the exclusion of certain foods, food groups, or macronutrients, are not effective in healthy, nonclinical populations. They are inappropriate for weight loss because:
   1. All diets will lead to weight loss if energy intake is sufficiently reduced.
   2. Loss of lean body mass may occur from lowered resting metabolic rate as a result of too low energy intake.
   3. Could be higher risk of nutritional deficiencies from reduction or elimination of certain foods or food groups.
   4. Long-term efficacy, safety, and maintenance are often unknown.
   5. Although some individuals may have initial success with fad or starvation diets, insufficient scientific evidence exists on their safety and efficacy to recommend them to the general public for long-term consumption.

V. ROLE OF DIET AND EXERCISE IN WEIGHT CONTROL

A. Regular, consistent physical activity appears to be required for long-term weight management and is the best predictor of successful weight loss management.
   1. Optimal weight control and health can be found by consuming a diet high in fruits and vegetables, three or more servings of whole grains, nonfat or low-fat dairy products, lean sources of protein, moderate amounts of healthy oils such as those found in certain types of fish and in nuts, keeping dietary fat <30% total energy, and including lean sources of protein along with regular, consistent physical activity or planned exercise.
   2. Energy intake for women should be a minimum of 1,200 kcal/day and for men a minimum of 1,800 kcal/day.
   3. The optimal mix of carbohydrates, protein, and fats for weight loss has not been determined by scientific studies.
   4. Aerobic exercise can help create sufficient energy deficit to lose 1–2 lb (0.5–1.0 kg) per week.
   5. Resistance training can be performed to maintain or increase lean body mass.

B. Gaining body weight may be indicated for persons who are underweight or with low BMI.
   1. Energy intake must be higher than energy expenditure for weight gain to occur; positive energy balance is required.
   2. Individuals should aim for 400–500 kcal/day more than the current energy intake.
   3. Consume larger portion sizes.
   4. Increase intake of foods with high-energy density, such as nuts, peanut butter, avocado, granola, dried fruits or breakfast bars, fruit smoothies, and shakes.
   5. Eat more frequent meals and snacks throughout the day.
   6. Resistance training may be integrated into exercise program to gain lean body mass.

VI. ESTIMATING ADEQUATE DAILY ENERGY INTAKE

A. **Total Energy Expenditure.**
   1. **Resting Metabolic Rate or Resting Energy Expenditure.**
      Amount of energy, usually expressed in kilocalories, required for the body's most basic vital functions in a quiet, resting state.
   2. **Thermic Effect of Food.**
      Energy required for digestion, absorption, and assimilation of nutrients.
   3. **Thermic Effect of Exercise.**
      Energy required for physical activity or exercise.

B. Measurement by indirect calorimetry is the gold standard measure for resting metabolic rate.
   1. Typically available in medical facilities or university research laboratories.
   2. May require overnight stay, or individual arrives very early morning.
   3. Usually some sort of fast (8–12 hours) is required.
   4. Assessed by either:
      a. Chamber or sealed room calorimeter.
      b. Metabolic cart. Measuring the amount of oxygen consumed and carbon dioxide produced can be used to calculate energy expenditure.

C. Prediction equations can give estimates of resting energy expenditure when used outside of laboratory settings.
   1. **Harris-Benedict Equation.**
      a. Resting metabolic rate (RMR) calculated as kilocalories per day.
      b. Males: RMR $= 88.32 + (4.799 \times$ height in cm$) + (13.397 \times$ weight in kg$) - (5.677 \times$ age in years$)$.
      c. Females: RMR $= 447.53 + (3.098 \times$ height in cm$) + (9.247 \times$ weight in kg$) - (4.33 \times$ age in years$)$.
      d. Use correction factors for physical activity levels:
         1) Sedentary: RMR $\times$ 1.4.
         2) Moderately active: RMR $\times$ 1.6.
         3) Highly active: RMR $\times$ 1.8.

2. Estimation of RMR based on fat-free mass:
   a. Obtain fat-free mass in kilogram by body composition assessment.
   b. RMR = 370 + (21.6 × fat free mass in kilograms).
   c. Use physical activity correction factors from Harris-Benedict equation.
3. These calculations allow exercise professionals to provide their individuals with reasonable energy intake and expenditure targets to help meet their goals for weight loss, weight maintenance, weight gain, or athletic performance. More valid resources exist to find energy expenditures of various physical activities for health, exercise, or sport.

TABLE 9-1. ENERGY NEEDS FOR WEIGHT MANAGEMENT

		ACTIVITY LEVEL		
GENDER	AGE (YEARS)	SEDENTARY	MODERATELY ACTIVE	ACTIVE
Child	2–3	1,000	1,000–1,400	1,000–1,400
Female	4–8	1,200	1,400–1,600	1,400–1,800
	9–13	1,600	1,600–2,000	1,800–2,200
	14–18	1,800	2,000	2,400
	19–30	2,000	2,000–2,200	2,400
	31–50	1,800	2,000	2,200
	51+	1,600	1,800	2,000–2,200
Male	4–8	1,400	1,400–1,600	1,600–2,000
	9–13	1,800	1,800–2,200	2,000–2,600
	14–18	2,200	2,400–2,800	2,800–3,200
	19–30	2,400	2,600–2,800	3,000
	31–50	2,200	2,400–2,600	2,800–3,000
	51+	2,000	2,200–2,400	2,400–2,800

Source: U.S. Department of Health and Human Services and U.S. Department of Agriculture. Dietary Guidelines for Americans, 2005. 6th Edition, Washington, DC: U.S. Government Printing Office, January 2005.

VII. DIETARY GUIDELINES FOR MANAGEMENT OF BODY WEIGHT

A. The *Dietary Guidelines for Americans*, developed by the United States Department of Agriculture (USDA) and Department of Health and Human Services (USDHHS), are modified every 5 years, most recently in 2005, to provide a more current, targeted approach on energy needs, macronutrient intake, and recommendations of food serving sizes for both health and weight management.
   1. Approximately 1,200 kcal/day for women and 1,800 kcal/day for men are considered the minimal energy intake requirements. When an individual drops below this minimum, there is increased risk of nutritional deficiency.
   2. Total energy needs for weight management in the *Dietary Guidelines for Americans* have been categorized by age, gender, and physical activity level based on recommendations from the Institute of Medicine (IOM) (*Table 9-1*).
      a. Sedentary: no additional physical activity other what is needed in typical day-to-day life.
      b. Moderately active: includes typical daily physical activity plus physical activity equivalent to walking approximately 1.5–3 miles/day at a 3- 4-mile/hour (mph) pace.
      c. Active: typical daily physical activity plus physical activity more than walking 1.5–3 miles/day at 3–4 mph.
   3. Carbohydrate intake is recommended at 45%–65% total energy.
      a. Dietary fiber, which helps with fullness, is recommended at 14 g/1,000 kcal. Most adults do not meet fiber targets.
      b. Eating whole fruits and vegetables and consuming whole grain breads, cereals, pastas, brown rice, and other whole grains such as popcorn versus their more processed varieties made from white flour will help an individual reach recommended fiber levels.
      c. Recommended: 2 cups of fruits and 2½ cups of vegetables per day for a 2,000 kcal diet, adjusted higher and lower depending on energy requirements.
      d. The color of the vegetable influences nutritional value. On a weekly basis, an individual should aim for at least 3 cups of dark green vegetables, 2 cups of orange vegetables, 3 cups of legumes or other dry beans, 3 cups of starchy vegetables such as potatoes, and 6½ servings of other vegetables.
      e. At least 3 servings of whole grain products are recommended per day.
      f. The terms "whole" or "whole grain" should appear as the first ingredient on the package nutrition label for an item to be classified as a whole grain.
      g. Individuals should aim to prepare foods with less added sugar, and minimize the amount of carbohydrates obtained from sugar, such as sodas and other sugar-sweetened drinks.
      h. It is difficult to maintain body weight when an individual consumes large amounts of sugar-sweetened foods and beverages because sugar provides large amounts of energy but little nutrients.
      i. Recommended: 2–3 cups of fat-free or low-fat milk is recommended per day. If an individual cannot tolerate milk, options include 1 cup fat-free or low-fat yogurt, cottage cheese, or 1.5 oz. of reduced fat or nonfat cheese. Soy-based beverages can also provide

carbohydrates and are typically fortified with calcium.

4. Protein Recommendations for Health and Weight Management.
   a. Up to 6 oz/day of cooked lean meats, fish, poultry, or vegetable-based meat alternatives.
   b. Other good sources of protein include 1-oz protein equivalents of:
      1) One egg, 1/4 cup egg whites, and 1/4 cup egg substitutes.
      2) Nonanimal sources, such 1/4 cup dry beans or 1/2 cup cooked beans, 1/4 cup tofu, 1 tablespoon peanut butter, 1/2 oz. nuts, or 1/2 oz. seeds.
5. For Weight Management and Health, Fat Intake recommendations.
   a. 20%–35% of total energy for adults.
   b. 30%–35% of total energy for children 2–3 years of age.
   c. 25%–25% of total energy for children ages 4–18 years.
   d. Saturated fat intake should be <10% total energy.
   e. Dietary cholesterol should be <300 mg/day.
   f. Reduction in consumption of *trans* fats found in many fried foods, salty snack foods, cookies, and pastries, although *trans* fats have been recently reduced or eliminated in many of these products.
   g. Leaner cuts of beef and pork, leaner protein sources, such as fish and poultry, and vegetable-based meat alternatives will lessen total daily fat intake.
   h. Healthy fats should comprise most fats in the diet.
      1) Polyunsaturated omega-3 fats: canola oil, soybean oil, flaxseed oil, walnuts, salmon, trout, and herring.
      2) Polyunsaturated omega-6 fats: soybean oil, corn oil, safflower oil.
      3) Monounsaturated fats: olive oil, high oleic safflower oil, canola, and sunflower oil.
   i. Fat intake at <20% of total energy may interfere with absorption of fat-soluble vitamins such as vitamin E and may lead to unfavorable changes in high-density lipoprotein (HDL) cholesterol and triglycerides.

VIII. MY PYRAMID

A. The original Food Guide Pyramid was introduced by the USDA in 1992. It very simply illustrated healthy food servings and portions in showing that foods at the base of the pyramid should make up most of the diet, with lesser amounts going up toward the top of the pyramid. Servings were based on USDA standard serving sizes.

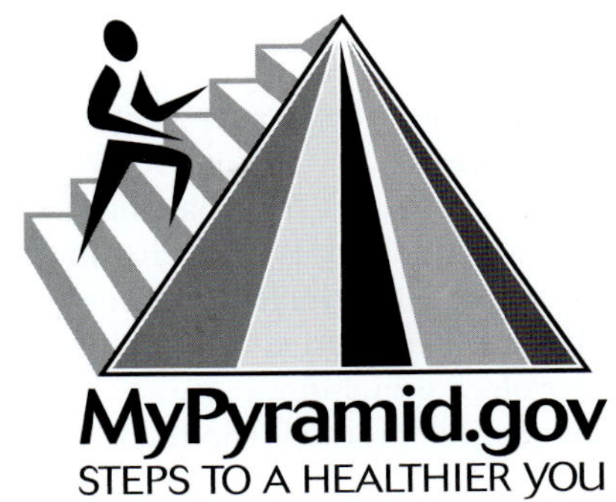

FIGURE 9-1. My Pyramid.

B. Since that time, there have been advances in nutrition research as well as increasing rates of obesity in all age groups. The Food Guide Pyramid was substantially revised in 2005 to become **My Pyramid** (*Fig. 9-1*), which provides a more individualized approach to nutrition and weight management.

C. My Pyramid is now a more interactive internet-based application. An individual can enter in his or her age, gender, weight, height, and minutes of physical activity per day and receive a personalized plan for either weight maintenance or weight loss.

D. Grains, with emphasis on whole grains, still are recommended to make up the largest portion of an individual's pyramid, followed by vegetables, milk, fruits, meat and beans, and, finally, oils and a small amount of discretionary calories.

E. Recommendations coincide with the *Dietary Guidelines for Americans*.

F. Serving sizes have been changed from USDA servings to either ounces for grains or meats and beans, or cups for fruits, vegetables, and milk, to help make it easier for consumers to understand portion sizes by actually using a measuring cup or visualizing the amount in a measuring cup.

G. **Grains:** Recommendations range from 3–8 oz, depending on gender, age, and physical activity level. At least half the servings should be whole grains as emphasized in the *Dietary Guidelines for Americans*.
   1. 1 oz. = 1 slice of bread, 1 cup cold cereal, 1/2 cup cooked rice, pasta, or cereal, 1/2 English muffin, 1/4 large bagel, one 6-inch corn or flour tortilla, 3 cups popped popcorn, one 4 1/2-inch pancake.

H. **Vegetables:** Consuming vegetables in a variety of colors is recommended as per the *Dietary Guidelines for Americans*.
   1. Recommended amounts begin at 1–3 cups for less physically active persons.

2. 1 cup = 1 cup cooked or raw vegetables or 2 cups leafy green vegetables.

I. **Fruits:** Recommended amounts begin at 1–2 cups for less physically active persons.
   1. 1 cup = 1 cup whole or cut fruit, large banana 8–9 inches in length, 1 small apple 2.5 inches in diameter, 1 large orange 3 1/16 inches in diameter 1 cup 100% fruit juice, 1/2 cup dried fruit, 1-inch thick small wedge of watermelon.

J. **Milk:** Fat-free or low-fat milk products should be chosen most often.
   1. Recommendations are 2–3 cups/day, depending on age.
   2. 1 cup = 1 cup fluid milk, 1 1/2 oz hard cheese, 1/3 cup shredded cheese, 1 cup yogurt, 2 cups cottage cheese, 1 cup ricotta cheese, 1 cup pudding made with milk.

K. **Meats and beans:** Recommendations vary by age, gender, and physical activity level, beginning at 2 oz for children ages 2–3 years up to 6 oz for men ages 31–50 years.
   1. Lean sources of meats are emphasized as in the *Dietary Guidelines for Americans*.
   2. 1 oz. = 1 oz cooked lean beef, poultry without skin, or fish; 1 egg, 1/2 oz nuts or seeds, 1 tablespoon peanut butter, 1/4 cup or 2 oz tofu, 1/4 cup beans, 2 tablespoons hummus.

L. **Oils:** Polyunsaturated and monounsaturated oils are emphasized as in the *Dietary Guidelines for Americans*.
   1. Allowances are based on gender, age, and physical activity level with ranges from 3–7 teaspoons/day.
   2. Portions vary depending on whether the item is an oil, such as canola or olive oil, or a food that contains oil, such as mayonnaise, peanut butter, or nuts.

M. **Discretionary calories:** Range from ~150–500 kcal/day depending on gender, age, and physical activity level.
   1. Can be used for additional portions of recommended foods, higher-fat meats or milk products, sugar-sweetened beverages, desserts and other sweets, and alcoholic beverages.

N. The left side of the pyramid shows a figure going up a staircase, to reinforce the importance of **physical activity every day or on most days of the week.**
   1. At least 30 minutes/day for health.
   2. 60 minutes/day to prevent weight gain.
   3. 60–90 minutes/day for weight loss or weight maintenance.
   4. 60 min/day for children and adolescents.
   5. All physical activity targets can be performed in multiple bouts throughout the day.

IX. MACRONUTRIENTS

A. CARBOHYDRATES

1. Made up of carbon, hydrogen, and oxygen.
2. Often abbreviated CHO.
3. Contain energy in the amount of 4 kcal/g.
4. Generally recommended to make up 45%–65% of total energy intake for healthy adults.
5. Athletes preparing for an endurance event may consume 70% carbohydrates.
6. Carbohydrates are stored and metabolized in the body for energy:
   a. Blood glucose is an immediately available source of carbohydrate lasting for a few seconds.
   b. Muscle glycogen is the primary substrate utilized for physical activity. Dependency on muscle glycogen increases with increasing exercise intensity.
   c. Liver glycogen is also another form of carbohydrate and is first in line when blood glucose falls.

B. PROTEIN

1. Composed of **amino acids.**
   a. In addition to C, H, and O amino acids contain an amino group (NH_2^+).
   b. Eight amino acids are considered essential because they cannot be synthesized in the body and must be consumed.
   c. Complete proteins, found in animal-based food products, contain all essential amino acids.
   d. Incomplete proteins are found in plant-based products and do not contain all essential amino acids. Consuming a variety of protein sources will ensure protein and amino acid needs are met.
2. Contains energy in the amount of 4 kcal/g.
3. Body proteins are continuously broken down and turned over, and the amino acids recycled in combination with amino acids consumed.
4. Despite myths to the contrary, protein is not a major energy source during either aerobic or anaerobic exercise.
5. Protein intake should be 10%–15% total energy or 0.8 g protein/kg body weight for most individuals.
6. Athletes may need 1.2–1.4 g protein/kg body weight for endurance athletes and 1.6–1.7 g protein/kg body weight for strength athletes.
7. Likely no benefit exists in exceeding a protein intake of 1.7 g/kg body weight, despite higher recommendations found in popular media which have not been scientifically supported.

C. FAT

1. **Triglycerides** are composed of a glycerol molecule combined with three fatty acids.
2. Contain energy in the amount of 9 kcal/g; more energy per weight than carbohydrate or protein.
3. Triglycerides represent the largest potential energy store in the body, found in:
   a. Bloodstream as free fatty acids.
   b. Subcutaneous fat.
   c. Intraabdominal fat that surrounds internal organs.
   d. Intramuscular fat, another readily available energy source.
4. An energy deficit of 3,500 kcal must be created to lose 1 lb (~0.5 kg) of body fat.
5. Fats are the primary substrate used in aerobic exercise, less so in anaerobic exercise, but they are always being metabolized for energy regardless of exercise intensity.

D. ALCOHOL

1. Is not a macronutrient, but may be source of excess energy in an individual's diet.
2. Catabolized (broken down) by the liver.
3. Alcohol provides energy at 7 kcal/g.
4. Research studies have reported health benefits, such as reduced risk of cardiovascular disease, may be associated with moderate alcohol use (up to 1 drink per day for women, up to 2 drinks per day for men). However, these findings are controversial.
5. Other studies have found risks of certain cancers may be increased with even moderate alcohol consumption, particularly breast cancer in women.
6. Serving sizes for alcohol are that 1 drink equals:
   a. 12 fluid ounces of beer.
   b. 5 fluid ounces of wine.
   c. 1.5 fluid ounces of 80-proof distilled spirits.

X. VITAMINS

A. Vitamins are organic compounds essential for life that are not produced by the body in amounts sufficient to meet physiologic needs and thus must be consumed from foods.
   1. Play key roles in metabolism; used in body functions, such as blood clotting, digestion, and enzyme reactions.
   2. Two classifications of vitamins: water-soluble and fat-soluble.
      a. Water-Soluble Vitamins (8 B Complex Vitamins and Vitamin C).
         1) Must be consumed on a frequent basis.
         2) Small excess amounts are easily excreted; however, large excesses may not be as readily excreted, and thus may cause detrimental effects.
         3) The effects of vitamins depend on dosage and, although water-soluble vitamins are less likely to reach toxic levels compared with the fat-soluble vitamins, it is possible to reach toxic levels from supplements.
      b. Fat-Soluble Vitamins (A, D, E, and K).
         1) Do not have to be consumed on a frequent basis as do water-soluble vitamins.
         2) Fat-soluble vitamins are less readily excreted and thus tend to be stored in body fat storage sites.
         3) Fat-soluble vitamins are likely to reach toxic levels if oversupplemented.

B. **Dietary Reference Intakes (DRI)** are new standards which include:
   1. **Estimated Average Requirements** (EAR): the average daily nutrient intake level estimated to meet the requirement of 50% of healthy individuals in a particular life stage and gender group.
   2. **Recommended Daily Allowances** (RDA).
      a. Categories by gender and age.
      b. Intake goals will meet nutrition of 97%–98% of individuals by life stage and gender.
   3. **Adequate Intake** (AI) for Age and Gender.
      a. Goal for intake based on covering needs for all individuals in a group.
      b. Not as much supporting scientific evidence as RDAs.
   4. **Upper Limits** (UL).
      a. Categories by gender and age.
      b. Toxicity is possible above these limits.
      c. Intake from food, water, and supplements combined.

C. A Registered Dietitian (R.D) should be consulted for persons at risk of deficiencies as a result of low energy intake or other chronic diseases.

XI. CALCIUM AND IRON IN HEALTH

A. Calcium is a mineral essential for:
   1. Bone formation and maintenance.
   2. Both formation and maintenance.
   3. Muscle contraction.
   4. Nerve conduction.
   5. Blood clotting.

B. Women are susceptible to calcium deficiencies because:
   1. Energy intake is less than men.
   2. Less dairy products consumed.

C. AIs for calcium:
   1. Male and female youths 9–18 years: 1,300 mg/day.
   2. Men and women 19–50 years: 1,000 mg/day.

3. Men and women 30–50 years: 1,000 mg/day.
4. Men and women >50 years: 1,200 mg/day.
5. Tolerable upper limits (UL) for all: 2,500 mg/day.
6. Women who may be pregnant or lactating: ≤18 years, 1,300 mg/day; >18 years, 1,000 mg/day.

D. Calcium deficiencies can progress so that bone loss occurs faster than it can be replaced (osteopenia), or bone loss occurs that is not replaced (osteoporosis).

E. Food Sources of Calcium.
1. All dairy products, such as milk, hard and soft cheeses, and yogurt.
2. Canned fish that includes bones, such as salmon and sardines.
3. Dark green vegetables, such as kale, broccoli, and some other greens.
4. Orange juice, certain breads, soy milk, and other foods may be calcium fortified; this is often clearly indicated on the package or label.

F. Iron is a mineral needed for:
1. Maintains hemoglobin in red blood cells.
2. Prevents some anemias.
3. Cofactor in enzymatic reactions.

G. Women are susceptible to deficiencies in iron because:
1. Energy intake is less than men.
2. Meat consumption is lower than men.
3. Losses through menstruation.

H. AI for Iron.
1. Male and female youths 9–13 years: 8 mg/day.
2. Males age 14–18 years: 11 mg/day.
3. Females age 14–18 years: 15 mg/day.
4. Men age 18 years and older: 8 mg/day.
5. Women age 19–50 years: 18 mg/day.
6. Women age 50 years and older: 8 mg/day.
7. Tolerable upper limit (UL) for all: 40–45 mg/day.

I. Iron deficiencies can cause anemia, which can manifest in fatigue and poor exercise or sport performance.

J. Iron can be found in the following foods:
1. Meats (beef, pork, or chicken).
2. Legumes.
3. Eggs.
4. Grains, breads, and cereals (often iron-fortified).
5. Dark green vegetables, such as broccoli, contribute some iron.

K. Vegetarian Needs.
1. AI intake needs to be adequate using nonmeat foods.
2. Vegetarian iron requirements may be double that of nonvegetarians.
3. The absorption of the nonheme iron found in plants eaten by vegetarians may be increased with a vitamin C source.

L. A Registered Dietitian (R.D.) should be consulted for women who could be at risk of calcium and iron deficiencies. Iron supplementation should only occur under the guidance of a physician because iron overload is possible.

XII. HYDRATION

A. WATER

1. An essential nutrient required for many bodily functions that makes up about 60% of total body mass (range 45%–75%).
   a. **Total body water** (TBW) is higher in persons with higher lean body mass versus those with higher fat mass.
   b. TBW normally regulated with 0.2%–0.5% of total body mass.
   c. Glycogen loading will increase TBW.
   d. TBW is replenished by water from liquids and food.
   e. TBW is lost by respiration, sweat, kidneys, and gastrointestinal tract.
2. Dehydration.
   a. Loss of body water at >2% of total body weight measured pre- and post-event.
   b. Leads to increased core temperature and increased risk of heat-related illnesses.
   c. Decreased aerobic exercise performance.
   d. Increased perceived exertion.
   e. Increased heart rate and cardiac strain.
   f. Can impair cognitive and mental capabilities.
   g. Dehydration by individuals, but influenced by:
      1) Body weight; higher body weight leads to more water loss.
      2) Genetic predisposition.
      3) Acclimatization to heat.
      4) Metabolic efficiency or economy for a particular activity.
      5) Type of position played within a sport.
3. Risk of dehydration is higher in:
   a. Prepubescent children, who have lower sweating rates than adults.
   b. Older adults, who have reduced thirst sensitivity and reduced ability to eliminate water and electrolytes.
   c. Athletes requiring reduced body weight for sports participation who may intentionally dehydrate before competition to "make weight."
   d. Athletes who participate in multiple workouts per day may not reach baseline hydration levels after the initial training session.
   e. Individuals who use prescription diuretics.
4. Water consumption recommendations:
   a. Healthy adults.

1) Normal hydration levels can be maintained by recommended healthy diet and water or beverage consumption.
2) General recommendations of 6–8 glasses (~250 ml, 8 fluid oz) of water or other beverages are sufficient for most individuals to replace daily water losses.

b. Active individuals.
1) Plain water meets hydration needs of nearly everyone.
2) Four hours prior to exercise, water can be consumed at 5–7 mL per kg of body weight.
3) Hyperhydration with special beverages is normally not recommended.
4) While exercising or during sports participation, water can be consumed as needed at the rate of 0.4–0.8 L/hour.
5) After exercise, ~1.5 L of fluid will replace 1 kg of body weight loss, and lost sodium should be replaced by either food or sports drinks.

B. SPORTS DRINKS

1. Typically contain carbohydrates in the form of glucose, which is easily absorbed without stomach irritation.
2. Typically contain the electrolytes sodium (Na^+) and potassium (K^+).
3. Most beneficial for higher-intensity exercise of longer duration (minimum 60 minutes), such as distance running, cycling, and sports team participation.
4. Also indicated for exercise in high temperature and/or humidity.
5. Electrolyte depletion can be dangerous in long-duration endurance events such as marathon running, distance cycling, triathlons, and sports team practices or events. Consuming large volumes of water can over-dilute electrolytes and lead to a life-threatening imbalance called hyponatremia (low blood sodium).

XIII. ERGOGENIC AIDS

Are substances reported to improve muscle size, strength, endurance, or athletic performance.

A. CARBOHYDRATE SUPPLEMENTS

1. A pre-event meal with adequate CHO (up to 70% CHO) is important for the maintenance of blood glucose levels during exercise.
   a. Maintenance of blood glucose during exercise may be achieved by drinking a 6%–8% carbohydrate or carbohydrate–electrolyte solution.
   b. Most persons should target 30–60 g CHO per hour.
   c. More than 17 g CHO/8 fluid oz may lead to stomach irritation and cramps.
2. Replenishing muscle glycogen after sport or exercise is highest when an athlete starts consuming 1.0–1.5 g CHO per kg body weight within 30–60 minutes after exercise, or at the latest within a 2-hour time period.
3. Any carbohydrate higher than the energy requirements will be converted to body fat.
4. Glucose or glucose polymer solutions are best because solutions containing fructose can lead to stomach upset.
5. Much scientific data support CHO efficacy and safety.

B. PROTEIN AND AMINO ACIDS

1. Not a major energy source during exercise.
2. No scientific evidence supports the effects of consuming >1.7 g protein/kg body weight.
3. Excessive use can cause dehydration and stress kidney function.
4. Protein requirements can easily be met through food versus supplements.
5. Scientific evidence is lacking to support benefit of supplementation of amino acids.

C. VITAMINS AND MINERALS

1. Reported to increase athletic performance by increasing energy availability or serving as cofactors in metabolism.
2. Toxicities of some vitamins are possible with oversupplmentation.
3. Athletes eating healthy diets and having adequate energy intake do not normally experience deficiencies.
4. Supplements cannot substitute for an inadequate diet; nutrient cofactors only found in whole foods are not present in supplements.
5. Supplementation of a particular vitamin or mineral may affect absorption or metabolism of other nutrients.

D. CREATINE AND CREATINE MONOHYDRATE

1. Mechanism of action is to raise the free creatine pool in muscle, which can facilitate creatine phosphate synthesis and lead to higher capacity to perform short bursts of high-intensity anaerobic exercise.
2. Good scientific evidence supports a possible ergogenic benefit in short-term, high-intensity anaerobic exercise.
3. Little or no benefit exists during aerobic activities.

4. No conclusions known regarding long-term effects of supplementation.

E. ANABOLIC STEROIDS

1. Used for promotion of muscle size and strength. Causes increased protein synthesis in muscle.
2. Banned by major collegiate, Olympic, and professional sports.
3. Classified as controlled substances, so illegal to possess and engage in trafficking to obtain in United States and many other countries, unless prescribed by physician for a very few medical conditions.
4. Available in oral and injectable forms.
5. Not recommended owing to many documented side effects:
    a. Increases lipid-related risk factors for cardiovascular disease.
    b. Alters secondary sex characteristics in both men and women.
    c. Promotes liver tumors and other liver abnormalities.
    d. Promotes aggressive behavior ("roid rage") and other psychological problems.
    e. Promotes altered glucose metabolism.

F. HERBAL SUPPLEMENTS

1. Most herbal supplements are used as stimulants to improve alertness, which may translate to increased exercise performance, or to suppress appetite, enhance weight loss, or increase metabolic rate.
2. Side effects can vary based on type, but typically include anxiety, headaches, lightheadedness, and increased physiologic measures, such as heart rate, blood pressure, and cardiac output.
3. Potential to lessen pain perception, fatigue, or reduce heat-related illness.
4. Manufacturers do not need to show scientific proof of safety or efficacy.
5. May interact with prescription or over-the-counter medications.
6. Could build up to toxic levels in the body.
7. Individuals need to inform their physician regarding use of any herbal supplements.
8. Examples of commonly-used herbs: Echinacea, Ginseng, and St. John's Wort.

G. CAFFIENE

1. Reported to spare glycogen by promoting use of fat stores during endurance exercise.
2. Demonstrated lower ratings of perceived exertion (RPE) during endurance exercise.
3. Legal by the International Olympic Committee (IOC) up to 1,000 mg (~8 cups of coffee), but athletes have failed drug tests with less than this amount because individual differences can affect caffeine metabolism.
4. Increased risk of dehydration.
5. Can cause insomnia and upset stomach.

H. DEHYDROEPIANDROSTERONE (DHEA)

1. Normally produced in adrenal gland as precursor to male and female androgens and estrogens.
2. Natural levels decrease after age 30 and may be low in some persons with chronic diseases, such as acquired immunodeficiency syndrome (AIDS), anorexia, and kidney disease.
3. Some scientific evidence for promotion of fat loss.
4. Conflicting scientific evidence on increased muscle strength.
5. Likely to increase risk of breast, prostate, and other hormone-related cancers.
6. Therefore, not recommended unless better safety and efficacy data emerge.

I. ANDROSTENEDIONE

1. Metabolic precursor to testosterone and estrogen.
2. Reported to increase muscle growth, size, and athletic performance as a result of conversion to testosterone.
3. Banned by the U.S. Food and Drug Administration (FDA) in 2004 because of safety concerns.
4. Reported associated side effects similar to anabolic steroids, such as changes in secondary sex characteristics and increased cardiac and liver disease risk factors.
5. Not recommended because of safety concerns.

XIV. THE FEMALE ATHLETE TRIAD

A. Despite the known benefits of exercise on women's health, within the last 15–20 years a medical condition called the "Female Athlete Triad" has been demonstrated in highly physically active women or athletes. This condition can cause serious medical complications and be life threatening. The triad is characterized by disordered eating, which manifests in a mismatch of too low energy taken combined with high-energy expenditure through exercise, disruption or total loss of menstrual cycle (amenorrhea), and reduced bone density resulting in osteoporosis.

B. Disordered eating could result from simple low-energy intake to fully diagnosed eating disorders, such as bulimia or anorexia nervosa.

C. Although low fat mass or lean body composition values have been associated with amenorrhea, the actual cause is believed to be high-energy expenditure combined with too low energy intake.

D. Osteoporosis.

1. Bone density levels well below normal levels expected for age.
2. Affected by low levels of estrogen.
3. Severity of osteoporosis is linked to severity and length of menstrual irregularity, nutritional status, particularly calcium and vitamin D intake, and amount of bone impact during exercise.

E. Treatment.
1. Medical and pharmaceutical intervention.
2. Counseling.
3. Daily calcium intake of 1,500 mg.
4. Oral contraceptives or other female hormone replacement.
5. Slight increases in energy intake by 250–350 kcal/day or reducing exercise training by 10%–20%.

F. Education and counseling for prevention.
1. Sensible nutrition practices, meet with a Registered Dietician if needed.
2. Reasonable goals for fitness or sport performance.
3. Appropriate targets for body composition.
4. Promotion of healthy body image.
5. Utilization of healthy female athlete role models.
6. Appropriate training for coaches and fitness professionals to recognize signs of the Female Athlete Triad.

XV. MAJOR POSITION STANDS: OBESITY, NUTRITION AND PHYSICAL PERFORMANCE, AND WEIGHT MANAGEMENT

A. National Institutes of Health (NIH)/National Heart, Lung and Blood Institute (NHLBI) Guidelines for the Identification, Evaluation, and Treatment of Overweight and Obesity in Adults: Key Points:
1. Assessment of body weight by BMI.
2. If assessment of body weight status indicates that weight loss is advisable, the patient's readiness to make lifestyle changes should be assessed. This should include:
   a. Reasons and motivation for weight loss.
   b. Previous attempts at weight loss.
   c. Support expected from friend and family.
   d. Understanding risks and benefits.
   e. Attitudes toward physical activity.
   f. Time availability.
   g. Potential barriers, including financial limitations.
3. The initial weight loss goal recommendation is 10% of initial body weight, achieved over a 6-month period (1–2 lb/wk). Further weight loss may be considered after a period of weight maintenance.
4. In some patients, prevention of further weight gain may be an appropriate goal.
5. Therapies should include diet modification, increased physical activity, and behavioral therapy.
6. Pharmacotherapy may be beneficial for some high-risk patients (BMI $\geq$30, or BMI $\geq$27 with obesity-related comorbid conditions).
7. Bariatric or weight loss surgery may be indicated for patients with extreme obesity (BMI $\geq$40), or with a BMI $\geq$35 and obesity-related comorbid conditions.

B. Joint Position of the American Dietetic Association, Dietitians of Canada, and the American College of Sports Medicine: Nutrition and Athletic Performance: Key Points:
1. Optimal nutrition enhances physical activity, athletic performance, and recovery from exercise.
2. Low-energy intakes can lead to loss of muscle mass, menstrual dysfunction, loss or failure to gain bone density, and increased risk of fatigue, injury, and illness.
3. Athletes should have sufficient energy intake during high-intensity training to maintain their weight, maximize training effects, and maintain health.
4. Optimal body fat levels vary with age, sex, sport, and heredity of the athlete.
5. If weight loss is desired, it should be undertaken before the competitive season and involve a trained health or nutrition professional.
6. Carbohydrate intake should be 6–10 g/kg body weight per day.
7. Fat intake should not be <15% total energy.
8. Protein requirements for endurance athletes are 1.2–1.4 g/kg body weight per day, and 1.6–1.7 g/kg body weight per day for strength and resistance-trained athletes.
9. Dehydration impairs athletic performance. Adequate fluid should be consumed as follows:
   a. 2–3 hours before exercise: 400–600 mL (14–22 oz).
   b. During exercise: 150–350 mL every 15–20 min (6–12 oz).
   c. After exercise: 450–675 mL for each pound of body weight lost (16–24 oz).
10. Nutrition recommendation for athletic events.
   a. Before exercise, a meal or snack should be consumed to provide fluid for hydration and carbohydrate to maximize maintenance of blood glucose, yet be limited in fat and fiber to avoid gastrointestinal (GI) distress.
   b. Enhanced performance has been seen in studies using 200–300 g of carbohydrate consumed 3–4 hours before exercise.

c. During exercise (particularly endurance events >1 hour), fluids should be consumed to maintain hydration and to provide carbohydrate (30–60 g/hour).
d. Following exercise, the consumption of a mixed meal (containing carbohydrates, protein, and fat) will facilitate recovery.

11. Vitamin or mineral supplementation should not be necessary if an athlete is consuming adequate energy and a nutritionally balanced diet. If an athlete is dieting, sick, or recovering from an injury, or eliminating foods or food groups, a multivitamin or mineral supplement may be indicated.
12. Vegetarian athletes may be at risk for low energy (inadequate calories), protein, or vitamin and mineral intake. Specific vitamins of concern include vitamin B_{12}, riboflavin, and vitamin D. Specific minerals of potential concern include iron, calcium, and zinc.

C. ACSM Position Stand: Appropriate Intervention Strategies for Weight Loss and Prevention of Weight Regain for Adults: Key Points:

1. Weight reduction should be achieved through a combination of a decrease in energy intake and an increase in energy expenditure.
2. Total energy deficit of 500–1,000 kcal/day is recommended.
3. A dietary fat intake of 30% total energy (kcal) may facilitate weight loss.
4. A minimum of 150 min/week (2.5 hours/week) of moderate intensity physical activity should be encouraged.
5. A progressive increase in activity to 200–300 minutes/week (3.3–3.5 hours/week) is recommended, because this may facilitate long-term weight control.
6. Resistance exercise may increase muscular strength and function, but may not prevent the loss of fat-free mass with weight loss.
7. Pharmacotherapy may be indicated, and is most effectively combined with other lifestyle modifications (e.g., increased activity and reduced energy intake).

XVI. NUTRITION AND EXERCISE FOR PERSONS WITH CHRONIC DISEASE

A. DIABETES

1. Sound nutrition and physical activity principles can help reduce risk of diabetes complications such as cardiovascular disease, neuropathy, obesity, hypertension, and dyslipidemia.
2. Cultural and individual preferences should be considered.
3. Research suggests that exercise promotes beneficial changes for those with type 2 diabetes.
   a. Exercising at an intensity of 50%–80% $\dot{V}O_2$ max for 30–60 minutes 3–4 times per week promotes carbohydrate metabolism and insulin sensitivity.
   b. Regular physical activity should be promoted through behavior modification.
   c. Increased insulin sensitivity leads to improved use of glucose during and after exercise.
   d. In addition, exercise blunts the effect of hormones that counter insulin, which leads to decreased glycogenolysis and gluconeogenesis, which can lead to better glucose control.
4. The glycemic response of persons with type 1 diabetes is affected by:
   a. Overall level of blood sugar control.
   b. Levels of insulin and glucose at the start of exercise.
   c. Previous diet.
   d. Training status.
   e. Timing, intensity, and duration of exercise.
5. Role of diet in diabetes management
   a. Carbohydrate consumption is portioned throughout the day to maintain glucose levels in normal ranges.
      1) Too little carbohydrate promotes hypoglycemia.
      2) Too much carbohydrate promotes hyperglycemia.
      3) Consumption of fruits, vegetables, and whole grains should be emphasized.
      4) Fiber intake recommendations are the same as for persons without diabetes.
   b. If high blood lipids are present or the diet suggests fat consumption in excess of those mentioned previously, the diabetic person may need to alter fat intake.
      1) Carbohydrate intake of 50% of total energy combined with primarily unsaturated fat intake up to 35% of total energy can help control blood glucose and blood lipids.
   c. Consuming additional kilocalories from fat can promote weight gain. If alcoholic beverages are consumed, they should be consumed with food. Men should not consume more than two, and women should not consume more than one alcoholic beverages per day.
   d. Protein needs in persons with diabetes may be only slightly higher than normal, but no special recommendations are needed, and protein should comprise 10%–15% of

total energy, the same recommendation for persons without diabetes.

e. There are often no special micronutrient needs.

f. Nutrition for persons with different life stages of diabetes:

1) Youths with type 1 diabetes need to ensure sufficient energy intake for normal growth and development; insulin monitoring should be integrated into daily meals and physical activity.

2) Youths with type 2 diabetes should focus on behavior modification changes in nutrition habits and physical activity to lower insulin resistance and improve metabolic control.

3) Pregnant and lactating women with diabetes need to ensure sufficient energy intake and micronutrients for their own health and the health of their baby.

4) Nutrition for older adults should address their individual nutritional and psychosocial needs.

5) Individuals currently receiving insulin or insulin secretagogues need education for self-management of blood glucose and prevention of hypoglycemia and other exercise-related blood glucose problems.

6) Persons at high risk of diabetes, such as those with metabolic syndrome, should focus on behavioral-based changes in nutrition and physical activity for weight loss or gain prevention to reduce their risk factors.

B. CARDIOVASCULAR DISEASE

1. The American Heart Association (AHA) 2006 Diet Recommendations for Cardiovascular Disease Risk Reduction include:

a. Energy balance to maintain healthy weight.

b. Recommended servings of fruits and vegetables.

c. Recommended levels of whole grains and dietary fiber.

d. Consumption of fish twice per week, especially oily fish.

e. Saturated fat should be limited to <7% of energy, *trans* fat to <1% of energy, and cholesterol to <300 mg/day by:

1) Choosing lean meats and vegetable alternatives.

2) Choosing fat-free and low-fat dairy products.

3) Minimizing intake of partially hydrogenated fats.

f. Minimize intake of beverages and foods with added sugars.

g. Foods should be prepared with no or little added salt.

h. Alcohol consumption in moderation.

i. Aim to follow the AHA guidelines when dining out.

C. CHRONIC HEART FAILURE

1. Persons whose hearts have the reduced ability to pump blood may have special nutrition needs.

a. Likely already following the American Heart Association recommendations.

b. May need to meet with a Registered Dietitian (R.D.) for individual needs.

c. Major aim is to control fluid retention (edema).

1) Weigh daily to monitor body weight and fluid.

2) Sodium should be limited to 2,000 mg/day and no more than 250 mg/food item.

3) Water and other fluids limited to 2.0 L/day.

D. PULMONARY DISEASE

1. Several types pulmonary diseases make it difficult, if not impossible, to discuss specific recommendations for everyone. However, there are general considerations that must be taken into consideration with each individual.

2. Some individuals may require increased energy intake.

3. Macronutrients may need to be balanced to provide for a satisfactory respiratory quotient (RQ).

4. Vitamin and mineral needs may need to be assessed, depending on type of disease.

5. Water and hydration needs may need to be addressed.

6. In some forms of pulmonary disease, such as cystic fibrosis, enzyme therapy is needed to correct maldigestion and malabsorption.

XVII. OTHER DIETARY PRACTICES FOR WEIGHT LOSS AND WEIGHT CONTROL

A. HIGH-PROTEIN AND LOW-CARBOHYDRATE DIETS

1. May limit foods that are an important source of nutrients while focusing on meat, eggs, and cheese, which are high in saturated fat.

a. Saturated fats are associated with heart disease, diabetes, stroke, and several types of cancer.

2. Some high protein diets limit cereals, grains, fruits, vegetables, and low-fat dairy products.
   a. Reduction in these foods could lead to micronutrient deficiencies.
   b. Because these foods help lower cholesterol when eaten as part of a nutritionally balanced diet, reducing consumption of them may have a negative effect on blood lipids.
3. Fat is incompletely oxidized, leading to formation of ketones, which can be potentially harmful because they can cause an acid build-up in the body.
4. Although weight loss may occur quickly, research is limited and more research is needed to evaluate long-term safety and efficacy.

B. MEDITERRANEAN DIETS

1. Although different Mediterranean countries have their own dietary habits, there are similarities relating to their food intake.
2. Common Dietary Features:
   a. Whole grains, potatoes, pasta.
   b. High in complex carbohydrates and fiber.
   c. Vegetables and legumes.
   d. Yogurt, feta, and mozzarella cheeses.
   e. Nuts.
   f. Fruits (grapes and figs).
   g. Little meat and egg consumption.
   h. Some seafood and poultry consumption.
   i. Sources of fat are olives, olive oil, nuts, and fish.
   j. High monounsaturated and polyunsaturated fat intake.
   k. Low saturated fat intake.
3. Research suggests that the Mediterranean diet leads to lower incidences of heart disease, certain cancers, and other diseases.
4. As might be expected, because of the lower incidences of disease, life expectancy is high.

C. VEGETARIAN DIETS

1. Vegetarians have lower rates of cancer, heart disease, and high blood pressure.
2. Although these benefits are associated with diet, vegetarians tend to have a lifestyle that differs from nonvegetarians.
3. Vegetarians tend to maintain a healthy body weight, are physically active, do not smoke, and drink little, if any alcohol.
4. Types of Vegetarian Diets.
   a. Vegan
      1) Excludes all animal-derived foods.
      2) Plant-based diet.
      3) Referred to as strict, pure, or total vegetarians.
   b. Lactovegetarian.
      1) In addition to plants, includes milk and milk products.
      2) Excludes other animal products.
   c. Lacto-ovo-vegetarian.
      1) In addition to plants, includes milk, milk products, and eggs.
      2) Excludes other animal products.

Review Test

1. Which of the following could be recommended as a safe and effective ergogenic aid?
   A) Herbal supplements.
   B) Carbohydrate.
   C) Amino acids.
   D) Androstenedione.

2. Vegetarian diets are associated with health, and there are several different types of vegetarian diets. What is the name for the type of vegetarian diet where absolutely no animal products are consumed?
   A) Lacto-ovo-vegetarian.
   B) Vegan.
   C) Lactovegetarian.
   D) None of the above.

3. Starting at which body mass index (BMI) level is an adult considered obese?
   A) 18.5.
   B) 24.9.
   C) 30.0.
   D) 40.0.

4. Which of the following assessments can be used to measure body composition?
   A) Weight measured on a digital scale.
   B) Dietary Reference Intakes (DRI).
   C) Skinfolds.
   D) Waist-hip ratio.

5. What are the correct of amounts of energy in carbohydrates, proteins, and fats, respectively, on a per gram basis (kcal/g)?
   A) 9, 4, 4.
   B) 4, 4, 9.
   C) 4, 7, 9.
   D) 9, 4, 9.

6. If you use the Harris-Benedict equation to estimate an individual's total daily enérgy requirements at 2,000 kcal, approximately how many fat grams should he or she consume using the recommend percentage of 30% of total daily energy from fat?
   A) 134 g.
   B) 67 g.
   C) 600 g.
   D) 44 g.

7. What happens to carbohydrates when consumed in amounts greater than required for energy?
   A) They are metabolized and then stored as body fat.
   B) Electrolyte imbalances can occur.
   C) They are stored as muscle glycogen only.
   D) They are excreted in the urine.

8. Which of the following fats is recommended as one of the healthy dietary fats?
   A) *Trans* fat.
   B) Monounsaturated fat.
   C) Saturated fat.
   D) None of the above.

9. What is the initial target for body weight reduction in a 6-month time frame according to the National Institutes of Health/National Heart, Lung, and Blood Institute (NIH/NHLBI)?
   A) 10%.
   B) 20%.
   C) 35%.
   D) None of the above.

10. Which of the following would indicate that an athlete could be dehydrated?
    A) Decreased exercise performance.
    B) Body weight loss >2%.
    C) Decreased cognitive abilities.
    D) All of the above.

11. Which of the following is correct regarding nutrition for a person with diabetes?
    A) Persons with diabetes have increased vitamin and mineral needs.
    B) More dietary fiber is required compared with a person without diabetes.
    C) The amount of carbohydrate consumed is more important than the type.
    D) There is no need for behavior modification programs.

12. Which of the following is a major symptom associated with the Female Athlete Triad?
    A) Fatigue.
    B) Amenorrhea.
    C) Excess carbohydrate intake.
    D) High body fat.

13. Which of the following pairs of waist circumference measurements in men and women are indicators of abdominal obesity?
    A) ≥0.95 inches (2.4 cm) for men; ≥0.86 inches (2.2 cm) for women.
    B) >40 inches (101.6 cm) for men; >35 inches (88.9 cm) for women.
    C) >40 inches (101.6 cm) for both men and women.

D) >39.9 inches (101.3 cm) for men; >29.9 inches (75.9 cm) for women.

14. Which of the following would you recommend for a person wishing to loss 7 kg of fat?
A) Reduction in total energy intake.
B) Proper regular aerobic exercise.
C) Behavior modification.
D) All of the above.

15. An athlete who needs to compete in a sport within a specific weight class, weight limit, or those participating in aesthetic sport would be at greatest risk for which eating disorder?
A) Bulimia.
B) Anorexia nervosa.
C) Obesity.
D) Metabolic syndrome.

16. The metabolic syndrome includes dyslipidemia, insulin resistance, elevated blood pressure, and what other component?
A) Amenorrhea.
B) Laxative use.
C) Abdominal obesity.
D) 25.0 BMI.

17. Which of the following would be recommended for a person who wishes to gain body weight?
A) Perform aerobic activity to create an energy deficit of 500 kcal/day.
B) Consume sport drinks, sodas, and other beverages high in sugar.
C) Avoid resistance training.
D) Choose energy-dense, but healthy snacks, such as dried fruit, nuts, and fruit smoothies.

18. For strength athletes, what would be the upper limit recommended for protein intake?
A) (A) 0.8 g/kg body weight.
B) 1.0 g/kg body weight.
C) 1.0 g/lb body weight.
D) 1.7 g/kg body weight.

19. The amount of energy required for the body's most basic vital functions is called:
A) Total daily energy expenditure.
B) Resting metabolic rate.
C) Thermic effect of food.
D) Thermic effect of exercise.

20. Women are likely to be deficient in both calcium and iron because they tend to consume less:
A) Food than men.
B) Fiber.
C) Protein from meat sources.
D) All of the above.

21. Which of the following foods would be recommended as a whole grain food item on My Pyramid?
A) Oatmeal.
B) White pasta.
C) Sugary "kids" breakfast cereal.
D) White rice.

22. All of the following chronic diseases are associated with abdominal obesity EXCEPT
A) Coronary artery disease.
B) Type 2 Diabetes.
C) Cancers of the reproductive system.
D) Lung cancer.

23. How much of a weekly energy deficit must be created by dietary changes or physical activity for a PERSON to lose 1 lb (~0.5 kg) of body fat?
A) 2,000 kcal.
B) 2,500 kcal.
C) 3,000 kcal.
D) 3,500 kcal.

24. Deficiency of which micronutrient can affect bone development?
A) Vitamin E.
B) Vitamin C.
C) Calcium.
D) Iron.

25. Which is the primary energy source for high-intensity aerobic exercise activity?
A) Muscle protein.
B) Creatine phosphate.
C) Fat.
D) Muscle glycogen.

ANSWERS AND EXPLANATIONS

1–B. Carbohydrate is well recognized as a safe and effective ergogenic aid. Consumption can improve athletic performance before and during endurance exercise. Protein and amino acid supplements are not major energy sources during exercise. Androstenedione is a proandrogenic hormone that has been banned since 2004 owing to its side effects.

2–B. Vegans are vegetarians who consume no animal products at all. Lactovegetarians consume milk products but no other animal products, whereas lacto-ovo-vegetarians consume milk products and eggs but no other animal products.

3–C. Body mass index (BMI) is calculated as: weight (kilograms) divided by height (meters squared). An adult with a BMI of 17.5 is considered underweight and could have an eating disorder. A BMI of 25.0–29.9 is considered overweight, whereas a BMI of 30.0–39.9 is considered obese. A BMI of 40.0 and higher is considered morbidly obese (class III obesity).

4–C. Skinfolds are the only measure listed that can estimate body composition. The waist-hip ratio can indicate abdominal obesity only. Body weight and BMI do not determine body composition.

5–B. Both carbohydrates and proteins contain 4 kcal/g, whereas fats are slightly more than double this amount at 9 kcal/g. The type of fat does not affect its energy. Alcohol provides 7 kcal/g.

6–B. First, take the daily total energy in kilocalories and multiply by 0.30 (convert 30% to decimal). This gives total kilocalories from fat alone, 600 kcal. Then, by knowing that fat contains 9 kcal/g, divide 600 kcal by 9 to get grams. This will be 67 g when the final answer is rounded.

7–A. When consumption of more calories, regardless of source, is more than the body's energy requirements, the excess energy is converted to body fat. Muscle glycogen is stored as well, but it is not the only storage if total energy intake is too high. Excess carbohydrate consumption has no effect on electrolyte balance, and carbohydrates would not be expected to be found in the urine of healthy persons.

8–B. Monosaturated and polyunsaturated fats, mostly found in plants, are recommended as healthy fats. These fats affect blood lipids in a positive, healthy manner. Both saturated fats, found in red meats and full-fat dairy, and trans fats, found in processed foods such as cakes, cookies, and salty snacks, have been associated with negatively affecting blood lipids, particularly low-density lipoprotein cholesterol (LDL-C) to increase heart disease risk.

9–A. Initial target for weight reduction in a 6-month time period is 10% of starting body weight at a rate of 1–2 lb/week, through changes in diet, increased physical activity, and behavior modification. At this level of weight loss, health benefits start to accrue, such as reduction in some coronary disease risk factors.

10–D. Signs of dehydration include body weight losses of >2%, decreased exercise performance, and decreased cognitive abilities in addition to increased heart rate and perceived exertion. Dehydration puts an athlete at risk of heat-related illnesses, such as heat exhaustion and heat stroke.

11–C. A person with diabetes has many similar nutritional needs as a person without diabetes. There are no or minimal differences in vitamin, mineral, fiber, and protein needs. However, a person with diabetes must monitor carbohydrate consumption to maintain healthy blood glucose levels.

12–B. A major symptom of the Female Athlete Triad is amenorrhea, or absence or disruption of the menstrual cycle. Other major components of the Triad include osteoporosis and disordered eating. Fatigue could occur in women with very low energy intakes, but it is not a specific component of the Triad. Because many female athletes have low energy intake, it is unlikely that they have excess carbohydrate consumption or higher body fat. Body fat could be below expected ranges.

13–B. Waist circumferences >40 inches in men and >35 inches in women are indicators of abdominal obesity. Waist-hip ratios ≥0.95 for men and ≥0.86 for women are also indicators of abdominal obesity.

14–D. An effective program for modifying body composition would include small reductions in energy intake, regular physical activity, and behavior modification to produce an energy deficit of 500 kcal/day and 1 lb (0.5 kg) of body fat loss per week.

15–A. Athletes who need to compete at a particular weight or in aesthetic sports could be at risk for bulimia. Bulimics typically binge on large amounts of food, purge by vomiting, using laxatives, exercising excessively, taking diuretics, or using sauna or sweat suits. Anorexia nervosa is an eating disorder marked by a very thin appearance and an obsession over weight, body image, and inability to eat or to eat certain foods. Obesity and metabolic syndrome are likely related to excess energy intake without purging behaviors.

16–C. Abdominal obesity is the major component of the metabolic syndrome and is a better predictor coronary artery disease. Amenorrhea is part of the Female Athlete Triad. Laxative use is common in bulimia.

17–D. Individuals trying to gain weight should be encouraged to consume healthy, nutrient-rich foods that are more energy dense versus consuming excess energy from sugar-laden sources. Aerobic exercise may need to be cut back to moderate levels to prevent large energy deficits. Resistance training should be emphasized and not avoided.

18–D. Nonathletes may require only 0.8 g/kg body weight, but strength athletes may need up to 1.7 g/kg body weight of protein. Fitness magazines and other popular media may recommend more protein, but amounts higher than 1.7 g/kg have not been verified as more effective in research studies. Athletes should be encouraged to get protein from healthy food sources, such as lean meats, low-fat dairy, and legumes.

19–B. Resting metabolic rate (RMR) is the amount of energy (usually expressed in kilocalories) needed for the body's most basic vital functions, such a respiration, circulation, and nerve conduction. The thermic effect of food is the amount of energy required for digestion, absorption, and assimilation of nutrients. The thermic effect of exercise is the amount of energy required for physical activity or exercise.

20–D. Women are likely to be at risk of both calcium and iron deficiencies because they tend to consume lower overall energy (kilocalories) than men, and they tend to consume fewer dairy products, which are a good source of calcium, as well as consume less meat, chicken, or pork which is higher in iron.

21–A. Oatmeal is a recommended whole grain food because it undergoes minimal chemical processing. White pasta would not be considered whole grain. Brown rice is a whole grain compared with white rice, which is highly polished and processed. Many breakfast cereals marketed to children are not considered to be good sources of whole grain even though the package may state that the cereal is made from whole grains. These breakfast cereals are often still highly refined, processed carbohydrates.

22–D. Lung cancer is not associated with abdominal obesity. Certain cancers, such as reproductive cancers in the prostate and breast, as well as colon and pancreatic cancer are associated with abdominal obesity. Abdominal obesity does increase risk of both heart disease and type 2 diabetes.

23–D. Whether it is from body fat stores or a dietary source, all fats contain energy at 3,500 kcal/lb. Reaching this energy deficit by a combination of small dietary changes and increased physical activity will likely be more acceptable to a person desiring weight loss.

24–C. Calcium is the mineral required for bone formation. Iron, vitamin E, and vitamin C do not play a major function in bone development.

25–C. Muscle glycogen is the primary fuel during physical activity and the body's dependency on glycogen as a fuel source increases with increasing exercise intensity. Protein from the diet or muscle breakdown is used during high-intensity exercise. Creatine phosphate (in the form of creatine monohydrate) is emphasized in high-intensity, brief duration anaerobic-type work.

Program and Administration/ Management

10 CHAPTER

I. GENERAL DESCRIPTION

A. Optimal program administration ensures the delivery of safe and efficacious programs and services while managing risk and reducing liability.
B. The program director/manager ensures appropriate staffing levels and support of exercise practitioners.
C. The program director/manager ensures that current legal and professional standards and practices for health/fitness and clinical exercise rehabilitation services are met.
D. The program director/manager understands basic management and financial principles.
E. The program director/manager coordinates all inter-related administrative functions and services.
F. The program director/manager solicits the input of upper management (e.g., executive leadership/ownership and medical director) as part of a continuous quality improvement process with respect to program development, implementation, administration, and evaluation.

II. WORKDAY ACTIVITIES OF A PROGRAM DIRECTOR/MANAGER

A. TO DESIGN AND MONITOR EXERCISE PROGRAMS BY

1. Accessing, organizing, and managing resources.
2. Ensuring appropriate staffing levels.
3. Supervising/mentoring staff.
4. Ensuring that equipment and inventory of supplies are maintained.
5. Overseeing performance improvement/quality assurance activities.
6. Participating in strategic planning.

B. TO ASSESS PROGRAM AND CLIENT NEEDS BY

1. Establishing program goals.
2. Monitoring program and facility safety.
3. Managing program outcomes.
4. Soliciting client feedback (e.g., formal and informal evaluations) and implementing changes when warranted.

C. TO ENSURE ADEQUATE STAFFING BY

1. Recruiting and hiring qualified staff.
2. Maintaining adequate service levels based on client or patient needs.
3. Developing and confirming appropriate workday schedules for staff.

D. TO DEVELOP AND MOTIVATE STAFF BY

1. Being accessible and receptive to issues and concerns.
2. Identifying opportunities for professional growth.
3. Providing informal and constructive feedback on a consistent and frequent basis.

E. TO OFFER CONTINIUING EDUCATION AND TRAINING BY

1. Demonstrating content expertise and strong teaching skills.
2. Developing and implementing staff training programs.
3. Encouraging peer mentoring and precepting.
4. Providing opportunities to attend professional conferences and workshops.

F. TO PROVIDE ROLE MODEL BEHAVIORS EXPECTED OF STAFF BY

1. "Living the Mission" of the program and leading by example.
2. Providing feedback on job performance.
3. Controlling situations and assuming a position of leadership.

G. TO MOTIVATE BOTH CLIENTS AND STAFF BY

1. Demonstrating strong communication skills.
2. Being persuasive and influential.
3. Demonstrating enthusiasm.
4. Being a catalyst and giving impetus to program activities and initiatives.

H. TO ACT AS A COUNSELOR BY

1. Practicing listening skills to better understand staff and client issues.
2. Expressing opinions openly and without offense.
3. Providing recommendations to improve a situation or resolve problems.

I. TO PROMOTE PROGRAMS BY

1. Encouraging participation.
2. Understanding the benefits of the program.
3. Demonstrating the ability to communicate effectively the benefits to staff and clients.

III. BASIC RESPONSIBILITIES OF A PROGRAM DIRECTOR/MANAGER

A. TO ASSESS CLIENT INTEREST AND SATISFACTION

Using surveys, focus groups, client and staff feedback, and observation of programs.

B. TO OBSERVE ALL ASPECTS OF THE PROGRAM, INCLUDING

1. Staff performance.
2. Efficiency of facility layout.
3. Operational efficiencies.
4. Efficacy of programs and services.
5. Cleanliness and environmental conditions.

C. TO IMPLEMENT POLICIES AND PROCEDURES

Including ensuring staff read, understand, and comply to policies and procedures (e.g., administrative, practice, emergency).

D. TO ENSURE AVAILABILITY OF RESOURCES, INCLUDING

1. Equipment.
2. Supplies.
3. Facilities or physical plant.
4. Personnel.

E. TO MANAGE THE FACILITY AND/OR PROGRAM FINANCIALS, INCLUDING

1. Developing operational budgets.
2. Providing cost-to-benefit analyses of specific programs.
3. Managing day-to-day spending based on Year-To-Date and Profit and Loss statements and explaining variances.

F. TO PROMOTE THE PROGRAM THROUGH MARKETING EFFORTS, INCLUDING

1. Designing promotional activities that attract clients.
2. Developing incentive programming that engages participants.

G. TO SCHEDULE SERVICES APPROPRIATELY

1. With target audience in mind.
2. With consideration of other programs.

H. TO MANAGE EMERGENCY PREPAREDNESS

1. Ensuring that staff maintain necessary credentials (e.g., basic life support [BLS], automatic external defibrillator [AED], advanced cardiac life support [ACLS]).
2. Ensuring that emergency equipment (e.g., emergency kits, defibrillator, AED) is operational.
3. Facilitating regular mock medical incidents and emergencies.

I. TO EVALUATE PROGRAM EFFICACY BY

1. Developing and identifying performance metrics and indicators.
2. Securing or devising validated survey tools.
3. Analyzing data and survey results.
4. Reporting outcomes to staff and executive leadership.

J. TO EVALUATE STAFF PERFORMANCE BY

1. Utilizing job task-based performance appraisal tools.
2. Conducting timely and regularly scheduled performance evaluations.
3. Soliciting and reviewing employee feedback.
4. Developing goals for improved performance.

IV. ORGANIZATIONAL STRUCTURE AND STAFFING

A major challenge facing the program director/manager is maintaining proper staffing levels. Levels of expertise as well as staff-to-client ratios need to be consistent with the organizational mission, service goals, budget, and desired outcomes as well as industry standards and guidelines.

A. DELINEATION OF ROLES

1. Considerations for role assignment from the perspective of staff include
   a. Individual staff expertise.
   b. **Credentials** (e.g., certifications and licenses).
   c. Desired staff-to-client ratios (considering medicolegal issues).
2. Considerations for role delineation from a business or programmatic perspective include
   a. Organizational mission.
   b. Clientele.
   c. Organizational structure.
   d. Program growth.

B. JOB DESCRIPTIONS

1. Each staff position should have a written **job description** that clearly details reporting relationships, responsibilities, minimal qualifications,

critical success factors, and physical work demands.

2. Each candidate seeking employment should have a clear understanding of the job expectations at the interview.
3. On both hire and during job orientation, employees should read and understand their respective job description and should be provided the opportunity to review and ask questions related to job expectations. Supervisors should document that employees understand their job responsibilities and performance expectations during the job orientation period with formal sign-off by employee and supervisor (via employment orientation form).
4. An effective job description is crafted to satisfy specific program needs and goals.
5. Because all possible duties and responsibilities cannot be detailed, some degree of flexibility and adaptability must be built into each job description.

C. ORGANIZATIONAL CHART

1. An organizational chart visually specifies the hierarchy of decision-making responsibility (i.e., chain of command) and lines of communication (*Figure 10-1*).
2. The chart should clearly reflect the relationship of employees within the overall organization.
3. The organizational chart should be readily accessible to all staff and be included within the policy and procedure manual.

D. STAFF COMPETENCY AND DEVELOPMENT

The program director/manager is responsible for generating and validating staff competencies.

1. Encouraging opportunities for professional development is essential to ensuring staff are prepared to perform their job.
2. In most preventive (e.g., commercial, corporate, private) and rehabilitative settings staffing is multidisciplinary.
   a. In clinical settings, this may include
      1) Clinical exercise physiologists and exercise specialists.
      2) Registered dietitians.
      3) Registered nurses.
      4) Respiratory therapists.
      5) Other allied health professionals.
   b. In fitness settings, this may include
      1) Applied exercise physiologists and fitness specialists.
      2) Personal trainers.
      3) Registered dietitians and nutritionists.
      4) Massage therapists.
      5) Other health and fitness professionals.

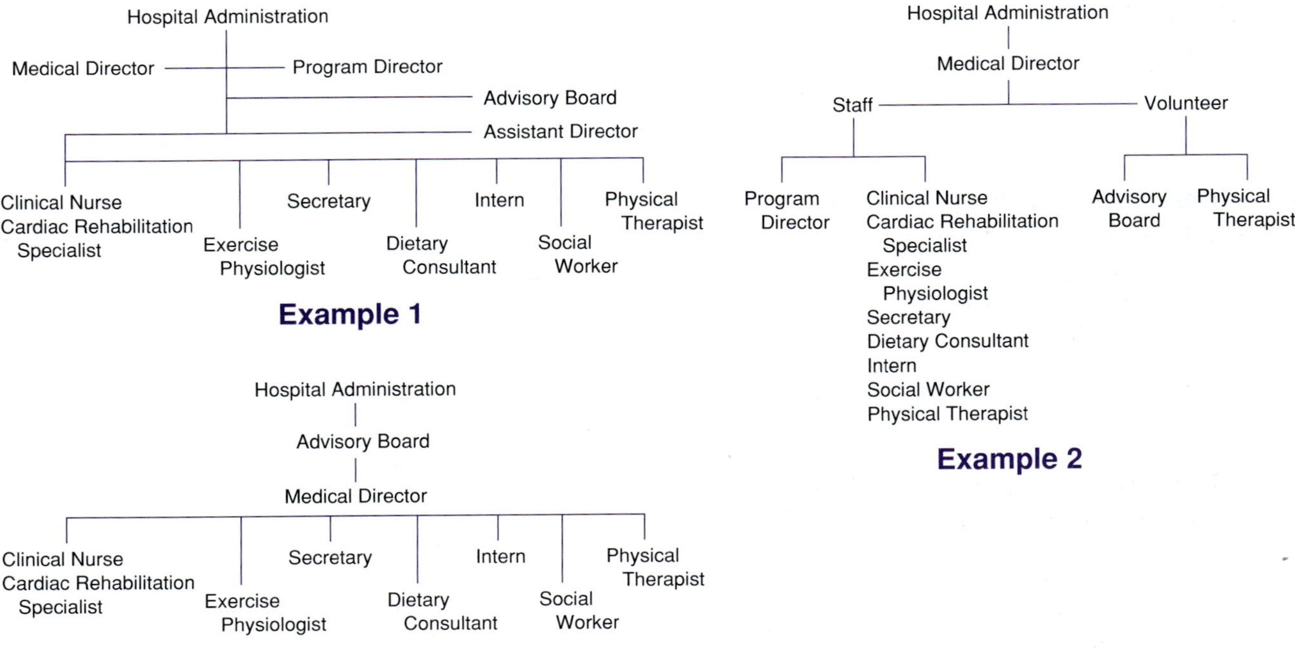

FIGURE 10-1. Organizational grids used for management of cardiopulmonary rehabilitation programs. (Redrawn with permission from Berra K, Hall LK. Administration of cardiac rehabilitation outpatient programs. In: Pollock ML, Schmidt DH. *Heart Disease and Rehabilitation*. Champaign (IL): Human Kinetics; 1995. p 188.).

3. Each respective discipline will have its own unique set of needs and opportunities for professional development; however, more generic needs may apply across disciplines.
   a. Staff training may focus on professional development issues that can be aimed at a particular group of staff (e.g., operation of a new exercise machine) or can encompass the entire staff (e.g., client service issues).
   b. **In-services** are excellent forums for professional development. In-services can be presented by staff within the organization with special expertise or by outside content experts.
   c. Encouraging staff to introduce skills and techniques acquired from learning opportunities outside the organization may provide advantages of broadening and enhancing service delivery. Such continuing education opportunities may include attending conferences or workshops, participating in web-based learning programs, or reading texts, journals, or other publications.
4. Effective **communication among staff members** is an essential component to advancing staff competencies. Strategies to foster communication include
   a. Following lines of communication depicted on the program's organizational chart.
   b. Holding regular staff meetings, both formal and informal, (including institutional, departmental, and service level meetings, depending on the agenda or purpose).
   c. Ensuring communication occurs in all directions of command, thus creating an "open door" policy.

E. PURSUIT OF PROFESSIONAL CREDENTIALS

Certification or licensure, for example, provides an opportunity to validate skills and competencies.

1. Credentialing should provide for standardized skills validation. Some disciplines or industries are regulated strictly by credentials (nursing, physical therapy, athletic training), whereas others are less regulated (e.g., exercise and fitness practitioners).
2. It is expected that credentialed professionals will be consistent in their delivery of service.
3. The program director/manager should be aware that credentialing in the fitness industry is voluntary (i.e., currently, there is no state or federal level regulation of professional practice). As a result, a wide range of knowledge, skills, and abilities (KSAs) exists among the varying credentials available. The program director/manager should become familiar with the minimum competency expectations of the available credentials in the industry, especially those with accreditation by either the National Commission for Certifying Agencies or the American National Standards Institute.

F. PROGRAM CERTIFICATION

1. The program director/manager should be able to determine the potential value impact of pursuing any third-party accreditation, certification, endorsement, or other type of formal recognition program.
2. The move toward program certification (e.g., American Association of Cardiovascular and Pulmonary Rehabilitation [AACVPR] program certification for cardiovascular and pulmonary rehabilitation programs) is relatively recent, although likely to become more widespread in the industry in the upcoming years.
3. The overall impact of program certification or endorsement on the fitness field is unknown.
4. Program accreditation in the clinical setting has been used to determine eligibility for **third-party reimbursement** (e.g., Centers for Medicare and Medicaid requirements for Center of Excellence status) and may be a requirement for cardiac and pulmonary rehabilitation programs in the future.
5. Program endorsement or accreditation of fitness facilities may help standardize care as well as provide the consumer with information related to determining the quality of the program or facility.

V. PROGRAM DEVELOPMENT

A. NEEDS ASSESSMENT

1. Involves gathering data to determine if a program or service is needed for a particular population within a community.
   a. Data may be obtained by surveying the community as well as members and staff within each facility.
   b. Demographic and health data available through local, state, and federal government may serve to provide additional information about need.
   c. Obtaining information about like-services offered within the surrounding communities should also be considered when determining need.
2. Includes a thorough market analysis for financial considerations and an analysis of staffing and facility needs.

3. Entails developing a cost-to-benefit analysis to help determine the financial impact of the program.

B. BUSINESS PLAN

1. The business plan is a detailed description of the mission statement, goals and objectives, program description, financial proforma, and marketing plan.
2. The business plan should include an analysis of strengths, weakness, opportunities, and threats (SWOT) of the products and services to be introduced.
3. The business plan also includes benchmarks for determining program success.

C. PROGRAM PLANNING

1. Scope Of Program Services

The scope of program services depends on various factors, including the needs of the target population, the existing or needed expertise of the care deliverers, and the market demand for particular services.

a. The needs of the target population change with innovations in the health/fitness industry. Thus, program directors/managers must be aware of the current evidence-based literature and industry trends, and must modify their program accordingly.

b. The expertise of the staff will define the services that can be offered. When existing staff are underprepared to deliver or do not customarily provide the level of care needed, contracted labor or services (i.e., external individuals or business that provide services or expertise on a limited basis) from specialized disciplines or practitioners may be utilized (e.g., registered dieticians, physicians, yoga instructors).

c. An identified market demand is strong justification for offering a particular program or service because of the likelihood of acceptance and ultimately financial success.

2. Financial and Budgetary Considerations

a. **Purposes of a budget** include
   1) Developing a financial plan for the program.
   2) Being accountable to expenses and resources available.
   3) Evaluating program financial performance.
   4) Determining program viability.
   5) Identifying variances to projections and responding accordingly.

b. Budget benchmarks should be realistic, clearly defined, and easily measured.

c. Program revenue (income) includes
   1) Direct billing to patient/clients (including self-payments and third-party reimbursements).
   2) Contracted services for specific client groups and managed care organizations.
   3) Sale of merchandise, including clothing, equipment, supplies, food and drink, nutritional supplements, and so forth.
   4) Grants for services or programs from educational, governmental, or other foundations.

d. Program expenses include
   1) **Capital expenses**: typically defined as large and extraordinary purchases (e.g., $\geq$\$1,000) of durable items with an extended useful life (e.g., $\geq$3 years). Capital expenses may include exercise equipment, furniture, and other tangible assets of the program.
   2) **Noncapital expenses**: typically defined as day-to-day operational expenses (e.g., medical and exercise supplies, minor equipment, forms and stationary, repairs and maintenance).
      a) **Fixed expenses** are those that are typically unchanged from month-to-month, including regular staff payroll, rent, maintenance agreements, and so forth.
      b) **Variable expenses** are those that vary based on utilization, including disposable supplies, per diem staff payroll, contract labor, and so forth.

e. **Profit-and-loss analyses**
   1) The profit-and-loss model of the particular program is based on factors such as financial expectations and mission statement (e.g., for-profit versus not-for-profit programs).
   2) Basic forms of profit and loss analyses.
      a) The break-even analysis is designed around the function of the program such that the revenue generated is sufficient to pay for the expenses incurred.
      b) The profitability analysis is an attempt to forecast future profits for the program based on potential revenue generation as well as predicted fixed and variable expenses.

f. A sample budget for a clinical exercise program is given in *Table 10-1*.
g. A sample budget for a health/fitness program is given in *Table 10-2*.

3. Marketing Plan

a. Assesses competition.
b. Provides a detailed description of marketing and promotional strategies.
c. Includes a projection of marketing impact on the business.

VI. PROGRAM IMPLEMENTATION

A. PROGRAM COMPONENTS

1. Patient/Client Care Plan and Exercise Prescription

a. The foundation for any clinical exercise program, the patient/client care plan, defines the specific intervention for rehabilitation as well as criteria and benchmarks for outcome assessment.
b. The foundation for any health/fitness exercise program, the exercise prescription (e.g., exercise modality, frequency, duration, intensity, and progression) provides a specific plan for improving fitness levels and health status, as well as attainment of patient/client goals.
c. The patient/client care plan and exercise prescription should be comprehensive, individualized, documented, reviewed by staff and a physician, and followed by the entire staff with regular reevaluation and modification as needed.
d. The patient/client care plan and exercise prescription should be reflected in, or be part of, periodic progress reports to the patient's/client's healthcare and fitness team.

2. Risk Stratification (Preparticipation Screening)

a. Can be modeled according to published criteria or guidelines, including those from
   1) The American College of Sports (clinical and health/fitness).
   2) The American Association for Cardiovascular and Pulmonary Rehabilitation (clinical).
   3) YMCA (health/fitness).
   4) The American College of Cardiology (clinical).
b. Can be useful for establishing
   1) Participant entry criteria.
   2) Exercise testing guidelines
   3) Electrocardiogram (ECG) monitoring and supervision guidelines (clinical program).
c. Is important in
   1) Determining participant eligibility and exclusion criteria to an exercise program.
   2) Evaluating the need for physician clearance or examination.
   3) Developing baseline fitness values.
   4) Designing a safe and effective exercise prescription.
d. May be tied to insurance reimbursement.

3. Other Program Components

a. Participant referral categories.
   1) Self-referral (participant identified a need or desire to enter the program voluntarily).
   2) Physician referral for disease prevention (e.g., improved fitness or weight management).
   3) Physician referral for disease management (e.g., rehabilitation or weight loss).
   4) Other healthcare provider referral.
b. Participant inclusion and exclusion criteria.
c. General exercise prescription guidelines.
d. Home exercise plans.
e. Medical supervision guidelines, including
   1) Participant-to-staff ratios.
   2) ECG and other medical monitoring needs (clinical).
f. Resistance exercise guidelines.
g. Intensive risk factor monitoring or counseling guidelines (clinical).
h. Periodic participant progress reports.
i. Communication with the patient's healthcare team.
j. Emergency plans and postemergency physician referral procedures.
k. Graduation procedures and guidelines from various program components or phases (clinical).
l. Guidelines for referral to other services or providers (e.g., psychological counseling, medical nutrition therapy) (clinical).
m. Program data analyses and outcome assessment.
n. Continuing client education.

B. INTERACTION WITH THE MEDICAL COMMUNITY

1. A client's participation in a clinical exercise rehabilitation program generally depends on referral from a physician. The program director/manager

TABLE 10-1. SAMPLE BUDGET FOR A CLINICAL EXERCISE PROGRAM

ENROLLMENT PROJECTIONS	EXISTING CLIENTS	MONTHLY FEE ($)	NEW CLIENTS	AVERAGE FEE ($)	CANCELLATIONS	TOTAL CLIENTS	TOTAL REVENUE ($)
Jan	700	45	0	150	0	750	42,120
Feb	750	45	75	150	23	803	44,320
March	803	45	75	150	24	853	46,640
Apr	853	45	65	150	26	893	47,380
May	893	45	55	150	27	921	47,620
June	921	45	50	150	28	943	48,110
July	943	45	50	150	28	965	49,100
Aug	965	45	50	150	29	986	50,060
Sept	986	45	60	150	30	1,017	52,480
Oct	1,017	45	65	150	30	1,051	54,580
Nov	1,051	45	70	150	32	1,090	56,850
Dec	1,090	45	50	150	33	1,107	55,540
TOTAL MEMBERSHIP REVENUE:							594,840

OTHER REVENUE	EXPENSE ($)
Smoking Cessation	1,200
Massage	16,200
Guest Fees	35,000
1-To-1 Training	32,400
Weight Management	12,000
Pro-Shop	1,200
Rest	3,000
Wellness Programs	1,200
Miscellaneous	10,000
Total Other Revenue	112,200
MEMBER REVENUE	594,840
OTHER REVENUE	112,200
TOTAL REVENUE	707,040
PAYROLL PROJECTIONS ($)	
General Manager	35,000
Sales 1	35,000
Administrator	20,000
Fitness Director	26,000
Full-Time Fitness 1	22,000
Full-Time Fitness 2	20,000
Part-Time Fitness	21,840
Receptionist	25,000
Aerobics	18,000
Nutrition	9,500
Cleaning	24,000
Bonus	8,000
Total Payroll	264,340
TAXES	34,364
BENEFITS	18,240
TOTAL SALARIES	316,944

PROJECTIONS	TOTAL OPERATING EXPENSES ($)
Salaries, Tax, and Benefits	316,944
Marketing	48,000
Maintenance/Repair	
HVAC	1,500
Equipment	2,400
Exterminating	1,200
Other	500
TOTAL MAINTENANCE	5,600
Operating supplies	
Cleaning Supplies	1200
Locker Room	3,000
Other Supplies	1,500
Towels	2,000
TOTAL SUPPLIES	7,700
Other Expenses	
Printing	3,600
Postage	3,000
Travel Seminars	2,000
Uniforms	6,000
Miscellaneous	1,000
Programs	500
Office Supplies	600
Telephone	7,200
TOTAL OTHER EXPENSES	10,800
TOTAL FIXED EXPENSES ($)	
Cam	24,000
Debt	10,000
Insurance	18,000
Leasing	8,400
Management Fees	48,000
Rent	70,705
Utilities	
Electricity	36,000
Gas	4,800
Water	2,000
TOTAL UTILITIES	42,800
TOTAL FIXED EXPENSES	264,705
TOTAL EXPENSES	653,749
NET PROFIT/(LOSS)	53,299

(With permission from McCarthy J: Fund allocation has become critical. *Club Business International*, 1990.)

TABLE 10-2. SAMPLE BUDGET FOR A HEALTH/FITNESS PROGRAM

ACSM FITNESS CENTER	EXISTING CLIENTS	MONTHLY FEE ($)	NEW CLIENTS	AVERAGE FEE ($)	CANCELLATIONS	TOTAL CLIENTS	TOTAL REVENUE ($)
Jan	700	45	50	150	0	750	39,000
Feb	750	45	75	150	22	803	44,010
Mar	803	45	75	150	25	853	46,260
Apr	853	45	65	150	25	893	47,010
May	893	45	55	150	27	921	47,220
June	921	45	50	150	28	943	47,685
July	943	45	50	150	28	965	48,675
Aug	965	45	50	150	29	986	49,620
Sept	986	45	60	150	29	1,017	52,065
Oct	1,017	45	65	150	31	1,051	54,120
Nov	1,051	45	70	150	31	1,090	56,400
Dec	1,090	45	50	150	33	1,107	55,065
TOTAL MEMBERSHIP REVENUE:							587,130

OTHER REVENUE ($)	
Smoking Cessation	1,200
Massage	16,200
Guest Fees	35,000
1-to-1 Training	32,400
Weight Management	12,000
Pro-Shop	1,200
Rest	3,000
Wellness Programs	1,200
Miscellaneous	10,000
TOTAL OTHER REVENUE	112,200
MEMBERSHIP REVENUE	587,130
TOTAL REVENUE	699,330

PAYROLL PROJECTIONS ($)	
General Manager	35,000
Sales 1	35,000
Administrator	20,000
Fitness Director	26,000
Full-Time Fitness 1	22,000
Full-Time Fitness 2	20,000
Part-Time Fitness	21,840
Receptionist	25,000
Aerobics	18,000
Nutrition	9,500
Cleaning	24,000
Bonus	8,000
TOTAL PAYROLL	264,340
TAXES	34,364
BENEFITS	18,240
TOTAL SALARIES	316,944

TOTAL OPERATING EXPENSES ($)	
Salary, Tax, & Benefits	316,944
Marketing	48,000
Maintenance/Repair	
VAC	1,500
Equipment	2,400
Exterminate	1,200
Other	500
TOTAL MAINTENANCE	5,600
Operating Supplies	
Cleaning	1,200
Locker Room	3,000
Other	1,500
Towels	2,000
TOTAL SUPPLIES	7,700
Utilities	
Electric	36,000
Gas	4,800
Water	2,000
TOTAL UTILITIES	42,800
Rent	70,705
Other Expenses	
Printing	3,600
Postage	3,000
Travel	2,000
Uniforms	6,000
Programs	500
Office Supplies	600
Telephone	7,200
Miscellaneous	1,000
TOTAL OTHER EXPENSES	23,900
Corporate Expenses	
Amortization/ Depreciation	24,000
Debt	
Insurance	
Leasing	
Management Fees	
TOTAL CORPORATE	108,400
TOTAL EXPENSES	624,049
NET PROFIT/(LOSS)	75,281

(With permission from McCarthy J: Fund allocation has become critical. *Club Business International*, 1990.)

(and medical director) should foster a positive working relationship with the local medical community.

a. This relationship can be fostered by
   1) Soliciting input from physicians (and other health professionals, as applicable) on planning and implementation.
   2) Maintaining regular communication through consultation and progress reports.

b. The program director/manager may consider establishing a medical advisory board to engage members of the medical community in program oversight.

2. A client's participation in a health/fitness program often does not require interaction or referral from a physician or health professional; however, an increasing number of fitness participants have medical issues that may require interaction with a health professional. The health/fitness program director/manager should consider implementing similar strategies noted above that are utilized for the medical/clinical setting.

C. PROGRAM MANAGEMENT

1. Program scheduling.
2. Staff scheduling, including accommodations for planned and unplanned time off (e.g., vacation, holiday and sick coverage).
3. Facility and equipment maintenance and cleaning.
   a. All equipment must be cleaned and disinfected regularly.
   b. All equipment must be in good repair and proper working condition.
   c. Routine documentation must be made related to equipment testing, cleaning and repairs.
   d. All walkways must be clear and floor surfaces safe.
4. Incident management.
   a. Immediate action must occur as defined in the program emergency plan.
   b. All administrative follow-up must be made in a timely manner (e.g., incident or accident reports).
   c. Debriefing of the incident must be conducted with the staff in a timely and confidential manner.

D. LEGAL AND ETHICAL CONSIDERATIONS

1. Risk Assessment and Management

a. The program director/manager must recognize all potential risk exposures in the program and make staff aware of these risks.

b. Identified risks should be minimized through appropriate means, including
   1) Procedures for dealing with malfunctioning equipment.
   2) Procedures for dealing with client injuries or incidents.

2. Standards of Care

a. Applicable standards of care must be defined in the program policies and procedures.

b. An example of an applicable standard of care is the most recent edition of the *ACSM's Guidelines for Exercise Testing and Prescription* (GETP), which may be used when performing various tasks in a clinical exercise rehabilitation program (e.g., exercise testing).

c. A program affiliated with a hospital or other care facility must adhere to the standard of care set by that institution.

d. A program that includes clinical exercise physiologists, nurses, respiratory therapists, and other healthcare professionals must take into account the standards of care for all involved professions.

e. All professional staff (and most ancillary staff) should be certified in cardiopulmonary resuscitation, and all clinical staff should be certified in Advanced Cardiac Life Support (ACLS).

3. Confidentiality

The Standards for Privacy of Individually Identifiable Health Information or the Privacy Rule creates national standards to protect patients'/clients personal health information and gives patients in a clinical setting access to their medical records. As required by the Health Insurance Portability and Accountability Act (HIPAA), for clinical settings, the Privacy Rule covers healthcare facilities, health plans and healthcare providers.

a. All client, patient and staff records are considered to be confidential and are to be kept secure as required by HIPAA; this includes both written and electronic health information.

b. Individuals who do not have a legitimate, program-related need to see data should not have access to that data.

4. Emergency Plans and Procedures

a. A plan for responding to emergency events should be outlined in the organization's policy and procedure manual. This emergency response plan must be well defined and well known to all staff members.

b. Emergency drills should be carried out on a regular basis (at least quarterly), involve all staff members, and be documented. To increase the effectiveness of such drills, scenarios that reflect common or "most likely" emergency situations should be presented and practiced.
c. **Emergency equipment should be calibrated and maintained on a regular basis.** Batteries should be tested and replaced to ensure optimal working order. Medications and supplies should be checked for expiration dates and replaced accordingly.

5. Accident and Injury Reporting

a. A process must be developed for the timely reporting of any and all accidents or injuries that may result from participation in a clinical exercise rehabilitation program.
b. The accident and injury reporting process should be specified in the organization's policy and procedure manual.
c. All forms used to document accidents and injuries and the responses to these events must be kept in a secure location.

6. Tort

a. A tort is a type of civil wrongdoing.
b. Negligence is failure to perform in a generally accepted standard.

7. Malpractice

a. Malpractice is a specific type of negligence.
b. Malpractice involves claims against a defined professional.
c. Malpractice is usually limited to those with public authority to practice arising from their responsibilities to a client.
d. Charges usually claim a breach of professional duties and responsibilities toward a client.
e. Generally, an injury has occurred, and a breach of duty preceded the injury.

8. State Laws and Regulations

The program director/manager must understand any written regulations or "practice acts" applicable to the programs and services offered.

E. MARKETING AND PROMOTION

1. Internal (within the facility) and external (outside the facility) marketing strategies should be developed.
2. Programs and the benefits of program participation should be promoted to various community and business organizations.
3. Marketing plans should be thorough and followed in compliance to the defined operational budget.

F. PROGRAM EVALUATION

1. Careful evaluation of a program's effectiveness is an essential extension of program development and implementation.
2. Subjective evaluation is accomplished through surveys of
   a. Program participants.
   b. Program staff.
   c. Referring physicians and healthcare providers.
   d. Other stakeholders involved in the program.
3. Program evaluation should be based on objective measures such as program statistics (e.g., attendance, net income, goal attainment rates) or client outcomes as outlined in the plan of care or exercise prescription.
   a. Standardized tools that are both reliable and valid can be used for outcome assessment.
   b. Outcome assessment tools should be easily administered and interpreted. For example, in a clinical program, the outcome assessment and program resources manual of the AACVPR can be used.
4. Continuous quality improvement (CQI), also known as Continuous Performance Improvement, is a systematic process of evaluation and implementation designed to maximize program effectiveness and safety.
5. Program evaluation criteria and process should be outlined in the organizational policy and procedure manual.
6. As an aspect of overall program evaluation, the program director/manager needs to take into account trends in healthcare and assess how well the program is adapting to these trends.

VII. DOCUMENTATION

A. THE MISSION STATEMENT

1. The mission statement is a simple statement of the program's main purposes (*Table 10-3*).
2. The mission statement forms the foundation of program planning, implementation, and evaluation.
3. The mission statement should be
   a. Worded clearly.
   b. Compatible with the parent organization's or institution's mission statement.
   c. Regularly reviewed and updated to reflect program changes.

TABLE 10-3. SAMPLE MISSION STATEMENTS

EXAMPLE 1	EXAMPLE 2
The mission of the Maintenance Cardiac Rehabilitation Component (MCRC) of the__________ complements the Mission Statements of the__________ and__________. Specifically, the mission of the MCRC has several facets and targeted groups for intervention. One group that the MCRC addresses through its services are the undergraduate and graduate students of__________ through its opportunities in research, service, and academic training in the rehabilitation of individuals with chronic diseases. The other important targeted group for the MCRC are those members of the community who have coronary artery disease (CAD) and other chronic diseases, as defined by the participant inclusion criteria of the MCRC. The MCRC provides educational, research, and service opportunities for those individuals with CAD in health and physical fitness assessment, exercise prescription, and exercise programming components as well as in other lifestyle management areas (e.g., smoking, nutrition).	The mission of XYZ Health and Fitness Center is to provide high quality exercise, health, and wellness programs to the community with the ultimate goal of improving the health of our community. Our staff will continually work to develop innovative services and programs will enhance one's fitness, be cost-effective to the consumer, and maintain profitability.

4. A central aspect of CQI is the evaluation of how a program is meeting its goals based on the mission statement.

B. GOALS AND OBJECTIVES

1. Program goals should be consistent with the program's mission statement.
2. Program goals should be defined by specific and measurable outcomes.
3. Program objectives should provide greater definition to the program goals and should provide specific means by which the goals are to be achieved.

C. POLICY AND PROCEDURES (P&P) MANUAL

1. The P&P provides documentation and dissemination of the program's specific protocols and practices.
2. The P&P should describe in detail the programs and services as well as the general rules and regulations of the program and facility.
3. The P&P should contain operational logistics, ranging from the organizational structure to the facility and equipment maintenance schedules.
4. The P&P should be readily accessible to all staff members.
5. The P&P should be updated regularly to reflect current practice and process of the program.
6. The P&P must be reviewed from a legal perspective, written in close collaboration with the program's general managers and directors, and approved by the parent organization's executive leadership.
7. The P&P should be consistent with the ever-changing standards and practices of applicable national, regional, and local organizations.

D. EMPLOYEE MANUAL

1. Provides basic rules and regulations for all staff positions.
2. Provides job descriptions, including reporting relationships, job responsibilities, minimum qualifications, critical success factors, and analysis of the physical demands.

E. PROGRAM DOCUMENTATION

A written record of agreements, waivers, releases, incidents, policies and procedures, and clearances is critical for an understanding of client activities and knowing who is protected if problems occur.

1. Agreements, releases, and consents should
   a. Clearly describe client participation, the rights and responsibilities of the client and the facility, as well as benefits to be expected and risks.
   b. Transfer appropriate levels of responsibility and risk associated with participation to the client (see Chapter 7, Figure 7-2, for an example of a participant agreement).
   c. Be created in clinical programs by the hospital or primary program management.
2. All fitness facilities are strongly encouraged to have program or service agreements and informed consents drafted and reviewed by a lawyer.
3. A client who does not meet the criteria for exercising within the scope of services or programming available or who does not comply with program policy should be excluded from participation, and referred to a more appropriate practitioner or facility.
4. A "Physician Clearance" requires a medical opinion of the client's risk with regard to exercise. This document places a level of shared risk on

the medical professional. A Physician's Clearance is recommended for

   a. A client who has considerable health risk with exercise, as indicated by a medical history questionnaire or Par-Q.
   b. A client who exhibits signs or symptoms during exercise that indicate increased risk if exercise continues.

5. Incident reports are used to document a problem or incident. These reports
   a. Provide a detailed description of the incident.
   b. List all witnesses.
   c. Include witness statements, if possible.
   d. State the results of the actions by the staff.
   e. Include a follow-up status of clients and staff involved in the incident.
   f. Provides corrective action to reduce recurrence of similar incidents.
6. **Malpractice and liability insurance** are necessary to provide coverage for staff and facility in cases of litigation for malpractice and accidents.

VIII. RECORDS

Records are important for the proper management of any program. Records are used for program evaluation, client motivation, understanding the success of the business, liability protection, and marketing. Types of records include

A. ATTENDANCE
B. EVALUATION AND SCREENING
C. WORKOUT AND TREATMENT
D. MEDICAL TESTS AND MEDICAL
E. SURVEYS
F. MAINTENANCE
G. EXPENSE

Review Test

DIRECTIONS: Carefully read all questions, and select the BEST single answer.

1. Which of the following is NOT an example of a variable expense for a clinical exercise rehabilitation program?
   A) ECG paper and electrodes.
   B) Heat and air conditioning.
   C) Rental fees for the facility space.
   D) Marketing.

2. Which of the following statements is NOT correct regarding a clinical exercise rehabilitation program's mission statement?
   A) Its clarity or understandability.
   B) It states the objectives of the organization or program.
   C) Each program should have a different mission statement.
   D) It should be compatible with the parent organization's mission statement.

3. Which of the following statements regarding a program's policy and procedures manual is NOT correct?
   A) It should be stored away for safekeeping.
   B) It is to be revised as the program's policies or procedures are modified.
   C) It should be viewed as a document in progress.
   D) It should contain program information ranging from the organizational structure to the facility's maintenance schedule.

4. Why is a comprehensive patient care plan necessary to provide effective program management?
   A) It is required by federal law.
   B) It provides a guide for individualized care and evaluation of care.
   C) It is a requirement for insurance reimbursement.
   D) It provides raw data for analysis in continuous quality improvement (CQI).

5. Which of the following statements is NOT correct regarding risk stratification?
   A) It can be modeled after AACVPR published criteria.
   B) It is useful for participant entry criteria, exercise testing guidelines, ECG monitoring, and supervision guidelines.
   C) It can be tied to insurance reimbursement.
   D) It is always used to determine the intensity of prescribed exercise.

6. Which of the following statements about confidentiality is NOT correct?
   A) All records must be kept by the program director/manager under lock and key.
   B) Data must be available to all individuals who need to see it.
   C) Data should be kept on file for at least 1 year before being discarded.
   D) Sensitive information (e.g., participant's name) needs to be protected.

7. Which of the following statements about injury reporting is NOT correct?
   A) A process for injury reporting, backed up with a form, should be developed.
   B) The process to be used and the accompanying forms must be part of the Policy and Procedure manual.
   C) Injury reporting forms must be kept under lock and key, just as are data records.
   D) A physician should sign every injury report form that is filed.

8. A personal trainer fails to spot a client performing heavy incline dumbbell presses and the client injures himself when the dumbbell is dropped on his face. Which of the following identify the appropriate type of negligence displayed in this scenario?
   A) Admission.
   B) Commission.
   C) Omission.
   D) Legal.

9. Which of the following best describes informed consent?
   A) It is a legal form.
   B) It is a process that is backed up by a form.
   C) It is something that only a lawyer can provide to an exercise program.
   D) It includes being an informed consumer to ensure that one undertakes the proper exercise program.

10. Which of the following elements is NOT part of an emergency plan for a clinical exercise program?
    A) Telephone number(s) needed to activate the emergency response system should be posted clearly on all phones.
    B) All personnel involved in exercise supervision should be trained in cardiopulmonary resuscitation (CPR).

C) Emergency drills should be carried out on a quarterly basis and documented.
D) Emergency equipment and supplies should be checked twice a year to make sure all equipment is in good working order.

11. Which of the following represents a fixed expense?
A) Office supplies.
B) Salaries.
C) Utilities (e.g., telephone).
D) Laboratory charge backs for blood work.

12. Which of the following financial analysis techniques would be the most appropriate for a not-for-profit program to determine the amount of revenue obtained from program fees required to meet the program's expenses without additional sources of income?
A) Break-down analysis.
B) Break-even analysis.
C) Profitability analysis.
D) Margin analysis.

13. Continuous quality improvement (CQI) is a systematic process of program evaluation that involves all of the following steps EXCEPT
A) Data analysis.
B) Goals assessment.
C) Outcomes assessment.
D) Budget assessment.

14. Which of the following statements about outcome assessment is NOT true?
A) The client care plan for each participant is not used in this process.
B) Data that are subjective or anecdotal in nature can be used in the assessment.
C) Periodic progress reports are valuable and should stimulate the need to collect objective data to support any subjective findings.
D) Standardized tools should be used for outcome assessment.

15. According to the AACVPR, which of the following would not be included as element for successful adult education?
A) Goal setting.
B) Rewards.
C) Contracts.
D) Knowledge testing.

16. Which one of the following statements concerning a needs assessment is NOT true?
A) It is a useful tool for gathering data and support for program implementation.
B) It often must be a creative tool developed in-house to meet the program's specific needs.
C) Given that the needs assessment may be developed in-house without the benefit of external validity, generalizing the results may be difficult.
D) Program planning is an essential step before needs assessment can be performed.

17. Which of the following is part of a comprehensive clinical exercise rehabilitation program?
A) The program is based on historical features of program administration.
B) The program adapts to changes in medical therapy based on clinical and scientific evidence.
C) The program is limited in scope and practice.
D) The program is the same for the entire client population served.

18. Do fitness specialists need management skills?
A) Only if they wish to become floor supervisors or program managers.
B) Yes, because of the natural progression of advancement into management.
C) Yes, because as instructors, they manage client programs and manage the floor with the clients.
D) No, because they will be trained in management if they become managers.

19. Which of the following statements are true regarding a facility fitness newsletter, fitness library, and bulletin boards?
A) They can be used as part of staff news.
B) They can be utilized for client and staff education.
C) They are a good source of facility marketing.
D) They all require considerable money and must be budgeted carefully.

20. Why would a fitness facility or rehabilitation program be interested in public relations?
A) To increase exposure for the facility and sell its services.
B) To become involved in local politics.
C) To improve staff morale.
D) To make the staff work harder.

21. In what way would tort laws affect a fitness specialist or clinical exercise physiologist?
A) Negligence is breaking a tort law and can ruin an instructor's career.
B) State taxes often are related to profit, which is governed by tort laws.
C) Tort laws are related to workers' compensation regulations.
D) They relate to the Americans with Disabilities Act (ADA).

22. Which of the following represents the best method for an administrator to educate the fitness staff?
A) Voicing his or her opinion.
B) Joining fitness organizations and subscribing to fitness journals.

C) Buying fitness videos.
D) Reading the newspaper.

23. Which of the following best represent the ideal manager involvement when developing fitness programs?
A) A hands-off approach should be maintained.
B) Involvement should only include the budgeting and final approval.
C) The manager should be the only person involved in program development.
D) The manager should be active as a program developer as well as a resource, supporter, and critic for programs developed by other staff.

24. Which of the following best describes the reason for designing a budget?
A) To make management happy.
B) To determine program viability.
C) To save money.
D) To teach managers about cost analysis.

25. Which of the following best describes the rules and regulations of a facility?
A) The law.
B) The client rights statement.
C) Policies and procedures.
D) Check and balance for management and clients.

26. Which of the following best describes a request by a fitness professional for physician's clearance?
A) It is not necessary if the client completes the medical history questionnaire.
B) It is a communication tool with little value.
C) It is necessary to provide information about the physician's attitude regarding your program.
D) It provides a medical opinion regarding the safety of the client to exercise.

27. Other than scheduling and implementing the policies and procedures, which of the following best represents a duty of the supervisor of a fitness facility?
A) Cleaning the equipment.
B) Maintaining emergency procedures and evaluations.
C) Marketing and promotions.
D) Managing the fitness billing.

28. What is the primary reason why a manager or director should conduct a needs assessment?
A) To determine the specific needs and interests of the target market.
B) To determine the quality of potential fitness specialists who could be hired in the area.
C) To determine the needs of management before developing the budget.
D) To identify a need for new or different exercise equipment.

29. Why are policies and procedures important in a fitness center?
A) They explain how to use the fitness equipment properly.
B) They clarify the rights of and risks in being a fitness member.
C) They are general guidelines for operating a fitness program or department.
D) They explain the employee insurance plans and how to use them.

30. What are some of the common sales "rules" in promoting a fitness program?
A) Selling memberships at any cost is key.
B) You know more than they do, so be aggressive.
C) Honesty and an understanding of the needs of the potential member important.
D) Long-term agreements make more money than short-term agreements.

31. Program description, resource availability, and client interest are examples of which of the following?
A) A business plan.
B) A survey.
C) Management factors.
D) Budget categories.

32. Which of the following is created or reduced by effective program administration and management?
A) Create problems with staff egos.
B) Reduce memberships.
C) Create successful programs and reduce problems.
D) Create more work for the staff and reduce feedback.

33. Why are incident reports important?
A) They inform the manager which employees are performing poorly.
B) They indicate which members are problematic and should be dismissed.
C) They document and give details of any incident or problem that occurs.
D) State laws often require them.

34. Why are records valuable to a fitness program?
A) They help in evaluation of a program.
B) They are useful for marketing purposes.
C) They help to provide facts in any legal issues.
D) They help the front desk to monitor paid and unpaid clients.

35. Which of the following is an example of a program record?
A) Client progress and outcomes.
B) Member needs.
C) Performance of clients on selected exercises.
D) Member suggestions and any actions taken regarding them.

36. Which of the following is an example of participant interaction as part of the supportive role of a manager?
    A) Offering a shoulder on which to cry.
    B) Conducting surveys and responding to client needs.
    C) Encouraging members to "let go" in exercise classes.
    D) Having members teach classes.

37. Which of the following statements best describe the manager's role in staff education?
    A) It looks good to the owners.
    B) It creates many opportunities for educating the staff.
    C) It lets the staff handle their own education but also to encourage it.
    D) It is not very valuable because member retention and sales are the key to any program.

38. Which of the following statements best describe staff certification?
    A) Not important, because members do not care.
    B) Important, primarily because it adds spice to marketing materials.
    C) Not a good idea, because certified staff will increase your payroll.
    D) Important, primarily because it adds a standard of knowledge and credibility to your facility.

39. Which of the following statements best describes capital budgets?
    A) Include the costs of equipment and building or facility expense.
    B) Include the costs to operate a program.
    C) Are not necessary with fitness programs.
    D) Are included as part of the balance sheet in financial reports.

40. What do budgets determine?
    A) Fitness equipment costs.
    B) If a company is making or losing money.
    C) Viability, identification of problems, and a plan for the future of a program.
    D) Assets and liabilities of the financial plan.

ANSWERS AND EXPLANATIONS

1–C. Rent is typically an agreed-on cost and, thus, is a fixed as opposed to a variable expense. Variable expenses vary based on program use; examples would include supplies (e.g., ECG electrodes) and utilities that may change with weather conditions, such as heat.

2–C. A mission statement can range from a very simple to a very complicated set of ideas about the organization's or a program's strategic goals. Once developed, missions statements serve to guide administration and staff when making strategic decisions. Although it may be necessary to create a mission statement for a particular program or department of an organization, a mission statement should not be created for multiple programs or components of a program. Too many mission statements within an organization begin to dilute the original, intended mission of the organization. Departments and programs of an organization should be guided by the parent organization's overall mission statement.

3–A. The P&P manual must be available to all staff and, thus, is kept in a readily accessible location and it not filed away. Also, the P&P manual is meant to be referred to and revised as needed.

4–B. A patient care plan is a thoughtfully produced document that plans for effective, individualized care of the patient. It should be used as a guide to implement a set of actions that address the patient's health or wellness problems.

5–D. Risk stratification is rarely used to determine the intensity of prescribed exercise. However, risk stratification can be an important tool for patient inclusion or exclusion criteria and, in some cases, it may be used for insurance reimbursement.

6–C. There is no accepted minimal or maximal amount of time that data should be stored. Clearly, however, data must be stored in a confidential (lock-and-key) manner, and discretion must be used when sharing data.

7–D. Legal advice suggests that the injury report form does not necessarily require a physician's signature. However, a process for injury reporting needs to be followed consistently and be described in the P&P manual.

8–C. Failure to spot or assist a participant may be considered negligence by omission.

9–B. Informed consent is a process, backed up by a form that, among other things, describes the risks and benefits of participation in certain activities (e.g., an exercise test). It is suggested that a legal expert be consulted regarding any informed consent procedures.

10–D. Emergency equipment should be checked frequently and on a routine basis. Defibrillators, suction and oxygen tanks, should be checked each work day to ensure proper functioning.

Supplies should be checked on a weekly basis for appropriate quantity and expiration date. Records should be kept documenting appropriate supply inventory and functioning of equipment. Practice sessions involving all staff members should be held at least quarterly. These sessions should be documented and may be most effective if scenarios are "played out" to mimic real emergencies.

11–B. Staff salaries usually are a fixed expense and not subject to change based on variable factors (e.g., number of program participants). As program use increases, so do expenses, such as blood work charge backs, telephone expenses, and office supplies. Thus, these latter expenses are known as variable expenses.

12–B. A break-even analysis is ideal for not-for-profit organizations that wish to understand how best to meet all of their expenses, including payroll. The for-profit sector will use a profitability analysis to determine how much, if any, money can be earned during a period.

13–D. Budget assessment is not necessarily a part of the CQI process, although it is a valuable step in program evaluation. Generally, CQI is an outcomes assessment based on the program's goals using data analysis of various measures.

14–A. The client care plan is a vital component of outcomes assessment. Outcomes assessment is driven by goals established for each client or patient.

15–D. According to the AACVPR, adult education can involve many techniques to foster education and behavior change, including goal setting, contracts, rewards, and support. Knowledge testing is a component of outcome analysis, however, and little justification exists for knowledge-based testing in promoting behavioral change.

16–D. Needs assessment should be done before the program planning and implementation phases to provide data on which to base these steps. Needs assessment is not a one-time measure. Successful programs perform frequent formal or informal needs assessments as they grow.

17–B. The justification for a clinical exercise rehabilitation program is based on its ability to adapt to changing practices and procedures for rehabilitation services. Thus, whereas history is important and interesting, flexibility is needed to adapt to an ever-changing healthcare model.

18–C. The definition of a manager is someone who designs, implements, and monitors programs, which is what fitness specialists are responsible for as a natural part of their job. Managing a client's program fits the basic definition of a manager, so the skills of managing a person and his or her program fit the need for management training. A fitness specialist does not naturally become a manager.

19–B. Educating a fitness client on the principles of exercise, proper nutrition, and good health is important, and this information can be communicated in a variety of ways. Newsletters, libraries, and bulletin boards are some of the recommended ways to communicate with and educate members. Staff news should not necessarily be within the library or posted on a board. Marketing strategies often do not include the library or bulletin boards. These forms of education usually are inexpensive to develop and maintain.

20–A. Public relations, a common form of promotion, is important for any business. It is very important to "get your name out" and increase exposure, and these activities can help people to learn who you are and how good you are. Public relations has nothing to do with politics when it involves your facility. It may improve the morale of your staff, but the intent is to generate exposure for your club. Public relations should not be considered a strategy for making the staff work harder.

21–A. A tort law refers to a civil wrong, such as negligence (failure to perform at a generally accepted standard). Negligence in fitness often refers to the instructor giving bad instruction or advice that leads to an injury or accident. Clients often sue instructors for negligence, which can be very damaging. Tort laws do not involve state taxes, are not regulated by workers compensation insurance, and do not involve the ADA.

22–B. Fitness organizations and journals offer excellent opportunities for staff and management to learn about many aspects of fitness. Most fitness organizations and journals work with experts in fitness and provide accurate and up-to-date information. An administrator's opinion may not be an educated or unbiased one, which can make for poor education. Newspapers and videos often present misinterpreted or inaccurate information.

23–D. The manager's job is to manage programs by being a program developer, to act as a resource for staff and clients, to evaluate programs, and to provide constructive input to staff. A hands-off approach is not recommended, because it often leads to poor program implementation and problems. Managing program development, not just budgeting, is an important role for managers. It is important to involve the staff in the design and implementation of the programs; otherwise, the manager does all of the work.

24–B. One of the primary goals of a fitness business is to make a profit. Budgeting helps a manager and the owner to understand if a program can make money and be successful (i.e., viable). Budgets are not designed to save money; the programs are designed to save money. Management is only happy if the budgets show a profit. Managers must learn cost analysis before developing budgets so that they know how to create a budget that will make management happy.

25–C. Policies and procedures are essentially the rules and regulations of a facility, plus the means of conducting and implementing the regulations correctly. Regulations can be considered to be the law, but they are not often labeled as such. The client rights statement is a different document. Management monitors the rules and makes sure that staff and members follow them; however, these regulations are not considered to be a balance measurement.

26–D. A fitness specialist will request or require a physician's clearance when concern exists regarding the risk of a medical crisis with exercise. The clearance is a medical opinion that it is safe for the client to exercise. The medical history will indicate if a concern with exercise is evident, but it will not assure the fitness specialist that it is safe for the client to exercise. A physician's clearance is a very important tool for the safety of the exercising client and should not be an opinion statement about your facility.

27–B. Evaluating staff members and developing emergency procedures are common duties in supervising staff. It is important that staff know how to implement emergency procedures, and the supervisor must train the staff. The staff, not the supervisors, handle the equipment cleaning. Marketing and billing are duties that are not involved with fitness staff supervision.

28–A. A needs assessment is designed to analyze a target market and determine what that market needs and wants. This assessment has nothing to do with assessing fitness staff, equipment, or management needs.

29–C. Policies and procedures provide general guidelines as well as how to enact those guidelines in implementing an exercise program. Policies and procedures help to establish control of the operations of programs. Use of fitness equipment may be a part of a P&P statement, but policies and procedures are much more than that. The rights and risks of a fitness member are written in the client rights statement. Insurance plans are presented in the employee handbook, not in the policies and procedures.

30–C. Honesty and understanding are always the best policy. It is very important to know what the client needs and wants. This information can help sell the programs that meet those needs and desires. Being honest enhances your reputation and client retention, because clients get what they were told they would get. Selling memberships at any cost often results in losing business over time, either because of dishonesty or because of giving away too much. Being aggressive and assuming the client does not know anything can alienate potential clients. Short-term agreements tend to improve client retention.

31–C. Managing involves many characteristics or factors. Developing programs, being a resource to staff and members, and monitoring client interest are some of the factors of management. A business plan explains the business in detail, the target market, and marketing strategies; it does not explain the resource availability. Surveys can assess client interest, but they do not assess program descriptions. These examples are not part of a budget.

32–C. Effective management should create a successful facility that meets the needs of the clients, staff, and owners. Problems should be reduced, membership should increase, and feedback and communication should be enhanced, not reduced.

33–C. Incident reports provide a detailed record of what happened in any incident at the fitness facility. These records may be critical for a physician or emergency medical unit if an accident occurs. The report also provides evidence, witnesses, and the results of actions taken by the staff. These reports are not intended to inform management of bad employees or members. State laws do not require incident reports, although they may recommend them.

34–A. Records help management in many ways, including in the evaluation of a program. Recording the workouts, client attendance, feedback, and more can help to determine if the program was successful. Records can help as evidence in a legal issue as well, but this value is not nearly as important as answer A. Records also help at the front desk, but they are not part of a fitness program. Instead, they are part of the facility management.

35–A. Program records refer to the specific evaluation of an individual or group program. The progress of clients throughout the program and the outcomes following the program are very important factors to assess. Specific exercise records are part of the data in the program records, which are then used to chart progress and outcomes. Member needs and suggestions usually are not part of program recordings; these usually are recorded as part of a survey.

36–B. Fitness facilities constantly seek information on what clients want, need, like, and dislike. Interacting with clients makes clients feel important and respected. Conducting surveys and responding to client input are two of the better ways to invite interaction. A shoulder to cry on is not a way to encourage interaction, nor do you want to increase the risk of a problem by letting clients "let go" or teach your classes.

37–B. Creating opportunities for educating the staff is very important, because it enhances their knowledge and provides a perk for them. A well-educated staff enhances the quality and safety of the programs, improves the facility's reputation, and increases the respect and acceptance of clients. It is not valuable to provide education only for the purpose of looking good to the owners or to ignore the need for education.

38–D. Certification shows the clients that staff members meet industry standards. The staff should have a certain level of skill and competency with certifications. Most members do care, and payroll should be a secondary factor to the choice of certifying staff. Certified staff should bring more members, which can justify the increased cost. The marketing also is secondary to the value to the clients and the program.

39–A. Capital budgets refer to the budgeting of program implementation or facility. How much does it cost to start the program and to implement the first stage? Capital budgets usually include equipment, facility expense, staffing, initial marketing, and so on in the start-up. Operating a program is part of the operating budget, not the capital budget. Capital budgets are critical in determining whether to start a program. Capital budgets are not included in the balance sheet.

40–C. Budgets show what it will cost to run a program and whether the program will be profitable. Managers can review a budget and determine if the program has financial problems. Budgets are a future look at a program and should be developed with the idea of making money. Budgets also present only a part of the financial statement of the facility. The facility must include other financial information (e.g., assets, liabilities) to determine if it is making or losing money.

Metabolic Calculations

11 CHAPTER

I. OVERVIEW

A. CONSIDERATIONS

1. Expect from 4 to 10 metabolic calculation questions on the examination. A few of these questions will be simple, requiring straightforward calculations. Some may be classified as moderately difficult, requiring simple mathematical substitution. One or two questions may be classified as difficult, requiring additional algebraic manipulation of these formulae.
2. The answer to any problem may be on either the right or left side of the metabolic formula. If you are trying to solve for oxygen cost or $\dot{V}O_2$ for the individual exercising at a particular workload (e.g., walking at 2.5 miles/hour on a treadmill) then the problem is a forward solving one with the final answer on the left side of the equation.

   For example: What is the oxygen cost ($\dot{V}O_2$) for a 160 pound person walking at 2.5 miles/hour on a level treadmill?

   However, you may be asked to calculate an appropriate workload on a piece of exercise equipment (e.g., treadmill speed or the resistance on a cycle ergometer). If so, then the problem is a backward solving one with the final answer on the right side of the equation.

   For example: At what speed should a 160 pound person walk on a level treadmill to achieve an oxygen cost of 24.5 $mL \cdot kg^{-1} \cdot min^{-1}$?

   Both types of problems can be solved with the use of the American College of Sports Medicine (ACSM) metabolic formulae. The forward-solving one is certainly more straightforward, with simple insertion of the relevant information (workload). The backward-solving one involves the use of higher mathematical skills with the simplification of the equation and the combination or elimination of like terms. You may or may not need to separate out the resting $\dot{V}O_2$ depending on the problem. Thus, backward-solving involves more steps and careful reading and interpretation of the problem.
3. A copy of the ACSM metabolic formulae (*Table 11-1*) is included in the written examination packet. You should be familiar with these formulae before you sit for the examination. Also familiarize yourself with Table 7.2 from the 8th edition of the ACSM Guidelines for Exercise Testing and Prescription, p. 158.
4. The unit conversion factors and the energy equivalency factors will NOT be provided with the examination. COMMIT THESE NUMBERS TO MEMORY.
5. The written examination might contain metabolic calculation questions that will not require the use of the ACSM metabolic formulae. However, a good understanding of energy expenditure and energy equivalency will be needed to arrive at the correct answer.

B. EXPRESSIONS OF ENERGY EXPENDITURE

Energy expenditure in humans can be expressed in many terms. Converting from one expression to another is simple. Be familiar with the following terms:

1. Absolute Oxygen Consumption

This is the rate at which oxygen is consumed by the whole person, expressed in liters per minute ($L \cdot min^{-1}$) or milliliters per minute ($mL \cdot min^{-1}$).

a. Resting absolute oxygen consumption for a 70-kg person is approximately 0.245 $L \cdot min^{-1}$.
b. In highly trained aerobic athletes, maximal absolute oxygen consumption as high as 5.5 $L \cdot min^{-1}$ may be expected.
c. Absolute oxygen consumption is useful because it allows for an estimation of caloric expenditure.
d. One liter of O_2 consumed expends 5 kilocalories (5 kcal), or 20.9 kilojoules (20.9 kJ).

2. Relative Oxygen Consumption

This is the rate of oxygen consumption relative to body weight, measured in $mL \cdot kg^{-1} \cdot min^{-1}$; in other words, the volume of oxygen consumed per kilogram of body weight every minute.

a. For the purpose of the ACSM examination, a given mass of lean body tissue requires the same amount of O_2 at rest, and at any

TABLE 11-1. SUMMARY OF METABOLIC CALCULATIONS[a]

Walking
$\dot{V}O_2 = (0.1 \cdot S) \cdot (1.8 \cdot S \cdot G) + 3.5$
Treadmill and Outdoor Running
$\dot{V}O_2 = (0.2 \cdot S) \cdot (0.9 \cdot S \cdot G) + 3.5$
Leg Ergometry
$\dot{V}O_2 = (10.8 \cdot W \cdot M^{-1}) + 7$
Arm Ergometry
$\dot{V}O_2 = (18 \cdot W \cdot M^{-1}) + 3.5$
Stepping
$\dot{V}O_2 = (0.2 \cdot f) \cdot (1.33 \cdot 1.8 \cdot H \cdot f) + 3.5$

[a] Where $\dot{V}O_2$ is gross oxygen consumption in mL · kg^{-1} · min^{-1}; S is speed in m · min^{-1}; M is body mass in kg; G is the percent grade expressed as a fraction; W is power in watts; f is stepping frequency in min^{-1}; H is step height in meters.

Note: These equations are presented in conventional units following each mode of exercise, simplifying the calculations.

(Modified from *ACSM's Guidelines for Exercise Testing and Prescription,* 8th ed. Philadelphia, Lippincott Williams & Wilkins; 2010.)

given work rate, irrespective of gender, race, age, and level of fitness. The resting relative oxygen consumption is always assumed to be 3.5 mL · kg^{-1} · min^{-1}.

b. In highly trained aerobic athletes, a maximal relative oxygen consumption ($\dot{V}O_{2\,max}$) may be as high as 75–80 mL · kg^{-1} · min^{-1}.

c. Relative $\dot{V}O_2$ is commonly used to compare oxygen consumption of individuals who vary in size. Because $\dot{V}O_{2\,max}$ is also used as an index of cardiopulmonary fitness, a higher value is indicative of greater aerobic fitness.

d. All ACSM formulae provide $\dot{V}O_2$ values in gross relative terms.

3. **Metabolic Equivalents (METs)**

Physicians and clinicians commonly use the term MET as an expression of energy expenditure or exercise intensity. One MET is equivalent to the relative oxygen consumption at rest. Therefore, 1 MET = 3.5 mL · kg^{-1} · min^{-1}. In clinical settings it is common for cardiac rehabilitation patients to begin with an initial MET prescription. The exercise specialist will then use the MET prescription to calculate initial walking and cycling workloads.

For Example: A phase II cardiac rehabilitation patient begins his first week. The exercise prescription calls for him to exercise using a level (0% grade) walking modality at 2.5 METs. Using the ACSM metabolic equations, the appropriate walking speed can be calculated from the MET value.

a. METs are calculated by dividing the relative oxygen consumption by 3.5. For example, an individual consuming 35 mL · kg^{-1} · min^{-1} during steady-state exercise is exercising at 10 METs.

b. A MET is a useful expression because it allows for an easy comparison of the amount of oxygen uptake during exercise with that at rest.

4. **Calorie (kilocalorie)**

A Calorie, also known as a kilocalorie (kcal), is an expression of energy intake and expenditure, which is commonly used to quantify the amount of energy derived from consumed foods as well as the amount of energy expended at rest and during physical activity.

5. **Fat Stores**

a. The human body stores most of its excess energy intake as fat.

b. It takes 3,500 calories to make and store 1 lb of body weight. Stated in reverse, 1 lb of body weight can provide the body with 3,500 calories. Because walking or running 1 mile expends 100 calories, you would need to walk or run about 35 miles to lose 1 lb of fat!

6. **Net Versus Gross $\dot{V}O_2$**

a. Humans require about 3.5 mL · kg^{-1} · min^{-1} (1 MET) of oxygen at rest. This amount of oxygen uptake is vital for the survival of the body's cells, tissues, and systems.

b. Physical activity elevates oxygen consumption above resting oxygen requirements. You will later note that at the end of each metabolic formula you will have to add 3.5 mL · kg^{-1} · min^{-1} (resting oxygen consumption) to what it costs to do work to calculate the total (gross) oxygen consumption.

   1) Gross $\dot{V}O_2$ is the sum of the oxygen cost of physical activity and the resting component.
   2) Net $\dot{V}O_2$ is the difference between the oxygen consumption value for exercise and the resting value. Net $\dot{V}O_2$ is used to assess the caloric cost of exercise.
   3) Hence,

$$\text{net } \dot{V}O_2 = \text{gross } \dot{V}O_2 - \text{resting } \dot{V}O_2$$

c. Net and gross oxygen uptake can be expressed in relative or absolute terms.

d. The ACSM metabolic formulae in *ACSM's Guidelines for Exercise Testing and Prescription*, 8th ed, and those described in this chapter, were designed to provide you with gross values.

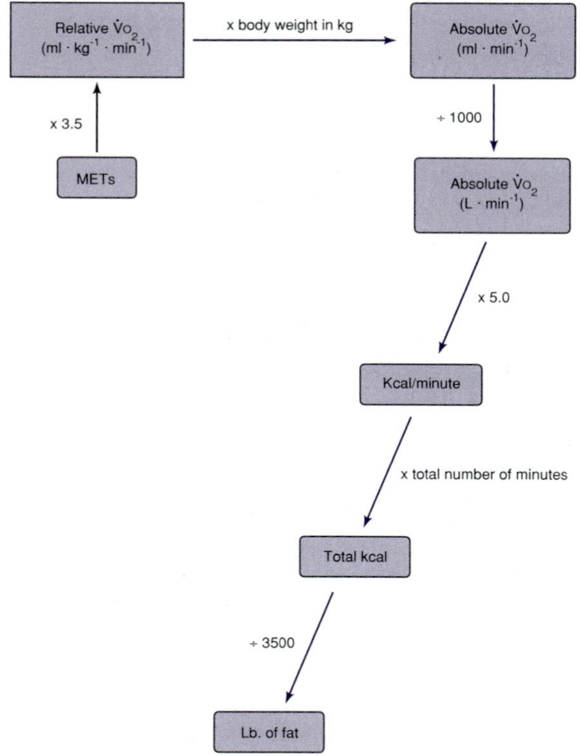

FIGURE 11-1. The energy equivalency chart: the 7 energy expressions.

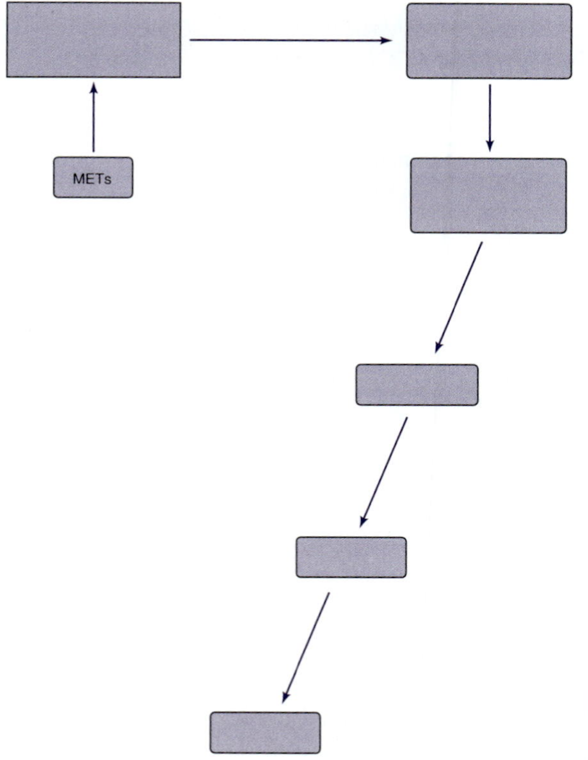

FIGURE 11-2. The energy equivalency chart practice sheet.

The ability to convert from one energy expression to another is fundamental. Do not proceed to the next section of this chapter until you master this task.

- Converting an expression merely requires the multiplication or division of that expression by a constant. For example, to convert from METs to relative oxygen consumption, multiply the MET value by 3.5. Conversely, to convert from relative oxygen consumption to METs, divide by 3.5 (*Figure 11-1*). Commit these constants to memory.
- *Figure 11-1*, the Energy Equivalency Chart, will help you to remember these conversions.
- *Figure 11-2* is a practice sheet. Duplicate this sheet and practice completing it from memory. Then answer the following questions.

CONVERTING ENERGY EXPRESSIONS PRACTICE QUESTIONS AND ANSWERS

Q1. What is the MET equivalent to 8.75 mL · kg^{-1} · min^{-1}?

A1. To convert from mL · kg^{-1} · min^{-1} to METs, divide 8.75 by 3.5. The correct answer is **2.5 METs.**

Q2. What is the absolute oxygen consumption equivalent to 10 METs for a 154-lb male?

A2. To convert from METs to absolute $\dot{V}O_2$, first multiply the MET value by 3.5 to convert METs to relative $\dot{V}O_2$ (mL · kg^{-1} · min^{-1}), then multiply the product (35 mL · kg^{-1} · min^{-1}) by body weight in kg (154 lb ÷ 2.2 = 70 kg). The correct answers are **2,450 mL · min^{-1}** or **2.45 L · min^{-1}.**

Q3. What is the equivalent total caloric expenditure of 2.5 lb of body weight?

A3. To convert from pounds of body weight to total kilocalories, multiply the body weight (in pounds) by 3,500. The correct answer is **8,750 kcal.**

Q4. A 70-kg male expends 7.5 kcal · min^{-1} while exercising. What is the equivalent MET value?

A4. To convert from kcal · min^{-1} to METs:

a. First, convert the value to absolute $\dot{V}O_2$ in L · min^{-1}: **7.5 kcal · min^{-1} ÷ 5.0 = 1.5 L · min^{-1}**

b. Then to absolute $\dot{V}O_2$ in mL · min^{-1}: **1.5 L · min^{-1} × 1,000 = 1,500 mL · min^{-1}**

c. Then to relative $\dot{V}O_2$: **1,500 mL · min^{-1} ÷ 70 kg = 21.4 mL · kg^{-1} · min^{-1}**

d. Then to METs: **21.4 mL · kg^{-1} · min^{-1} ÷ 3.5 = 6.1 METs**

Q5. How many pounds of body weight will a 50-kg woman lose after 4 weeks of training if she exercises at a frequency of 3 days per week, a duration of 45 minutes per session, and an energy expenditure of 6.5 kcal · min^{-1}? Assume no modifications were made in her eating habits during the 4 weeks of training.

TABLE 11-2. CONVERSION FACTORS

TO CONVERT FROM:	TO:	DO THIS:
Centimeters (cm)	Meters (m)	÷ by 100
Inches (in)	Meters (m)	× by 0.0254
Inches (in)	Centimeters (cm)	× by 2.54
$kg \cdot m \cdot min^{-1}$	Watts (W)	÷ by 6.0
Liters (L)	Milliliters (mL)	× by 1,000
Miles per hour (mph)	Meters per minute ($m \cdot min^{-1}$)	× by 26.8
Pounds (lbs)	Kilograms (kg)	÷ by 2.2
Revolutions per minute (rpm) on a	Meters per minute ($m \cdot min^{-1}$)	
• Monark arm ergometer		× by 2.4
• Monark leg ergometer		× by 6
• Tunturi or BodyGuard cycle ergometer		× by 3

A5. The first step to solving this conversion question is to calculate the total number of minutes spent exercising during the 4 weeks.

a. Because she trained for 45 minutes per session, three times per week, she accumulated a total of 540 minutes of exercise during the 4 weeks:

$$45 \text{ minutes/session} \times 3 \text{ sessions/week} \times 4 \text{ weeks} = 540 \text{ minutes}$$

b. The second step is to calculate the total number of calories expended during exercise throughout the 4 weeks (540 minutes) of training:

$$6.5 \text{ kcal} \cdot \text{min}^{-1} \times 540 \text{ minutes of exercise} = 3{,}510 \text{ kcal}$$

c. Finally, find the body weight equivalent to the expended calories:

$$3\ 510 \text{ kcal} \div 3\ 500 = 1\ 0 \text{ lb of body weight}$$

Q6. Using the ACSM walking formula, you calculate a gross $\dot{V}O_2$ of 13.0 $mL \cdot kg^{-1} \cdot min^{-1}$. What is the net oxygen uptake?

A6. Because gross $\dot{V}O_2$ = net $\dot{V}O_2$ + resting $\dot{V}O_2$, then net $\dot{V}O_2$ = gross $\dot{V}O_2$ – resting $\dot{V}O_2$:

$$\begin{aligned} \text{Net } \dot{V}O_2 &= 13\ 0 \text{ mL} \cdot kg^{-1} \cdot min^{-1} \\ &\ -3\ 5 \text{ mL} \cdot kg^{-1} \cdot min^{-1} \\ \text{Net } \dot{V}O_2 &= 9\ 5 \text{ mL} \cdot kg^{-1} \cdot min^{-1} \end{aligned}$$

OTHER CONVERSION FACTORS

You must also commit to memory some other important conversions. Practice writing out the conversions in Table 11-2 from memory.

PRACTICE QUESTIONS: OTHER CONVERSION FACTORS

Convert the following values to the desired units:

1. 1.5 meters to cm.
2. 59.1 inches to meters.
3. 70 kg to pounds.
4. 6.0 mph to meters per minute.
5. 50 RPM on the Monark leg ergometer to meters per minute.

SOLUTIONS

1. 1.5 meters × 100 = 150 cm.
2. 59.1 inches × 0.0254 = 1.5 meters.
3. 70 kg × 2.2 = 154 lb.
4. 6.0 mph × 26.8 = 160.8 $m \cdot min^{-1}$.
5. 50 RPM × 6 = 300 $m \cdot min^{-1}$.

C. RATIONALE FOR USE OF THE ACSM METABOLIC FORMULAE

Fundamental to the application of proper exercise testing or prescription is the ability to measure or estimate energy expenditure (see Chapter 8).

1. Direct measurement of energy expenditure is impractical.

a. The actual rate of oxygen consumption ($\dot{V}O_2$), as determined using open-circuit spirometry, provides the best measure of the energy cost of physical activity.

b. The rate of oxygen uptake during maximal exercise ($\dot{V}O_{2\,max}$) is commonly used as an index of cardiopulmonary fitness.

c. Actual $\dot{V}O_2$ measurement using open-circuit spirometry is arduous and costly, making it impractical for nonclinical purposes.

2. Energy expenditure can be estimated using the ACSM metabolic formulae.

The ACSM introduced metabolic formulae to provide health/fitness practitioners with a practical method to estimate the energy cost of the most common exercises expressed in terms of the rate of oxygen uptake. Practical uses for the ACSM metabolic formulae include the following:

a. Estimating the rate of oxygen uptake during exercise ($\dot{V}O_2$) allows for an estimate of the energy expenditure and caloric expenditure associated with exercise.

b. An estimate of the rate of oxygen uptake during maximal exercise ($\dot{V}O_{2\,max}$) indicates the maximal capacity for aerobic work, allowing for fitness categorization, and inter- and intrasubject comparisons.

c. Calculating the appropriate exercise intensity (work rate) needed to elicit the desired oxygen consumption will allow the health/fitness professional to develop more effective exercise prescriptions.

II. THE ACSM METABOLIC FORMULAE

Remember, all ACSM formulae yield gross oxygen uptake in relative terms. In other words, each formula calculates

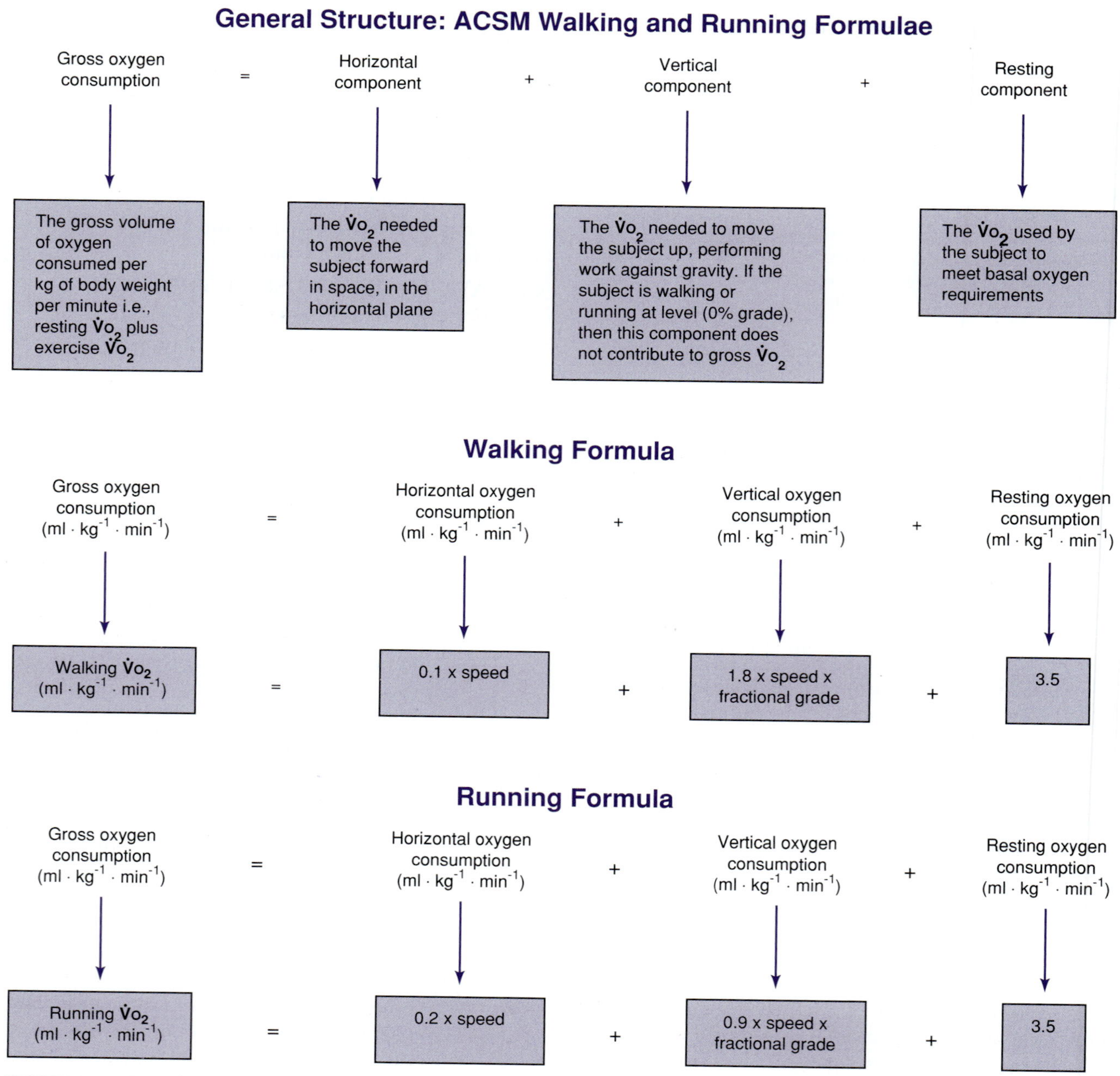

General Structure: ACSM Walking and Running Formulae

Gross oxygen consumption	=	Horizontal component	+	Vertical component	+	Resting component
The gross volume of oxygen consumed per kg of body weight per minute i.e., resting $\dot{V}O_2$ plus exercise $\dot{V}O_2$		The $\dot{V}O_2$ needed to move the subject forward in space, in the horizontal plane		The $\dot{V}O_2$ needed to move the subject up, performing work against gravity. If the subject is walking or running at level (0% grade), then this component does not contribute to gross $\dot{V}O_2$		The $\dot{V}O_2$ used by the subject to meet basal oxygen requirements

Walking Formula

Gross oxygen consumption ($ml \cdot kg^{-1} \cdot min^{-1}$)	=	Horizontal oxygen consumption ($ml \cdot kg^{-1} \cdot min^{-1}$)	+	Vertical oxygen consumption ($ml \cdot kg^{-1} \cdot min^{-1}$)	+	Resting oxygen consumption ($ml \cdot kg^{-1} \cdot min^{-1}$)
Walking $\dot{V}O_2$ ($ml \cdot kg^{-1} \cdot min^{-1}$)	=	0.1 x speed	+	1.8 x speed x fractional grade	+	3.5

Running Formula

Gross oxygen consumption ($ml \cdot kg^{-1} \cdot min^{-1}$)	=	Horizontal oxygen consumption ($ml \cdot kg^{-1} \cdot min^{-1}$)	+	Vertical oxygen consumption ($ml \cdot kg^{-1} \cdot min^{-1}$)	+	Resting oxygen consumption ($ml \cdot kg^{-1} \cdot min^{-1}$)
Running $\dot{V}O_2$ ($ml \cdot kg^{-1} \cdot min^{-1}$)	=	0.2 x speed	+	0.9 x speed x fractional grade	+	3.5

FIGURE 11-3. General structure of the walking and running formulae.

the amount of oxygen needed to do the work, including resting oxygen needs, per kilogram of body weight.

A. WALKING AND RUNNING FORMULAE (*Figure 11-3*)

1. Walking Formula

This formula applies to speeds of 50 to 100 $m \cdot min^{-1}$ (1.9 to 3.7 mph).

a. Gross $\dot{V}O_2$ is calculated in relative terms ($mL \cdot kg^{-1} \cdot min^{-1}$).

b. The horizontal component is the product of the speed of the treadmill, in meters per minute ($m \cdot min^{-1}$), multiplied by 0.1 (the O_2 cost of walking). The product, the $\dot{V}O_2$ of walking forward, is in $mL \cdot kg^{-1} \cdot min^{-1}$.

c. The vertical component is the product of the fractional grade of the treadmill multiplied by the speed of the treadmill ($m \cdot min^{-1}$) multiplied by 1.8 (the O_2 cost of walking uphill). The product, the $\dot{V}O_2$ of walking uphill, is in $mL \cdot kg^{-1} \cdot min^{-1}$.

Do not confuse the percent grade of the treadmill with the degree angle of inclination. Percent grade of the treadmill is the amount of vertical rise for 100 units of belt travel. For example, a client walking on a treadmill at a 12% grade travels 12 meters vertically for every 100 meters of belt travel. (In this example, the fractional grade = 12 m ÷ 100 m = 0.12).

d. The **resting component** is 3.5 $mL \cdot kg^{-1} \cdot min^{-1}$.

2. **Running Formula**

This formula applies to treadmill and outdoor running speeds exceeding 134 $m \cdot min^{-1}$ (5.0 mph) and for true jogging speeds above 80.4 $m \cdot min^{-1}$ (3.0 mph).

This formula may also be used for off-the-treadmill level running, but not for running on a graded track.

a. **Gross $\dot{V}O_2$** is calculated in **relative terms** ($mL \cdot kg^{-1} \cdot min^{-1}$).
b. The **horizontal component** is the product of the speed of the treadmill, in $m \cdot min^{-1}$ multiplied by 0.2 (the O_2 cost of running). The product, the $\dot{V}O_2$ of running forward, is in $mL \cdot kg^{-1} \cdot min^{-1}$.
c. The **vertical component** is the product of the fractional grade of the treadmill multiplied by the speed of the treadmill ($m \cdot min^{-1}$) multiplied by 0.9 (the O_2 cost of running uphill). The product, the $\dot{V}O_2$ of running uphill, is in $mL \cdot kg^{-1} \cdot min^{-1}$.
d. The **resting component** is 3.5 $mL \cdot kg^{-1} \cdot min^{-1}$.

Examination Note: Work Rate

The work rate may be provided to you in the question. You may also be expected to derive it from the cadence of the cycle ergometer and the resistance set on the flywheel.

- Work rate, also known as the **power output** or **workload**, is the product of the resistance set on the cycle ergometer and the speed of cycling (velocity):

  Work rate = force (resistance set on the flywheel in kgf) × velocity (in $m \cdot min^{-1}$)

- For the units for the resistance set on the flywheel, **kilogram-force (kgf) and kilopond (kp), can be used interchangeably**: 1 kgf = 1 kp.
- **Calculate velocity from revolutions per minute (rpm)** by multiplying the rpm value by **6 $m \cdot rev^{-1}$ for a Monark cycle ergometer, or 3 $m \cdot rev^{-1}$ for either a Tunturi or a BodyGuard.** For example, an individual cycling at 50 rpm on a Monark leg ergometer is pedaling at a velocity of 300 $m \cdot min^{-1}$. If the same individual works against a resistance of 2 kp, then the work rate will be 2 kp × 50 rpm × 6 $m \cdot rev^{-1}$ = 600 $kg \cdot m \cdot min^{-1}$.
- **Work rate can also be expressed in watts:**

  1 watt = 6.0 $kg \cdot m \cdot min^{-1}$

Examination Note: Work Rate–Arm Erogometer

The work rate may be provided to you in the question. You also may be expected to derive it from the cadence of the cycle ergometer and the resistance set on the flywheel.

- Work rate, also known as the power output or workload, is the product of the resistance set on the flywheel and the speed of cycling (velocity):

  Work rate = Force (resistance set on the flywheel in kg) · Velocity ($m \cdot min^{-1}$)

- Calculate velocity from rpm by multiplying the rpm value by **2.4 for a Monark arm ergometer.** The units for the resistance set on the flywheel, kilogram-force (kgf) and kilopond (kp), can be used interchangeably (1 kgf = 1 kp).

For example, an individual arm cycling at 50 rpm on a Monark arm ergometer is pedaling at a velocity of 120 $m \cdot min^{-1}$. If the same individual works against a resistance of 2 kp, then the work rate will be 2 · 50 · 2.4 = 240 $kg \cdot m^{-1} \cdot min^{-1}$.

- Work rate can also be expressed in watts:

  1 W = 6.0 · $kg \cdot m^{-1} \cdot min^{-1}$

B. LEG AND ARM ERGOMETRY FORMULAE (*Figure 11-4*)

1. **Leg Cycling**

This formula applies to work rates between 300 and 1,200 $kg \cdot m \cdot min^{-1}$, or 50 to 200 watts (50 to 200 W).

a. **Gross O_2** consumption is calculated in **relative terms** ($mL \cdot kg^{-1} \cdot min^{-1}$).
b. **Oxygen cost of loaded leg cycling.** This is the product of the cost of cycling (1.8) multiplied by the work rate ($kg \cdot m \cdot min^{-1}$) divided by body weight (kg). The O_2 cost of loaded leg cycling may also be calculated using the following expression:

10.8 × work rate (in watts) ÷ body weight (in kg)

or

1.8 × work rate (in $kg \cdot m^{-1} \cdot min^{-1}$) ÷ body weight (in kg)

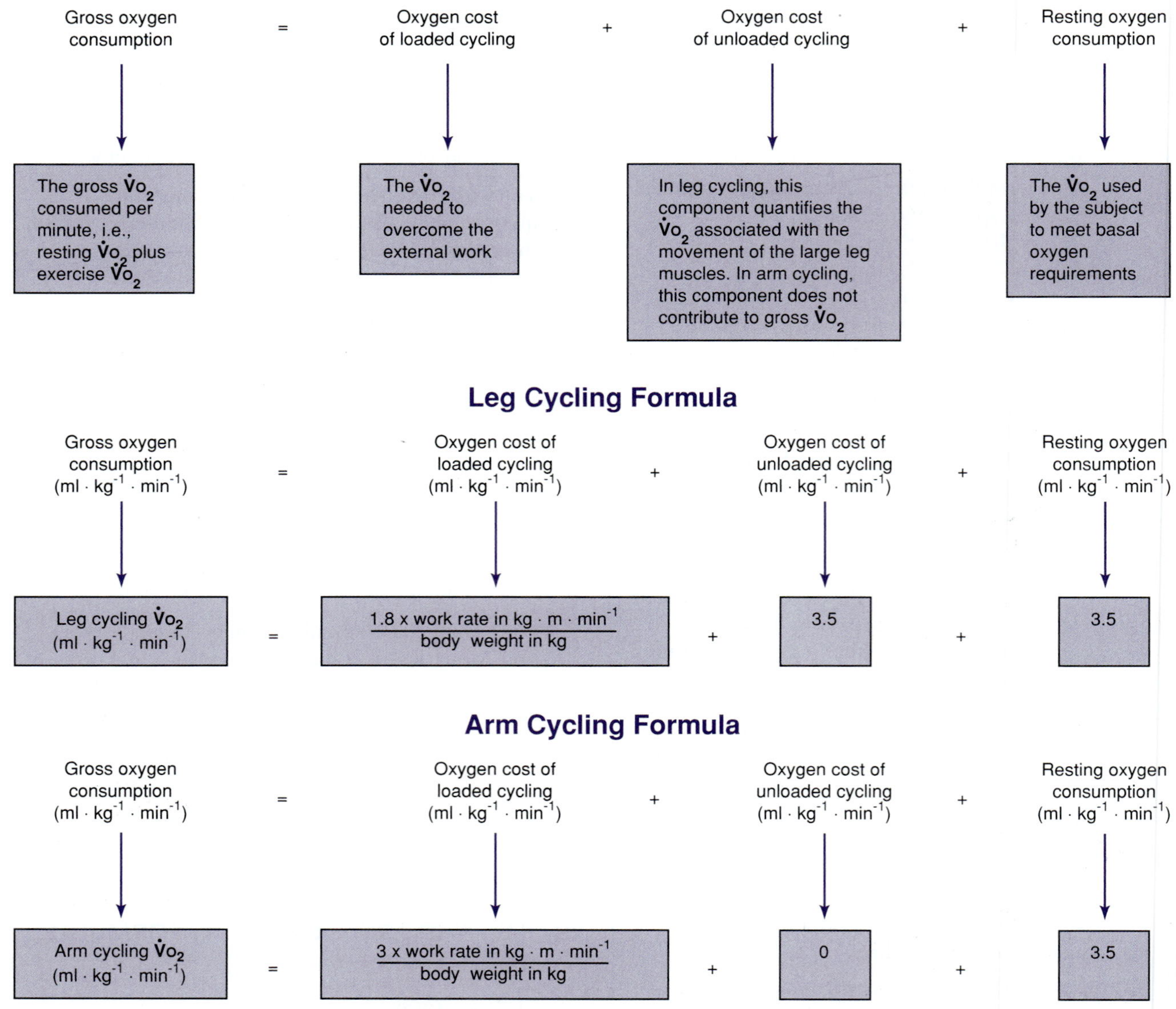

FIGURE 11-4. General structure of the leg and arm ergonometry formulae.

c. Oxygen cost of unloaded leg cycling. Leg cycling incurs a small oxygen cost of 3.5 $mL \cdot kg^{-1} \cdot min^{-1}$ for the movement of the legs in space.

d. The resting O_2 component is 3.5 $mL \cdot kg^{-1} \cdot min^{-1}$.

2. **Arm Cycling**

This formula applies to work rates between 150 and 750 $kg \cdot m \cdot min^{-1}$ (25 to 125 W).

a. Gross O_2 consumption is calculated in relative terms ($mL \cdot kg^{-1} \cdot min^{-1}$).

b. Oxygen cost of loaded arm cycling. This is the product of the cost of cycling (3) multiplied by the work rate ($kg \cdot m \cdot min^{-1}$) divided by body weight (kg). The O_2 cost of loaded arm cycling may also be calculated using the following expression:

18 × work rate (in watts) ÷ body weight (in kg)

or

3 × work rate (in $kg \cdot m^{-1} \cdot min^{-1}$) ÷ body weight (in kg)

c. Oxygen cost of unloaded arm cycling. Arm cycling does not incur an oxygen cost of unloaded cycling.

d. The resting component is 3.5 $mL \cdot kg^{-1} \cdot min^{-1}$.

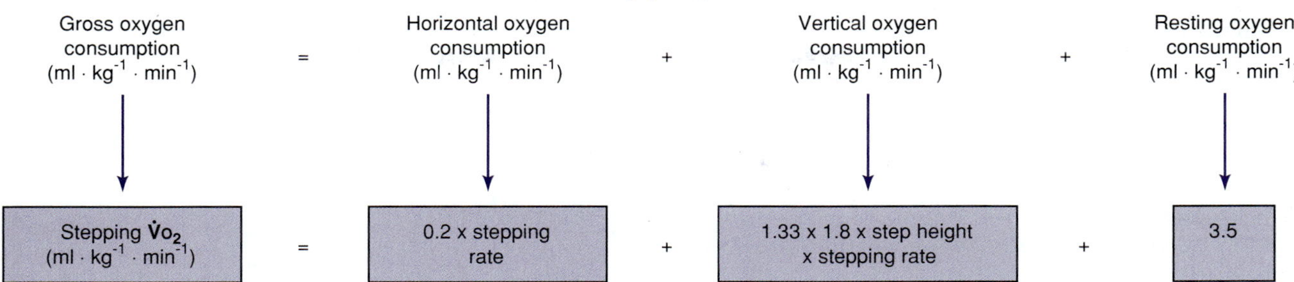

FIGURE 11-5. American College of Sports Medicine (ACSM) stepping formula.

C. STEPPING FORMULA (*Figure 11-5*)

This formula applies to stepping performed on a step box, a bleacher, or a similar stepping object where both concentric contractions (moving up against gravity) and eccentric contractions (moving down with gravity) are involved.

The formula is appropriate for stepping rates between 12 and 30 steps $\cdot$ min^{-1}, and heights between 0.04 and 0.4 m (1.6 to 15.7 inches).

1. **Gross O_2 consumption** is calculated in **relative terms** (mL $\cdot$ kg^{-1} $\cdot$ min^{-1}).
2. **Horizontal component.** This is the product of the rate of stepping per minute multiplied by 0.2. The product is O_2 consumption in mL $\cdot$ kg^{-1} $\cdot$ min^{-1}.
3. **Vertical component.** This is the product of the height of each step (in meters) multiplied by the rate of stepping per minute multiplied by 1.33 multiplied by 1.8. The product is O_2 consumption in mL $\cdot$ kg^{-1} $\cdot$ min^{-1}.
4. **Resting component** is 3.5 mL $\cdot$ kg^{-1} $\cdot$ min^{-1}.

III. SOLVING THE ACSM METABOLIC FORMULAE

A. USING A SYSTEMATIC APPROACH

The task of solving the ACSM formulae is made much easier using a systematic approach, which will help you avoid small but costly mistakes.

1. Read each question carefully and do not proceed until you know what you are expected to calculate. Remember that some questions may be solved without the use of a metabolic formula.
2. Extract the required information. Do not be misled with extraneous information. If, for example, a question wants you to calculate the $\dot{V}O_2$ for walking on a treadmill, volunteered data about the height, age, or the gender of the subject are irrelevant.
3. Select the correct metabolic equation. A common error committed by many candidates is choosing the wrong formula.
4. Write down each step. *Avoid shortcuts.* Going through all the steps once is faster than two shortcut attempts!
5. On the top left corner of a clean sheet of paper, write the known values and indicate what is unknown.
6. Where needed, convert all values to the appropriate units (see *Table 11-2*).
   a. Convert the treadmill speed or cycling cadence to meters per minute (m $\cdot$ min^{-1}).
   b. Convert body weight to kilograms (kg).
   c. Convert step height to meters (m).
   d. Convert work rate to kg $\cdot$ m $\cdot$ min^{-1}.
7. Write down the formula and plug in the known values and constants. Write clearly and place units after all variables.
8. Solve for the unknown. If the unknown is on the left side of the equation (i.e., the $\dot{V}O_2$ value), simply calculate the sum of the three components of the appropriate equation. If the unknown is on the right side of the equation, substitute and solve for the unknown. More on solving linear equations later.
9. Examine the answer. Is the answer logical? Does it fall within expected "normal" values and human abilities?
10. Examine the choices. Make sure that your answer is in the same units as the answer on the examination, especially if a question does not specify what energy expression is needed (i.e., relative or absolute $\dot{V}O_2$, METs, kcal).

> To solve an equation with an unknown on the right side of the equation, you must simplify the expression so that the unknown stands by itself on one side of the equation and all the known numbers on the other.

B. SOLVING LINEAR EQUATIONS

The ACSM metabolic formulae are simple linear equations.

The process of arriving at an answer to a metabolic calculation question is greatly simplified if the unknown is the $\dot{V}O_2$ value.

In instances where the $\dot{V}O_2$ value is known, you might be expected to calculate an unknown value on the right side of the equation, such as the resistance on the cycle ergometer, the speed of the treadmill, the height of the step bench, and so on.

1. **Example 1**
   Solve for χ in the following equation:

$$\chi - 4 = 10$$

Solution: Add 4 to both sides of the equation:

$$\chi - 4 + 4 = 10 + 4$$
$$\chi = 14$$

2. **Example 2**
   Solve for α in the following equation:

$$2\alpha + 7 = 3$$

Solution: Subtract 7 from both sides of the equation:

$$2\alpha = -4$$

Divide both sides by 2:

$$\alpha = -2$$

3. **Example 3**
   Solve for β in the following equation:

$$4\beta - 3/4 = 7/9$$

Solution: Add 3/4 to both sides of the equation:

$$4\beta = 55/36$$

Divide both sides by 4:

$$\beta = 55/144$$

4. **Helpful hint:** Substitute your answer for the unknown value in the original equation. If the left side equals the right side after the substitution, your answer is correct. For example, in the previous problem, plugging in 55/144 in the place of β yields 7/9. Hence, 55/144 is the correct answer.

C. SOLVING LINEAR EQUATIONS: Q & A

1. What is the gross oxygen cost of walking on a treadmill at 3.5 mph and a 10% grade?

   Solution: Choose the walking equation.

   a. On the top left corner of a clean sheet of paper, write down the knowns and convert all numbers to the appropriate units:

$$\textbf{Speed in m} \div \textbf{min}^{-1} = \textbf{3.5 mph} \times \textbf{26.8} = \textbf{93.8 m} \cdot \textbf{min}^{-1}$$

> **Math Remainder**
> *Multiply and divide* numbers **before** *adding or subtracting*. For example, in the following expression:
>
> $$Y = 5 + 2 \times 5 + 7 \times 2$$
>
> Multiply the 2 by the 5 (= 10), the 7 by the 2 (= 14), and then add the 10, the 14, and the 5 together. The correct answer is Y = 29, not 84.

   b. Write down the ACSM walking formula:

$$\text{Walking } \dot{V}O_2\ (\text{mL} \cdot \text{kg}^{-1} \cdot \text{min}^{-1}) = (0.1 \times \text{speed}) + (1.8 \times \text{speed} \times \text{fractional grade}) + (3.5\ \text{mL} \cdot \text{kg}^{-1} \cdot \text{min}^{-1})$$

   c. Substitute the variable name with the known values:

$$\text{Walking } \dot{V}O_2\ (\text{mL} \cdot \text{kg}^{-1} \cdot \text{min}^{-1}) = (0.1 \times \mathbf{93.8}\ \text{m} \cdot \text{min}^{-1}) + (1.8 \times \mathbf{93.8}\ \text{m} \cdot \text{min}^{-1} \times \mathbf{0.1}) + 3.5\ \text{mL} \cdot \text{kg}^{-1} \cdot \text{min}^{-1}$$

   d. Multiply values:

$$\text{Walking } \dot{V}O_2\ (\text{mL} \cdot \text{kg}^{-1} \cdot \text{min}^{-1}) = 9.38\ \text{mL} \cdot \text{kg}^{-1} \cdot \text{min}^{-1} + 16.88\ \text{mL} \cdot \text{kg}^{-1} \cdot \text{min}^{-1} + 3.5\ \text{mL} \cdot \text{kg}^{-1} \cdot \text{min}^{-1}$$

   e. Then add numbers:

$$\text{Gross walking } \dot{V}O_2 = \mathbf{29.76 mL} \cdot \mathbf{kg}^{-1} \cdot \mathbf{min}^{-1}$$

2. A 176-lb client set the treadmill at 3.0 mph and 2% grade. While exercising, his heart rate was 140 beats · min^{-1} and his blood pressure was 160/80 mm Hg. What was his estimated oxygen consumption in relative terms?

   Solution: The question is clearly asking for $\dot{V}O_2$ in relative terms ($\text{mL} \cdot \text{kg}^{-1} \cdot \text{min}^{-1}$).

   a. Extract the information you need (speed and elevation of the treadmill) and ignore extraneous information (HR and BP).
   b. Choose the walking equation.
   c. On the top left corner of a clean sheet of paper, write down the knowns and convert all numbers to the appropriate units:

$$\text{Weight} = 176\ \text{lb} \div 2.2 = 80.0\ \text{kg}$$

$$\text{Speed} = 3.0\ \text{mph} \times 26.8 = 80.4\ \text{m} \cdot \text{min}^{-1}$$

$$\text{Treadmill elevation} = 2\%\ \text{grade} = 2/100 = 0.02$$

d. Plug the knowns into the formula and calculate the answer:

$$\text{Walking } \dot{V}O_2 \ (mL \cdot kg^{-1} \cdot min^{-1}) = (0.1 \times \text{speed}) + (1.8 \times \text{speed} \times \text{fractional grade}) + (3.5\ mL \cdot kg^{-1} \cdot min^{-1})$$

$$\text{Walking } \dot{V}O_2 \ (mL \cdot kg^{-1} \cdot min^{-1}) = (80.4\ m \cdot min^{-1} \times 0.1) + (1.80 \times 80.4\ m \cdot min^{-1} \times 0.02) + (3.5\ mL \cdot kg^{-1} \cdot min^{-1})$$

$$\text{Walking } \dot{V}O_2 \ (mL \cdot kg^{-1} \cdot min^{-1}) = 8.04\ mL \cdot kg^{-1} \cdot min^{-1} + 2.89\ mL \cdot kg^{-1} \cdot min^{-1} + 3.5\ mL \cdot kg^{-1} \cdot min^{-1}$$

$$\text{Relative } \dot{V}O_2 = 14.43\ mL \cdot kg^{-1} \cdot min^{-1}$$

3. What resistance should you set a Monark cycle ergometer at to elicit a $\dot{V}O_2$ value of 2,250 mL · min^{-1} while cycling at 50 RPM? The subject is 65 inches tall and weighs 110 lb.

Solution: Read the question carefully; know what the question is asking for. The question is providing you with the oxygen consumption (2,750 mL · min^{-1}), but expects you to calculate the resistance (F) to be set on the cycle ergometer.

a. Extract the information you need. Only the weight of the subject and the speed of the cycle are needed.
b. Convert the known units:

$$110\ lb = 50.0\ kg$$

c. Select the leg ergometer equation.
d. Calculate the gross relative $\dot{V}O_2$ from the given information:

$$\dot{V}O_2\ mL \cdot kg^{-1} \cdot min^{-1} = 2{,}250\ mL \cdot min^{-1} \div 50.0\ kg = 45.0\ mL \cdot kg^{-1} \cdot min^{-1}$$

e. Now, write out the leg ergometer formula

$$\text{Leg cycling } \dot{V}O_2 \ (mL \cdot kg^{-1} \cdot min^{-1}) = (1.8 \times \text{work rate} \div \text{body weight}) + (3.5\ mL \cdot kg^{-1} \cdot min^{-1}) + (3.5\ mL \cdot kg^{-1} \cdot min^{-1})$$

f. Note that the unknown (F = resistance in kg) is part of the work rate. Write out the work rate as force (in kg) × speed (in m · min^{-1}):

$$45\ mL \cdot kg^{-1} \cdot min^{-1} = (1.8 \times \boxed{F \times \text{velocity}} \div \text{body weight}) + (3.5\ mL \cdot kg^{-1} \cdot min^{-1}) + (3.5\ mL \cdot kg^{-1} \cdot min^{-1})$$

g. From the given information, we also know that the velocity of cycling is 300 m · min^{-1} (50 RPM × 6). Plug all the knowns into the equation:

$$45\ mL \cdot kg^{-1} \cdot min^{-1} = (1.8 \times F \times 300\ m \cdot min^{-1} \div 50\ kg) + (3.5\ mL \cdot kg^{-1} \cdot min^{-1}) + (3.5\ mL \cdot kg^{-1} \cdot min^{-1})$$

h. Move the unknown F to one side of the equation, all the knowns to the other side, and calculate for the unknown:

$$45\ mL \cdot kg^{-1} \cdot min^{-1} = (1.8 \times F \times 300\ m \cdot min^{-1} \div 50\ kg) \boxed{+ (3.5\ mL \cdot kg^{-1} \cdot min^{-1}) + (3.5\ mL \cdot kg^{-1} \cdot min^{-1})}$$

$$45\ mL \cdot kg^{-1} \cdot min^{-1} - 3.5\ mL \cdot kg^{-1} \cdot min^{-1} - 3.5\ mL \cdot kg^{-1} \cdot min^{-1} = 1.8 \times F \times 300\ m \cdot min^{-1} \div 50\ kg$$

$$38\ mL \cdot kg^{-1} \cdot min^{-1} = 1.8 \times F \times 300\ m/min \div 50\ kg$$

$$38 \times 50 \div 1.8 \div 300 = F$$
$$3.52\ KG = F$$

Review Test

DIRECTIONS: Carefully read all questions and select the BEST single answer.

1. What is the relative oxygen consumption of walking on a treadmill at 3.5 mph and 0% grade?
   A) 9.38 mL · kg^{-1} · min^{-1}.
   B) 12.88 mL · kg^{-1} · min^{-1}.
   C) 18.76 mL · kg^{-1} · min^{-1}.
   D) 22.26 mL · kg^{-1} · min^{-1}.

2. A client is walking on a treadmill at 3.4 mph up a 5% grade. What is her $\dot{V}O_2$ in relative terms?
   A) 9.11 mL · kg^{-1} · min^{-1}.
   B) 11.9 mL · kg^{-1} · min^{-1}.
   C) 24 mL · kg^{-1} · min^{-1}.
   D) 20.81 mL · kg^{-1} · min^{-1}.

3. A 70-kg client is running on a treadmill at 5 mph set at a 5% grade. What is his caloric expenditure rate?
   A) 12.7 kcal · min^{-1}.
   B) 1.271 kcal · min^{-1}.
   C) 3.633 kcal · min^{-1}.
   D) 36.33 kcal · min^{-1}.

4. What is the relative oxygen consumption of walking on a treadmill at 3.5 mph up a 10% grade?
   A) 181.72 mL · kg^{-1} · min^{-1}.
   B) 18.17 mL · kg^{-1} · min^{-1}.
   C) 29.76 mL · kg^{-1} · min^{-1}.
   D) 27.96 mL · kg^{-1} · min^{-1}.

5. What is the MET equivalent to level walking on a treadmill at 3.0 mph?
   A) 5.59 METs.
   B) 3.30 METs.
   C) 2.30 METs.
   D) 3.02 METs.

6. What is the relative oxygen consumption of running on a treadmill at 6.5 mph and 0% grade?
   A) 34.84 mL · kg^{-1} · min^{-1}.
   B) 34.48 mL · kg^{-1} · min^{-1}.
   C) 38.34 mL · kg^{-1} · min^{-1}.
   D) 43.83 mL · kg^{-1} · min^{-1}.

7. What is the relative oxygen consumption of running on a treadmill at 5.5 mph and 12% grade?
   A) 29.48 mL · kg^{-1} · min^{-1}.
   B) 45.4 mL · kg^{-1} · min^{-1}.
   C) 47.2 mL · kg^{-1} · min^{-1}.
   D) 48.9 mL · kg^{-1} · min^{-1}.

8. A 150-lb man sets the treadmill speed at 5.0 mph and a 5.2% grade. Calculate his MET value.
   A) 36.57 METs.
   B) 10.45 METs.
   C) 12.25 METs.
   D) Not enough information to answer the question.

9. What is a subject's work rate in watts if he pedals on a Monark cycle ergometer at 50 rpm at a resistance of 2.0 kiloponds?
   A) 50 watts.
   B) 100 watts.
   C) 200 watts.
   D) 300 watts.

10. A 110-lb woman pedals a Monark cycle ergometer at 50 rpm against a resistance of 2.5 kiloponds. Calculate her absolute oxygen consumption.
    A) 300 mL · min^{-1}.
    B) 750 mL · min^{-1}.
    C) 1.25 L · min^{-1}.
    D) 1.7 L · min^{-1}.

11. How many calories will a 110-lb woman expend if she pedals on a Monark cycle ergometer at 50 rpm against a resistance of 2.5 kiloponds for 60 minutes?
    A) 12.87 calories.
    B) 31.28 calories.
    C) 510 calories.
    D) 3,500 calories.

12. A 55-kg woman trains on a cycle ergometer by pedaling at 60 rpm against a resistance of 1.5 kiloponds. What is her absolute oxygen consumption?
    A) 1.36 L · min^{-1}.
    B) 2.47 L · min^{-1}.
    C) 3.62 L · min^{-1}.
    D) 3,600 mL · min^{-1}.

13. The same 55-kg woman also trains on a Monark arm ergometer at 60 rpm against a resistance of 1.5 kiloponds. What is her absolute oxygen consumption?
    A) 1.52 L · min^{-1}.
    B) 773.0 mL · min^{-1}.
    C) 0.840 L · min^{-1}.
    D) 0.774 L · min^{-1}.

14. If a 70-kg man runs on a treadmill at 8 mph and 0% grade for 45 minutes, what is his caloric expenditure?
    A) 1,067.07 calories,
    B) 392.18 calories.
    C) 730.48 calories.
    D) Not enough information to answer the question.

15. What is the relative oxygen cost of bench stepping at a rate of 24 steps per minute up a 10-inch stepping box? The individual weighs 140 lb.
    A) 12.91 mL · kg^{-1} · min^{-1}.
    B) 14.61 mL · kg^{-1} · min^{-1}.
    C) 16.41 mL · kg^{-1} · min^{-1}.
    D) 22.89 mL · kg^{-1} · min^{-1}.

16. What stepping rate should a client use if she wishes to exercise at 5 METs? The step box is 6 inches high and she weighs 50 kg.
    A) 12 steps per minute.
    B) 32 steps per minute.
    C) 25 steps per minute.
    D) 96 steps per minute.

17. A 143-lb woman regularly exercises on a treadmill at a speed of 5.5 mph and a 2% elevation. What is her caloric expenditure?
    A) 6.78 kcal · min^{-1}.
    B) 11.58 kcal · min^{-1}.
    C) 20.85 kcal · min^{-1}.
    D) 25.47 kcal · min^{-1}.

18. A 143-lb woman regularly exercises on a treadmill at a speed of 5.5 mph and a 2% elevation. How much weight will she lose weekly if she exercises for a duration of 45 minutes per session, a frequency of three sessions per week?
    A) 1.5 kg.
    B) 2.07 kg.
    C) 0.25 lb.
    D) 0.45 lb.

19. What resistance would you set a cycle ergometer at if your 80-kg client needs to train at 6 METs? Assume a 50 rpm cycling cadence.
    A) 1.5 kg.
    B) 2.07 kg.
    C) 0.25 lb.
    D) 0.45 lb.

20. What running speed would you set a level treadmill at to elicit an oxygen consumption of 40 mL · kg^{-1}· min^{-1}?
    A) 5.0 mph.
    B) 6.8 mph.
    C) 18.25 m · min^{-1}.
    D) 18.25 mph.

21. If a 70-kg healthy young man exercises at an intensity of 45 mL · kg^{-1}· min^{-1} three times per week for 45 minutes each session, how long would it take him to lose 10 lb of fat?
    A) 4 weeks.
    B) 7.14 weeks.
    C) 16.5 weeks.
    D) 19 weeks.

22. A 35-year-old woman reduced her caloric intake by 1,200 kcal per week. How much weight will she lose in 26 weeks?
    A) 8.9 lb.
    B) 12.0 lb.
    C) 26.0 lb.
    D) 34.3 lb.

23. From question 22, how much weight will she lose in 26 weeks if she integrated a 1-mile walk three times per week into her weight loss program?
    A) 3 lb.
    B) 6 lb.
    C) 11 lb.
    D) 15 lb.

CASE I. A 75-kg man cycles at 120 watts on the leg ergometer.

1. His training $\dot{V}O_2$ is:
    A) 24 METs.
    B) 17.06 mL · kg^{-1} · min^{-1}.
    C) 12.5 mL · kg^{-1} · min^{-1}.
    D) 7 METs.

2. His energy expenditure during a 30 minute ride is:
    A) 273 kcal.
    B) 9.2 kcal.
    C) 1,050 kcal.
    D) 300 kcal.

3. If he chooses to walk up a 10% grade, what would be the appropriate walking speed to get the same energy expenditure?
    A) 211 m · min^{-1}.
    B) 3.4 mph.
    C) 2.8 mph.
    D) 100 m · min^{-1}.

CASE II. During an aerobic dance class, Lisa, who weighs 58 kg, is stepping on a 9-inch step at a rate of 20 steps per minute.

4. How many kilocalories will she expend in 20 minutes?
    A) 107.
    B) 160.
    C) 5.4.
    D) 185.

5. What is an equivalent work rate on the leg ergometer?
    A) 300 watts.
    B) 2,264 watts.
    C) 120 kg · m · min^{-1}.
    D) 370 kg · m · min^{-1}.

CASE III. An 80-kg male is running on a level track at 9.0 mph.

6. He has a $\dot{V}O_2$ of:
   A) 51.7 mL · kg^{-1} · min^{-1}.
   B) 10 METs.
   C) 27.6 mL · kg^{-1} · min^{-1}.
   D) 42.3 mL · kg^{-1} · min^{-1}.

7. How many kilocalories per minute (kcals · min^{-1}) is he expending?
   A) 0.11.
   B) 50.
   C) 20.5.
   D) 7.5.

CASE IV. John's $\dot{V}O_2$ max is 32.0 mL · kg^{-1} · min^{-1}. He weighs 74 kg.

8. What is his work rate on the Monark arm ergometer at 40% of $\dot{V}O_2$ max?
   A) 703 kg · m · min^{-1}.
   B) 688 kg · m · min^{-1}.
   C) 100 kg · m · min^{-1}.
   D) 229 kg · m · min^{-1}.

9. John's leg ergometer work rate at 80% of $\dot{V}O_{2\,RESERVE}$ is:
   A) 764 kg · m · min^{-1}.
   B) 793 kg · m · min^{-1}.
   C) 195 watts.
   D) 110 watts.

10. How many calories are expended at an exercise intensity of 60% of $\dot{V}O_{2\,MAX}$?
    A) 7.1 kcal · min^{-1}.
    B) 11.8 kcal · min^{-1}.
    C) 7.6 kcal · min^{-1}.
    D) 9.2 kcal · min^{-1}.

CASE V. Nichole, a 54-kg woman, wants to begin a crosstraining program.

11. What is her $\dot{V}O_2$ at 2.5 mph and a 12% grade?
    A) 1,525 L · min^{-1}.
    B) 6 METs.
    C) 12 METs.
    D) 24.7 mL · kg^{-1}· min^{-1}.

12. What is the equivalent work rate on the cycle ergometer?
    A) 30 watts.
    B) 531 kg · m · min^{-1}.
    C) 575 kg · m · min^{-1}.
    D) 87 kg · m · min^{-1}.

13. If she steps on a 12-inch step, what step rate is required to elicit the same $\dot{V}O_2$?
    A) 23 steps per minute.
    B) 20 steps per minute.
    C) 27 steps per minute.
    D) 30 steps per minute.

ANSWERS AND EXPLANATIONS

1–B. The steps are as follows:

a. Choose the ACSM walking formula.

b. Write down your knowns and convert the values to the appropriate units:

Knowns: 3.5 mph × 26.8 m · min^{-1} = 93.8 m · min^{-1}0% grade = 0.0

c. Write down the ACSM walking formula:

$$\text{Walking } \dot{V}O_2\ (\text{mL} \cdot \text{kg}^{-1} \cdot \text{min}^{-1}) = (0.1 \times \text{speed}) + (1.8 \times \text{speed} \times \text{fractional grade}) + (3.5\ \text{mL} \cdot \text{kg}^{-1} \cdot \text{min}^{-1})$$

d. Substitute the known values for the variable name:

$$\text{mL} \cdot \text{kg}^{-1} \cdot \text{min}^{-1} = (0.1 \times 93.8) + (1.8 \times 93.8 \times 0) + (3.5)$$
$$\text{mL} \cdot \text{kg}^{-1} \cdot \text{min}^{-1} = (9.38) + (0) + (3.5)$$

e. Solve for the unknown:

$$\text{mL} \cdot \text{kg}^{-1} \cdot \text{min}^{-1} = (9.38) + (3.5)$$
$$\text{Gross walking } \dot{V}O_2 = 12.88\ \text{mL} \cdot \text{kg}^{-1} \cdot \text{min}^{-1}$$

2–D. The steps are as follows:

a. Choose the ACSM walking formula.

b. Write down your knowns and convert the values to the appropriate units:

Knowns: 3.4 mph × 26.8 m · min^{-1} = 91.12 m · min^{-1}
5% grade = 0.05

c. Write down the ACSM walking formula:

$$\text{Walking } \dot{V}O_2\ (\text{mL} \cdot \text{kg}^{-1} \cdot \text{min}^{-1}) = (0.1 \times \text{speed}) + (1.8 \times \text{speed} \times \text{fractional grade}) + (3.5\ \text{mL} \cdot \text{kg}^{-1} \cdot \text{min}^{-1})$$

d. Substitute the known values for the variable name:

$$\text{mL} \cdot \text{kg}^{-1} \cdot \text{min}^{-1} = (0.1 \times 91.12) + (1.8 \times 91.12 \times .05) + (3.5\ \text{mL} \cdot \text{kg}^{-1} \cdot \text{min}^{-1}) = (9.112) + (8.2008) + (3.5)$$

e. Solve for the unknown:

$$mL \cdot kg^{-1} \cdot min^{-1} = (9.112) + (8.2008) + (3.5)$$

$$\text{Gross walking } \dot{V}O_2 = 20.81\ mL \cdot kg^{-1} \cdot min^{-1}$$

3–A. The steps are as follows:

a. Choose the ACSM running formula.
b. Write down your knowns and convert the values to the appropriate units:

Knowns: 5 mph × 26.8 = 134 m · min^{-1}

5% grade = 0.05

c. Write down the ACSM running formula:

$$\text{Running } \dot{V}O_2\ (mL \cdot kg^{-1} \cdot min^{-1}) = (0.2 \times \text{speed}) + (0.9 \times \text{speed fractional grade}) + (3.5\ mL \cdot kg^{-1} \cdot min^{-1})$$

d. Substitute the known values for the variable name:

$$mL \cdot kg^{-1} \cdot min^{-1} = (0.2 \times 134) + (0.9 \times 134 \times .05) + (3.5)$$

$$mL \cdot kg^{-1} \cdot min^{-1} = (26.8) + (6.03) + (3.5)$$

e. Solve for the unknown:

$$mL \cdot kg^{-1} \cdot min^{-1} = (26.8) + (6.03) + (3.5)$$

$$\text{Gross running } \dot{V}O_2 = 36.33\ mL \cdot kg^{-1} \cdot min^{-1}$$

f. You are asked to find the client's caloric expenditure rate, which means that you need to first determine his O_2 consumption in absolute terms:

$$\text{Absolute } \dot{V}O_2\ (mL \cdot min^{-1}) = \text{relative } \dot{V}O_2\ (mL \cdot kg^{-1} \cdot min^{-1}) \times \text{body weight (kg)}$$

$$mL \cdot min^{-1} = 36.33\ mL \cdot kg^{-1} \cdot min^{-1} \times 70\ kg$$

$$\text{Absolute } \dot{V}O_2\ (mL \cdot min^{-1}) = 2{,}543.1\ mL \cdot min^{-1}$$

Now, divide by 1,000 to get L · min^{-1}:

$$2{,}543.1 \div 1{,}000 = 2.54\ L \cdot min^{-1}$$

g. Multiply absolute $\dot{V}O_2$ in L · min^{-1} by 5.0 to determine his caloric expenditure rate:

$$2.54\ L \cdot min^{-1} \times 5.0 = 12.7\ kcal \cdot min^{-1}$$

4–C. The steps are as follows:

a. Choose the ACSM walking formula.
b. Write down your knowns and convert the values to the appropriate units:

Knowns: ×3.5 mph 26.8 = 93.8 m · min^{-1}
10% grade = 0.10

c. Write down the ACSM walking formula:

$$\text{Walking } \dot{V}O_2\ (mL \cdot kg^{-1} \cdot min^{-1}) = (0.1 \times \text{speed}) + (1.8 \times \text{speed} \times \text{fractional grade}) + (3.5\ mL \cdot kg^{-1} \cdot min^{-1})$$

d. Substitute the known values for the variable name:

$$mL \cdot kg^{-1} \cdot min^{-1} = (0.1 \times 93.8) + (1.8 \times 93.8 \times 0.1) + (3.5)\ mL \cdot kg^{-1} \cdot min^{-1} = (9.38) + (16.884) + (3.5)$$

e. Solve for the unknown:

$$mL \cdot kg^{-1} \cdot min^{-1} = (9.38) + (16.884) + (3.5)$$

$$\text{Gross walking } \dot{V}O_2 = 29.76\ mL \cdot kg^{-1} \cdot min^{-1}$$

5–B. The steps are as follows:

a. Choose the ACSM walking formula.
b. Write down your knowns and convert the values to the appropriate units:

Knowns: 3.0 mph × (26.8) = 80.4 m·min^{-1}
0% grade (level walking) = 0.0

c. Write down the ACSM walking formula:

$$\text{Walking } \dot{V}O_2\ (mL \cdot kg^{-1} \cdot min^{-1}) = (0.1 \times \text{speed}) + (1.8 \times \text{speed} \times \text{fractional grade}) + (3.5\ mL \cdot kg^{-1} \cdot min^{-1})$$

d. Substitute the known values for the variable name:

$$mL \cdot kg^{-1} \cdot min^{-1} = (0.1 \times 80.4) + (1.8 \times 80.4 \times 0) + (3.5)$$

e. Solve for the unknown:

$$mL \cdot kg^{-1} \cdot min^{-1} = (8.04) + (0) + (3.5)$$

$$\text{Gross walking } \dot{V}O_2 = 11.54\ mL \cdot kg^{-1} \cdot min^{-1}$$

f. Because this question wants you to find the MET equivalent, you must divide the gross walking $\dot{V}O_2$ by the constant 3.5:

$$\text{METs} = \text{relative } \dot{V}O_2\ (mL \cdot kg^{-1} \cdot min^{-1}) \div 3.5$$

$$\text{METs} = 11.54\ mL \cdot kg^{-1} \cdot min^{-1} \div 3.5 = 3.30\ \text{METs}$$

6–C. The steps are as follows:

a. Choose the ACSM running formula.
b. Write down your knowns and convert the values to the appropriate units:

Knowns: 6.5 mph × 26.8 = 174.2 m · min^{-1}
0% grade = 0.0

c. Write down the ACSM running formula:

$$\text{Running } \dot{V}O_2 \ (mL \cdot kg^{-1} \cdot min^{-1}) = (0.2 \times \text{speed}) + (0.9 \times \text{speed} \times \text{fractional grade}) + (3.5\ mL \cdot kg^{-1} \cdot min^{-1})$$

d. Substitute the known values for the variable name:

$$mL \cdot kg^{-1} \cdot min^{-1} = (0.2 \times 174.2) + (0.9 \times 174.2 \times 0) + (3.5)$$

e. Solve for the unknown:

$$mL \cdot kg^{-1} \cdot min^{-1} = (34.84) + (0) + (3.5)$$
$$\text{Gross running } \dot{V}O_2 = 38.34\ mL \cdot kg^{-1} \cdot min^{-1}$$

7–D. The steps are as follows:

a. Choose the ACSM running formula.
b. Write down your knowns and convert the values to the appropriate units:

Knowns: $5.5\ mph \times 26.8 = 147.4\ m \cdot min^{-1}$
12% grade = 0.12

c. Write down the ACSM running formula:

$$\text{Running } \dot{V}O_2 \ (mL \cdot kg^{-1} \cdot min^{-1}) = (0.2 \times \text{speed}) + (0.9 \times \text{speed} \times \text{fractional grade}) + (3.5\ mL \cdot kg^{-1} \cdot min^{-1})$$

d. Substitute the known values for the variable name:

$$mL \cdot kg^{-1} \cdot min^{-1} = (0.2 \cdot 147.4) + (0.9 \cdot 147.4 \cdot 0.12) + (3.5)$$

e. Solve for the unknown:

$$mL \cdot kg^{-1} \cdot min^{-1} = (29.48) + (15.92) + (3.5)$$
$$\text{Gross running } \dot{V}O_2 = 48.9\ mL \cdot kg^{-1} \cdot min^{-1}$$

8–B. The steps are as follows:

a. Choose the ACSM running formula.
b. Write down your knowns and convert the values to the appropriate units:

Knowns: $5.0\ mph \times 26.8 = 134\ m \cdot min^{-1}$
5.2% grade = 0.052
(Body weight is irrelevant in this problem.)

c. Write down the ACSM running formula:

$$\text{Running } \dot{V}O_2 \ (mL \cdot kg^{-1} \cdot min^{-1}) = (0.2 \times \text{speed}) + (0.9 \times \text{speed} \times \text{fractional grade}) + (3.5\ mL \cdot kg^{-1} \cdot min^{-1})$$

d. Substitute the known values for the variable name:

$$mL \cdot kg^{-1} \cdot min^{-1} = (0.2 \times 134) + (0.9 \times 134 \times 0.052) + (3.5)$$

e. Solve for the unknown:

$$mL \cdot kg^{-1} \cdot min^{-1} = (26.8) + (3.5)$$
$$\text{Gross running } \dot{V}O_2 = 36.57\ mL \cdot kg^{-1} \cdot min^{-1}$$

f. You are asked for his MET value so, you must divide his gross funning $\dot{V}O_2$ ($mL \cdot kg^{-1} \cdot min^{-1}$) by the constant 3.5:

$$\text{METs} = \text{relative } \dot{V}O_2 \ (mL \cdot kg^{-1} \cdot min^{-1}) \div 3.5$$
$$\text{METs} = 36.57\ mL \cdot kg^{-1} \cdot min^{-1} \div 3.5 = 10.45 \text{ METs}$$

9–B. This question does not require the use of a metabolic formula because it is asking for the subject's work rate. The steps are as follows:

a. Write down your knowns and convert the values to the appropriate units:

Knowns: $50\ rpm \times 6\ m = 300\ m \cdot min^{-1}$
(Each revolution on a Monark cycle ergometer = 6 m.)
2.0 kiloponds = 2.0 kilograms

b. Write down the formula for work rate:

$$\text{Work rate} = \text{force} \times \text{distance} \div \text{time}$$

c. Substitute the known values for the variable name:

$$\text{Work rate} = 2.0\ kg \times 300\ m \cdot min^{-1}$$
$$\text{Work rate} = 600\ kg \cdot m \cdot min^{-1}$$

d. You are asked for watts, so you must divide the work rate ($kg^{-1} \cdot m \cdot min^{-1}$) by 6:

$$W = kg \cdot m \cdot min^{-1} \div 6 = 600\ kg \cdot m \cdot min^{-1} \div 6 = 100\ W$$

10–D. The steps are as follows:

a. Choose the ACSM leg cycling formula.
b. Write down your knowns and convert the values to the appropriate units:

Knowns: Body weight = 110 lb ÷ 2.2 = 50 kg
$50\ rpm \times 6\ m = 300\ m \cdot min^{-1}$
2.5 kp = 2.5 kg

c. Write down the ACSM leg cycling formula:

$$\text{Leg cycling } \dot{V}O_2 \ (mL \cdot kg^{-1} \cdot min^{-1}) = (1.8 \times \text{work rate} \div \text{body weight}) + (3.5) + (3.5\ mL \cdot kg^{-1} \cdot min^{-1})$$

d. Calculate work rate:

$$\text{Work rate } (kg \cdot m \div min) = 2.5\ kg \times 300\ m \cdot min^{-1} = 750\ kg \cdot m \cdot min^{-1}$$

e. Substitute the known values for the variable name:

$$mL \cdot kg^{-1} \cdot min^{-1} = (1.8 \times 750 \div 50) + (3.5) + (3.5)$$

f. Solve for the unknown:

$$mL \cdot kg^{-1} \cdot min^{-1} = (27) + (3.5) + (3.5)$$

$$\text{Gross leg cycling } \dot{V}O_2 = 34\ mL \cdot kg^{-1} \cdot min^{-1}$$

g. This question asks for her absolute oxygen consumption, so you must multiply her gross $\dot{V}O_2$ (in relative terms) by her body weight:

$$\text{Absolute } \dot{V}O_2\ (mL \cdot min^{-1}) = \text{relative } \dot{V}O_2\ (mL \cdot kg^{-1} \cdot min^{-1}) \times \text{body weight (kg)} = 34\ mL \cdot kg^{-1} \cdot min^{-1} \times 50\ kg = 1{,}700\ mL \cdot min^{-1}$$

h. Convert $mL \cdot min^{-1}$ to $L \cdot min^{-1}$ by dividing by 1,000:

$$1{,}700\ mL \cdot min^{-1} \div 1{,}000 = 1.7\ L\ min^{-1}$$

11–C. The steps are as follows:

a. Choose the ACSM leg cycling formula.

b. Write down your knowns and convert the values to the appropriate units:

Knowns: Body weight = 110 lb ÷ 2.2 = 50 kg
50 RPM × 6 m = 300 m · min^{-1}
2.5 kp = 2.5 kg
60 minutes of cycling

c. Write down the ACSM formula:

$$\text{Leg cycling } \dot{V}O_2\ (mL \cdot kg^{-1} \cdot min^{-1}) = (1.8 \times \text{work rate} \div \text{body weight}) + (3.5) + (3.5\ mL \cdot kg^{-1} \cdot min^{-1})$$

d. Calculate work rate:

$$\text{Work rate } (kg \cdot m^{1} \cdot min^{-1}) = 2.5\ kg \cdot 300\ m \cdot min^{-1} = 750\ kg^{-1} \cdot m \cdot min^{-1}$$

e. Substitute the known values for the variable name:

$$mL \cdot kg^{-1} \cdot min^{-1} = (1.8 \times 750 \div 50) + (3.5) + (3.5)$$

f. Solve for the unknown:

$$\text{Gross leg cycling } \dot{V}O_2 = 34 mL \cdot kg^{-1} \cdot min^{-1}$$

g. To find out how many calories she expends, we must first convert her relative oxygen consumption to absolute terms:

$$\text{Absolute } \dot{V}O_2 (mL \cdot min^{-1}) = \text{relative } \dot{V}O_2\ (mL \cdot kg^{-1} \cdot min^{-1}) \times \text{body weight (kg)} = 34\ mL \cdot kg^{-1} \cdot min^{-1} \times 50\ kg = 1{,}700\ mL \cdot min^{-1}$$

h. Convert $mL \cdot min^{-1}$ to $L \cdot min^{-1}$ by dividing by 1,000:

$$1{,}700\ mL \cdot min^{-1} \div 1{,}000 = 1.7\ L \cdot min^{-1}$$

i. Next, to see how many calories she expends in 1 minute, multiply her absolute $\dot{V}O_2$ (in $L \cdot min^{-1}$) by the constant 5.0:

$$1.7\ L \cdot min^{-1} \times 5.0 = 8.5\ kcal \cdot min^{-1}$$

j. Finally, multiply the number of calories she expends in 1 minute by the number of minutes she cycles:

$$8.5\ kcal \cdot min^{-1} \times 60\ min = 510 \text{ total kcal}$$

12–A. The steps are as follows:

a. Choose the ACSM leg cycling formula.

b. Write down your knowns and convert the values to the appropriate units:

Knowns: Body weight = 55 kg
60 rpm × 6 m = 360 m · min^{-1}
1.5 kp = 1.5 kg

c. Write down the ACSM formula:

$$\text{Leg cycling } \dot{V}O_2 (mL \cdot kg^{-1} \cdot min^{-1}) = (1.8 \times \text{work rate} \div \text{body weight}) + (3.5) + (3.5 mL \cdot kg^{-1} \cdot min^{-1})$$

d. Calculate work rate:

$$\text{Work rate } (kg \cdot m \cdot min^{-1}) = 1.5\ kg \times 360\ m \cdot min^{-1} = 540\ kg \cdot m \cdot min^{-1}$$

e. Substitute the known values for the variable name:

$$mL \cdot kg^{-1} \cdot min^{-1} = (1.8 \times 540 \div 55) + (3.5) + (3.5)$$

f. Solve for the unknown:

$$mL \cdot kg^{-1} \cdot min^{-1} = (17.67) + (3.5) + (3.5)$$

$$\text{Gross leg cycling } \dot{V}O_2 = 24.67 mL \cdot kg^{-1} \cdot min^{-1}$$

g. To get her absolute oxygen consumption, multiply by her body weight:

$$\text{Absolute } \dot{V}O_2\ (mL \cdot min^{-1}) = \text{relative } \dot{V}O_2\ (mL \cdot kg^{-1} \cdot min^{-1}) \times \text{body weight (kg)} = 24.67\ mL \cdot kg^{-1} \cdot min^{-1} \times 55\ kg = 1{,}356.85\ mL \cdot min^{-1}$$

h. Convert $mL \cdot min^{-1}$ to $L \cdot min^{-1}$ by dividing by 1,000:

$$1{,}356.85\ mL \cdot min^{-1} \div 1{,}000 = 1.36\ L \cdot min^{-1}$$

13–C. The steps are as follows:

a. Choose the ACSM arm cycling formula.

b. Write down your knowns and convert the values to the appropriate units:

Knowns: Body weight = 55 kg
60 rpm × 2.4 ms (each revolution on a

Monark arm ergometer = 2.4 m)
$= 144\ \text{m} \cdot \text{min}^{-1}$
$1.5\ \text{kp} = 1.5\ \text{kg}$

c. Write down the ACSM formula:

$$\text{Arm cycling } \dot{V}O_2(\text{mL} \cdot \text{kg}^{-1} \cdot \text{min}^{-1}) = (3 \times \text{work rate} \div \text{body weight}) + (0) + (3.5\ \text{mL} \cdot \text{kg}^{-1} \cdot \text{min}^{-1})$$

d. Calculate work rate:

$$\text{Work rate (kg} \cdot \text{m} \cdot \text{min}^{-1}) = 1.5\ \text{kg} \times 144\ \text{m} \cdot \text{min}^{-1} = 216\ \text{kg} \cdot \text{m} \cdot \text{min}^{-1}$$

e. Substitute the known values for the variable name:

$$\text{mL} \cdot \text{kg}^{-1} \cdot \text{min}^{-1} = (3 \times 216 \div 55) + (0) + (3.5)$$

f. Solve for the unknown:

$$\text{mL} \cdot \text{kg}^{-1} \cdot \text{min}^{-1} = (11.78) + (0) + (3.5)$$
$$\text{Gross arm cycling } \dot{V}O_2 = 15.28\ \text{mL} \cdot \text{kg}^{-1} \cdot \text{min}^{-1}$$

g. To get her absolute oxygen consumption, multiply her relative oxygen consumption by her body weight:

$$\text{Absolute } \dot{V}O_2(\text{mL} \cdot \text{min}^{-1}) = \text{relative } \dot{V}O_2 (\text{mL} \cdot \text{kg}^{-1} \cdot \text{min}^{-1}) \times \text{body weight (kg)} = 15.28\ \text{mL} \cdot \text{kg}^{-1} \cdot \text{min}^{-1} \times 55\ \text{kg} = 840.4\ \text{mL} \cdot \text{min}^{-1}$$

h. Convert $\text{mL} \cdot \text{min}^{-1}$ to $\text{L} \cdot \text{min}^{-1}$ by dividing by 1,000:

$$840.4\ \text{mL} \cdot \text{min}^{-1} \div 1{,}000 = 0.8404\ \text{L} \cdot \text{min}^{-1}$$

14–C. The steps are as follows:

a. Choose the ACSM running formula.
b. Write down your knowns and convert the values to the appropriate units:

Knowns: 8 mph × 26.8 = 214.4 $\text{m} \cdot \text{min}^{-1}$
Body weight = 70 kg
45 minutes of running
0% grade = 0.0

c. Write down the ACSM running formula:

$$\text{Running } \dot{V}O_2 (\text{mL} \cdot \text{kg}^{-1} \cdot \text{min}^{-1}) = (0.2 \times \text{speed}) + (0.9 \times \text{speed} \times \text{fractional grade}) + (3.5\ \text{mL} \cdot \text{kg}^{-1} \cdot \text{min}^{-1})$$

d. Substitute the known values for the variable name:

$$\text{mL} \cdot \text{kg}^{-1} \cdot \text{min}^{-1} = (0.2 \times 214.4) + (0.9 \times 214.4 \times 0) + (3.5)$$

e. Solve for the unknown:

$$\text{mL} \cdot \text{kg}^{-1} \cdot \text{min}^{-1} = (42.88) + (0) + (3.5)$$
$$\text{Gross running } \dot{V}O_2 = 46.38\ \text{mL} \cdot \text{kg}^{-1} \cdot \text{min}^{-1}$$

f. To find out his total caloric expenditure, first put his gross running $\dot{V}O_2$ in absolute terms by multiplying by his body weight:

$$\text{Absolute } \dot{V}O_2 (\text{mL} \cdot \text{min}^{-1}) = \text{relative } \dot{V}O_2 (\text{mL} \cdot \text{kg}^{-1} \cdot \text{min}^{-1}) \times \text{body weight (kg)} = 46.38\ \text{mL} \cdot \text{kg}^{-1} \cdot \text{min}^{-1} = 3{,}246.6\ \text{mL} \cdot \text{min}^{-1}$$

g. Convert $\text{mL} \cdot \text{min}^{-1}$ to $\text{L} \cdot \text{min}^{-1}$ by dividing by 1,000:

$$3{,}246.6\ \text{mL} \cdot \text{min}^{-1} \div 1{,}000 = 3.2466\ \text{L} \cdot \text{min}^{-1}$$

h. Then multiply $\text{L} \cdot \text{min}^{-1}$ by the constant 5.0 to get $\text{kcal} \cdot \text{min}^{-1}$:

$$3.2466\ \text{L} \cdot \text{min}^{-1} \times 5.0 = 16.233\ \text{kcal} \cdot \text{min}^{-1}$$

i. Finally, multiply $\text{kcal} \cdot \text{min}^{-1}$ by the total number of minutes to get total caloric expenditure:

$$16.233\ \text{kcal} \cdot \text{min}^{-1} \times 45\ \text{min} = 730.48\ \text{calories}$$

15–D. The steps are as follows:

a. Choose the ACSM stepping formula.
b. Write down your knowns and convert the values to the appropriate units:

Knowns: Rate = 24 steps per minute
Step height = 10 in × 0.0254 = 0.254 meters
(Body weight is irrelevant in this problem.)

c. Write down the ACSM stepping formula:

$$\text{Stepping } \dot{V}O_2 (\text{mL} \cdot \text{min}^{-1}) = (0.2 \times \text{stepping rate}) + (1.33 \times \text{step height} \times 1.8 \times \text{stepping rate}) + (3.5\ \text{mL}^{-1} \times \text{kg}^{-1} \times \text{min}^{-1})$$

d. Substitute the known values for the variable name:

$$\text{mL} \cdot \text{kg}^{-1} \cdot \text{min}^{-1} = (0.2 \times 24) + (1.33 \times 1.8 \times 0.254 \times 24) + (3.5)$$

e. Solve for the unknown:

$$\text{mL} \cdot \text{kg}^{-1} \cdot \text{min}^{-1} = (4.8) + (14.59) + (3.5)$$
$$\text{Gross stepping } \dot{V}O_2 = 22.89\ \text{mL} \cdot \text{kg}^{-1} \cdot \text{min}^{-1}$$

16–C. The steps are as follows:

a. Choose the ACSM stepping formula.
b. Write down your knowns and convert the values to the appropriate units:

Knowns: 5 METs × 3.5 = 17.5 $\text{mL} \cdot \text{kg}^{-1} \cdot \text{min}^{-1}$

(This gives us the relative $\dot{V}O_2$ equivalent, which you will need for the stepping formula.)

Step height = 6 in × 0.0254 = 0.1524 ms (Body weight is irrelevant in this problem.)

c. Write down the ACSM stepping formula:

$$\text{Stepping } \dot{V}O_2\ (\text{mL} \cdot \text{min}^{-1}) = (0.2 \times \text{stepping rate}) + (1.33 \times \text{step height} \times 1.8 \times \text{stepping rate}) + (3.5\ \text{mL} \cdot \text{kg}^{-1} \cdot \text{min}^{-1})$$

d. Substitute the known values for the variable name:

$$17.5 = (0.2 \times \text{stepping rate}) + (1.33 \times 0.1524 \times 1.8 \times \text{stepping rate}) + (3.5)$$

e. Move all of the knowns on one side of the equation and keep the unknown on the other:

$$17.5 - 3.5 = (0.2 \times \text{stepping rate}) + (0.365 \times \text{stepping rate})$$
$$14 = 0.565\ (\text{stepping rate})$$

f. Divide by 0.565 to get the stepping rate:

$$24.78 = \text{stepping rate}$$

The stepping rate is about 25 steps per minute.

17–B. The steps are as follows:

a. Choose the ACSM running formula.

b. Write down your knowns and convert the values to the appropriate units:

Knowns: Body weight = 143 lb ÷ 2.2 = 65 kg
5.5 mph × 26.8 = 147.4 m · min^{-1}
2% grade = 0.02

c. Write down the ACSM running formula:

$$\text{Running } \dot{V}O_2\ (\text{mL} \cdot \text{kg}^{-1} \cdot \text{min}^{-1}) = (0.2 \times \text{speed}) + (0.9 \times \text{speed} \times \text{fractional grade}) + (3.5\text{mL} \cdot \text{kg}^{-1} \cdot \text{min}^{-1})$$

d. Substitute the known values for the variable name:

$$\text{mL} \cdot \text{kg}^{-1} \cdot \text{min}^{-1} = (0.2 \times 147.4) + (0.9 \times 147.4 \times 0.02) + (3.5)$$

e. Solve for the unknown:

$$\text{mL} \cdot \text{kg}^{-1} \cdot \text{min}^{-1} = (29.48) + (2.65) + (3.5)$$
$$\text{Gross running } \dot{V}O_2 = 35.63\text{mL} \cdot \text{kg}^{-1} \cdot \text{min}^{-1}$$

f. To find out how many calories per minute she is expending, first convert her gross running $\dot{V}O_2$ (in relative terms) to absolute $\dot{V}O_2$ by multiplying by her body weight:

$$\text{Absolute } \dot{V}O_2\ (\text{mL} \cdot \text{min}^{-1}) = \text{relative } \dot{V}O_2\ (\text{mL} \cdot \text{kg}^{-1} \cdot \text{min}^{-1}) \times \text{body weight (kg)}$$
$$= 35.63\ \text{mL} \cdot \text{kg}^{-1} \cdot \text{min}^{-1} \times 65\ \text{kg}$$
$$= 2{,}315.95\ \text{mL} \cdot \text{min}^{-1}$$

g. Convert mL · min^{-1} to L · min^{-1} by dividing by 1,000:

$$2{,}315.95\ \text{mL} \cdot \text{min}^{-1} \div 1{,}000 = 2.31595\ \text{L} \cdot \text{min}^{-1}$$

h. Finally, to find out how many calories she is expending per minute, multiply 2.31595 by the constant 5.0:

$$2.31595\ \text{L} \cdot \text{min}^{-1} \times 5.0 = 11.58\ \text{kcal} \cdot \text{min}^{-1}$$

18–D. This problem expands on problem #17. We established that she is expending 11.58 kcal · min^{-1}. The steps are as follows:

a. Multiply 11.58 kcal · min^{-1} by the total number of minutes she exercises (45 minutes × 3 sessions per week = 135 total minutes):

$$11.58\ \text{kcal} \cdot \text{min}^{-1} \times 135 \text{ total minutes} = 1{,}563.3 \text{ total calories expended}$$

b. To find out how many pounds of fat she will lose per week, divide the total calories expended by 3,500 (because there are 3,500 kcal in 1 lb of fat):

$$1{,}563.3\ \text{kcal} \div 3{,}500 = 0.4466 \text{ lb of fat per week of exercise}$$

19–B. The steps are as follows:

a. Choose the ACSM leg cycling formula.

b. Write down your knowns and convert the values to the appropriate units:

Knowns: 6 METs × 3.5 = 21 mL · kg^{-1} · min^{-1}
Body weight = 80 kg
Cycling cadence = 50 RPM × 6 m (each revolution on a Monark leg cycle ergometer = 6 m) = 300 m · min^{-1}

c. Write down the ACSM leg cycling formula:

$$\text{Leg cycling } \dot{V}O_2\ (\text{mL} \cdot \text{kg}^{-1} \cdot \text{min}^{-1}) = (1.8 \times \text{work rate} \div \text{body weight}) + (3.5) + (3.5\ \text{mL} \cdot \text{kg}^{-1} \cdot \text{min}^{-1})$$

d. Substitute the known values for the variable name:

$$21 = (1.8 \times \text{work rate} \div 80) + 7$$

e. Move all of the knowns to one side of the equation and solve for the unknown:

$$21 - 7 = 1.8 \times \text{work rate} \div 80$$
$$14 \times 80 = 1.8 \times \text{work rate}$$
$$1{,}120 \div 1.8 = \text{work rate}$$
$$622.22\ (\text{kg} \cdot \text{m} \cdot \text{min}^{-1}) = \text{work rate}$$

f. Next, substitute in the formula for work rate:

$$622.22\ (\text{kg} \cdot \text{m} \cdot \text{min}^{-1}) = \text{force (kg)} \times \text{velocity } (\text{m} \cdot \text{min}^{-1})$$

Assuming that he cycles at a cadence of 50 RPM, or 300 m · min^{-1}: Convert mL · min^{-1} to L · min^{-1} by dividing by 1,000:

$$622.22\ (\text{kg} \cdot \text{m} \cdot \text{min}^{-1}) = \text{force (resistance kgf)} \times 300\ \text{m} \cdot \text{min}^{-1})$$
$$622.22 \div 300 = \text{force}$$
$$2.07\ \text{kg} = \text{force}$$

About 2.1 kg of force (F) is needed.

20–B. The steps are as follows:

a. Choose the ACSM running formula.

b. Write down your knowns and convert the values to the appropriate units:

Knowns: 40 mL · kg^{-1} · min^{-1} = relative $\dot{V}O_2$
Level treadmill = 0% grade

c. Write down the ACSM running formula:

$$\text{Running } \dot{V}O_2\ (\text{mL} \cdot \text{kg}^{-1} \cdot \text{min}^{-1}) = (0.2 \times \text{speed}) + (0.9 \times \text{speed} \times \text{fractional grade}) + (3.5\text{mL} \cdot \text{kg}^{-1} \cdot \text{min}^{-1})$$

d. Substitute the known values for the variable name:

$$40 = (0.2 \times \text{speed}) + (0) + (3.5)$$

e. Solve for the unknown:

$$36.5 = 0.2\ (\text{speed})$$
$$182.5\ \text{m} \cdot \text{min}^{-1} = \text{speed}$$

f. Convert m · min^{-1} to mph by dividing m · min^{-1} by 26.8:

$$182.5\ \text{m} \cdot \text{min}^{-1} \div 26.8 = 6.8\ \text{mph}$$

21–C. The steps are as follows:

a. Convert relative $\dot{V}O_2$ to absolute $\dot{V}O_2$ by multiplying relative $\dot{V}O_2$ (mL · kg^{-1} · min^{-1}) by his body weight.

b. Given that his body weight is 70 kg:

$$\text{Absolute } \dot{V}O_2\ (\text{mL} \cdot \text{min}^{-1}) = \text{relative } \dot{V}O_2\ (\text{mL} \cdot \text{kg}^{-1} \cdot \text{min}^{-1}) \times \text{body weight (kg)}$$
$$= 45\ \text{mL} \cdot \text{kg}^{-1} \cdot \text{min}^{-1} \times 70\ \text{kg}$$
$$= 3{,}150\ \text{mL} \cdot \text{min}^{-1}$$

c. Convert mL · min^{-1} to L · min^{-1} by dividing by 1,000:

$$3{,}150\ \text{mL} \cdot \text{min}^{-1} \div 1{,}000 = 3.15\ \text{L} \cdot \text{min}^{-1}$$

d. Multiply 3.150 L · min^{-1} by the constant 5.0 to get kcal · min^{-1}:

$$3.15\ \text{L} \cdot \text{min}^{-1} \times 5.0 = 15.75\ \text{kcal} \cdot \text{min}^{-1}$$

e. Multiply 15.75 kcal · min^{-1} by the total number of minutes he exercises (45 minutes × 3 times per week = 135 total minutes) to get the total caloric expenditure:

$$15.75\ \text{kcal} \cdot \text{min}^{-1} \times 135\ \text{minutes} = 2{,}126.25\ \text{total kcal per week}$$

f. Divide by 3,500 to get pounds of fat:

$$2{,}126.25\ \text{kcal} \div 3{,}500 = 0.6075\ \text{lb of fat per week}$$

g. Divide 10 lb by 0.6075 lb of fat per week to get how many weeks it will take him to lose 10 lb of fat:

$$10 \div 0.6075 = 16.46\ \text{weeks } (\sim 16.5\ \text{weeks})$$

22–A. No metabolic formula is needed. The steps are as follows:

a. Multiply the number of calories per week she is eliminating by the number of weeks:

$$1{,}200\ \text{kcal per week} \times 26\ \text{weeks} = 31{,}200\ \text{total kcal}$$

b. Now divide by 3,500 to get the total pounds she will lose:

$$31{,}200 \div 3{,}500\ \text{total kcal} = 8.9\ \text{or about 9 lb over 26 weeks}$$

23–C. No metabolic formula is needed. The steps are as follows:

a. One mile of walking or running expends about 100 kcal. Because she walks 1 mile three times per week, she expends about 300 kcal per week. Multiply 300 kcal by 26 weeks to determine the total amount of calories she expends by walking:

$$300\ \text{kcal per week} \times 26\ \text{weeks}$$
$$= 7{,}800\ \text{kcal}$$

b. Divide 7,800 kcal by 3,500 to see how many pounds of fat this represents:

$$7{,}800\ \text{kcal} \div 3{,}500 = 2.22\ \text{lb or about 2 lb}$$

So she would lose about 11 lb (9 lb from question 22 + 2 lb from adding the walking) over 26 weeks if she incorporated walking into her weight loss program.

ANSWERS TO CASE QUESTIONS

Case I

1–D. The steps are as follows:

a. Choose the ACSM leg cycling formula.
b. Write down your knowns and convert the values to the appropriate units:

Knowns: Body weight = 75 kg
Work rate = 120 W = 720 kg · m · min^{-1}
(multiply W by 6.0 to get kg · m · min^{-1})

c. Write down the ACSM leg cycling formula:

$$\text{Leg cycling } \dot{V}O_2 \text{ (mL} \cdot \text{kg}^{-1} \cdot \text{min}^{-1}) = (1.8 \times \text{work rate} \div \text{body weight}) + (3.5) + (3.5 \text{ mL} \cdot \text{kg}^{-1} \cdot \text{min}^{-1})$$

d. Substitute the known values for the variable name:

$$\text{mL} \cdot \text{kg}^{-1} \cdot \text{min}^{-1} = (1.8 \times 720 \div 50) + (3.5) + (3.5)$$

e. Solve for the unknown:

$$\text{mL} \cdot \text{kg}^{-1} \cdot \text{min}^{-1} = (17.28) + (3.5) + (3.5)$$
$$\text{Gross } \dot{V}O_2 = 24.28 \text{ mL} \cdot \text{kg}^{-1} \cdot \text{min}^{-1}$$

f. Because the *24.28 mL · kg^{-1} · min^{-1}* does not match any of the choices, and the remaining choices are in MET equivalents, you must divide gross walking $\dot{V}O_2$ by the constant 3.5:

$$\text{METs} = \text{relative } \dot{V}O_2 (\text{mL} \cdot \text{kg}^{-1} \cdot \text{min}^{-1}) \div 3.5$$
$$\text{METs} = 24.28 \text{ mL} \cdot \text{kg}^{-1} \cdot \text{min}^{-1} \div 3.5 = 6.94 \text{ METs, or about 7 METs}$$

2–A. The steps are as follows:

a. First convert the gross $\dot{V}O_2$ (in relative terms) calculated in step "e" of the previous question (24.28 mL · kg^{-1} · min^{-1}) to absolute $\dot{V}O_2$ by multiplying by body weight:

$$\text{Absolute } \dot{V}O_2 (\text{mL} \cdot \text{min}^{-1}) = \text{relative } \dot{V}O_2 (\text{mL} \cdot \text{kg}^{-1} \cdot \text{min}^{-1}) \times \text{body weight (kg)} = 24.28 \text{ mL} \cdot \text{kg}^{-1} \cdot \text{min}^{-1} \times 75 \text{ kg} = 1{,}821 \text{ mL} \cdot \text{min}^{-1}$$

b. Convert mL · min^{-1} to L · min^{-1} by dividing by 1,000:

$$1{,}821 \text{ mL} \cdot \text{min}^{-1} \div 1{,}000 = 1.821 \text{ L} \cdot \text{min}^{-1}$$

c. Then multiply L · min^{-1} by the constant 5.0 to get kcal · min^{-1}:

$$1.821 \text{ L} \cdot \text{min}^{-1} \times 5.0 = 9.105 \text{ kcal} \cdot \text{min}^{-1}$$

d. Finally, multiply kcal · min^{-1} by the total number of minutes to get total caloric expenditure:

$$9.105 \text{ kcal} \cdot \text{min}^{-1} \times 30 \text{ min} = 273 \text{ kcal}$$

3–C. The steps are as follows:

a. Choose the ACSM walking formula.
b. Write down your knowns and convert the values to the appropriate units:

Knowns: $\dot{V}O_2$ = 24.28 mL · kg^{-1} · min^{-1}
(from question no. 1)
10% grade = 0.10

c. Write down the ACSM walking formula:

$$\text{Walking } \dot{V}O_2 (\text{mL} \cdot \text{kg}^{-1} \cdot \text{min}^{-1}) = (0.1 \times \text{speed}) + (1.8 \times \text{speed} \times \text{fractional grade}) + (3.5 \text{ mL} \cdot \text{kg}^{-1} \cdot \text{min}^{-1})$$

d. Substitute the known values for the variable name:

$$24.28 = (0.1 \times \text{speed}) + (1.8 \times \text{speed} \times 0.10) + (3.5 \text{ mL} \cdot \text{kg}^{-1} \cdot \text{min}^{-1})$$

e. Solve for the unknown:

$$24.28 - 3.5 = (0.1 \times \text{speed}) + (0.18 \times \text{speed})$$
$$20.78 = 0.28 \times \text{speed}$$
$$20.78 \div 0.28 = \text{speed}$$
$$74.2 \text{ m} \cdot \text{min}^{-1} = \text{speed}$$

f. The speed calculated above did not match any of the choices, so next you have to convert the speed in m · min^{-1} to mph by dividing by 26.8:

$$74.2 \text{ m} \cdot \text{min}^{-1} \div 26.8 = 2.77 \text{ mph, or approximately 2.8 mph.}$$

Case II

4–A. The steps are as follows:

a. Choose the ACSM stepping formula.
b. Write down your knowns and convert the values to the appropriate units:

Knowns: Rate = 20 steps per minute
Step height = 9 inches × 0.0254 = 0.2286 m
Body weight = 58 kg

c. Write down the ACSM stepping formula:

$$\text{Stepping } \dot{V}O_2 (\text{mL} \cdot \text{min}^{-1}) = (0.2 \times \text{stepping rate}) + (1.33 \times \text{step height} \times 1.8 \times \text{stepping rate}) + (3.5 \text{ mL} \cdot \text{kg}^{-1} \cdot \text{min}^{-1})$$

d. Substitute the known values for the variable name:

$$mL \cdot kg^{-1} \cdot min^{-1} = (0.2 \times 20) + (1.33 \times 0.2286 \times 1.8 \times 20) + (3.5)$$

e. Solve for the unknown:

$$mL \cdot kg^{-1} \cdot min^{-1} = (4.0) + (10.945) + (3.5)$$
$$\text{Gross stepping } \dot{V}O_2 = 18.5\ mL \cdot kg^{-1} \cdot min^{-1}$$

f. Next, convert the gross stepping $\dot{V}O_2$ (in relative terms) calculated in the previous question ($18.4\ mL \cdot kg^{-1} \cdot min^{-1}$) to absolute $\dot{V}O_2$ by multiplying by body weight:

$$\text{Absolute } \dot{V}O_2\ (mL \cdot min^{-1}) = \text{relative } \dot{V}O_2\ (mL \cdot kg^{-1} \cdot min^{-1}) \times \text{body weight (kg)} = 18.5\ mL \cdot kg^{-1} \cdot min^{-1} \times 58\ kg = 1{,}073\ mL \cdot min^{-1}$$

g. Convert $mL \cdot min^{-1}$ to $L \cdot min^{-1}$ by dividing by 1,000:

$$1{,}073\ mL \cdot min^{-1} \div 1{,}000 = 1.073\ L \cdot min^{-1}$$

h. Then multiply $L \cdot min^{-1}$ by the constant 5.0 to get $kcal \cdot min^{-1}$:

$$1.067\ L \cdot min^{-1} \times 5.0 = 5.365\ kcal \cdot min^{-1}$$

i. Finally, we multiply $kcal \cdot min^{-1}$ by the total number of minutes to get total caloric expenditure:

$$5.365\ kcal \cdot min^{-1} \times 20\ min = 107.3\ kcal, \text{ or approximately } 107\ kcal.$$

5–D. The steps are as follows:

a. Choose the ACSM leg cycling formula.

b. Write down the ACSM leg cycling formula:

$$\text{Leg cycling } \dot{V}O_2 (mL \cdot kg^{-1} \cdot min^{-1}) = (1.8 \times \text{work rate} \div \text{body weight}) + (3.5) + (3.5\ mL \cdot kg^{-1} \cdot min^{-1})$$

c. Substitute the known values for the variable name:

$$18.4\ mL \cdot kg^{-1} \cdot min^{-1} \text{ (from step "e" in previous problem)} = (1.8 \times \text{work rate} \div 58) + (3.5) + (3.5)$$

d. Solve for the unknown:

$$18.5 - 7 = 1.8 \times \text{work rate} \div 58$$
$$11.5 \times 58 \div 1.8 = \text{work rate}$$
$$\text{work rate} = 370.5\ kg \cdot m^{-1} \cdot min^{-1}, \text{ or approximately } 370\ kg \cdot m^{-1} \cdot min^{-1}$$

Case III

6–A. The steps are as follows:

a. Choose the ACSM running formula.

b. Write down your knowns and convert the values to the appropriate units:

Knowns: 9 mph × 26.8 = 241.2 $m \cdot min^{-1}$
Level track = 0% grade = 0.0
Body weight = 80 kg

c. Write down the ACSM running formula:

$$\text{Running } \dot{V}O_2 (mL \cdot kg^{-1} \cdot min^{-1}) = (0.2 \times \text{speed}) + (0.9 \times \text{speed} \times \text{fractional grade}) + (3.5\ mL \cdot kg^{-1} \cdot min^{-1})$$

d. Substitute the known values for the variable name:

$$(mL \cdot kg^{-1} \cdot min^{-1}) = (0.2 \times 241.2) + (0.9 \times 241.2 \times 0.0) + (3.5)$$

e. Solve for the unknown:

$$(mL \cdot kg^{-1} \cdot min^{-1}) = (48.2) + (0) + (3.5)$$
$$\text{Running } \dot{V}O_2 = 51.7\ mL \cdot kg^{-1} \cdot min^{-1}$$

7–C. The steps are as follows:

a. First convert the gross $\dot{V}O_2$ (in relative terms) calculated in the previous question ($51.7\ mL \cdot kg^{-1} \cdot min^{-1}$) to absolute $\dot{V}O_2$ by multiplying by body weight:

$$\text{Absolute } \dot{V}O_2\ (mL \cdot min^{-1}) = \text{relative } \dot{V}O_2\ (mL \cdot kg^{-1} \cdot min^{-1}) \times \text{body weight (kg)} = 51.7\ mL \cdot kg^{-1} \cdot min^{-1} \times 80\ kg = 4{,}136\ mL \cdot min^{-1}$$

b. Convert $mL \cdot min^{-1}$ to $L \cdot min^{-1}$ by dividing by 1,000:

$$4{,}136\ mL \cdot min^{-1} \div 1{,}000 = 4.136\ L \cdot min^{-1}$$

c. Then multiply $L \cdot min^{-1}$ by the constant 5.0 to get $kcal \cdot min^{-1}$:

$$4.136\ L \cdot min^{-1} \times 5.0 = 20.7\ kcal \cdot min^{-1}$$

Case IV

8–D. The steps are as follows:

a. Choose the ACSM arm cycling formula.

b. Write down your knowns and convert the values to the appropriate units:

Knowns: Body weight = 74 kg
$\dot{V}O_2max = 32.0\ mL \cdot kg^{-1} \cdot min^{-1}$

c. Calculate 40% of $\dot{V}O_2$ max:

$$40\% \text{ of } \dot{V}O_2max = \dot{V}O_2max \times 0.4 = 32.0\ mL \cdot kg^{-1} \cdot min^{-1} \times 0.4 = 12.8\ mL \cdot kg^{-1} \cdot min^{-1}$$

d. Write down the ACSM arm cycling formula:

$$\text{Arm cycling } \dot{V}O_2 (mL \cdot kg^{-1} \cdot min^{-1}) = (3 \times \text{work rate} \div \text{body weight}) + (0) + (3.5\ mL \cdot kg^{-1} \cdot min^{-1})$$

e. Substitute the known values for the variable name:

$$12.8\ \text{mL} \cdot \text{kg}^{-1} \cdot \text{min}^{-1} = (3 \times \text{work rate} \div 74) + (0) + (3.5)$$

f. Solve for the unknown:

$$12.8 - 3.5 = 3 \times \text{work rate} \div 74$$
$$9.3 \div 3 \times 74 = \text{work rate}$$
$$229\ \text{kg} \cdot \text{m}^{-1} \cdot \text{min}^{-1} = \text{work rate}$$

9–B. The steps are as follows:

a. Choose the ACSM leg cycling formula.

b. Write down your knowns and convert the values to the appropriate units:
Knowns: Body weight = 74 kg

$$\dot{V}o_2max = 32.0\ \text{mL} \cdot \text{kg}^{-1} \cdot \text{min}^{-1}$$
$$\dot{V}o_2rest = 3.5\ \text{mL} \cdot \text{kg}^{-1} \cdot \text{min}^{-1}$$

c. Calculate 80% of $\dot{V}o_{2RESERVE}$:

$$80\%\ \text{of}\ \dot{V}o_{2RESERVE} = (\dot{V}o_2max - \dot{V}o_2rest) \times 0.8 = (32.0 - 3.5) \times 0.8 = (28.5) \times 0.8 = 23\ \text{mL} \cdot \text{kg}^{-1} \cdot \text{min}^{-1}$$

d. Write down the ACSM leg cycling formula:

$$\text{Leg cycling}\ \dot{V}o_2\ (\text{mL} \cdot \text{kg}^{-1} \cdot \text{min}^{-1}) = (1.8 \times \text{work rate} \div \text{body weight}) + (3.5) + (3.5\ \text{mL} \cdot \text{kg}^{-1} \cdot \text{min}^{-1})$$

e. Substitute the known values for the variable name:

$$23\ \text{mL} \cdot \text{kg}^{-1} \cdot \text{min}^{-1} = (1.8 \times \text{work rate} \div 74) + (3.5) + (3.5)$$

f. Move all of the knowns to one side of the equation and solve for the unknown:

$$23 - 7 = 1.8 \times \text{work rate} \div 74$$
$$16 \times 74 \div 1.8 = \text{work rate}$$
$$658\ \text{kg} \cdot \text{m}^{-1} \cdot \text{min}^{-1} = \text{work rate}$$

g. Because this did not match any of the choices, next you have to convert the work rate in $\text{kg} \cdot \text{m}^{-1} \cdot \text{min}^{-1}$ to watts by dividing by 6:

$$658\ \text{kg} \cdot \text{m} \cdot \text{min}^{-1} \div 6 = 109.6\ \text{watts, or approximately 110 watts.}$$

10–A. The steps are as follows:

a. No formula is necessary. This problem involves only converting between different expressions of energy.

b. Write down your knowns and convert the values to the appropriate units:
Knowns: Body weight = 74 kg

$$\dot{V}o_2max = 32.0\ \text{mL} \cdot \text{kg}^{-1} \cdot \text{min}^{-1}$$

c. Calculate 60% of $\dot{V}o_2$ max:

$$60\%\ \dot{V}o_2max = \dot{V}o_2max \times 0.6 = 32.0\ \text{mL} \cdot \text{kg}^{-1} \cdot \text{min}^{-1} \times 0.6 = 19.2\ \text{mL} \cdot \text{kg}^{-1} \cdot \text{min}^{-1}$$

d. Next, convert the gross $\dot{V}o_2$ (in relative terms) to absolute $\dot{V}o_2$ by multiplying by body weight:

$$\text{Absolute}\ \dot{V}o_2\ (\text{mL} \cdot \text{min}^{-1}) = \text{relative}\ \dot{V}o_2\ (\text{mL} \cdot \text{kg}^{-1} \cdot \text{min}^{-1}) \times \text{body weight (kg)} = 19.2\ \text{mL} \cdot \text{kg}^{-1} \cdot \text{min}^{-1} \times 74\ \text{kg} = 1{,}420\ \text{mL} \cdot \text{min}^{-1}$$

e. Convert $\text{mL} \cdot \text{min}^{-1}$ to $\text{L} \cdot \text{min}^{-1}$ by dividing by 1,000:

$$1{,}420\ \text{mL} \cdot \text{min}^{-1} \div 1{,}000 = 1.42\ \text{L} \cdot \text{min}^{-1}$$

f. Then multiply $\text{L} \cdot \text{min}^{-1}$ by the constant 5.0 to get $\text{kcal} \cdot \text{min}^{-1}$:

$$1.42\ \text{L} \cdot \text{min}^{-1} \times 5.0 = 7.1\ \text{kcal} \cdot \text{min}^{-1}$$

Case V

11–D. The steps are as follows:

a. Choose the ACSM walking formula.

b. Write down your knowns and convert the values to the appropriate units:
Knowns: Body weight = 54 kg

$$2.5\ \text{mph} \times 26.8 = 67\ \text{m} \cdot \text{min}^{-1}$$
$$12\%\ \text{grade} = 0.12$$

c. Write down the ACSM walking formula:

$$\text{Walking}\ \dot{V}o_2\ (\text{mL} \cdot \text{kg}^{-1} \cdot \text{min}^{-1}) = (0.1 \times \text{speed}) + (1.8 \times \text{speed} \times \text{fractional grade}) + (3.5\ \text{mL} \cdot \text{kg}^{-1} \cdot \text{min}^{-1}$$

d. Substitute the known values for the variable name:

$$\text{mL} \cdot \text{kg}^{-1} \cdot \text{min}^{-1} = (0.1 \times 67) + (1.8 \times 67 \times 0.12) + (3.5)$$

e. Solve for the unknown:

$$\text{mL} \cdot \text{kg}^{-1} \cdot \text{min}^{-1} = (6.7) + (14.5) + (3.5)$$
$$\text{Gross walking}\ \dot{V}o_2 = 24.7\ \text{mL} \cdot \text{kg}^{-1} \cdot \text{min}^{-1}$$

12–B. The steps are as follows:

a. Choose the ACSM leg cycling formula.

b. Write down your knowns and convert the values to the appropriate units:
Knowns: Body weight = 54 kg

$$\dot{V}o_2(\text{mL} \cdot \text{kg}^{-1} \cdot \text{min}^{-1}) = 24.7\ \text{mL} \cdot \text{kg}^{-1} \cdot \text{min}^{-1}\ \text{(from previous problem)}$$

c. Write down the ACSM leg cycling formula:

$$\text{Leg cycling}\ \dot{V}o_2\ (\text{mL} \cdot \text{kg}^{-1} \cdot \text{min}^{-1}) = (1.8 \times \text{work rate} \div \text{body weight}) + (3.5) + (3.5\ \text{mL} \cdot \text{kg}^{-1} \cdot \text{min}^{-1})$$

d. Substitute the known values for the variable name:

$$24.7\ \text{mL} \cdot \text{kg}^{-1} \cdot \text{min}^{-1} = (1.8 \times \text{work rate} \div 54) + (3.5) + (3.5)$$

e. Solve for the unknown:

$$24.7 - 3.5 - 3.5 = (1.8 \times \text{work rate} \div 54)$$
$$17.7 \div 1.8 \times 54 = \text{work rate}$$
$$7531\ \text{kg} \cdot \text{m} \cdot \text{min}^{-1} = \text{work rate}$$

13–A. The steps are as follows:

a. Choose the ACSM stepping formula.

b. Write down your knowns and convert the values to the appropriate units:
Knowns: Body weight = 54 kg

$$\text{Step height} = 12\ \text{in} \times 0.0254 = 0.3048\ \text{m}$$
$$\dot{V}O_2\ (\text{mL} \cdot \text{kg}^{-1} \cdot \text{min}^{-1}) = 24.7\ \text{mL} \cdot \text{kg}^{-1} \cdot \text{min}^{-1}\ \text{(from problem no. 11)}$$

c. Write down the ACSM stepping formula:

$$\text{Stepping } \dot{V}O_2\ (\text{mL} \cdot \text{min}^{-1}) = (0.2 \times \text{stepping rate}) + (1.33 \times \text{step height} \times 1.8 \times \text{stepping rate}) + (3.5\ \text{mL} \cdot \text{kg}^{-1} \cdot \text{min}^{-1})$$

d. Substitute the known values for the variable name:

$$24.7\ \text{mL} \cdot \text{kg}^{-1} \cdot \text{min}^{-1} = (0.2 \times \text{stepping rate}) + (1.33 \times 0.3048 \times 1.8 \times \text{stepping rate}) + (3.5)$$

e. Solve for the unknown:

$$24.7 - 3.5 = (0.2 \times \text{stepping rate}) + (0.73 \times \text{stepping rate})$$
$$21.2 = 0.93 \times \text{stepping rate}$$
$$21.2 \div 0.93 = \text{stepping rate}$$
$$22.8\ \text{steps per minute} = \text{stepping rate}$$

Approximately 23 steps per minute.

CHAPTER 12

Electrocardiography

I. ELECTRICAL ACTIVITY OF THE HEART AND BASIC ELECTROCARDIOGRAM WAVES

The electrocardiogram (ECG) records differences in electrical potential (voltage) between two electrodes placed on the skin. The electrical conduction system is shown in *Figure 12-1*.

A. PRINCIPLES OF ELECTROPHYSIOLOGY

1. Myocardial cells can be excited in response to external electrical, chemical, and mechanical stimuli.
2. The myocardium comprises ordinary contractile cells located in the atria and ventricles, as well as specialized cells that conduct electrical impulses.
3. Cardiac impulses normally arise in the sinoatrial (SA), or sinus node, located in the right atrium near the opening of the superior vena cava.
4. From the SA node, impulses travel through the right atrium into the left atrium. Thus, the SA node functions as the normal pacemaker.
5. The first phase of cardiac activation involves electrical stimulation of the right and left atria. This, in turn, signals the atria to contract and to pump blood simultaneously through the tricuspid and mitral valves into the right and left ventricles.
6. The electrical stimulus then spreads to specialized conduction tissues in the atrioventricular (AV) junction, which includes the AV node and the bundle of His, and then into the left and right bundle branches, which transmit the stimulus to the ventricular muscle cells.
7. During the resting period of the myocardial cell, the inside of the cell membrane is negatively charged and the outside of the cell membrane is positively charged. As such, the term "polarized cell" is reserved for the normal resting myocardial cell and describes the presence of electrical potential across the cell membrane owing to separation of electrical charges.
8. When an electrical impulse is generated in a particular area in the heart, the outside of the cell in this area becomes negative, and the inside of the cell in the same area becomes positive. This excited state of the cell, which is caused by change in polarity, is called **depolarization**.
   a. Cardiac impulses originate in the SA node and spread to both atria, causing **atrial depolarization**, represented on the ECG by a P wave.
   b. **Ventricular depolarization** is represented on the ECG by the QRS complex.
9. **Repolarization** is the return of the stimulated myocardial cells to their resting state.
   a. **Atrial repolarization** is not usually seen on ECG, because it is obscured by ventricular potentials.
   b. **Ventricular repolarization** is represented on the ECG by the ST segment, T wave, and U wave.

B. PRINCIPLES OF ELECTROCARDIOGRAPHY

1. The movement of ions inside and across the membrane of myocardial cells constitutes a flow of electrical charge (ionic current) that is recorded on the ECG.
2. Cardiac electrical potentials are recorded on special ECG graph paper that, under standard conditions, travels at a speed of 25 mm/second.
   a. **Horizontally, the ECG measures duration;** each small square is 0.04 second in duration, and each large square is 0.20 second in duration.
   b. **Vertically, the ECG measures voltages.** Because ECGs are standardized, 1 mV of electrical potential registers a deflection of 10 mm in amplitude.

C. ELEMENTS OF ECG WAVEFORMS (*Figure 12-2*)

1. The **P wave** is a small positive (or negative) deflection preceding the QRS complex.
2. A **QRS complex** may be composed of a Q wave, an R wave, and an S wave.
   a. A **Q wave** is a negative deflection of the QRS complex preceding an R wave.
   b. An **R wave** is the first positive deflection of the QRS complex.
   c. An **S wave** is a negative deflection of the QRS complex following an R wave.

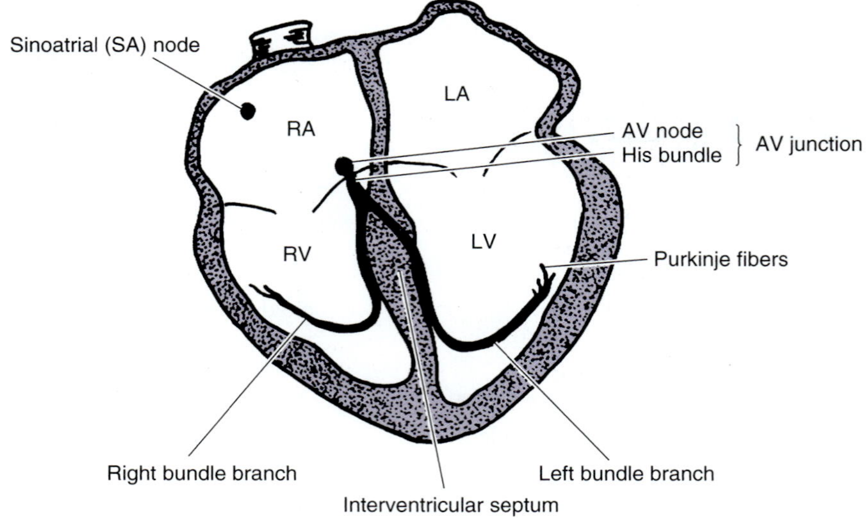

FIGURE 12-1. Conduction system of the heart. Normally the cardiac stimulus is generated in the *sinoatrial (SA) node,* which is located in the *right atrium (RA).* The stimulus then spreads through the *RA* and *left atrium (LA).* Next it spreads through the *atrioventricular (AV) node* and the *bundle of His,* which comprise the *AV junction.* The stimulus then passes into the *left* and *right ventricles (LV* and *RV)* by way of the *left* and *right bundle branches,* which are continuations of the bundle of His. Finally, the cardiac stimulus spreads to the ventricular muscle cells through the *Purkinje fibers.* (From Goldberger AL: *Clinical Electrocardiography: A Simplified Approach,* 6th ed. St. Louis: Mosby; 1999, p 4.)

3. The **ST segment** is that portion of the ECG from the point where the S wave of the QRS ends (**J point**) to the beginning of the T wave.
   a. The ST segment should be isoelectric.
   b. The ST segment is considered a sensitive indicator of myocardial ischemia or infarction.
4. The **PR interval** is measured from the beginning of the P wave to the beginning of the QRS complex, and reflects the time needed for the impulse to spread through the atria and to pass through the AV junction.
   a. The normal PR interval is 0.12–0.20 second.
   b. A PR interval prolonged for >0.20 second with all P waves being conducted and all PR intervals the same indicates first-degree AV block.
5. The **QRS interval** is measured from the beginning of the first wave of the QRS complex to the end of the last wave of the QRS complex.
   a. The normal range is 0.04–0.11 second.
6. The **QT interval** is measured from the beginning of the QRS complex to the end of the T wave.
   a. Normal QT intervals depend on heart rate (HR).
   b. Prolonged QT interval may be related to certain drugs, electrolyte disturbances, and myocardial ischemia and infarction.
7. The **T wave** represents ventricular repolarization.
   a. Normal T waves lack symmetry.
   b. Prominent peaked T waves may indicate myocardial infarction or hyperkalemia.
   c. Deep, symmetrically inverted T waves suggest myocardial ischemia.
8. The **U wave** represents the last phase of ventricular repolarization.
   a. The U wave is frequently hard to detect in a normal ECG, but may appear as a small deflection after the T wave.
   b. U waves are prominent in hypokalemia and left ventricular hypertrophy.
   c. Inverted U waves suggest ischemia.

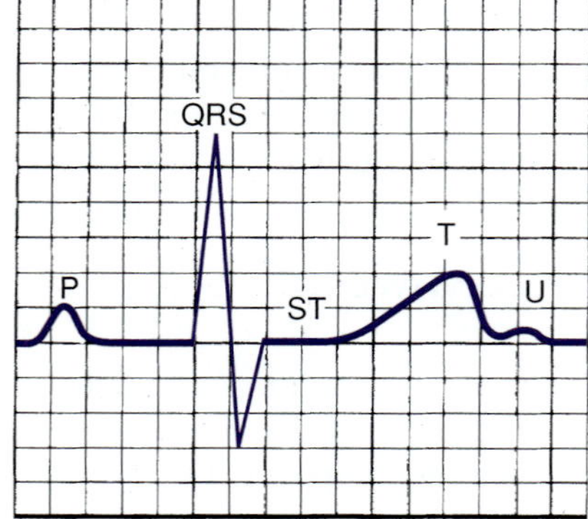

FIGURE 12-2. Basic ECG complexes. The P wave represents atrial depolarization. The PR interval is the time from initial stimulation of the atria to initial stimulation of the ventricles. The QRS represents ventricular depolarization. The ST segment, T wave, and U wave are produced by ventricular repolarization. (From Goldberger AL: *Clinical Electrocardiography: A Simplified Approach,* 6th ed. St. Louis: Mosby; 1999, p 8.)

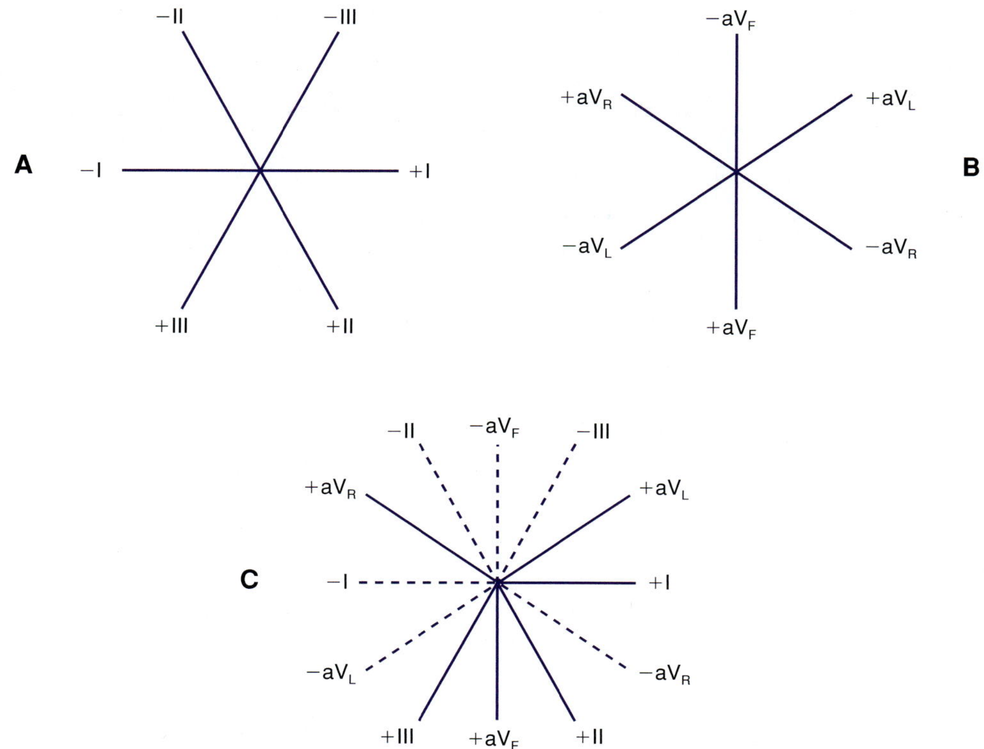

FIGURE 12-3. Derivation of hexaxial lead diagram. **A.** Triaxial diagram of the bipolar leads (I, II, and III). **B.** Triaxial diagram of the unipolar leads (aV_R, aV_L, and aV_F). **C.** The two triaxial diagrams can be combined into a hexaxial diagram that shows the relationship of all six extremity leads. The negative pole of each lead is now indicated by a dashed line. (From Goldberger AL: *Clinical Electrocardiography: A Simplified Approach,* 6th ed. St. Louis: Mosby; 1999, p 26.)

D. THE 12-LEAD ECG

Represents 12 electrically different views of the heart recorded on special ECG paper.

1. The 12 leads can be subdivided into three groups (*Figure 12-3*):
   a. **Bipolar standard leads I, II, and III.**
   b. **Unipolar augmented leads aVR, aVL, and aVF.**
   c. **Unipolar precordial leads V_1–V_6.**
2. Leads i, ii, iii, aVR, aVL, and aVF are collectively called limb leads because they record potential differences through electrodes placed on limbs.
   a. Lead I records the difference in electrical potential between the left arm (positive) and right arm (negative) electrodes.
   b. Lead II records the difference in electrical potential between the left leg (positive) and right arm (negative) electrodes.
   c. Lead III records the difference in electrical potential between the left leg (positive) and left arm (negative) electrodes.
   d. The augmented unipolar leads record electrical potentials at one site relative to zero potential. Electrical potentials are augmented electronically by the ECG.
      1) For lead **aVR**, the positive electrode is placed on the right arm.
      2) For lead **aVL**, the positive electrode is placed on the left arm.
      3) For lead **aVF**, the positive electrode is placed on the left foot.
3. The six **unipolar precordial leads** view electrical activity of the heart in the horizontal plane. An electrode is placed on six different positions on the chest.
   a. V_1: at the fourth intercostal space on the right sternal border.
   b. V_2: at the fourth intercostal space on the left sternal border.
   c. V_3: at the midpoint of a straight line between leads V_2 and V_4.
   d. V_4: at the fifth intercostal space, on the left midclavicular line.
   e. V_5: on the anterior axillary line and horizontal to lead V_4.
   f. V_6: on the midaxillary line and horizontal to leads V_4 and V_5.

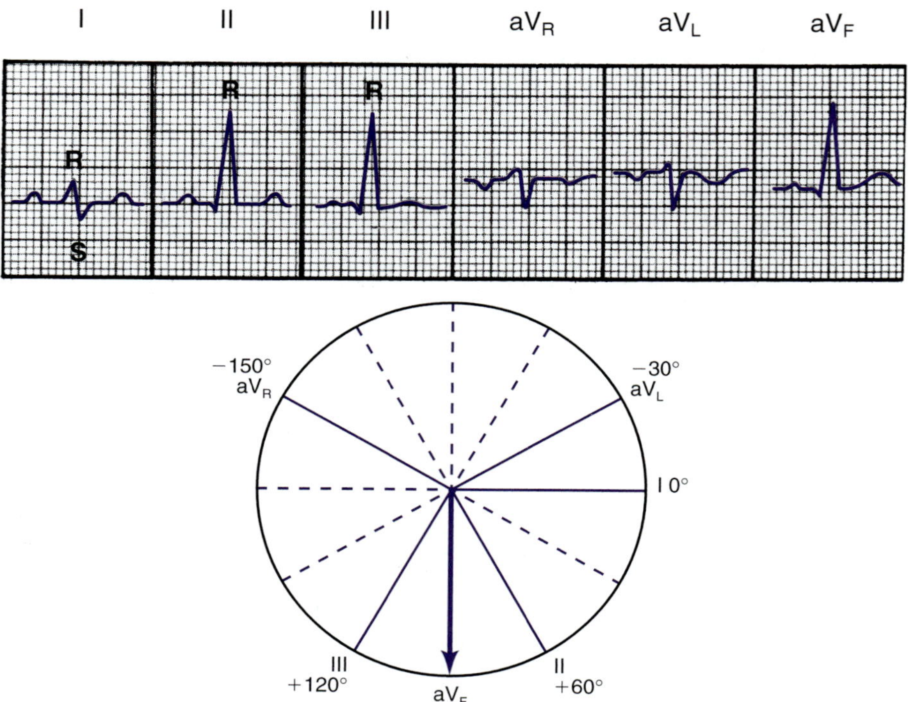

FIGURE 12-4. Mean QRS axis of +90°. (From Goldberger AL: *Clinical Electrocardiography: A Simplified Approach,* 6th ed. St. Louis: Mosby; 1999, p 46.)

4. The **mean QRS axis** represents the average direction of depolarization as it travels through the ventricles, resulting in excitation and contraction of myocardial fibers.
   a) The mean QRS axis can be calculated by simply inspecting leads I, II, III, aVR, aVL, and aVF and applying the following general rules:
   1) The mean QRS axis is directed midway between two leads that register tall R waves of equal amplitude.
   2) The mean QRS axis is directed at right angles (90°) to any extremity lead that registers a biphasic isoelectric complex; for example, in *Figure 12-4*, the mean QRS axis is +90°.
      a) Axes between −30° and +100° are normal.
      b) An axis more negative than −30° is considered **left axis deviation** (LAD).
      c) An axis more positive than +100° is considered **right axis deviation** (RAD).
5. **Heart rate** is the number of times that the myocardium depolarizes and contracts (beats) in 1 minute.
   a. Several techniques are available for determining HR.
   b. If the HR is regular, then the constant 300 is divided by number of large boxes between two consecutive QRS complexes.
   c. If HR is irregular, then the number of cardiac cycles (cardiac cycle: unit between two consecutive R waves) over a 6-second period is multiplied by 10. For example, in *Figure 12-5*, the HR is 100 beats/minute.
6. Alternative lead arrangements.
   a. Many problems with the reading of the electrical signal occur during and exercise ECG, including electrode movement, muscular activity and respiration. The **Mason Likar** modification is a commonly utilized approach to minimize these problems.
   b. Left and right arm electrodes are moved to the upper half of the torso, specifically, at a point in the infraclavicular fossa medial to the border of the deltoid muscle, 2 cm below the lower border of the clavicle.
   c. The leg electrodes are moved to the lower half of the torso, specially, at the iliac crest.

II. ARRHYTHMIAS AND CONDUCTION DISTURBANCES

A. SINUS ARRHYTHMIAS (*Figure 12-6*)

1. **Sinus bradycardia** is characterized by a normal sinus rhythm but with an HR <60 beats/minute.

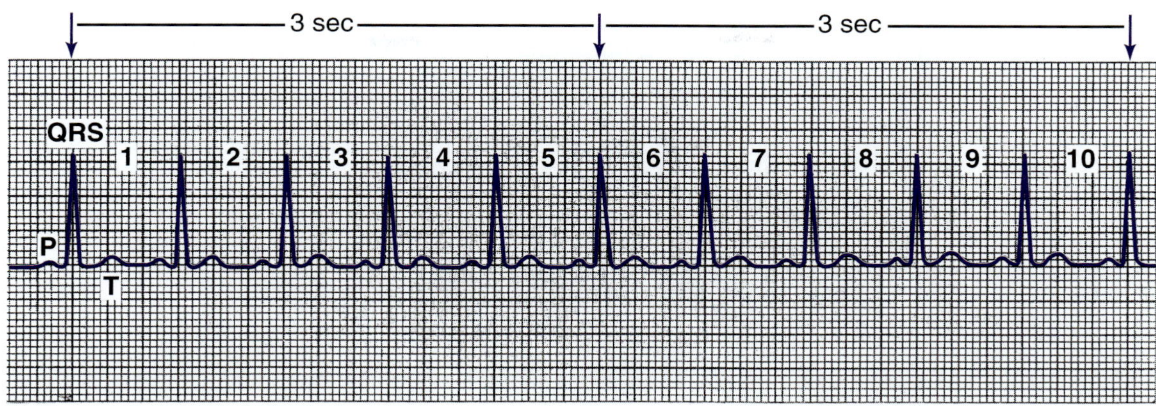

FIGURE 12-5. Measurement of heart rate (beats per minute) by counting the number of cardiac cycles in a 6-second interval and multiplying this number by 10. In this example, 10 cardiac cycles occur in 6 seconds. Therefore the heart rate is 10 · 10 = 100 beats/min. The *arrows* point to 3-second markers. (From Goldberger AL: *Clinical Electrocardiography: A Simplified Approach,* 6th ed. St. Louis: Mosby; 1999, p 16.)

2. **Sinus tachycardia** is characterized by a normal sinus rhythm but with an HR of 100–180 beats/minute.
3. Under certain circumstances, the SA node does not maintain a regular sinus rate from beat to beat. This condition is called **sinus arrhythmia** (i.e., respiratory arrhythmia).
4. **Sinus pause (sinus arrest).** The SA node may fail to depolarize the atria for pathologic reasons. This condition, differentiated by the absence of P wave or QRS complex, is termed **sinus pause** or **sinus arrest.** This condition can lead to cardiac arrest unless the AV node or some other focus assumes the role as pacemaker.

B. ATRIAL ARRHYTHMIAS

1. Atrial Flutter and Atrial Fibrillation (*Figure 12-7*)

a. In these arrhythmias, the atria are stimulated not from the SA node, but rather from some ectopic focus or foci.
b. The rate of atrial contraction varies from 250–350 beats/minute for atrial flutter and from 400–600 beats/minute for atrial fibrillation.
c. With either atrial flutter or atrial fibrillation, the rate of ventricular depolarization depends on the rate at which the AV node conducts the supraventricular stimuli.

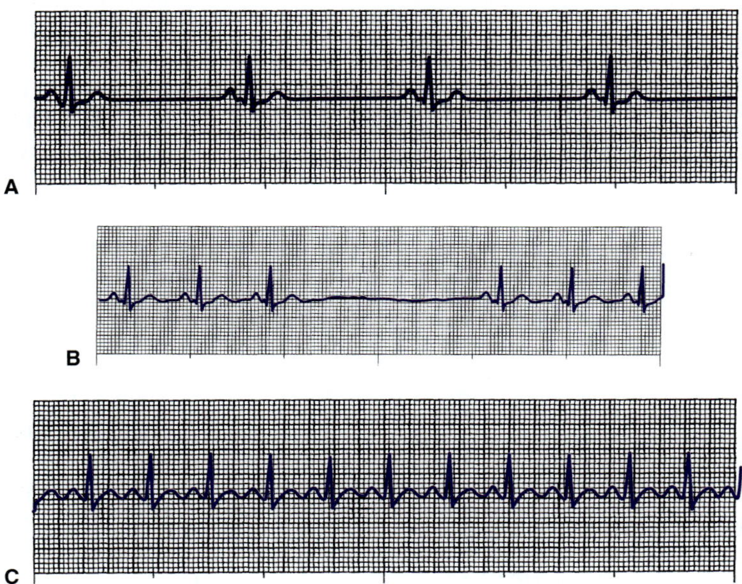

FIGURE 12-6. A. Sinus bradycardia. **B.** Sinus arrest. **C.** Sinus tachycardia. (From Aehlert B: *ECGs Made Easy Pocket Reference.* St. Louis: Mosby; 1995, pp 25, 29, 26.)

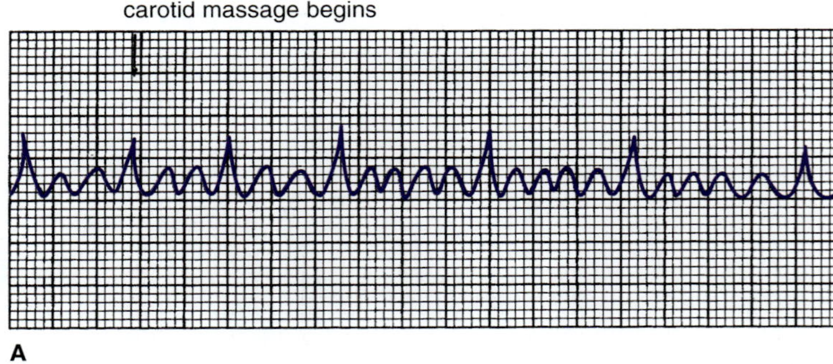

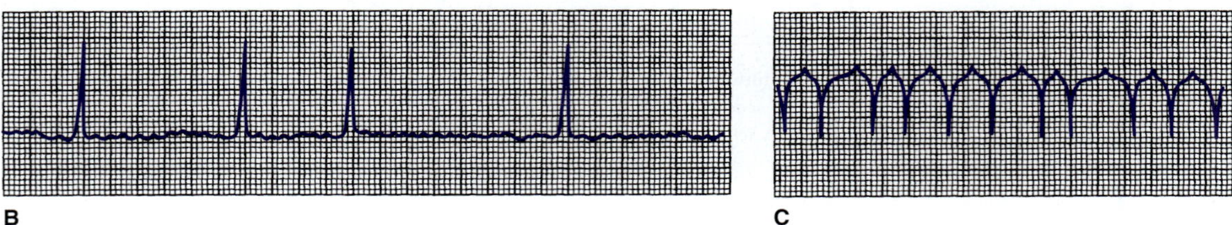

FIGURE 12-7. A. Atrial flutter. Carotid massage increases the block from 3:1 to 5:1. **B.** Atrial fibrillation with a slow, irregular ventricular rate. **C.** Another example of atrial fibrillation. In the absence of a clearly fibrillating baseline, the only clue that this rhythm is atrial fibrillation is the irregularly irregular appearance of the QRS complex. (From Thaler MS: *The Only EKG Book You'll Ever Need,* 3rd ed. Philadelphia: Lippincott Williams & Wilkins; 1999, pp 125–126.)

d. The presence of characteristic "saw-tooth" waves differentiates atrial flutter, and the absence of P waves and irregular ventricular response characterizes atrial fibrillation.

e. Atrial flutter and atrial fibrillation can occur in otherwise healthy people as well as in those with heart disease.

2. Supraventricular tachycardia (SVT) (*Figure 12-8*)

a. Supraventricular ectopic rhythm with an HR of 140–250 beats/minute.

b. Distinguishing features include a regular HR, ectopic P waves, a PR interval that may be normal, and a QRS complex that is typically normal.

C. JUNCTIONAL ARRHYTHMIA (*Figure 12-9*)

1. Supraventricular ectopic rhythm that results from a focus of automaticity located in the bundle of His.
2. ECG waveform characteristics include a regular rhythm, HR of 100–140 beats/minute, normal QRS interval, and P waves (when present) possibly appearing upright or retrograde.

D. VENTRICULAR ARRHYTHMIAS

1. Premature Ventricular Complexes (PVCs)

a. Premature ventricular depolarizations that occur in one of the ventricles and spread to the other ventricle with some delay owing to slow conduction through the ventricular myocardial fibers. The ventricles are not depolarized simultaneously, and the duration of the QRS is = 0.12 second.

b. PVCs are common in both apparently healthy individuals and in patients with pathologic heart disease. Common causes include emotional stress, electrolyte abnormalities, drug therapy, and myocardial ischemia or infarction.

c. Decreased ectopy during exercise testing may be benign. However, increased ectopy or onset of ventricular tachycardia may be related to underlying pathology or other cardiac disorder.

d. PVCs linked to acute myocardial infarction are sometimes the forerunners of ventricular tachycardia and ventricular fibrillation.

e. PVCs may occur with varying frequency:

1) Two PVCs occurring in a row is referred to as a **ventricular couplet**.
2) Three or more PVCs in a row constitute **ventricular tachycardia** (*Figure 12-10*).
3) The repetitive pattern of one normal beat and one PVC is called **ventricular bigeminy**.
4) The repetitive pattern of two normal beats and a PVC is called **ventricular trigeminy**.

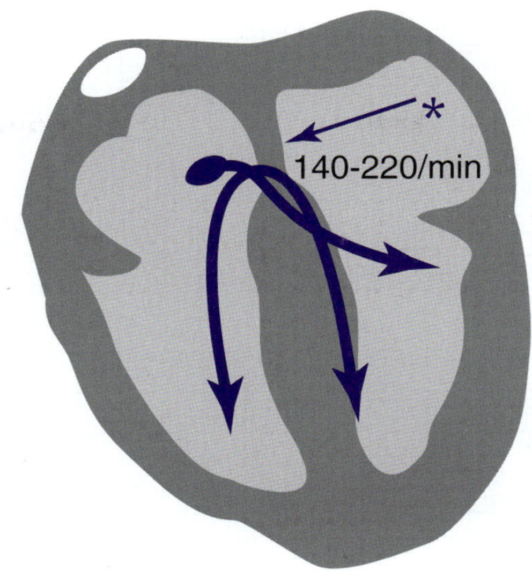

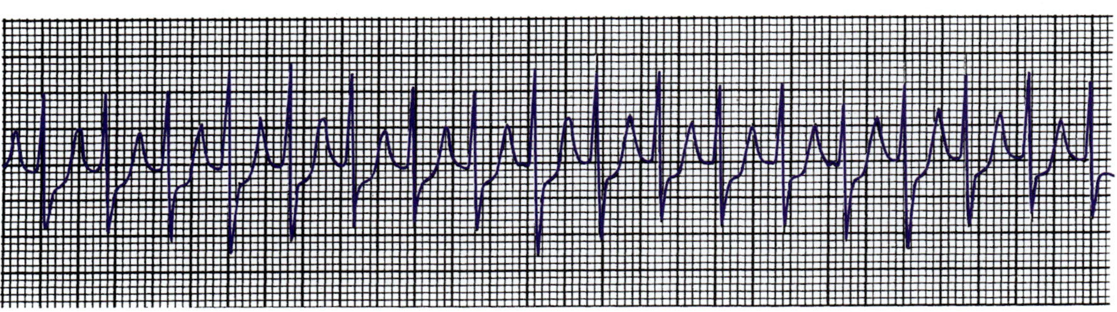

FIGURE 12-8. Atrial tachycardia. (From Davis D: *Quick and Accurate 12-Lead ECG Interpretation,* 3rd ed. Philadelphia: Lippincott Williams & Wilkins, 2001, p 412.)

5) Short, frequent bursts of nonsustained ventricular tachycardia are called "salvos".
6) **Monomorphic ventricular tachycardia** produces ventricular beats of similar morphology (appearance). **Polymorphic tachycardia** is defined by multiple forms of ventricular beats. Polymorphic tachycardias are often related to electrolyte imbalance or myocardial ischemia.

2. Ventricular Escape

a. Ventricular beats occurring late in relation to the normal R–R cycle with a wide QRS.

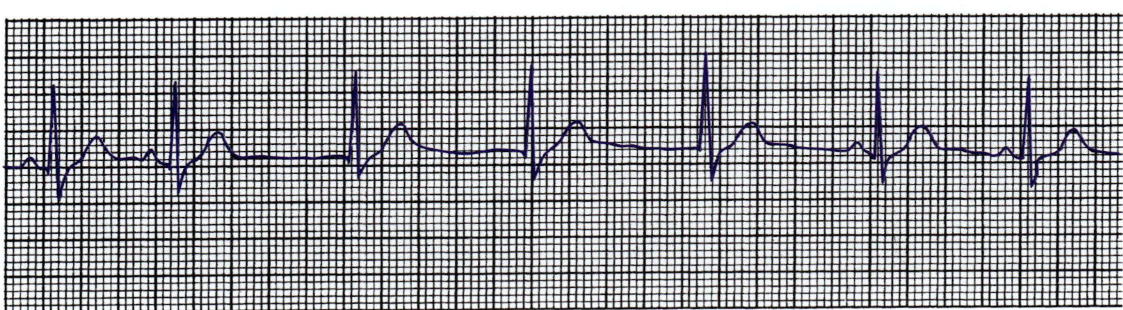

FIGURE 12-9. Sinus rhythm with three junctional escape beats. (From Davis D: *Quick and Accurate 12-Lead ECG Interpretation,* 3rd ed. Philadelphia: Lippincott Williams & Wilkins, 2001, p 408.)

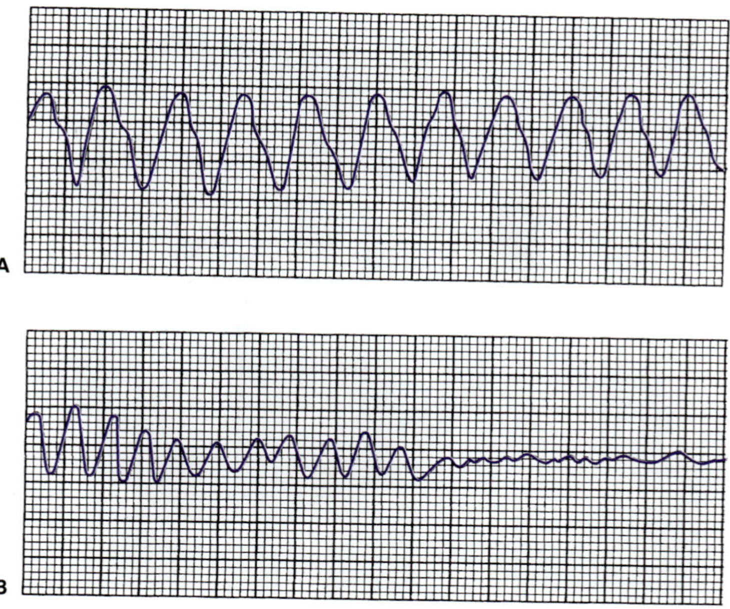

FIGURE 12-10. A. Ventricular tachycardia. The rate is about 200 beats per minute. **B.** Ventricular tachycardia degenerates into ventricular fibrillation. (From Thaler MS: *The Only EKG Book You'll Ever Need,* 3rd ed. Philadelphia: Lippincott Williams & Wilkins; 1999, pp 132, 133.)

3. Ventricular Fibrillation

a. Often triggered by the simultaneous conduction of ischemic ventricular cells with enhanced automaticity in multiple locations of the ventricles.

b. Distinguishing features include a regular rhythm, a ventricular rate of 150–500 beats/minute, fibrillatory waves, and the absence of a distinct QRS complex.

c. Ventricular fibrillation can occur spontaneously in patients with pathologic heart disease and is considered the most common cause of sudden cardiac death in patients during an acute myocardial infarction.

d. Treatment of ventricular fibrillation requires defibrillation.

E. ATRIOVENTRICULAR (AV) BLOCKS (*Figure 12-11*)

Result when supraventricular impulses are delayed or blocked in the AV node or intraventricular conduction system.

1. First-Degree AV Block

a. Characterized by a delay in the conduction of the impulse through the AV junction to the ventricles.

b. Does not impair cardiac function.

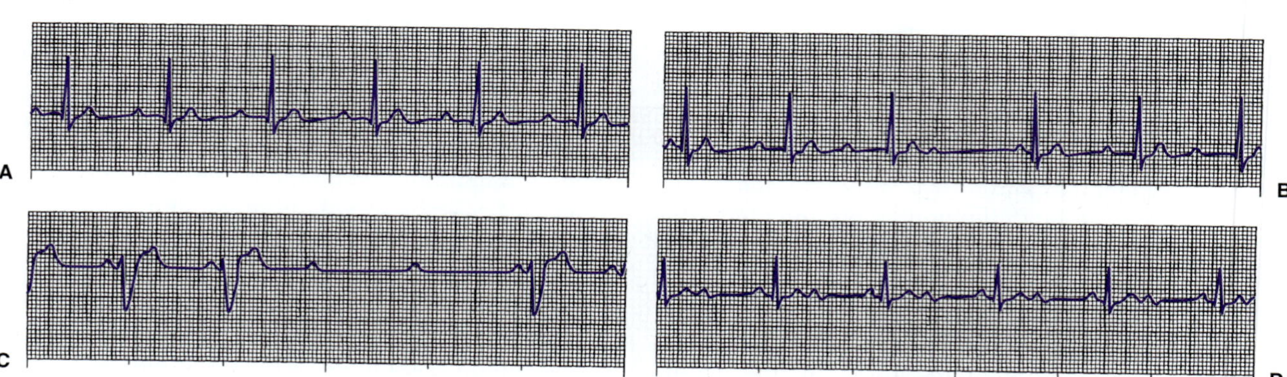

FIGURE 12-11. A. Sinus rhythm (borderline sinus bradycardia) at 60 beats per minute with a first-degree AV block. **B.** Second-degree AV block type I. **C.** Second-degree AV block type II. **D.** Second-degree AV block, 2:1 conduction, probably type I. (From Aehlert B: *ECGs Made Easy Pocket Reference.* St. Louis: Mosby; 1995, pp 61, 62, 63, 64.)

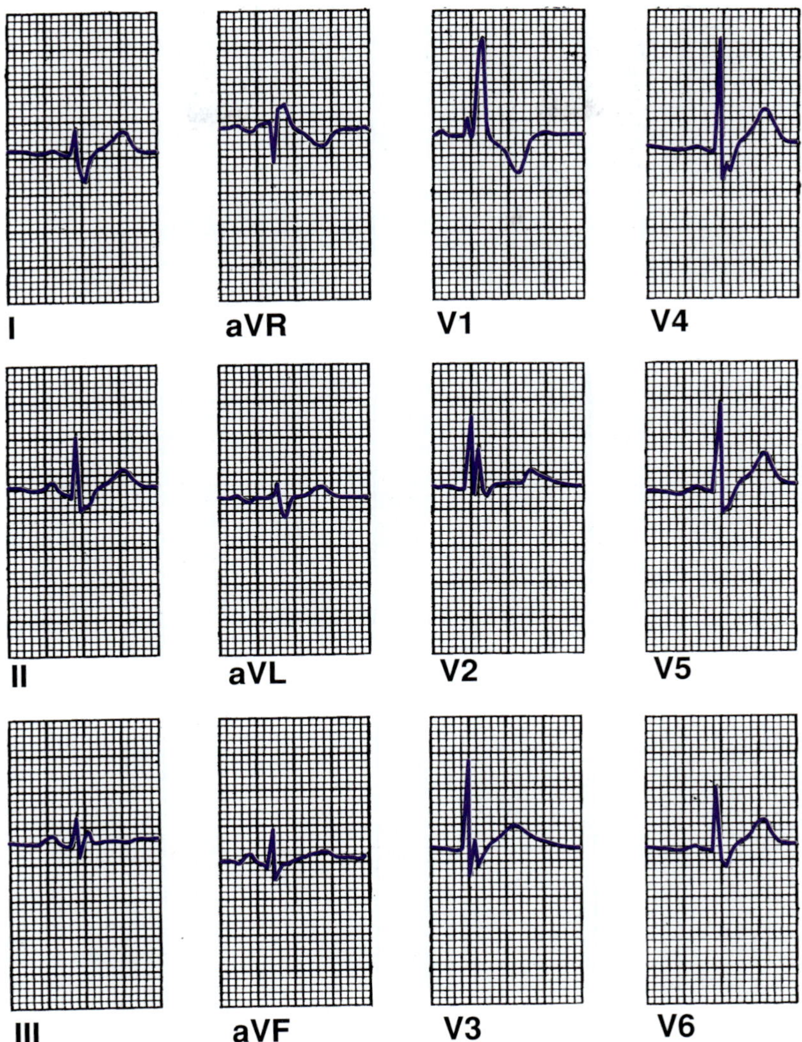

FIGURE 12-12. Right bundle branch block. (From Davis D: *Quick and Accurate 12-Lead ECG Interpretation,* 3rd ed. Philadelphia: Lippincott Williams & Wilkins; 2001, p 155.)

c. The PR interval is >0.20 seconds.

d. Causes include hyperkalemia, quinidine, digitalis, and ischemic heart disease.

2. Second-Degree AV Block

a. Subdivided into two types: Mobitz I and Mobitz II.

1) **Mobitz I (Wenckebach AV) block.**

a) Impulse conduction through the AV junction becomes increasingly more difficult, causing a progressively longer PR interval until a P wave is not conducted. As such, the ECG shows a P wave not followed by a QRS complex, which indicates that the AV junction failed to conduct the impulse from the atria to the ventricles. However, this pause allows the AV node to recover, and the following P wave is conducted with a normal or slightly shorter PR interval.

(i) This may be a normal physiological finding in a young athlete and usually disappears with the onset of exercise.

(ii) Causes include certain drugs (digitalis, calcium-channel blockers), ischemic heart disease, and inferior wall myocardial infarction.

2) **Mobitz II block.**

a) A delay in AV conduction at the level of the bundle branches.

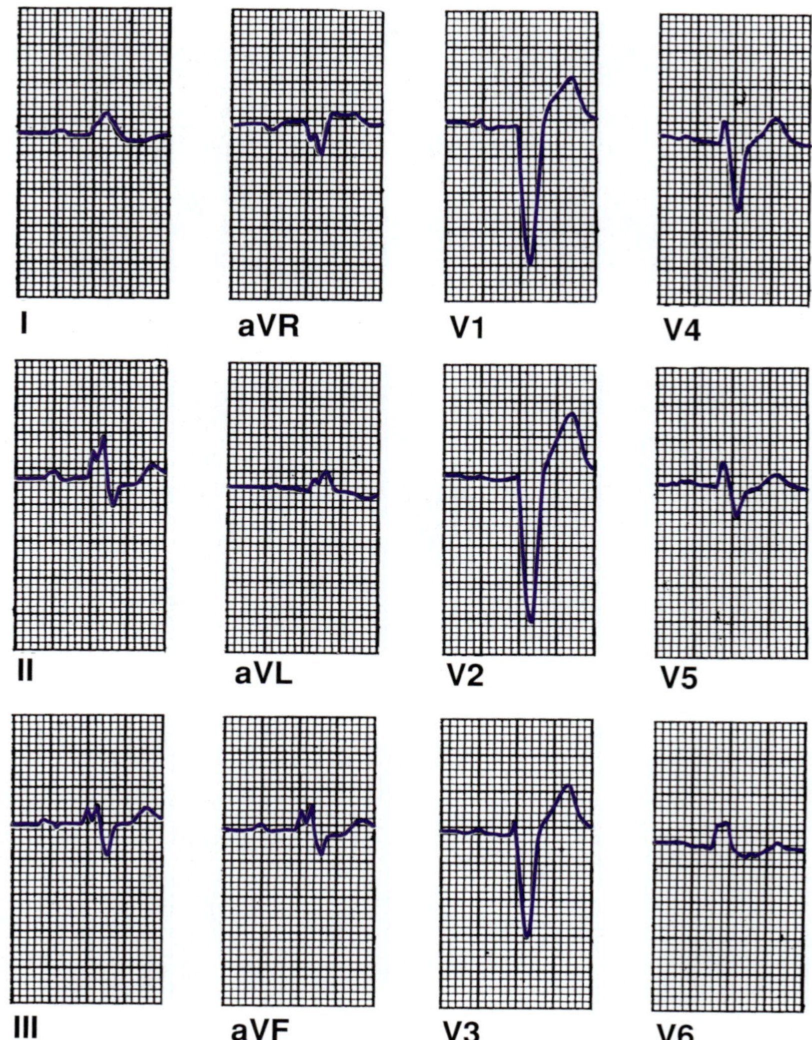

FIGURE 12-13. Left bundle branch block. (From Davis D: *Quick and Accurate 12-Lead ECG Interpretation,* 3rd ed. Philadelphia: Lippincott Williams & Wilkins, 2001; p 159.)

b) Characterized by fixed, normal PR intervals, broad QRS complexes, and nonconducted P waves (dropped beats).
   (i) Causes include anterior wall myocardial infarction and severe conduction system disease.
   (ii) Patients with Mobitz II may be considered candidates for a pacemaker.

3. **Third-Degree AV Block**
   a. Also called **complete heart block,** because there is no conduction of impulses from the atria to the ventricles.
   b. The PR interval changes continually because there is no relationship between the P waves and the QRS complexes.
   c. The atria are usually under the control of the sinus node, so that P waves are present with a normal atrial rate.
   d. The ventricles are paced by a pacemaker located below the point of blockage in the AV junction, so that QRS complexes are seen with a ventricular rate of 30–60 beats/minute. These QRS complexes are of normal or prolonged duration, depending on the pacemaker location.

TABLE 12-1. LOCALIZATION OF MYOCARDIAL INFARCTIONS (MIS)

Anterior infarction: Q waves in leads V_1, V_2, V_3, and V_4
Inferior infarction: Q waves in leads II, III, and aVF
Lateral infarction: Q waves in leads I, aVL, V_5, and V_6
Posterior infarction: Tall R waves in leads V_1 and V_2

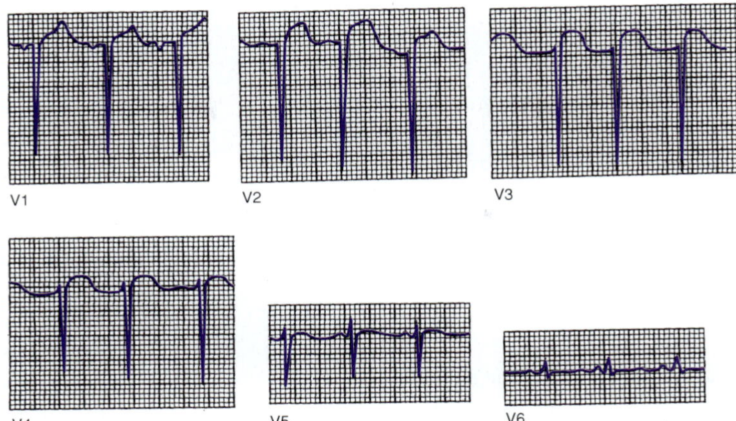

FIGURE 12-14. An anterior infarction with poor R wave progression across the precordium. (From Thaler MS: *The Only EKG Book You'll Ever Need,* 3rd ed. Philadelphia: Lippincott Williams & Wilkins; 1999, p 221.)

e. Third-degree AV block can occur because of advanced age, digitalis intoxication, or myocardial infarction.

f. Patients with third-degree AV block that is not transient (i.e., caused by digitalis intoxication) are good candidates for pacemaker implantation.

4. Bundle Branch Blocks

a. Right Bundle Branch Block (RBBB)

1) Represents a delay in impulse conduction through the right bundle branch (*Figure 12-12*).

2) The QRS complex is widened (>0.12 second) as a result of

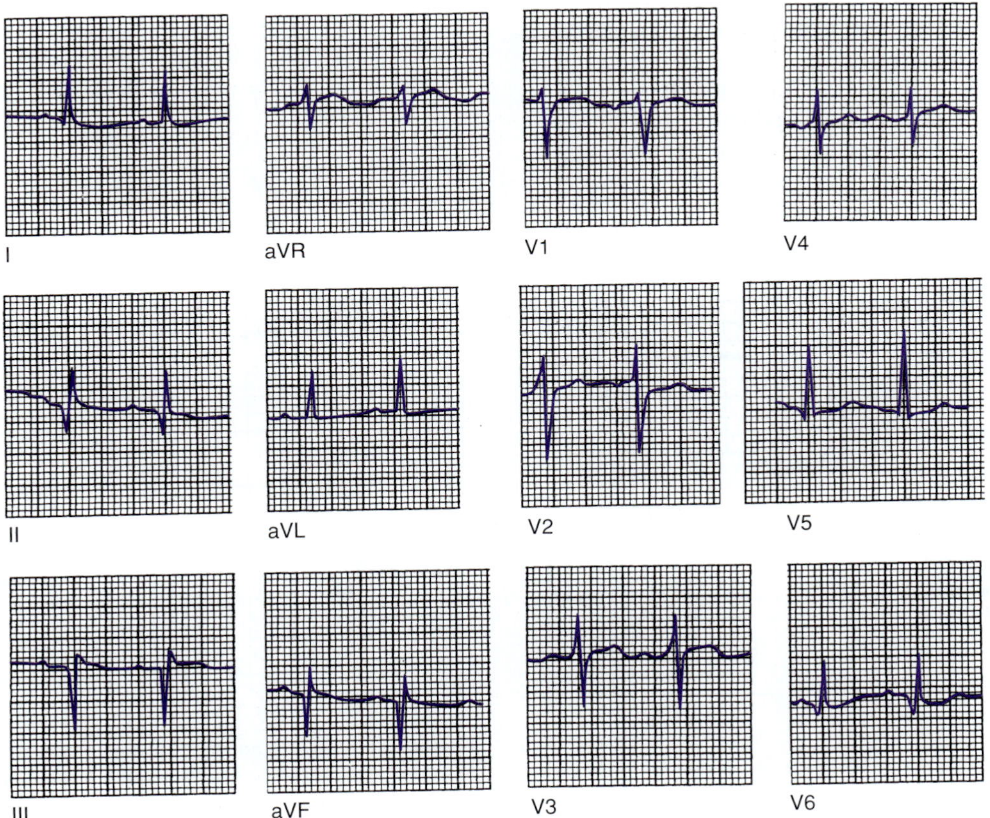

FIGURE 12-15. A fully evolved inferior infarction. Deep Q waves can be seen in leads II, III, and AVF. (From Thaler MS: *The Only EKG Book You'll Ever Need,* 3rd ed. Philadelphia: Lippincott Williams & Wilkins; 1999, p 219.)

delayed depolarization of the right ventricle.

3) An rSR′ with a wide R wave in V_1 is a characteristic ECG change associated with RBBB.

4) Although RBBB may be caused by heart disease, it can also be present in the absence of heart disease.

b. **Left Bundle Branch Block (LBBB)**

1) Represents a delay in impulse conduction through the left bundle branch (*Figure 12-13*).

2) The impulse travels through the right bundle branch and then across the septum and depolarizes the left ventricle.

3) The QRS complex is widened (>0.12 second as a result of delayed depolarization of the left ventricle.

4) A wide negative deflection (QS) is present in lead V_1; lead V_6 shows a wide and tall R wave.

5) LBBB is commonly associated with heart disease (e.g., coronary artery disease, hypertension, cardiomyopathy, left ventricular hypertrophy).

5. Hemiblocks

a. Blocks involving the anterior or posterior fascicle of the main left bundle branch of the bundle of His.

1) **Left Anterior Fascicular Block**

a) Blocked conduction through the anterior fascicle of the main left bundle branch so that the impulse continues down the posterior fascicle.

b) A mean QRS axis of $>-45°$ coupled with a QRS duration of <0.12 second suggests left anterior hemiblock.

2) **Left Posterior Fascicular Block**

a) Blocked conduction through the posterior fascicle of the main left bundle branch, so that the impulse continues to travel down the posterior fascicle of the main left bundle branch.

b) A mean QRS axis of $>+120°$ coupled with a QRS duration of <0.12 second suggest left posterior hemiblock.

III. ECG PATTERNS IN SELECTED DISORDERS

A. CORONARY ARTERY DISEASE (CAD)

1. In exercise ECG, usually performed on a treadmill or cycle ergometer, a horizontal or downsloping ST depression of at least 1 mm lasting for 0.08 second is considered an abnormal test finding and may signify CAD. T-wave abnormalities also may be seen in patients with CAD.

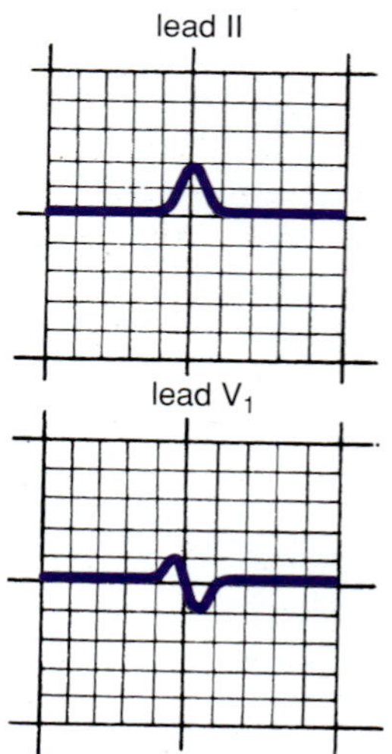

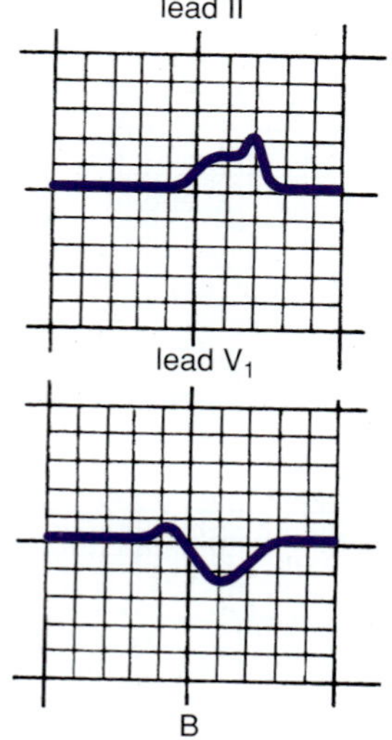

FIGURE 12-16. A. The normal P wave in leads II and V_1. **B.** Left atrial enlargement. Note the increased amplitude and duration of the terminal, left atrial component of the P wave. (From Thaler MS: *The Only EKG Book You'll Ever Need,* 3rd ed. Philadelphia: Lippincott Williams & Wilkins; 1999, p 80.)

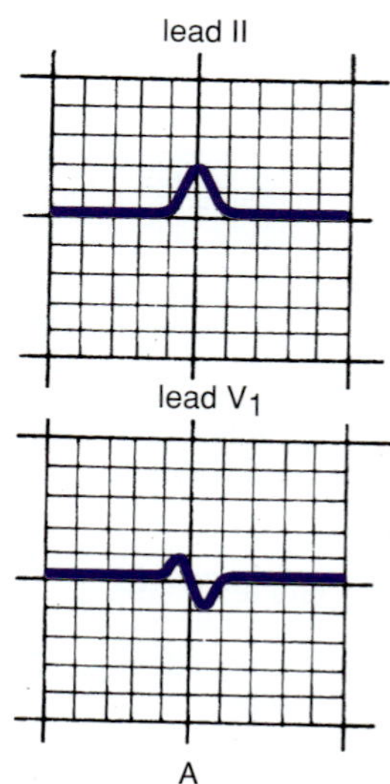

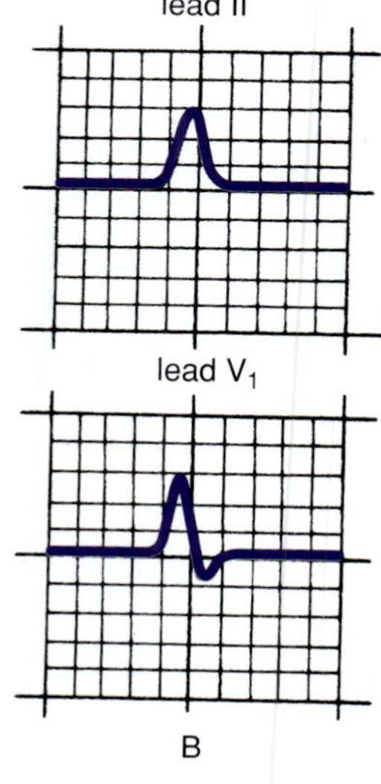

FIGURE 12-17. A. The normal P wave in leads II and V_1. **B.** Right atrial enlargement. Note the increased amplitude of the early, right atrial component of the P wave. The terminal left atrial component, and hence the overall duration of the P wave, is essentially unchanged. (From Thaler MS: *The Only EKG Book You'll Ever Need,* 3rd ed. Philadelphia: Lippincott Williams & Wilkins; 1999, p 79.)

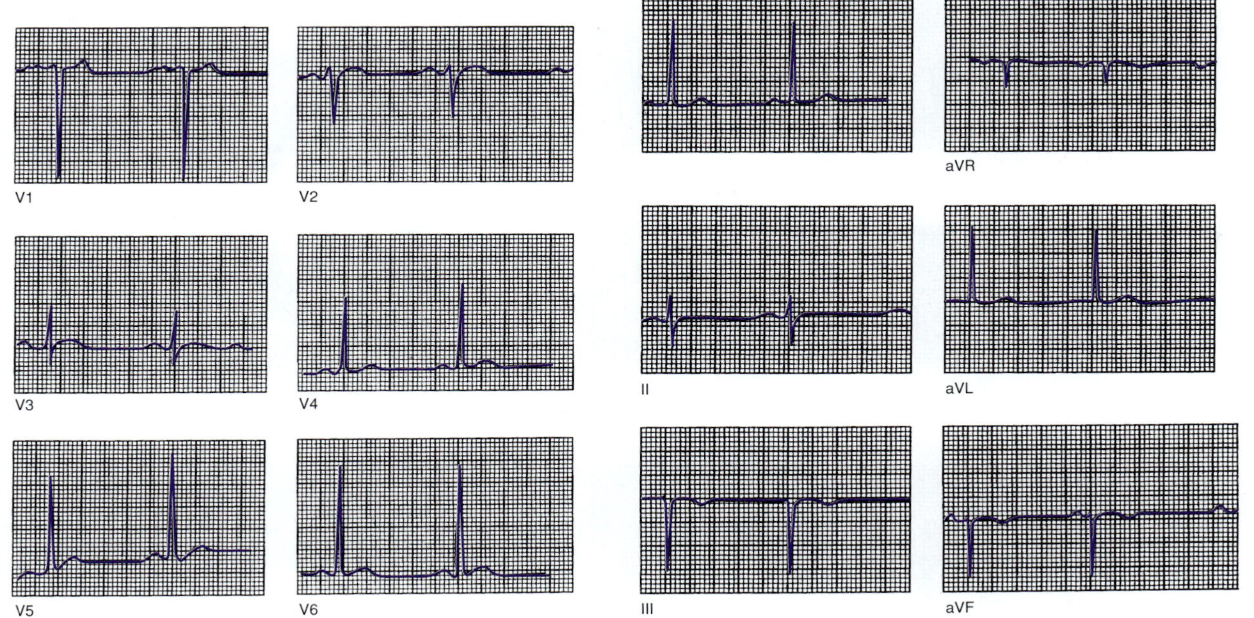

FIGURE 12-18. A. Left ventricular hypertrophy in the precordial leads. Three of the four criteria are met: the R wave amplitude in V_5 plus the S wave amplitude in V_1 exceeds 35 mm, the R wave amplitude in V_6 exceeds 18 mm, and the R wave amplitude in lead V_6 slightly exceeds the R wave amplitude in lead V_5. The only criterion not met is for the R wave in lead V_5 to exceed 26 mm. **B.** Left ventricular hypertrophy in the limb leads. Criteria 1, 3, and 4 are met; only criterion 2, regarding the R wave amplitude in lead AVF, is not met. (From Thaler MS: *The Only EKG Book You'll Ever Need,* 3rd ed. Philadelphia: Lippincott Williams & Wilkins; 1999, pp 85, 86.)

B. MYOCARDIAL ISCHEMIA AND INFARCTION

1. Myocardial ischemia can occur transiently and be limited to the inner myocardial layer (subendocardial ischemia) or affect the entire ventricular wall (transmural ischemia).
   a. If the myocardial oxygen supply remains inadequate, injury (necrosis) will occur.
2. **Myocardial infarction (MI)** is myocardial injury caused by severe or prolonged ischemia.
3. *Table 12-1* summarizes the ECG leads associated with various areas of myocardial injury. *Figures 12-14* and *12-15* illustrate anterior and inferior infarction, respectively.
4. **Transmural Ischemia with MI.**
   a. Transmural MI is associated with changes in both the QRS and ST-T complexes.
      1) ST elevation, or tall, upright T waves, is the earliest sign of transmural MI.
      2) ST elevations may persist for a few hours to a few days. Over this period, Q waves formin leads with ST-segment elevations.
      3) During the evolving phase, ST-segment elevations may return to baseline, and T waves may become inverted.
      4) Q waves may persist for years following a transmural MI; however, their amplitude decreases and in some cases they may disappear.
      5) In most cases, inverted T waves persist indefinitely over the infarcted area following a transmural MI.
         a) Transmural MIs are localized to a specific portion of the left ventricular wall supplied by one of the coronary arteries: left anterior descending artery (LAD), right coronary artery (RCA), and left circumflex (LCx).
         b) A transmural MI can be diagnosed by the presence of abnormal Q waves (>—0.04 second and at least 25% of the height of the R wave).
         c) Q waves in leads V_1 and V_2 should be examined carefully, because they can be a normal variant or may signify anteroseptal MI.
         d) Myocardial infarction can be determined and localized by viewing certain ECG leads; for example, tall R waves in leads V_1 and V_2 may suggest posterior wall MI or right ventricular hypertrophy.

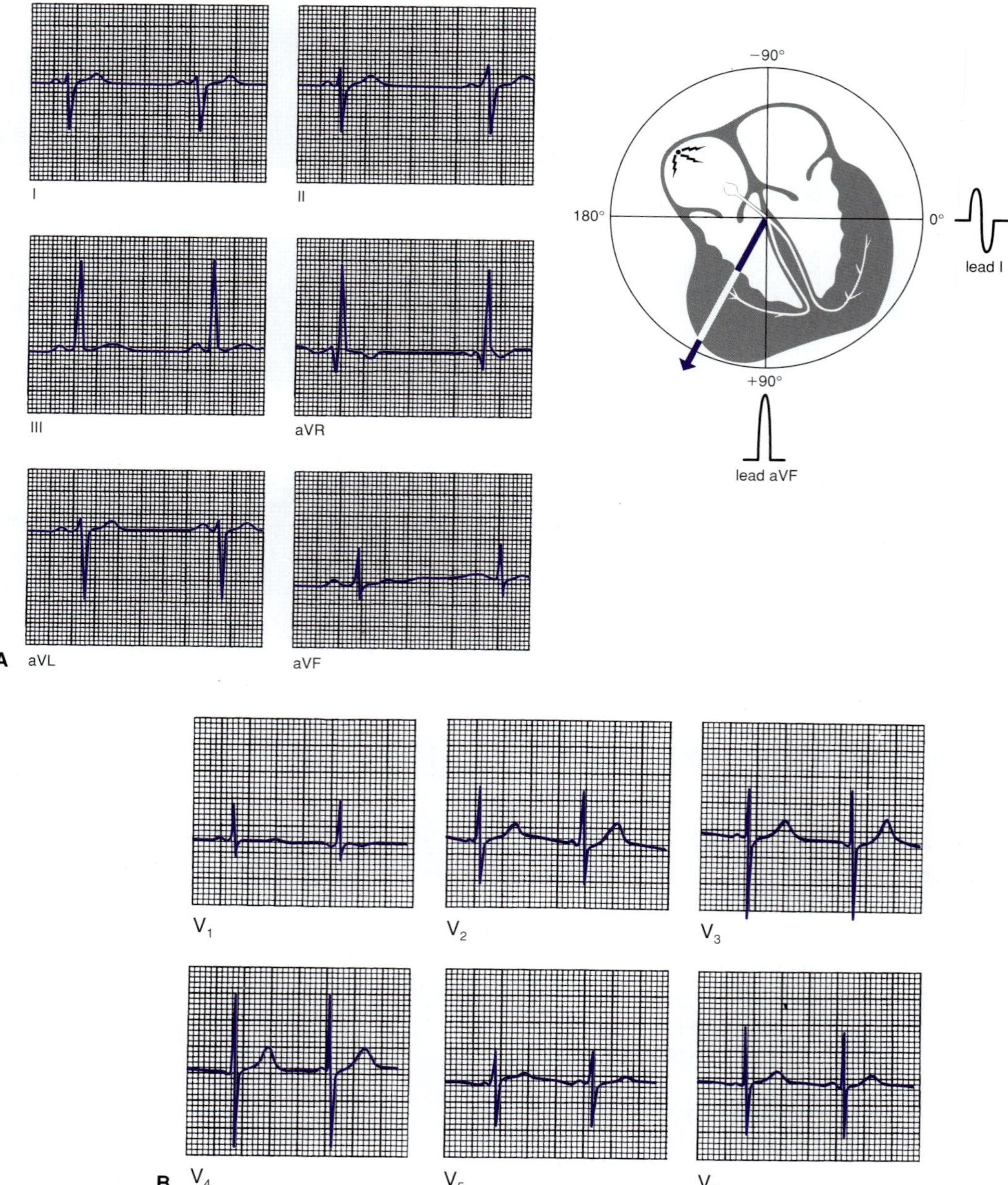

FIGURE 12-19. A. Right ventricular hypertrophy shifts the axis of the QRS complex to the right. The ECG tracings confirm right axis deviation. In addition, the QRS complex in lead I is slightly negative, a criterion that many believe is essential for properly establishing the diagnosis of right ventricular hypertrophy. **B.** In lead V_1, the R wave is larger than the S wave. In lead V_6, the S wave is larger than the R wave. (From Thaler MS: *The Only EKG Book You'll Ever Need,* 3rd ed. Philadelphia: Lippincott Williams & Wilkins; 1999, pp 82, 83.)

5. **Subendocardial Ischemia and Infarction.**
   a. Subendocardial ischemia usually produces ST-segment depression in anterior leads, inferior leads, or both, commonly during attacks of typical angina pectoris.
   b. A horizontal or downsloping ST depression of $\geq$1 mm lasting 0.08 second is considered an abnormal response during exercise ECG and constitutes a positive exercise test.
   c. Severe subendocardial ischemia may lead to **subendocardial infarction**, marked by persistent ST depression, possible T wave inversion, and usually normal Q waves.
6. Ischemia or Infarction Location.
   The location of ischemia or the area of infarction can be identified by previously mentioned ECG changes as follows:

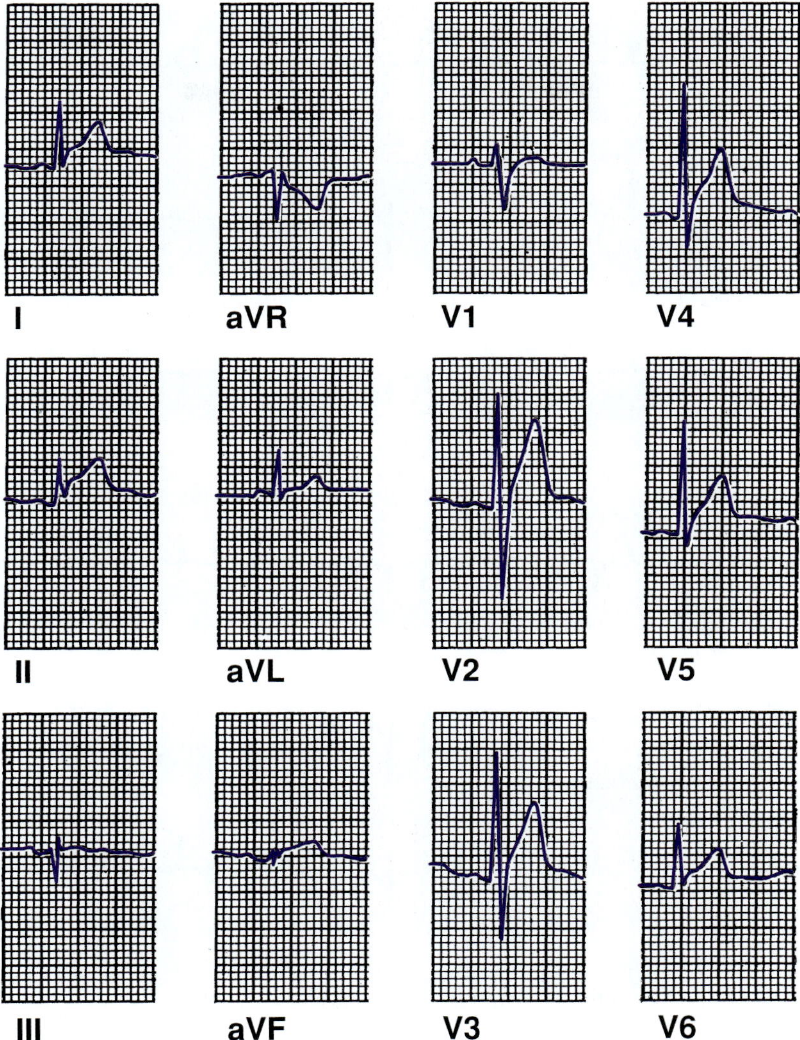

FIGURE 12-20. Pericarditis. (From Davis D: *Quick and Accurate 12-Lead ECG Interpretation,* 3rd ed. Philadelphia: Lippincott Williams & Wilkins; 2001, p 248.)

a. Inferior infarction: leads II, III, aVF.
b. Anteroseptal infarction: leads V_1, V_2.
c. Anterior infarction: leads V_2-V_5.
d. Anterolateral infarction: leads V_2-V_6, aVL, I.
e. Lateral infarction: leads I, aVL.

7. Differentiation Between Q-Wave and Non–Q-Wave MI (NQWMI).
   a. NQWMI is a clinical syndrome of acute chest pain, enzyme evidence of infarction, but lack of Q-waves on the surface ECG.
   b. Q-wave MI is demonstrated and diagnosed by Q-waves on the surface ECG.

C. ATRIAL ENLARGEMENT

1. **Left atrial enlargement** is best demonstrated in lead V_1.
   a. A wide P wave of >0.12 second is seen in *Figure 12-16B*.
   b. P-wave voltage is normal or slightly increased.
   c. Sometimes the terminal portion of the P wave, which represents left atrial depolarization, shows a distinct wide negative deflection. As such, lead V_1 may show a biphasic P wave.
   d. Wide P waves are often referred to as **P mitrale**, because they are often seen in patients with rheumatic mitral valve disease.
2. **Right atrial enlargement** is best detected in lead II (*Figure 12-17B*).
   a. P-wave amplitude may be increased to >2.5 mm.
   b. P wave duration may be normal.
   c. The tall P wave seen in right atrial enlargement is called **P pulmonale**, because it is

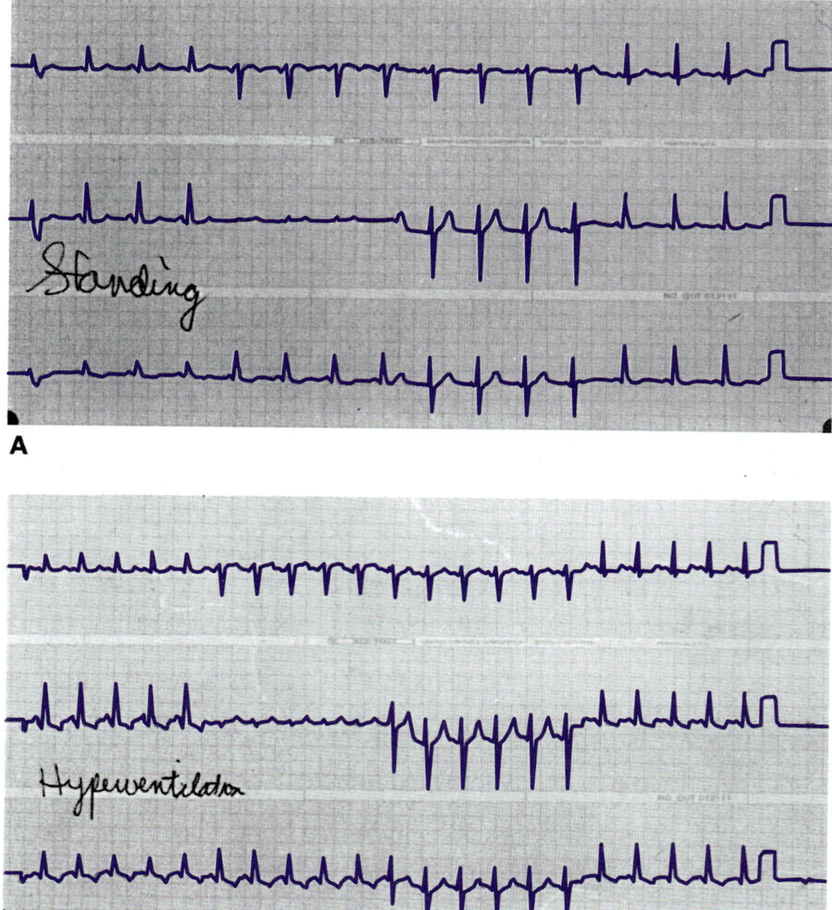

FIGURE 12-21. **A.** Resting ECG. **B.** ECG showing results of hyperventilation (i.e., inverted T waves).

common in patients with pulmonary disease.

D. VENTRICULAR HYPERTROPHY

1. An increase in the size of either ventricular wall may produce high voltages in the leads over the hypertrophied area.
   a. Left Ventricular Hypertrophy (LVH) (*Figure 12-18*).
      1) Usually associated with abnormally tall R waves in the left chest leads and abnormally deep S waves in the right chest leads.
      2) Voltage criteria for the diagnosis of LVH are S wave in lead V_1 + R wave in lead V_5 or $V_6 > 35$ mm, or R wave in lead aVL >11 mm.
      3) ST changes and T-wave inversions are usually present in leads with tall R waves.
      4) LVH is commonly associated with conditions such as aortic stenosis and systemic hypertension.
   b. Right Ventricular Hypertrophy (RVH) (*Figure 12-19*).

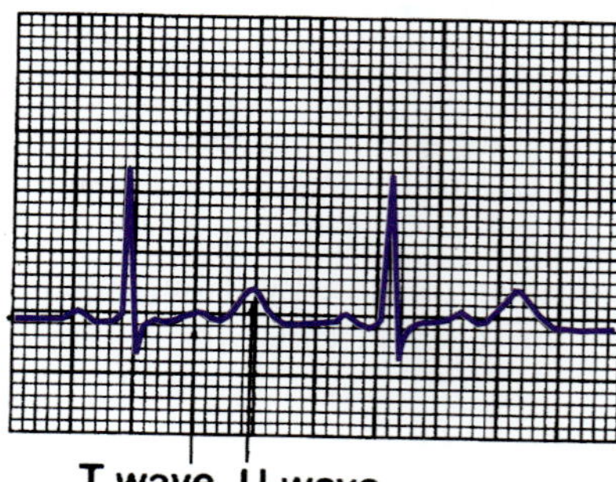

FIGURE 12-22. Hypokalemia. The U waves are even more prominent than the T waves. (From Thaler MS: *The Only EKG Book You'll Ever Need*, 3rd ed. Philadelphia: Lippincott Williams & Wilkins; 1999, p 247.)

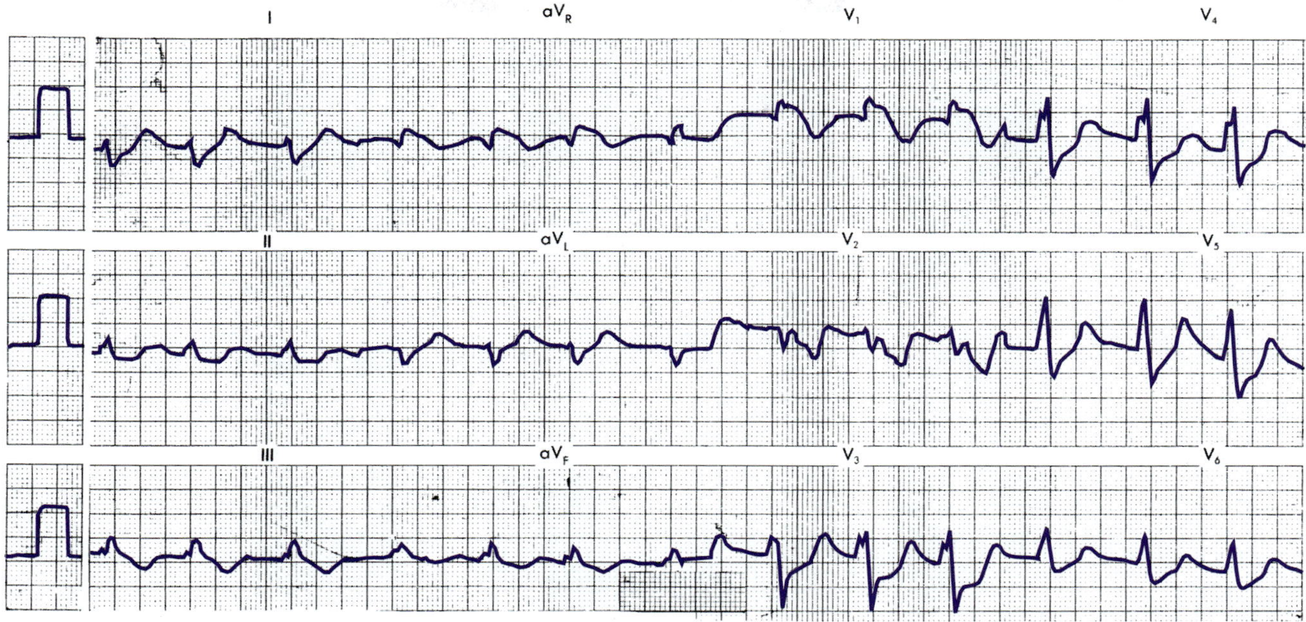

FIGURE 12-23. Marked hyperkalemia: ECG of a patient with a serum potassium concentration of 8.5 mEq/L. Notice the absence of P waves and the presence of bizarre, wide QRS complexes. (From Goldberger AL: *Clinical Electrocardiography: A Simplified Approach,* 6th ed. St. Louis: Mosby; 1999, p 118.)

1) Associated with high voltages in leads V_1 and V_2 and possibly an R wave greater than the S wave in these leads.
2) RVH also causes right axis deviation and ST changes and T-wave inversions in right chest leads.

E. PERICARDITIS

1. Acute pericarditis (inflammation of the pericardium) is associated with diffuse ST-segment elevation (in contrast to the localized ST-segment elevation seen in acute MI), possibly followed by T wave inversion (*Figure 12-20*).

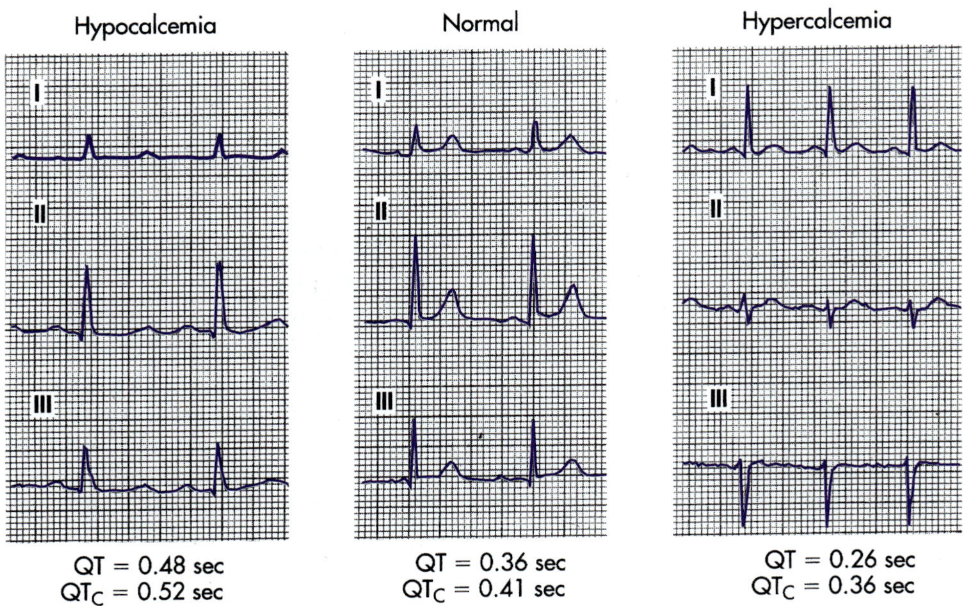

FIGURE 12-24. Hypocalcemia prolongs the QT interval by stretching out the ST segment. Hypercalcemia decreases the QT interval by shortening the ST segment so that the T wave seems to take off directly from the end of the QRS complex. (From Goldberger AL: *Clinical Electrocardiography: A Simplified Approach,* 6th ed. St. Louis: Mosby; 1999, p 120.)

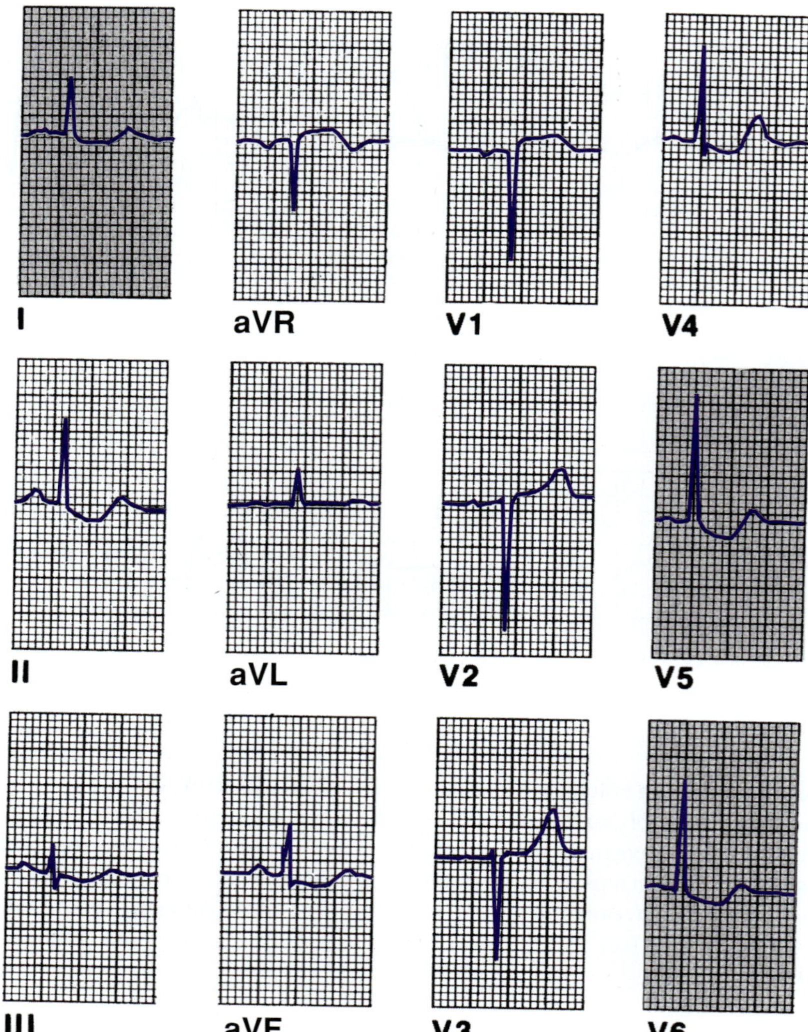

FIGURE 12-25. Digitalis effect. (From Davis D: *Quick and Accurate 12-Lead ECG Interpretation,* 3rd ed. Philadelphia: Lippincott Williams & Wilkins; 2001, p 263.)

F. PULMONARY DISEASE

1. Patients with emphysema (chronic lung disease) often exhibit such ECG changes as low voltage, poor R wave progression in chest leads, and a vertical or rightward QRS axis.

G. HYPERTENSIVE HEART DISEASE

1. Commonly causes left ventricular hypertrophy that eventually leads to left atrial enlargement.
2. Patients with long-standing hypertensive disease often develop LBBB and, in some cases, atrial fibrillation.

H. HYPERVENTILATION

1. Fast, deep breathing for approximately 20 seconds. This procedure is performed before or after a stress test, and any ECG changes are noted. Typical changes may include ST-segment and T-wave abnormalities in all leads (*Figure 12-21*).

I. ELECTROLYTE ABNORMALITIES

1. **Hypokalemia** produces ST depression with prominent U waves and flattened T waves (*Figure 12-22*).
2. **Hyperkalemia** produces predictable ECG changes depending on severity (*Figure 12-23*).
   a. Mild hyperkalemia causes narrowing and peaking of T waves.
   b. Moderate hyperkalemia is marked by prolonged PR intervals and small or sometimes absent P waves.
   c. Severe hyperkalemia produces wide QRS complexes and asystole.
3. **Hypocalcemia** produces prolonged QT intervals (*Figure 12-24*).

4. **Hypercalcemia** shortens ventricular repolarization and thus shortens the QT interval (see *Figure 12-24*).

J. DRUG THERAPY

1. **Digitalis**, used to treat heart failure and arrhythmias, can produce a shortened QT interval and scooped ST-T complex (*Figure 12-25*). Digitalis toxicity often results in arrhythmias and conduction disturbances.
2. **Quinidine**, **procainamide**, and **disopyramide**, used to treat arrhythmias, can produce prolonged QT intervals and flattened T waves.

Review Test

DIRECTIONS: Carefully read all questions, and select the BEST single answer.

1. Slow conduction in the atrioventricular node is associated with which of the following?
   A) Prolonged PR interval.
   B) Prolonged QRS interval.
   C) Shortened QT interval.
   D) Elevated ST segment.

2. Examine the six extremity leads shown in the figure below. What is the appropriate mean QRS axis?
   A) −30°.
   B) 60°.
   C) 90°.
   D) 120°.

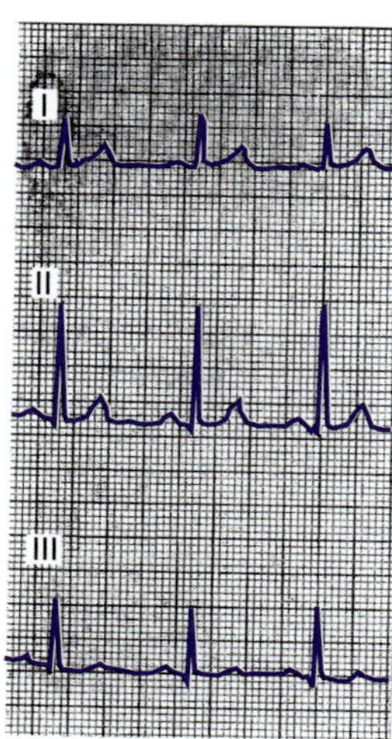

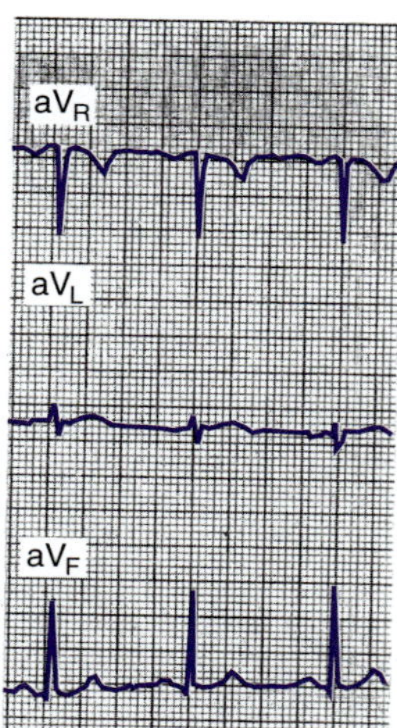

(From Goldberger AL. *Clinical Electrocardiography: A Simplified Approach*, 6th ed. St. Louis: Mosby; 1999; p 55.)

3. In the following ECG, which of the following conduction abnormalities is indicated?
   A) Right bundle branch block.
   B) Third-degree atrioventricular block.
   C) First-degree atrioventricular block.
   D) Mobitz I.

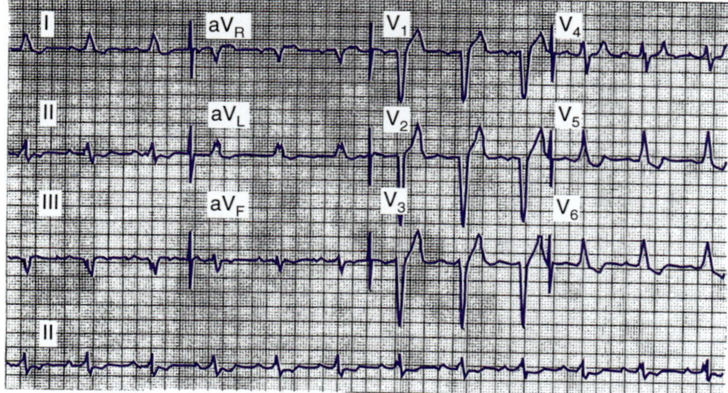

(From Goldberger AL. *Clinical Electrocardiography: A Simplified Approach*, 6th ed. St. Louis: Mosby; 1999, p 80.)

4. Which of the following conditions can cause ST-segment elevation?
   A) Digitalis toxicity.
   B) Hypocalcemia.
   C) Hypokalemia.
   D) Acute pericarditis.

5. In the ECG strip shown below, which of the following disorders is indicated?
   A) Acute pericarditis.
   B) Old inferior myocardial infarction.
   C) Old posterior myocardial infarction.
   D) Anterior myocardial infarction.

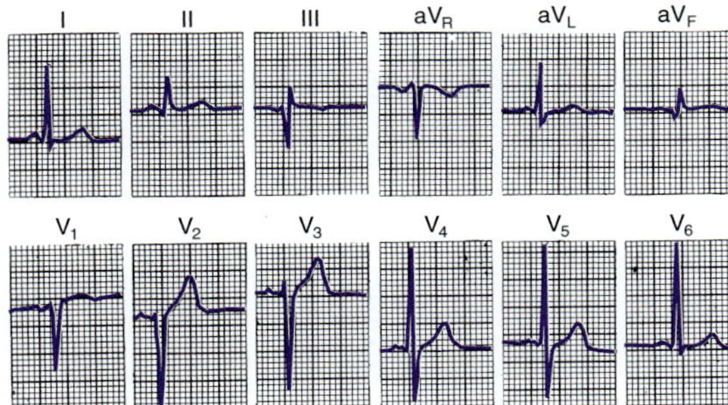

(From Goldberger AL. *Clinical Electrocardiography: A Simplified Approach*, 6th ed. St. Louis: Mosby; 1999, p 91.)

6. In the ECG strip shown below, which of the following disorders is indicated?
   A) Subendocardial ischemia.
   B) Transmural ischemia.
   C) Acute inferior myocardial infarction.
   D) Posterior myocardial infarction.

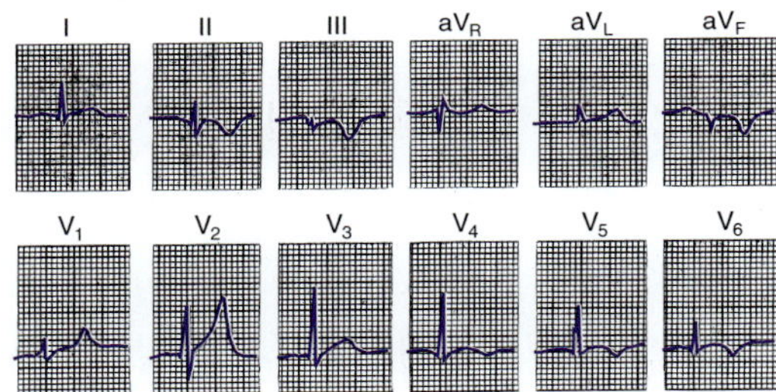

(From Goldberger AL. *Clinical Electrocardiography: A Simplified Approach*, 6th ed. St. Louis: Mosby; 1999, p 91.)

7. In the ECG strip shown below, which of the following abnormalities is indicated?
   A) Left bundle branch block.
   B) Posterior wall myocardial infarction.
   C) Right bundle branch block.
   D) Left ventricular hypertrophy.

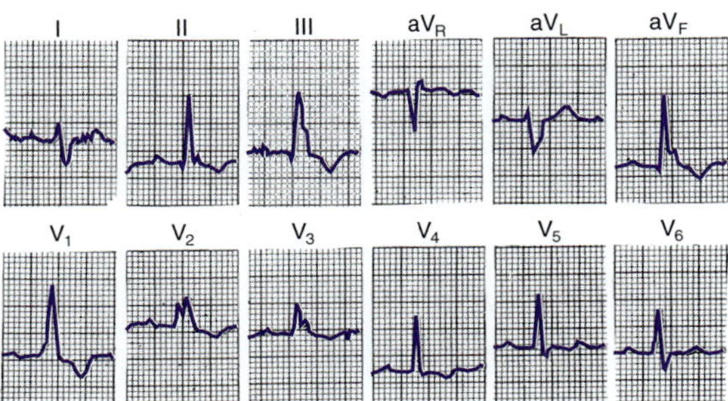

(From Goldberger AL. *Clinical Electrocardiography: A Simplified Approach*, 6th ed. St. Louis: Mosby; 1999, p 70.)

8. Which of the following is usually produced by subendocardial ischemia?
   A) ST elevation.
   B) ST depression.
   C) Q waves.
   D) U waves.

9. In the ECG strip shown below, which of the following arrhythmias is present?
   A) Premature ventricular contractions.
   B) Ventricular tachycardia.
   C) Ventricular trigeminy.
   D) Ventricular bigeminy.

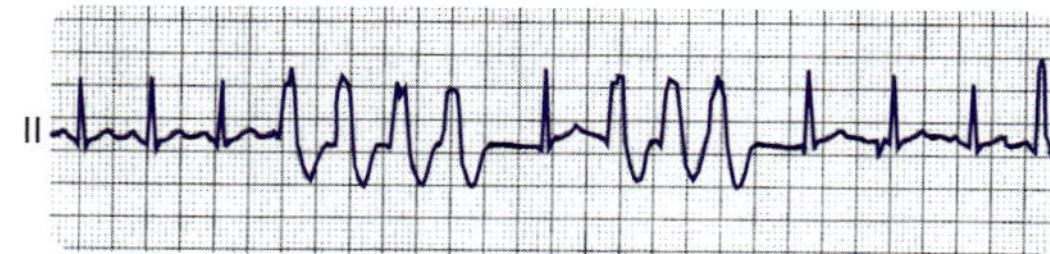

(From Goldberger AL. *Clinical Electrocardiography: A Simplified Approach*, 6th ed. St. Louis: Mosby; 1999, p 167.)

10. In the ECG strip shown below, which of the following arrhythmias is indicated?
    A) Atrial flutter.
    B) Atrial fibrillation.
    C) Premature atrial contractions.
    D) Atrial tachycardia.

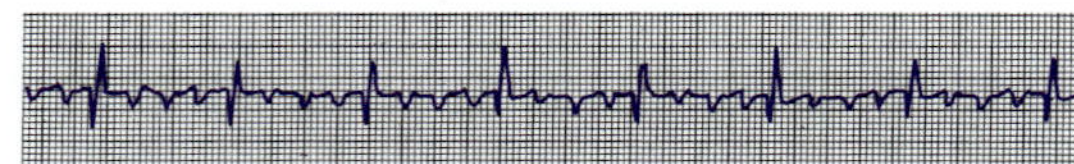

(From Goldberger AL. *Clinical Electrocardiography: A Simplified Approach*, 6th ed. St. Louis: Mosby; 1999, p 164.)

11. Abnormally tall and peaked T waves suggest which of the following?
    A) Hypercalcemia.
    B) Acute pericarditis.
    C) Acute myocardial infarction.
    D) Hypokalemia.

12. Which of the following conditions can prolong the QT interval?
    A) Hypokalemia and hypercalcemia.
    B) Hyperkalemia and hypercalcemia.
    C) Hypocalcemia and hypokalemia.
    D) Hypocalcemia and hyperkalemia.

13. Differentiation between supraventricular and ventricular rhythm is often made on the basis of which of the following?
    A) Duration (width) of the QRS complex and presence or absence of P waves.
    B) Appearance of the ST segment.
    C) Amplitude of the U wave.
    D) Duration of the PR interval.

14. Which of the following is one cause of a wide QRS complex?
    A) Hypokalemia.
    B) Defective intraventricular conduction.
    C) Right atrial enlargement.
    D) Abnormal ST segment.

15. Which of the following is the process by which movements of ions occur in response to various stimuli, causing the rapid loss of the internal negative potential?
    A) Polarization.
    B) Repolarization.
    C) Automaticity.
    D) Depolarization.

16. Which of the following refers the digitalis effect?
    A) Scooped-out depression of the ST segment.
    B) Elevation of the PR interval.
    C) Shortening of the QT interval.
    D) Prolongation of the QRS complex.

17. Tall positive T waves may be caused by all of the following EXCEPT
    A) Hyperacute phase of myocardial infarction.
    B) Left ventricular hypertrophy.
    C) Acute pericarditis.
    D) Hypocalcemia.

18. In the ECG strip shown below, what abnormalities are indicated?
    A) Left atrial enlargement and left ventricular hypertrophy.
    B) Right atrial enlargement and right ventricular hypertrophy.
    C) Left anterior fascicular block and left posterior fascicular block.
    D) Subendocardial ischemia and infarction.

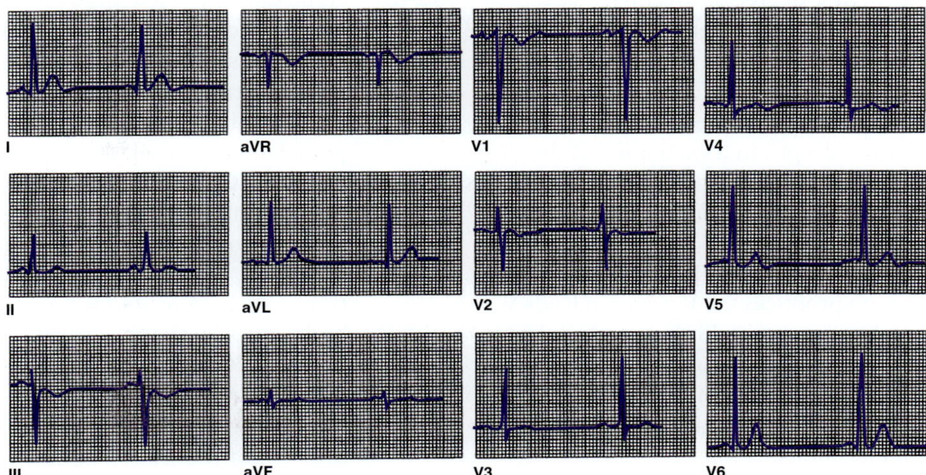

(From Thaler MS. *The Only EKG Book You'll Ever Need*, 3rd ed. Philadelphia: Lippincott Williams & Wilkins; 1999, p 87.)

19. Which of the following may be indicated by right axis deviation?
    A) Acute pericarditis.
    B) Right atrial enlargement.
    C) Chronic obstructive pulmonary disease.
    D) Cardiomyopathy.

20. In atrial flutter, which of the following represents the approximate atrial stimulation rate?
    A) 75 beats/minute.
    B) 125 beats/minute.
    C) 200 beats/minute.
    D) 300 beats/minute.

21. Myocardial cells can be excited in response to all of the following stimuli EXCEPT
    A) Electrical.
    B) Chemical.
    C) Mechanical.
    D) Emotional.

22. Which of the following is correct regarding the P-wave deflection on an ECG?
    A) Negative.
    B) Positive.
    C) Isoelectric.
    D) Either positive or negative.

ANSWERS AND EXPLANATIONS

1–A. The PR interval represents the time that it takes for the stimulus to spread through the atria and pass through the atrioventricular (AV) junction. As such, slow conduction in the AV node affects the PR interval. Slow conduction through the AV node is not associated with the duration of either the QRS complex or the QT interval.

2–B. The mean QRS axis is 60°. Notice the biphasic QRS complex in lead aVL. As such, the mean QRS axis must point at a right angle to –30°. Obviously, it points at 60°, because leads II, III, and aVF show positive QRS complexes.

3–C. Notice the QS in lead V_1 and the wide R wave in lead V_6. The PR interval is prolonged (>0.20 second). As such, first-degree atrioventricular block is present. There is no progressive PR prolongation with a nonconducted P wave; therefore, Mobitz I is not present.

4–D. Acute pericarditis is associated with ST-segment elevations. Digitalis produces scooping of the ST-T complex. Hypokalemia produces ST depression, and hypocalcemia prolongs the QT interval.

5–B. Notice the Q waves in leads II, III, and aVF. Posterior infarction produces tall R waves in leads V_1 and V_2. Anterior myocardial infarction results in the loss of R-wave progression in the precordial leads and pathologic waves in one or more of the chest leads. Acute pericarditis produces diffuse ST-segment elevations.

6–D. Notice the tall R waves in leads V_1 and V_2. Also notice the Q waves in leads III and aVF. Acute inferior myocardial infarction produces ST-segment elevation in leads II, III, and aVF.

7–C. Notice the wide notched R wave in lead V_2 and the secondary T-wave inversions in leads V_1, V_2, II, III, and aVF. Left bundle branch block produces a wide QS in lead V_1 and a wide R wave in lead V_6. Posterior wall myocardial infarction produces tall R waves in leads V_1 and V_2 with ST-segment depression in the same leads. Left ventricular hypertrophy produces high voltages, marked by tall R waves in lead V_5 or V_6 and deep S waves in lead V_1 or V_2.

8–B. Subendocardial ischemia usually produces ST depression. ST elevations usually appear in transmural ischemia, pericarditis, and acute myocardial infarction (MI). Q waves appear following transmural MI, and U waves are often seen in hypokalemia.

9–B. Ventricular tachycardia is defined as a run of three or more consecutive premature ventricular contractions (PVCs). In ventricular bigeminy, each normal sinus impulse is followed by a PVC. In ventricular trigeminy, a PVC is seen after every two sinus impulses.

10–A. Atrial flutter is characterized by "sawtooth" flutter waves instead of P waves, with a constant or variable ventricular rate. Atrial fibrillation shows fibrillatory waves instead of P waves and an irregular ventricular rate. Atrial tachycardia is defined as three or more consecutive premature atrial beats.

11–A. Hyperkalemia and acute myocardial infarction often show abnormally tall and peaked T waves. Hypokalemia often produces ST depressions with prominent U waves.

12–D. Hypokalemia often produces low-amplitude T waves and sometimes large U waves, which merge, resulting in a prolonged QT interval. Hypocalcemia primarily prolongs the ST segment, resulting in a prolonged QT interval. Hyperkalemia causes narrowed and peaked T waves.

13–A. A narrow QRS complex (<0.1 second) indicates that the entire ventricular myocardium was depolarized quickly. This can occur only if electrical activation spreads along the ventricular conduction system. A wide QRS complex (>0.10 second) suggests that electrical activation required considerable time to spread. As such, the impulse did not use the ventricular conduction system to travel. The duration of the PR interval is an indication of the time required for the impulse to travel from the SA node down to the AV node. The ST segment represents the beginning of ventricular repolarization, and U waves are characteristic of hypokalemia or drug therapy.

14–B. A lesion in the ventricular conduction system will cause a slower spread of activation throughout the ventricles, leading to a wide QRS complex. Hypokalemia does not affect the duration of the QRS complex. Hypokalemia produces ST depressions and prominent U waves. The ST segment represents the beginning of ventricular repolarization and is not related to the duration of the QRS complex.

15–D. In response to various stimuli, cations (mainly sodium) move inward, causing rapid loss of the internal negative potential. This process is known as depolarization. Polarization refers to the resting state of cardiac muscle cells where the interior of a cell is more negative compared with the exterior. Repolarization is the return of cardiac muscle cells to their resting negative potential. Automaticity refers to the ability of the heart to initiate its own beat.

16–A. Digitalis effect refers to the characteristic scooped-out depression of the ST segment produced by therapeutic doses of digitalis. A therapeutic dose of digitalis does not produce ST-segment elevation. ST-segment elevations are often observed in myocardial ischemia or infarction, acute pericarditis, hyperkalemia, and left ventricular hypertrophy. Hypercalcemia is often associated with shortening of the QT interval owing to shortening of the ST segment.

17–D. The hyperacute phase of a myocardial infarction often produces tall positive T waves. Tall positive T waves are also seen in left ventricular hypertrophy (left precordial leads). Acute pericarditis is occasionally associated with tall T waves.

18–A. Left atrial enlargement is manifested by P-wave duration of >0.11 second, P-wave notching, and a negative P-wave deflection in V_1. Left ventricular hypertrophy is demonstrated by large R waves (>27 mm) in lead V_5 plus deep waves in lead V_1. Left anterior hemiblock is associated with a mean QRS axis of $-45°$ and a QRS width of <0.12 second.

19–C. Chronic obstructive pulmonary disease causes right axis deviation because of right ventricular overload. Any cause of right ventricular hypertrophy, such as pulmonic stenosis or primary pulmonary hypertension, is also associated with right axis deviation. Cardiomyopathy is associated with dilation and usually with diffuse fibrosis.

20–D. With atrial flutter, the atrial stimulation rate is about 300 beats/minute and the ventricular rate varies, depending on the ability of the atrioventricular junction to transmit stimuli from the atria to the ventricles. In atrial flutter, the ventricular rate may not vary.

21–D. All myocardial cells can be stimulated by external electrical, chemical, and mechanical stimuli. The myocardium comprises ordinary contractile cells located in the atria and ventricles as well as specialized cells that conduct the impulses.

22–D. The P wave on the electrocardiogram can be either positive or negative, depending on the lead. For example, the P wave is always negative in a normal aVR lead, and always positive in a normal V_6 lead.

APPENDIX

A Health and Fitness Comprehensive Examination

DIRECTIONS: Each of the numbered items or incomplete statements in this section is followed by answers or by completions of the statement. Select the ONE lettered answer or completion that is BEST in each case.

1. Which of the following exercise modes allows buoyancy to reduce the potential for musculoskeletal injury?
   A) Cycling.
   B) Walking.
   C) Skiing.
   D) Water exercise.

2. In the first 2 seconds of a 100-m race, on which of the following energy systems does skeletal muscle rely most heavily?
   A) ATP-PC.
   B) Anaerobic glycolysis.
   C) Oxidative phosphorylation.
   D) Free fatty acid metabolism.

3. Which of the following medications is designed to modify blood cholesterol levels?
   A) Nitrates.
   B) β-blockers.
   C) Antihyperlipidemics.
   D) β-Blockers

4. Which of the following represents more than 90% of the fat stored in the body and is composed of a glycerol molecule connected to three fatty acids?
   A) Phospholipids.
   B) Cholesterol.
   C) Triglycerides.
   D) Free fatty acids.

5. Limited flexibility of which of the following muscle groups increases the risk of low back pain?
   A) Quadriceps.
   B) Hamstrings.
   C) Hip flexors.
   D) Biceps femoris.

6. Calcium, phosphorus, magnesium, potassium, sulfur, sodium, and chloride are examples of ___.
   A) Macrominerals.
   B) Microminerals.
   C) Proteins.
   D) Vitamins.

7. Which of the following terms represents an imaginary horizontal plane passing through the midsection of the body and dividing it into upper and lower portions?
   A) Sagittal.
   B) Frontal.
   C) Transverse.
   D) Superior.

8. Which of the following is a function of bone?
   A) Provides structural support for the entire body.
   B) Serves as a lever that can change the magnitude and direction of forces generated by skeletal muscles.
   C) Protects organs and tissues.
   D) All of the above.

9. Which of the following blood pressure readings would characterize hypertension in the adult?
   A) 100/60 mmHg.
   B) 110/70 mmHg.
   C) 120/80 mmHg.
   D) 140/90 mmHg.

10. The term **risk stratification** refers to ___.
    A) The risk for the client to travel by airplane.
    B) The ability of the client to perform high-intensity exercise.
    C) The placing of clients into categories based on risk factors and disease identification.
    D) The identification of latent or overt coronary artery disease.

11. Uncoordinated gait, headache, dizziness, vomiting, and elevated body temperature are signs and symptoms of
    A) Acute exposure to the cold.
    B) Hypothermia.
    C) Heat exhaustion and heat stroke.
    D) Acute altitude sickness.

12. Moving the hand from palm up to palm down with the elbow flexed at 90 degrees
    A) Adducts the ulna.

B) Internally rotates the radius.
C) Internally rotates the humerus.
D) Flexes the ulna.

13. Which of the following energy systems is capable of using all three fuels (carbohydrates, fats, and proteins)?
A) Anaerobic glycolysis.
B) Lactic acid system.
C) Phosphagen system.
D) Aerobic system.

14. What is a subject's work rate in watts if he pedals on a Monark cycle ergometer at 5 revolutions per minute (RPM) at a resistance of 2.0 kiloponds? Assume that one revolution of the cycle ergometer flywheel is 6 m long.
A) 10 W.
B) 50 W.
C) 100 W.
D) 200 W.

15. Relative proportions of fat and fat-free (lean) tissue can be reported as
A) Percentage body fat.
B) Relative composition.
C) Body mass index.
D) Weight-to-waist circumference ratio.

16. How many calories are contained in a food bar that contains 5 g of fat, 30 g of carbohydrates including 4 g of fiber, and 3 g of protein?
A) 161 kcal.
B) 168 kcal.
C) 177 kcal.
D) 193 kcal.

17. The interconnected sacs and tubes surrounding each myofibril in which calcium ions are stored are referred to as
A) Terminal cisternae.
B) Sarcomeres.
C) Myofilaments.
D) Sarcoplasmic reticulum.

18. Anaerobic glycolysis also is known as the
A) Phosphagen system.
B) Aerobic metabolism.
C) Lactic acid system.
D) None of the above.

19. Regular exercise will result in what chronic adaptation in cardiac output during exercise at the same workload?
A) Increase.
B) Decrease.
C) No change.
D) Increase during dynamic exercise only.

20. Which of the following conditions is characterized by a decrease in bone mass and density, producing bone porosity and fragility?
A) Osteoarthritis.
B) Osteomyelitis.
C) Epiphyseal osteomyelitis.
D) Osteoporosis.

21. Studies designed to measure the success of a program based on some quantifiable data that can be analyzed examine
A) Incomes.
B) Outcomes.
C) Client progress notes.
D) Attendance records.

22. When using the original Borg scale (6–20) for the general public, intensity should be maintained between
A) 7 and 10.
B) 12 and 16.
C) 17 and 18.
D) 19 and 20.

23. Muscle fibers that can produce a large amount of tension in a very short period of time but fatigue quickly are referred to as
A) Slow-twitch glycolytic.
B) Fast-twitch glycolytic.
C) Fast-twitch oxidative.
D) Slow-twitch oxidative.

24. Rotation of the anterior surface of a bone toward the midline of the body is called
A) Medial rotation.
B) Lateral rotation.
C) Supination.
D) Pronation.

25. The smallest, narrowest passage within the bronchial system is called the
A) Lobe.
B) Trachea.
C) Bronchiole.
D) Nasopharynx.

26. Cardiac output can be calculated by multiplying
A) Heart rate and stroke volume.
B) Stroke volume and the difference between the oxygen-carrying capacity of the arterial blood and venous blood.
C) Oxygen consumption and heart rate.
D) Heart rate and blood volume.

27. A source of intimal injury thought to initiate the process of atherogenesis is
A) Dyslipidemia.
B) Hypertension.

C) Turbulence of blood flow within the vessel.
D) All of the above.

28. At what level is high-density lipoprotein considered a risk factor in the development of cardiovascular disease?
A) <200 mg/dL.
B) <110 mg/dL.
C) <60 mg/dL.
D) <35 mg/dL.

29. Which of the following health history combinations would place an individual into the MODERATE RISK category for coronary artery disease?
A) HDL <40 mg/dL; current smoker; female waist-to-hip ratio <0.86.
B) HDL >60 mg/dL; current smoker; male waist girth >102 cm.
C) HDL <40 mg/dL; current smoker; BMI <28.
D) HDL >60 mg/dL; current smoker; fasting blood glucose >100.

30. What could be an alternative to the contraindicated, high-risk plough exercise?
A) Squats to 90 degrees.
B) Flexion with rotation.
C) Double knee to chest.
D) Lateral neck stretches.

31. Which of the following water-soluble vitamins must be consumed on a daily basis?
A) Vitamins A and C.
B) Vitamins A, D, E and K.
C) Vitamins B complex and C.
D) Vitamins A, B complex, D, and K.

32. What muscles of the heart contract to tighten the chordae tendinea, and are connected on the inner surface of the ventricle?
A) Myocardial muscles.
B) Papillary muscles.
C) Endocardial muscles.
D) Epicardial muscles.

33. An individual's maximal oxygen consumption ($\dot{V}O_{2max}$) is a measure of the power of the aerobic energy system. This value is generally regarded as the best indicator of aerobic fitness. At what percentage of one's $\dot{V}O_{2max}$ does the anaerobic threshold occur in untrained individuals?
A) 55%.
B) 65%.
C) 75%.
D) 85%.

34. What type of muscle tissue is the most abundant in the body?
A) Arteries.
B) Cardiac.
C) Skeletal.
D) Smooth.

35. Which of the following is NOT true regarding the psychological benefits of regular exercise in the elderly?
A) Self-concept.
B) Life satisfaction.
C) Stimulate appetite.
D) Self-efficacy.

36. What is angina pectoris?
A) Discomfort associated with myocardial ischemia.
B) Discomfort associated with hypertension.
C) Discomfort associated with heartburn.
D) Discomfort associated with papillary necrosis.

37. To determine program effectiveness, psychological theories provide a conceptual framework for assessment and
A) Management of programs or interventions.
B) Application of cognitive-behavioral or motivational principles.
C) Measurement.
D) All of the above.

38. Information gathered by way of an appropriate health screening allows the health/fitness specialist to develop specific exercise programs that are appropriate to the individual needs and goals of the client. This is called the
A) Physical Activity Readiness Questionnaire (PAR-Q).
B) Heart rate.
C) Exercise prescription.
D) Graded exercise test.

39. To maximize safety during a physical fitness assessment, which of the following items should be addressed?
A) Hospital emergency room services.
B) Cardiopulmonary resuscitation training of the assessment administrator.
C) Emergency plan.
D) All of the above.

40. Some externally applied forces, such as exercise pulleys, do not act in a vertical direction as do weights attached to the body because
A) Weights applied to the body behave as weights of body segments, thus changing the torque and altering the difficulty of an exercise when weight is applied.
B) A distractive force sometimes is used to promote normal joint movement.
C) The angle of application changes in different parts of the range of motion, causing a change in the magnitude of the rotary component of the force and, thus, the torque.

D) The force of the pulley is applied through an arc rather than in a straight trajectory.

41. During contraction of skeletal muscle, the force generated by the whole muscle is a function of
A) The size of the myofibers within the muscle that are twitching and the rate at which the twitches occur.
B) The number of myofibers within the muscle that are twitching and the rate at which the twitches occur.
C) The number of myofibers within the muscle that are twitching and the strength of the action potential.
D) The size of the myofibers within the muscle that are twitching and the strength of the action potential.

42. Heart rate can be measured by counting the number of pulses in a specified time period at one of several locations, including the radial, femoral, and carotid arteries. Which of the following is a special precaution when taking the carotid pulse?
A) When the heart rate is measured by palpation, the first two fingers should be used and not the thumb, because the thumb has its own pulse.
B) Heart rates taken during exercise sometimes exceed 200 bpm, making it too difficult to count at the carotid artery.
C) If the heart rate is taken at the carotid artery, do not press too hard, or a reflex slowing of the heart can occur and cause dizziness.
D) The heart rate should never be taken at the carotid artery.

43. As a result of regular exercise training, which of the following is NOT affected during maximal exercise?
A) Cardiac output.
B) Stroke volume.
C) Maximal heart rate.
D) None of the above.

44. When exercise training children,
A) Exercise programs should increase physical fitness in the short term and strength and stamina in the long term.
B) Strength training should be avoided for safety reasons.
C) Increasing the rate of training intensity more than approximately 10% per week increases the likelihood of overuse injuries of bone.
D) Children with exercise-induced asthma are often unable to lead active lives.

45. Which of the following risk factors for the development of coronary artery disease has the greatest likelihood of being influenced by regular exercise?
A) Smoking.
B) Cholesterol.
C) Type I diabetes.
D) Hypertension.

46. At minimum, professionals performing fitness assessments on others should possess which combination of the following?
A) Cardiopulmonary resuscitation (CPR) and ACSM Health/Fitness Specialist.
B) Advanced cardiac life support and ACSM Exercise Specialist.
C) Advanced cardiac life support and ACSM Registered Clinical Exercise Physiologist.
D) Only physicians can perform fitness assessments.

47. Which of the following components of the exercise prescription work inversely with each other?
A) Intensity and duration.
B) Mode and intensity.
C) Mode and duration.
D) Mode and frequency.

48. Which of the following types of muscle stretching can cause residual muscle soreness, is time consuming, and typically requires a partner?
A) Static.
B) Ballistic.
C) Proprioceptive neuromuscular facilitation.
D) All of the above.

49. Glucose, fructose, and sucrose commonly are referred to as
A) Proteins.
B) Complex carbohydrates.
C) Simple carbohydrates.
D) Fats.

50. Failure of a health/fitness specialist to perform in a generally acceptable standard is called
A) Malpractice.
B) Malfeasance.
C) Negligence.
D) None of the above.

51. All energy for muscular contraction must come from the breakdown of a chemical compound called
A) Adenosine triphosphate (ATP).
B) Guanosine triphosphate (GTP).
C) Nicotinamide adenine dinucleotide (NAD).
D) Flavin adenine dinucleotide ($FADH_2$).

52. What two regulatory proteins are found within the actin complex of skeletal muscle?
A) Epimysium and perimysium.
B) Perimysium and endomysium.
C) Troponin and tropomyosin.
D) Myosin and troponin.

53. From rest to maximal exercise, the systolic blood pressure should ______ with an increasing workload.
A) Increase.

B) Decrease.
C) Stay the same.
D) Decrease with isometric or increase with isotonic contractions.

54. Most sedentary people who begin an exercise program are likely to stop within
A) 1 to 2 days.
B) 3 to 6 weeks.
C) 1 month.
D) 3 to 6 months.

55. Reasons for fitness testing of the older adult include
A) Evaluation of progress.
B) Exercise prescription.
C) Motivation.
D) All of the above.

56. A body weight of 15% less than expected, a morbid fear of fatness, a preoccupation with food, and an abnormal body image are symptoms of
A) Bulimia nervosa.
B) Dieting.
C) Anorexia nervosa.
D) Obesity.

57. The process of adding a second stimulus to a muscle fiber that has already been excited is known as
A) Twitch.
B) Tetanus.
C) Summation.
D) Motor unit.

58. What is the energy cost of running at 6.5 mph up a grade of 5%?
A) 8.2 METs.
B) 10.2 METs.
C) 13.2 METs.
D) 15.2 METs.

59. Feeling good about being able to perform an activity or skill, such as finally being able to run a mile or to increase the speed of walking a mile, is an example of an:
A) Extrinsic reward.
B) Intrinsic reward.
C) External stimulus.
D) Internal stimulus.

60. Albuterol, terbutaline, glucocorticosteroids, cromolyn sodium, and theophylline are effective drugs that prevent or reverse
A) Coronary artery disease.
B) Emphysema.
C) Asthma.
D) Cancer.

61. An important safety consideration for exercise equipment in a fitness center includes
A) Flexibility of equipment to allow for different body sizes.
B) Size of equipment to accommodate small and large clients.
C) Affordability of equipment to allow for changing out equipment periodically.
D) Mobility of equipment to allow for easy rearrangement.

62. The ACSM recommendation for intensity, duration, and frequency of cardiorespiratory exercise for apparently healthy individuals includes
A) Intensity of 60% to 90% maximal heart rate, duration of 20 to 60 minutes, and frequency of 3 to 5 days a week.
B) Intensity of 85% to 90% maximal heart rate, duration of 30 minutes, and frequency of 3 days a week.
C) Intensity of 50% to 70% maximal heart rate, duration of 15 to 45 minutes, and frequency of 5 days a week.
D) Intensity of 60% to 90% maximal heart rate reserve, duration of 20 to 60 minutes, and frequency of 7 days a week.

63. A method of strength and power training that involves an eccentric loading of muscles and tendons followed immediately by an explosive concentric contraction is called
A) Plyometrics.
B) Periodization.
C) Super-sets.
D) Isotonic reversals.

64. Which of the following personnel is responsible for program design as well as implementation of that program?
A) Administrative assistant.
B) Exercise specialist.
C) Manager/director.
D) Health/fitness specialist.

65. What is the purpose of agreements, releases, and consent forms?
A) To inform the client of participation risks, as well as the rights of the client and the facility.
B) To inform the client what he or she can and cannot do in the facility.
C) To define the relationship between the facility operator and the health/fitness specialist.
D) To detail the rights and responsibilities of the club owner to reject an application by a prospective client.

66. Sufficient ATP is stored in a given skeletal muscle to fuel how many seconds of activity?
A) 2 to 3.
B) 5 to 10.
C) 10 to 20.
D) 45 to 60.

67. The sliding filament theory of muscle contraction depends on the interaction of the contractile proteins actin and myosin. At rest, no interaction occurs. When called on to contract, these two proteins create an interdigitation, and the muscle then contracts. This process is dependent on the presence of
   A) Magnesium.
   B) Manganese.
   C) Creatine.
   D) Calcium.

68. After 30 years of age, skeletal muscle strength begins to decline, primarily because of which of the following?
   A) A gain in fat tissue.
   B) A gain in lean tissue.
   C) A loss of muscle mass caused by a loss of muscle fibers.
   D) Myogenic precursor cell inhibition.

69. At what rate does an acute cardiovascular event occur in men during exercise?
   A) 1 in 20,000 hours.
   B) 1 in 57,000 hours.
   C) 1 in 187,500 hours.
   D) 1 in 1 million hours.

70. Which of the following is a complex carbohydrate that is not digestible by the body and passes straight through the digestive system?
   A) Triglycerides.
   B) Proteins.
   C) Sugars.
   D) Fiber.

71. The Health Belief Model assumes that people will engage in a behavior, such as exercise, when
   A) There is a perceived threat of disease.
   B) External motivation is provided.
   C) Optimal environmental conditions are met.
   D) Internal motivation outweighs external circumstances.

72. The informed consent document
   A) Is a legal document.
   B) Provides immunity from prosecution.
   C) Provides an explanation of the test to the client.
   D) Legally protects the rights of the client.

73. A measure of muscular endurance is
   A) One-repetition maximum.
   B) Three-repetition maximum.
   C) Number of curl-ups in 1 minute.
   D) Number of curl-ups in 3 minutes.

74. If a client exercises too much without rest days or develops a minor injury and does not allow time for the injury to heal, what can occur?
   A) An overuse injury.
   B) Shin splints.
   C) Sleep deprivation.
   D) Decreased physical conditioning.

75. The ACSM recommends that exercise intensity be prescribed within what percentage of maximal heart rate range?
   A) 40% and 60%.
   B) 50% and 80%.
   C) 60% and 90%.
   D) 70% and 100%.

76. The ACSM recommends how many repetitions of each exercise for muscular strength and endurance?
   A) 5 to 6.
   B) 8 to 12.
   C) 12 to 20.
   D) More than 20.

77. For higher intensity activities
   A) The benefit outweighs any potential risk.
   B) The risk of orthopedic and cardiovascular complications are increased.
   C) The risk of orthopedic and cardiovascular complications are minimal.
   D) There is no increased risk of orthopedic and cardiovascular complications.

78. Auscultation of the heart rate refers to
   A) Feeling the pulse at the radial artery.
   B) Listening to the sounds of the heart through the chest.
   C) Feeling the pulse at the carotid artery.
   D) Counting the pulse rate at the carotid, radial, or femoral arteries.

79. Which of the following are changes seen as a result of regular, chronic exercise?
   A) Decreased heart rate at rest.
   B) Increased stroke volume at rest.
   C) No change in cardiac output at rest.
   D) All of the above.

80. The heart (unlike skeletal muscle) has its own capability to produce an action potential. If an electrical impulse is not received from higher-level brain centers, cardiac muscle will stimulate itself. This is called
   A) Tetany.
   B) Simulated contraction.
   C) Diastole.
   D) Autorhythmicity.

81. Maximal exercise testing has been labeled by some medical experts as a dangerous situation for most people. Actually, the death rate during maximal exercise testing is approximately
   A) 0.01%.
   B) 1%.
   C) 10%.
   D) 5%.

82. While assessing the behavioral changes associated with an exercise program, which of the following would be categorized under the cognitive process of the Transtheoretical Model?
   A) Stimulus control.
   B) Reinforcement management
   C) Self-reevaluation.
   D) Self-liberation.

83. Fitness assessment is an important aspect of the training program because it provides information for which of the following?
   A) Developing the exercise prescription.
   B) Evaluating proper nutritional choices.
   C) Diagnosing musculoskeletal injury.
   D) Developing appropriate billing categories.

84. Following an acute musculoskeletal injury, the appropriate action calls for stabilization of the area and incorporating the RICE treatment method. RICE is the acronym for which of the following?
   A) Recovery, Ibuprofen, Compression, Education.
   B) Rest and Ice for injury Care.
   C) Rest, Ice, Compression, Elevation.
   D) Rotate, Ice, Care, Evaluate.

85. A resistance training program that starts with light weights and high repetitions for the first set and then gradually moves to heavier weights and fewer repetitions for each successive set, would be an example of which of the following training style?
   A) Circuits.
   B) Super-sets.
   C) Split routines.
   D) Pyramids.

86. For individuals undertaking nonmedically supervised weight loss initiatives to reduce energy intake, the ACSM recommends weight loss of approximately:
   A) 1 to 2 lb per week (0.5–1 kg).
   B) 5 to 8 lb per week (2.3–4 kg).
   C) 8 to 10 lb per week (4–4.5 kg).
   D) 10 to 15 lb per week (4.5–7 kg).

87. A client with scoliosis exhibits which of the following conditions?
   A) A chronic, inflammatory, demyelinating disease.
   B) An abnormal curvature of the spine.
   C) Softening of the articular cartilage.
   D) Inflammation of the growth plate at the tibial tuberosity.

88. Which of the following assumes that a person will adopt appropriate health behaviors if they feel the consequences are severe and feel personally vulnerable?
   A) Learning theories.
   B) Health Belief Model.
   C) Transtheoretical Model.
   D) Stages of Motivational Readiness.

89. Identify the appropriate self-directed evaluation tool used as a quick health screening before beginning any exercise program.
   A) Minnesota Multiphasic Personality Inventory (MMPI).
   B) Ratings of Perceived Exertion (RPE-Borg scale).
   C) Physical Activity Readiness Questionnaire (PAR-Q).
   D) Exercise Electrocardiogram (E-ECG).

90. You have examined your patient's health-screening documents and obtained physiologic resting measurements and you decide to proceed with a single session of fitness assessments. Identify the recommended order of administration.
   A) Flexibility, cardiorespiratory fitness, body composition, and muscular fitness.
   B) Flexibility, body composition, muscular fitness, and cardiorespiratory fitness.
   C) Body composition, cardiorespiratory fitness, muscular fitness, and flexibility.
   D) Body composition, flexibility, cardiorespiratory fitness, and muscular fitness.

91. Implementing emergency procedures must include the fitness center's
   A) Management.
   B) Staff.
   C) Clients.
   D) Management and staff.

92. Which of the following is a possible medical emergency that a client can experience during an exercise session?
   A) Hypoglycemia.
   B) Hypotension.
   C) Hyperglycemia.
   D) All of the above.

93. During a graded exercise test, blood pressure must be taken at least how often?
   A) Twice.
   B) Twice during each stage.
   C) Once during each stage.
   D) Every minute.

94. Which of the following muscle actions occurs when muscle tension increases but the length of the muscle does not change?
   A) Concentric isotonic.
   B) Eccentric isotonic.
   C) Isokinetic.
   D) Isometric.

95. Which macronutrient should comprise 45% to 65% of an individual's total energy intake?
   A) Fats.

B) Proteins.
C) Carbohydrates.
D) Alcohol.

96. Which of the following activities provides the greatest improvement in aerobic fitness for someone who is beginning an exercise program?
A) Weight training.
B) Downhill snow skiing.
C) Stretching.
D) Walking.

97. In commercial settings, clients should be more extensively screened for potential health risks. The information solicited should include which of the following?
A) Personal medical history.
B) Present medical status.
C) Medication.
D) All of the above.

98. Generally, low-fit or sedentary persons may benefit from
A) Shorter duration, higher intensity, and higher frequency of exercise.
B) Longer duration, higher intensity, and higher frequency of exercise.
C) Shorter duration, lower intensity, and higher frequency of exercise.
D) Shorter duration, higher intensity, and lower frequency of exercise.

99. What is the planning tool that addresses the organization's short- and long-term goals, identifies the steps needed to achieve the goals, and gives the timeline, priority, and allocation of resources to each goal?
A) Financial plan.
B) Strategic plan.
C) Risk management plan.
D) Marketing plan.

ANSWERS AND EXPLANATIONS

1–D. Water exercise has gained in popularity, because the buoyancy properties of water help to reduce the potential for musculoskeletal injury and may even allow injured people an opportunity to exercise without further injury. A variety of activities may be offered in a water-exercise class. Walking, jogging, and dance activity all may be adapted for water. Water-exercise classes typically should combine the benefits of the buoyancy properties of water with the resistive properties of water. In this regard, both an aerobic stimulus as well as activity to enhance muscular strength and endurance may be provided.
[Chapter 8]

2–A. Because the number of reactions is small (basically two), the ATP-PC system can provide ATP at a very fast rate. Sufficient PC is stored in skeletal muscle for approximately 25 seconds of high-intensity work. Therefore, the ATP-PC system will last for approximately 30 seconds (5 seconds for stored ATP, and 25 seconds for PC).
[Chapter 2]

3–C. Nitrates and nitroglycerine are antianginals (used to reduce chest pain associated with angina pectoris). β-Blockers are antihypertensives (used to reduce blood pressure by inhibiting the action of adrenergic neurotransmitters at the β-receptor, thereby promoting peripheral vasodilation). β-Blockers also are designed to reduce blood pressure by inhibiting the action of adrenergic neurotransmitters at the β-receptors, thereby decreasing cardiac output. Antihyperlipidemics control blood lipids, especially cholesterol and LDL.
[Chapter 4]

4–C. Dietary fats include triglycerides, sterols (e.g., cholesterol), and phospholipids. Triglycerides represent more than 90% of the fat stored in the body. A triglyceride is a glycerol molecule connected to three fatty acid molecules. The fatty acids are identified by the amount of "saturation" or the number of single or double bonds that link the carbon atoms. Saturated fatty acids only have single bonds. Monounsaturated fatty acids have one double bond, and polyunsaturated fatty acids have two or more double bonds.
[Chapter 9]

5–B. An adequate range of motion or joint mobility is requisite for optimal musculoskeletal health. Specifically, limited flexibility of the low back and hamstring regions may relate to an increased risk for development of chronic low back pain and disability. Activities that will enhance or maintain musculoskeletal flexibility should be included as a part of a comprehensive preventive or rehabilitative exercise program.

6–A. Minerals are inorganic substances that perform a variety of functions in the body. Many play an important role in assisting enzymes (or coenzymes) that are necessary for the proper functioning of body systems. They also are found in cell membranes, hormones, muscles, and connective tissues as well as electrolytes in body fluids. Minerals are considered to be either macrominerals (needed in relatively large doses), such

as calcium, phosphorus, magnesium, potassium, sulfur, sodium, and chloride; or microminerals (needed in very small amounts), such as iron, zinc, selenium, manganese, molybdenum, iodine, copper, chromium, and fluoride.
[Chapter 9]

7–C. The body has three cardinal planes, and each individual plane is perpendicular to the other two. Movement occurs along these planes. The sagittal plane divides the body into right and left parts, and the midsagittal plane is represented by an imaginary vertical plane passing through the midline of the body, dividing it into right and left halves. The frontal plane is represented by an imaginary vertical plane passing through the body, dividing it into front and back halves. The transverse plane represents an imaginary horizontal plane passing through the midsection of the body and dividing it into upper and lower portions.
[Chapter 1]

8–D. The bones of the skeletal system perform five functions: They provide structural support for the entire body, serve as levers that can change the magnitude and direction of forces generated by skeletal muscles, protect organs and tissues, provide storage of minerals, and produce red blood cells and other elements within the bone marrow.
[Chapter 1]

9–D. To be classified as hypertensive, the systolic blood pressure must equal or exceed 140 mm Hg or the diastolic pressure must equal or exceed 90 mm HG as measured on two separate occasions, preferably days apart. An elevation of either the systolic or diastolic pressure is classified as hypertension.
[Chapter 4]

10–C. The purpose of risk stratification is to identify high-risk individuals (persons with contraindications leading to potential exclusion from testing or exercise, individuals with disease symptoms or risk factors that require medical evaluation before testing or exercise, individuals with clinically significant disease that requires medical supervision during testing or exercise, or individuals with special testing or exercise needs) and to select the appropriate activities for those persons. Risk categories include apparently healthy, low risk, moderate risk, and high risk.
[Chapter 6]

11–C. Heat exhaustion and heat stroke are serious conditions that result from a combination of the metabolic heat generated from exercise accompanied by dehydration and electrolyte loss from sweating. Signs and symptoms include uncoordinated gait, headache, dizziness, vomiting, and elevated body temperature. If these conditions are present, exercise must be stopped. Attempts to rehydrate, perhaps intravenously, should be attempted, and the body must be cooled by any means possible. The person should be placed in the supine position, with the feet elevated.

12–B. Rotation is a movement of long bones about their long axis. Angular movements decrease or increase the joint angle produced by the articulating bones. The four types of angular movements are flexion (a movement that decreases the joint angle, bringing the bones closer together), extension (the movement opposite to flexion decreasing the joint angle between two bones), abduction (the movement of a body part away from the midline in a lateral direction), and adduction (the opposite of abduction, the movement toward the midline of the body).
[Chapter 1]

13–D. The oxygen system is capable of using all three fuels (carbohydrate, fat, and protein). Significant amounts of protein, however, are not used as a source of ATP energy during most types of exercise. Although all three fuels can be used, the two most important are carbohydrate and fat. When fat is used as a fuel, significantly more energy is released; however, this requires that more oxygen be supplied to produce this energy. If proteins are used, the amount of energy is comparable to that of carbohydrate. The carbohydrate, fat, and small amount of protein used by this energy system during exercise are metabolized completely, leaving only carbon dioxide (which is exhaled) and water. The nitrogen found in the protein is excreted as urea.
[Chapter 2]

14–A. This question does not require the use of a metabolic formula because it is asking for the subject's work rate. The steps to answering this question are: Write down the known values and convert those values to the appropriate units: 5 RPM $\times$ 6 meters $= 30\ \text{m} \cdot \text{min}^{-1}$ (each revolution on a Monark cycle ergometer $= 6$ m); 2.0 kiloponds $= 2.0$ kg. Write down the formula for work rate: Work rate $=$ force $\times$ distance/time. Substitute the known values for the variable name: Work rate $= 2.0\ \text{kg} \times 30\ \text{m} \cdot \text{min}^{-1}$; Work rate $= 60\ \text{kg m} \cdot \text{min}^{-1}$. The question asks for watts, so divide the work rate ($\text{kg}^{-1\cdot}\ \text{m} \cdot \text{min}^{-1}$) by 6. W $= \text{kg} \cdot \text{m} \cdot \text{min}^{-1}/6$ watts $= 600\ \text{kg} \cdot \text{m} \cdot \text{min}^{-1}/6$ $= 10$ W
[Chapter 11]

15–B. Body composition refers to the relative proportions of fat and fat-free (lean) tissue in the body. To determine the relative proportion of fat mass

or fat-free mass, each is divided into the total body mass.
[Chapter 6]

16–A. There are 4 calories per gram of carbohydrate and protein and 9 calories per gram of fat.
5 g × 9 calories = 45 calories from fat
3 g × 4 calories = 12 calories from protein
26 g × 4 calories = 104 calories from carbohydrate
Total calories in the bar is 161 calories.
Fiber is a carbohydrate but, because it is not absorbed, there are no absorbable carbohydrates and it should not be used in determining calorie content of food.

17–D. Surrounding each myofibril is the sarcoplasmic reticulum, specialized endoplasmic reticulum consisting of a series of interconnected sacs and tubes. Calcium is stored in portions of the sarcoplasmic reticulum called **terminal cisternae**. Myofibrils contain the myofilaments, which are contractile proteins consisting primarily of actin and myosin.
[Chapter 1]

18–C. Anaerobic glycolysis also is known as the lactic acid system. A human stores carbohydrate in the body as muscle (or liver) glycogen. Glycogen is simply a long string of glucose molecules hooked end-to-end. Anaerobic glycolysis can use only carbohydrate, not fat or protein, as fuel. This system will use muscle glycogen, which is broken down to glucose and then enters anaerobic glycolysis. Only a small amount of ATP is produced, and the end-product is lactic acid (or lactate). If lactate is allowed to accumulate significantly in the muscle, it eventually will cause fatigue. Because no oxygen is required, this system is anaerobic.
[Chapter 2, Chapter 5]

19–C. Cardiac output does not change significantly, primarily because the person is performing the same amount of work and, thus, responds with the same cardiac output. It should be noted, however, that the same cardiac output is now being generated with a lower heart rate and higher stroke volume compared with when the person was untrained.
[Chapter 2]

20–D. Every population that has been studied exhibits a decline in bone mass with aging. Therefore, bone loss is considered by most clinicians to be an inevitable consequence of aging. Osteoporosis refers to a condition that is characterized by a decrease in bone mass and density, producing bone porosity and fragility, and it refers to the clinical condition of low bone mass and the accompanying increase in susceptibility to fracture from minor trauma. The age at which bone loss begins and the rate at which it occurs vary greatly between males and females. Risk factors for age-related bone loss and development of clinical osteoporosis include being a white or Asian female, being thin-boned or petite, having a low peak bone mass at maturity, having a family history of osteoporosis, premature or surgically induced menopause, alcohol abuse and/or cigarette smoking, sedentary lifestyle, and inadequate dietary calcium intake.
[Chapter 3]

21–B. Outcomes are designed to measure the success of a program based on the outcome for a patient or client. Outcome studies require quantifiable data that can be analyzed, data that study the success of a program in terms of quantifiable measures (e.g., change in body composition). Measuring client satisfaction, level of change, length of time for change to occur, or percentage of clients who reach their goals are other examples of outcomes. Outcomes can be very helpful in marketing programs as well as in comparing one facility with another.

22–B. Although some learning is required on the part of the participant, the rating of perceived exertion (RPE) should be considered an adjunct to heart rate measures. The RPE can be used as a reliable barometer of exercise intensity. The RPE is particularly useful when participants are incapable of monitoring their pulse accurately or when medications such as β-blockers alter the heart rate response to exercise. The ACSM recommends an exercise intensity that will elicit an RPE within a range of 12 to 16 on the original Borg scale of 6 to 20.

23–B. Fast-twitch (type II) muscle fibers can be subdivided into fast-twitch aerobic (type IIa) and fast-twitch glycolytic (type IIb). Although classified as a fast-twitch fiber, the type IIa fiber has the capability to perform some amounts of aerobic work. The motor nerve supplying fast-twitch fibers is larger than slow-twitch muscle fibers. Fast-twitch fibers are recruited when performing high-intensity, short-duration activities. Examples include weightlifting, sprints, jumping, and other similar activities. These fibers can produce large amounts of tension in a very short period; however, they fatigue quickly.
[Chapter 2]

24–A. Rotation is the turning of a bone around its own longitudinal axis or around another bone. Rotation of the anterior surface of the bone toward the midline of the body is medial rotation, whereas rotation of the same bone away from the midline is lateral rotation. Supination is a specialized rotation of the forearm that results in the palm of the hand being turned forward (anteriorly). Pronation (the opposite of supination) is the rotation of the forearm that results in the palm of the hand being directed backward (posteriorly). *[Chapter 1]*

25–C. The trachea branches within the mediastinum to form the right and left primary bronchi. As each primary bronchus enters the lung, secondary bronchi branch off, with smaller and smaller branches continuing to branch until the smallest narrow passage is formed, which is called the bronchiole. Terminal bronchioles, the smallest-diameter bronchioles, supply air to the lobules of the lung. Varying the diameter of the bronchioles gives control over the resistance to airflow and distribution of air to the lungs. *[Chapter 1]*

26–A. Cardiac output is calculated by multiplying heart rate and stroke volume. During dynamic exercise, cardiac output increases with increasing exercise intensity. Stroke volume increases only until approximately 40% to 50% of $\dot{V}O_{2max}$. Above this point, increases in cardiac output are accounted for only by an increase in heart rate. During static exercise, cardiac output may fall as a result of a drop in venous return. When the contraction is released, a rapid increase in cardiac output occurs as the venous return increases. *[Chapter 2]*

27–D. Initial causes of coronary artery disease are thought to be an irritation of, or an injury to, the tunica intima (the innermost of the three layers in the wall) of the blood vessel. Sources of this initial injury are thought to be caused by dyslipidemia (elevated total blood cholesterol), hypertension (chronic high blood pressure, either an elevation of systolic blood pressure or diastolic blood pressure measured on two different days), immune responses, smoking, tumultuous and nonlaminar blood flow in the lumen of the coronary artery (turbulence), vasoconstrictor substances (chemicals that cause the smooth muscle cells in the walls of the vessel to contract, resulting in a reduction in the diameter of the lumen), and viral infections. *[Chapter 4]*

28–C. Risk factors that contribute to the development of coronary artery disease include age (men, >45 years; women, >55 years), a family history of myocardial infarction or sudden death (male first-degree relatives <55 years and female first-degree relatives <65 years), cigarette smoking, hypertension (arterial blood pressure >140/90 mm Hg measured on two separate occasions), hypercholesterolemia (total cholesterol >200 mg/dL or 5.2 mmol/L, or high-density lipoprotein <35 mg/dL or 0.9 mmol/L), diabetes mellitus in individuals older than 30 years or in individuals who have had type 1 diabetes more than 15 years or type 2 diabetes in individuals older than 35 years. Other risk factors contribute to the development of coronary artery disease but are not primary risk factors. *[Chapter 4]*

29–B. The low-risk category is asymptomatic and has one or no major risk factor for coronary artery disease. A person is placed in the moderate-risk category if he or she has two or more major risk factors for coronary artery disease. A person in the high-risk category is someone with signs, symptoms of, or known cardiac disease, pulmonary disease, and metabolic disease. If a person has high serum HDL cholesterol, (>60 mg $\cdot$ dL^{-1}), subtract one risk factor from the sum of positive risk factors because high HDL levels decrease the risk of coronary artery disease. *[Chapter 6]*

30–C. Double knee to chest stretches are a safe alternative to the plough. Squats to 90 degrees and lateral neck stretches are considered safe alternative exercises to full squats and full neck rolls, respectively. Flexion with rotation is considered a contraindicated high-risk exercise and is not recommended. An alternative to the flexion with rotation is supine curl ups with flexion followed by rotation. *[Chapter 8]*

31–B. Fat-soluble vitamins are composed of vitamins A, D, E, and K and are stored in body fat after consumption. Vitamins C and B complex are water-soluble vitamins, must be consumed on a regular basis, and excess amounts are excreted. Water-soluble vitamins are found in citrus fruits, broccoli, cauliflower, brussel sprouts, whole grain breads and cereals, and organ meats. They serve as antioxidants as well as coenzymes in carbohydrate metabolism, metabolic pathways, amino acid metabolism, and nucleic acid metabolism. *[Chapter 9]*

32–B. Each atrium communicates with the ventricle on the same side via an AV valve, which allows one-way flow of blood from the atrium to the ventricle. The right AV valve also is known as the tricuspid valve because of the three cusps, or flaps, of fibrous tissue that constitute the valve. The left AV valve is called the bicuspid valve (or mitral valve), because it contains a pair of cusps rather than a trio. Each cusp is braced by tendinous fibers called chordae tendinea, which, in

turn, are connected to papillary muscles on the inner surface of the ventricle.
[Chapter 1]

33–A. The oxygen system is complicated and involves many reactions. The oxygen system takes 2 to 3 minutes to adjust to a new exercise intensity. This system is ranked third in power. An individual's $\dot{V}O_{2max}$ is a measure of the power of the aerobic energy system. This value generally is regarded as the best indicator of aerobic fitness. Training adaptations are evident in the exercise intensity at which the anaerobic threshold occurs. In untrained individuals, anaerobic threshold occurs at 55% of a person's $\dot{V}O_{2max}$. In well-trained endurance athletes, the anaerobic threshold occurs at 80%–85% of their $\dot{V}O_{2max}$.
[Chapter 2]

34–C. Skeletal muscle tissue enables movement of the body and is composed of individual cells known as myocytes or myofibers. Skeletal muscle tissue accounts for nearly 50% of the body's muscle mass and is the most abundant muscle tissue in the body. Cardiac muscle tissue also known as heart muscle pumps blood through the circulatory system. Smooth muscle tissue assists in the regulation of blood flow to various parts of the body.
[Chapter 2]

35–C. Older people who exercise regularly report greater life satisfaction (older people who exercise regularly have a more positive attitude toward their work and generally are in better health than sedentary persons), greater happiness (strong correlations have been reported between the activity level of older adults and self-reported happiness), higher self-efficacy (older persons taking part in exercise programs commonly report that they can do everyday tasks more easily than before they began exercising), improved self-concept and self-esteem (older adults improve their score on self-concept questionnaires following participation in an exercise program), and reduced psychological stress (exercise is effective in reducing psychological stress without unwanted side effects).
[Chapter 3]

36–A. Angina pectoris is a heart-related chest pain caused by ischemia, which is insufficient blood flow that results from a temporary or permanent reduction of blood flow in one or more coronary arteries. Angina-like symptoms often are felt in the chest area, neck, shoulder, or arm.
[Chapter 4]

37–B. Psychological theories are the foundation for effective use of strategies and techniques of effective counseling and motivational skill-building for exercise adoption and maintenance. Theories provide a conceptual framework for development, rather than management, of programs or interventions. Psychological theories facilitate evaluation of program effectiveness, not just measurement of outcomes. Within the field of behavioral change, a theory is a set of assumptions that accounts for the relationships between certain variables and the behavior of interest.
[Chapter 5]

38–A. A-well designed health screening provides the exercise leader or health/fitness specialist with information that can lead to identification of those individuals for whom exercise is contraindicated. From that information, a proper exercise prescription also can be developed. The Physical Activity Readiness Questionnaire (PAR-Q) is a commonly used health screening tool. A graded exercise test can be useful to measure the heart rate response.
[Chapter 6]

39–D. Regularly scheduled practices of responses to emergency situations, including a minimum of one announced and one unannounced drill, should take place. Emergency plans should include written, posted emergency plans and posted emergency numbers. Contact information for the nearest hospital emergency room may be included in the emergency plan. Maintenance of certifications, such as cardiopulmonary resuscitation training, is an accepted professional practice.
[Chapter 6]

40–C. Some externally applied forces do not act in a vertical direction, as do weights attached to the body. The forces exert effects that vary according to their particular angle of application. In the case of exercise pulleys, the angle of application changes in different parts of the range of motion. Each change in angle or force causes a change in magnitude of the rotary component of the force and, thus, the torque. In addition to the rotary component, weights applied to the extremities frequently exert traction on joint structures. This is known as a distractive force.
[Chapter 1]

41–B. Both regulatory and contractile filaments are essential to the generation of the myofiber twitch. The force generated by the whole muscle is a function both of the number of myofibers within that muscle that are twitching and of the rate at which these twitches occur. The size of the myofibers that are twitching and the strength of the action potential do not affect the force generated by the whole muscle.
[Chapter 2]

42–C. If heart rate is taken at the carotid artery, take care not to press too hard, or a reflex slowing of the heart may occur and cause dizziness. Using the thumb to count the carotid pulse may result in an inaccurate count, but this is less of a safety concern than causing dizziness by pressing too hard. Heart rates exceeding 200 bpm are no more difficult to count at the carotid artery than at other sites.
[Chapter 2]

43–C. Maximal heart rate does not change significantly with exercise training, although it declines with age. Maximal stroke volume increases after training as a result of an increase in contractility or in the size of the heart. Because maximal heart rate is unchanged and maximal stroke volume increases, maximal cardiac output must increase.
[Chapter 2]

44–C. Increasing the rate of progression of training more than approximately 10% per week is a risk factor for overuse injuries of bone. Exercise programs for children and adolescents should increase physical fitness in the short term and lead to adoption of a physically active lifestyle in the long term. Strength training in youth carries no greater risk of injury than comparable strength training programs in adults if proper instruction, exercise prescription, and supervision are provided. Children who have exercise-induced asthma often are physically unfit because of restriction of activity imposed by the child, parents, or physicians.
[Chapter 3]

45–D. Regular exercise will decrease systolic and diastolic blood pressure. Exercise has no effect on age and family history of heart disease and no direct effect on cigarette smoking, although some individuals may choose to quit smoking after beginning to exercise. Regular endurance exercise does increase high-density lipoprotein, but it has limited influence on total cholesterol. Exercise has no direct effect on type 1 diabetes, but it can promote weight loss and improve glucose tolerance for those with type 2 diabetes.
[Chapter 4]

46–A. At minimum, professionals performing fitness assessments on others should possess CPR and ACSM Health/Fitness Specialist certification.
[Chapter 6]

47–A. Intensity and duration of exercise must be considered together and are inversely related. Similar improvements in aerobic fitness may be realized if a person exercises at a low intensity for a longer duration or at a higher intensity for less time.

48–C. Three different stretching techniques typically are practiced and have associated risks and benefits. Static stretching is the most commonly recommended approach to stretching. It involves slowly stretching a muscle to the point of individual discomfort and holding that position for a period of 10 to 30 seconds. Minimal risk of injury exists and it has been shown to be effective. Ballistic stretching uses repetitive bouncing-type movements to produce muscle stretch. These movements can produce residual muscle soreness or acute injury. Proprioceptive neuromuscular facilitation stretching alternates contraction and relaxation of both agonist and antagonist muscle groups. This technique is effective, but it can cause residual muscle soreness and is time-consuming. Additionally, a partner typically is required, and the potential for injury exists when the partner-assisted stretching is applied too vigorously.

49–C. Carbohydrates are compounds made of carbon, hydrogen, and oxygen. They are commonly known as simple carbohydrates (sugars) or complex carbohydrates (starch). Glucose, fructose, and sucrose are examples of sugars or simple carbohydrates. Some sources are refined sugar (white or brown) and fruits. Food sources for complex carbohydrates are grains, breads, cereals, pastas, potatoes, beans, and legumes. Proteins have nitrogen in them as well as carbon, hydrogen, and oxygen and may be found in such food sources as meats and nuts. Fats are found in foods such as butter and oils.
[Chapter 9]

50–C. Legal issues abound for fitness professionals involved in exercise testing, exercise prescription, and program administration. Legal concerns can develop with the instructor–client relationship, the exercises involved, the exercise setting, the purpose of the programs and exercises used, and the procedures used by the staff. A tort law is simply a type of civil wrong. Negligence is the failure to perform on the level of a generally accepted standard. Fitness professionals have certain documented and understood responsibilities to ensure the client's safety and to succeed in reaching predetermined goals. If these responsibilities are not followed, it is possible that a person could be considered negligent.

51–A. All energy for muscular contraction must come from the breakdown of ATP. The energy is stored in the bonds between the last two phosphates. When work is performed (e.g., a biceps curl), the last phosphate is split (forming ADP), releasing heat energy. Some (but not all) of this heat energy is converted to mechanical energy to perform the curl. Because humans are not 100% efficient at converting this heat energy to mechanical

energy, the rest of the heat is released to the environment.
[Chapter 2]

52–C. A muscle is composed of muscle fibers (or cells). Each muscle fiber is composed of many myofibrils. Each myofibril is composed of sarcomeres. The sarcomere is the smallest part of muscle that can contract. The contractile (or muscle) proteins are contained in the sarcomere. Actin is a muscle protein (sometimes called the thin filament) that can be visualized as a twisted strand of beads. Actin also contains two other proteins, troponin and tropomyosin. Tropomyosin is a long, stringlike molecule that wraps around the actin filament. Troponin is a specialized protein found at the ends of the tropomyosin filament.
[Chapter 2]

53–A. Systolic blood pressure is an indicator of cardiac output (the amount of blood pumped out of the heart in 1 minute) in a healthy vascular system. Cardiac output normally increases as workload increases, because the peripheral and central stimuli that control cardiac output normally increase with an increase in workload. Thus, systolic blood pressure should increase with an increase in workload. Failure of the systolic blood pressure to increase as workload increases indicates that cardiac output is not increasing, which, in turn, indicates an abnormal response to increasing workload. Additionally, an abnormally elevated systolic blood pressure response to aerobic exercise indicates an unhealthy vascular system.
[Chapter 4]

54–D. Most sedentary people are not motivated to initiate exercise programs and, if exercise is initiated, they are likely to stop within 3 to 6 months. In general, participants in earlier stages benefit most from cognitive strategies, such as listening to lectures and reading books without the expectation of actually engaging in exercise, whereas individuals in later stages depend more on behavioral techniques, such as reminders to exercise and developing social support to help them establish a regular exercise habit and be able to maintain it.
[Chapter 5]

55–D. Fitness testing is conducted in older adults for the same reasons as in younger adults, including exercise prescription, evaluation of progress, motivation, and education.
[Chapter 6]

56–C. Disordered eating covers a continuum from the preoccupation with food and body image to the syndromes of anorexia nervosa and bulimia. Anorexia nervosa is defined by symptoms that include a body weight that is 15% less than expected, a morbid fear of being or becoming fat, a preoccupation with food, and an abnormal body image (the thin person feels "fat"). Bulimia nervosa is defined by symptoms that include binge eating twice a week for at least 3 months, loss of control over eating, purging behavior, and being overly concerned with body weight. Although specific psychiatric criteria must be met for a diagnosis to be made by a specialist, any degree of disordered eating can affect the eating pattern of the exerciser and place her or him at risk for nutritional deficiencies.
[Chapter 9]

57–C. A motor unit consists of the efferent (motor) nerve and all muscle fibers supplied (or innervated) by that nerve. The total number of motor units varies between different muscles. In addition, the total number of fibers in each motor unit varies between and within muscles. Different degrees of contraction can be achieved by varying the total number of motor units stimulated (or recruited) in a particular muscle. The major determinants of how much force is produced when a muscle contracts are the number of motor units that are recruited and the number of muscle fibers in each motor unit. When a motor unit is stimulated by a single nerve impulse, it responds by contracting one time and then relaxing. This is called a twitch. If a motor unit is continuously stimulated without adequate time for relaxation to occur, tetanus occurs. If a motor unit receives a second stimulation before it is allowed to relax, the two impulses are added (or summated), and the tension developed is greater.
[Chapter 2]

58–A. The steps are as follows:

a. Write out the running equation (accurate for speeds in excess of 5 mph):

$$\dot{V}O_2\ (mL \cdot kg^{-1} \cdot min^{-1}) = \text{horizontal} + \text{vertical} + \text{resting}$$

$$\dot{V}O_2\ (mL \cdot kg^{-1} \cdot min^{-1}) = (\text{speed} \times 0.2) + (\text{speed} \times \text{grade} \times 0.9) + 3.5$$

b. Convert speed (6.5 mph) to meters per minute:

$$6.5 \times 26.8 = 174.2\ m \cdot min^{-1}$$

c. Solve for the unknown:

$$\dot{V}O_2\ (mL \cdot kg^{-1} \cdot min^{-1}) = (174.2 \times 0.2) + (174.2 \times 0.05 \times 0.9) + 3.5\dot{V}O_2\ (mL \cdot kg^{-1} \cdot min^{-1}) = 46.18\ mL \cdot kg^{-1} \cdot min^{-1}$$

d. Convert 46.18 $mL \cdot kg^{-1} \cdot min^{-1}$ to MET:

$$1\,MET = 3.5\,mL \cdot kg^{-1} \cdot min^{-1}$$
$$46.18 \div 3.5 = 13.2\,MET$$

[Chapter 11]

59–B. Reinforcement is the positive or negative consequence for performing or not performing a behavior. Positive consequences are rewards that motivate behavior. This can include both intrinsic and extrinsic rewards. Intrinsic rewards are the benefits gained because of the rewarding nature of the activity. Extrinsic or external rewards are the positive outcomes received from others, which may include encouragement and praise or material reinforcements such as T-shirts and money.
[Chapter 5]

60–C. Exercise-induced asthma is a reversible airway obstruction that results directly from the ventilatory response to exercise. Hyperventilation causes an individual to breathe more through the mouth than through the nose and actually inhale deconditioned (cool, dirty, dry) air. The nose serves to warm, clean, and humidify the air. Deconditioned air triggers an immune or allergic response primarily in the small- and medium-sized airways in some individuals and may manifest in bronchoconstriction or bronchospasm. Medications are available that may prevent or reverse asthma attacks. These usually are administered in a tablet or aerosol form. Albuterol, terbutaline, glucocorticosteroids, cromolyn sodium, and theophylline are effective drugs to prevent or reverse asthma.

61–A. Creating a safe environment in which to exercise is a primary responsibility for any fitness facility. In developing and operating facilities and equipment for use by exercisers, the managers and staff are obligated to meet a standard of care for exerciser safety. The equipment to be used not only includes testing, cardiovascular, strength, and flexibility pieces, but also rehabilitation, pool, locker room, and emergency equipment. You must evaluate a number of criteria when selecting equipment. These criteria include correct anatomic positioning, ability to adjust to different body sizes, quality of design and materials, durability, repair records, and then price.
[Chapter 7]

62–A. The ability to take in and to utilize oxygen is depends on the health and integrity of the heart, lungs, and circulatory systems. Efficiency of the aerobic metabolic pathways also is necessary to optimize cardiorespiratory fitness. The degree of improvement that may be expected in cardiorespiratory fitness relates directly to the frequency, intensity, duration, and mode or type of exercise. Maximal oxygen uptake may improve between 5% and 30% with training. The exercise prescription can be altered for different populations to achieve the same results. However, for an apparently healthy person, the ACSM recommends an intensity of 60% to 90% maximal heart rate, duration of 20 to 60 minutes, and frequency of 3 to 5 days a week.

63–A. Plyometrics is a method of strength and power training that involves an eccentric loading of muscles and tendons followed immediately by an explosive concentric contraction. This stretch–shortening cycle may allow an enhanced generation of force during the concentric (shortening) phase. Most well-controlled studies have shown no significant difference in power improvement when comparing plyometrics with high-intensity strength training. The explosive nature of this type of activity may increase the risk for musculoskeletal injury. Plyometrics should not be considered a practical resistance exercise alternative for health/fitness applications, but may be appropriate for select athletic or performance needs.

64–C. The characteristics of a good manager or director include designing programs and monitoring the implementation of programs. He or she also guides the staff or clients through the program. He or she is a good communicator who also purchases equipment and supplies. A good manager monitors the safety of the program or facility and surveys clients and staff to assess the success and value of the program.

65–A. Agreements, releases, and consents are documents that clearly describe what the client is participating in, the risks involved, and the rights of the client and the facility. If signed by the client, he or she is accepting some of the responsibility and risk by participating in this program. All fitness facilities are strongly encouraged to have program or service agreements and informed consents drafted by a lawyer for their protection.

66–B. The stores of ATP energy in skeletal muscle are very limited (5 to 10 seconds of high-intensity work). After this time, another high-energy source, PC, which has only one high-energy phosphate band, begins to break down. The energy from the breakdown of PC is used to re-form ATP, which then breaks down to provide energy for exercise. Only energy released from the breakdown of ATP, however, can provide energy for biologic work such as exercise.
[Chapter 2]

67–D. The sliding filament theory defines how skeletal muscles are believed to contract. These steps can best be described as what occurs during rest, stimulation, contraction, and then relaxation of the muscle. At rest, no nerve activity (except normal resting tone) occurs. Calcium is stored in a network of tubes in the muscle called the sarcoplasmic reticulum. If no calcium is present, the active sites (where the myosin cross-bridges can attach) are kept covered. If the active sites are uncovered, the enzyme that causes ATP to break down and release energy is kept inactive. During conditions when a nerve impulse is present, this impulse causes calcium to be released. The calcium binds to the troponin on the actin filament. When this occurs, the active sites are uncovered. Now, the myosin cross-bridges bind the active sites and form actomyosin (a connection between the actin and myosin proteins), and contraction occurs.
[Chapter 2]

68–C. After 30 years of age, skeletal muscle strength begins to decline. However, the loss of strength is not linear, with most of the decline occurring after 50 years of age. By 80 years of age, strength loss usually is in the range of 30% to 40%. The loss of strength with aging results primarily from a loss of muscle mass, which, in turn, is caused by both the loss of muscle fibers and the atrophy of the remaining fibers.
[Chapter 3]

69–C. Specific risks are associated with exercise for men and for women (although the statistics for women are not yet known). The rate of acute cardiovascular events is 1 in 187,500 hours of exercise. The rate of death during exercise for men is 1 in 396,000 hours. In addition, deaths during exercise are more common among men who have more than one risk factor for coronary artery disease. The risk of cardiovascular events or death is lower among men who are habitually active.
[Chapter 4]

70–D. Fiber is a type of complex carbohydrate that is indigestible by the body. This means that it will pass straight through the digestive system and is commonly referred to as “adding bulk to the diet.” Fiber can be either water-soluble (pectin or gums) or water-insoluble (cellulose, hemicellulose, and lignin). Dietary fiber has been linked to the prevention of certain diseases.
[Chapter 9]

71–A. The Health Belief Model assumes that people will engage in a behavior (e.g., exercise) when exist a perceived threat of disease and a belief of susceptibility to disease, and the threat of disease is severe. This model also incorporates cues to action as critical to adopting and maintaining behavior. The concept of self-efficacy (confidence) is also added to this model. Motivation and environmental considerations are not a part of the Health Belief Model.
[Chapter 5]

72–C. Informed consent is not a legal document. It does not provide legal immunity to a facility or individual in the event of injury to a client, nor does it legally protect the rights of the client. It simply provides evidence that the client was made aware of the purposes, procedures, and risks associated with the test or exercise program. The consent form does not relieve the facility or individual of the responsibility to do everything possible to ensure the safety of the client. Negligence, improper test administration, inadequate personnel qualifications, and insufficient safety procedures all are items that are not expressly covered by informed consent. Because of the limitations associated with informed consent documents, legal counsel should be sought during the development of the document.
[Chapter 6]

73–C. Three common assessments for muscular endurance include the bench press, for upper body endurance (a weight is lifted in cadence with a metronome or other timing device; the total number of lifts performed correctly and in time with the cadence); the push-up, for upper body endurance (the client assumes a standardized beginning position with the body held rigid and supported by the hands and toes for men and the hands and knees for women; the body is lowered to the floor, then pushed back up to the starting position; the score is the total number of properly performed push-ups completed without a pause by the client, with no time limit); and the curl-up (crunch), for abdominal muscular endurance (the client begins in the bent-knee sit-up with knees at 90 degrees, the arms at the side, palms facing down with middle fingers touching masking tape. A second piece of tape is placed 10 cm apart. OR set a metronome to 50 bpm and the client performs slow, controlled curl-ups to lift the shoulder blades off the mat with the trunk making a 30-degree angle, in time with the metronome at a rate of 25 per minute done for 1 minute. OR the client performs an many curl-ups as possible in 1 minute.
[Chapter 4 GETP]

74–A. Overuse injuries become more common when people participate in more cardiovascular exercise by increasing time, duration, or intensity too quickly. A client exercises too much without time

for rest and recovery or develops a minor injury and does not reduce or change that exercise allowing the injury to heal.
[Chapter 7]

75–C. Several methods are available to define exercise intensity objectively. The ACSM recommends that exercise intensity be prescribed within a range of 64% to 70% and 94% of maximal heart rate or between 40% to 50% and 85% of oxygen uptake reserve ($\dot{V}O_{2MAX}R$). Lower intensities will elicit a favorable response in individuals with very low fitness levels. Because of the variability in estimating maximal heart rate from age, it is recommended that, whenever possible, an actual maximal heart rate from a graded exercise test be used. Factors to consider when determining appropriate exercise intensity include age, fitness level, medications, overall health status, and individual goals.
[Chapter 7 GETP]

76–B. The ACSM recommends that one set of 8 to 12 repetitions of each exercise should be performed to volitional fatigue for healthy individuals. Choose a range of repetitions between 3 and 20 (i.e., 3 to 5, 8 to 10, 10 to 15) that can be performed at a moderate repetition duration (~3 seconds concentric, ~3 seconds eccentric) based on age, fitness level, assessment, ability. The ACSM recommends exercising each muscle group 2 to 3 nonconsecutive days per week.
[Chapter 7 GETP]

77–B. The risk of orthopedic and, perhaps, cardiovascular complications can be increased with high-intensity activity. Factors to consider when determining exercise intensity include the individual's level of fitness, presence of medications that may influence exercise performance, risk of cardiovascular or orthopedic injury, and individual preference for exercise and individual program objectives.

78–B. During auscultation, a stethoscope is placed over the left aspect of the midsternum, or just under the pectoralis major. Care must be taken to avoid placing the stethoscope bell over fat or muscle tissue because this can interfere with the clarity of the sound. When measuring heart rate by auscultation, the initial sound is counted as zero. The longer the time for which heart sounds are counted, the less the error introduced by inadvertently missing a single beat yet the greater the risk of miscounting. The heart rate is typically counted in a specific period of time (10 to 30 seconds).
[Chapter 6]

79–D. The effects of regular (chronic) exercise can be classified or grouped into those that occur at rest, during moderate (or submaximal) exercise, and during maximal effort work. For example, you can measure an untrained individual's resting heart rate, train the person for several weeks or months, and then measure resting heart rate again to see what change has occurred. Resting heart rate declines with regular exercise, probably because of a combination of decreased sympathetic tone, increased parasympathetic tone, and decreased intrinsic firing rate of the sinoatrial node. Stroke volume increases at rest as a result of increased time for ventricular filling and an increased myocardial contractility. Little or no change occurs in cardiac output at rest, because the decline in heart rate is compensated for by the increase in stroke volume.
[Chapter 2]

80–D. Heart muscle has the capability of producing its own action potential (autorhythmicity). In other words, if an impulse is not received from higher-level brain centers, cardiac muscle will stimulate itself.
[Chapter 2]

81–A. The rate of death, either during or immediately after exercise testing, is 0.5 in 10,000 (~0.01%). The rate of myocardial infarction during or immediately after exercise testing is 3.6 in 10,000 (~0.04%). Complications during testing that require hospitalization are approximately 0.1%.
[Chapter 4; Chapter 1 GETP]

82–C. Key components of the Transtheoretical Model are the Processes of Behavioral Change. These processes include five cognitive processes (consciousness raising, dramatic relief, environmental reevaluation, self-reevaluation, and social liberation) and five behavioral processes (counterconditioning, helping relationships, reinforcement management, self-liberation, and stimulus control).
[Chapter 5]

83–A. The purpose of the fitness assessment is to develop a proper exercise prescription (the data collected through appropriate fitness assessments assist the health/fitness specialist in developing safe, effective programs of exercise based on the individual client's current fitness status), to evaluate the rate of progress (baseline and follow-up testing indicate progression toward fitness goals), and to motivate (fitness assessments provide information needed to develop reasonable, attainable goals). Progress toward or attainment of a goal is a strong motivator for continued participation in an exercise program.
[Chapter 6]

84–C. Basic principles of care for musculoskeletal injuries include the objectives for care of

exercise-related injuries, which are to decrease pain, reduce swelling, and prevent further injury. These objectives can be met in most cases by following "RICE" guidelines. "RICE" stands for "Rest, Ice, Compression, Elevation." Rest will prevent further injury and ensure that the healing process will begin. Ice is used to reduce swelling, bleeding, inflammation, and pain. Compression also helps to reduce swelling and bleeding. Compression is achieved by the use of elastic wraps or tape. Elevation helps to decrease the blood flow and excessive pressure to the injured area.
[Chapter 7]

85–D. Various systems of resistance training exist that differ in their combinations of sets, repetitions, and resistance applied, all in an effort to overload the muscle. Circuit weight training uses a series of exercises performed in succession with minimal rest between exercises. Various health benefits as well as modest improvements in aerobic capacity have been demonstrated as a result of circuit weight training. Super-sets refer to consecutive sets for antagonistic muscle groups with no rest between sets or multiple exercises for a specific muscle group with little or no rest. Split routines entail exercising different body parts on different days or during different sessions. Pyramids are performed either in ascending (increasing the resistance within a set of repetitions or from one set to the next) or descending (decreasing the resistance within a set of repetitions or from one set to the next) fashion.

86–A. The goal of the exercise component of a weight reduction program should be to maximize caloric expenditure. Frequency, intensity, and duration must be manipulated in conjunction with a dietary regimen in an attempt to create a caloric deficit of 500 to 1,000 calories per day. The recommended maximal rate for weight loss is 1 to 2 lb per week.
[ACSM position stand]

87–B. Scoliosis is a lateral deviation in the alignment of the vertebrae. Kyphosis is a posterior thoracic curvature. Lordosis is an anterior lumbar curvature. A chronic, inflammatory, demyelinating disease describes multiple sclerosis. Softening of the articular cartilage describes chondrosis. Inflammation of the growth plate at the tibial tuberosity is a condition known as Osgood-Schlatter disease.
[Chapter 1]

88–B. The Health Belief Model is a theoretical framework to help explain and predict interventions to increase physical activity. The model originated in the 1950's based on work by Rosenstock. Learning theories assume that an overall complex behavior arises from many small simple behaviors. By reinforcing partial behaviors and modifying cues in the environment, it is possible to shape the desired behavior.
[Chapter 5]

89–C. The PAR-Q is a screening tool for self-directed exercise programming. The MMPI is a psychological scale. The RPE Borg scale is used to measure or to rate perceived exertion during exercise or during an exercise test. The E-ECG would involve continuous electrical heart monitoring during exercise stress test utilized in a clinical setting when deemed appropriate by a physician.
[Chapter 6]

90–C. To get the best and most accurate information, the following order of testing is recommended: resting measurements (e.g., heart rate, blood pressure, blood analysis), body composition, cardiorespiratory fitness, muscular fitness and flexibility. Some methods of body composition assessment are sensitive to hydration status and some tests of cardiorespiratory and muscular fitness may affect hydration, so it is inappropriate to administer those before the body composition assessment. Assessing cardiorespiratory fitness often utilizes measures of heart rate. Some tests of muscular fitness and flexibility affect heart rate, so they are inappropriate to administer before cardiorespiratory fitness testing, because the elevated heart rate from those assessments may, in turn, affect the cardiorespiratory fitness testing results.
[Chapter 6]

91–D. When an emergency or injury occurs, safe and effective management of the situation will assure the best care for the individual. Implementing emergency procedures is an important part of the training of the staff. In-services, safety plans, and emergency procedures should be a part of the staff training. In addition, all exercise staff should be CPR certified and knowledgeable of first aid. Therefore, the fitness center management and staff all are included in the implementation of an emergency plan.
[Chapter 50 RM]

92–D. Possible medical emergencies during exercise include heat exhaustion or heat stroke, fainting, hypoglycemia, hyperglycemia, simple or compound fractures, bronchospasm, hypotension or shock, seizures, bleeding, and other cardiac symptoms.
[Chapter 50 RM]

93–C. During most graded exercise tests, the blood pressure should be measured and recorded during the last 45 seconds of each stage or 2-minute

time period. ECG, heart rate, signs or symptoms and gas exchange are monitored continuously. ECG is recorded during the last 15 seconds of each stage or 2-minute time period; heart rate and RPE are recorded during the last 5 seconds of each minute; and signs and symptoms are recorded as observed.
[Chapter 5 GETP]

94–D. Isometric muscle action, also known as static muscle action, occurs when muscle tension increases with no overt muscular or limb movement; the length of the muscle does not change. These actions occur when with an attempt to push or pull against an immovable object. Measures of static strength are specific to both the muscle group and joint angle being tested, therefore these tests' usefulness to generalize overall muscular strength is limited.
[Chapter 4 GETP]

95–C. A good balance of energy is important within consuming the proper amount of energy within a person's daily food intake. Carbohydrates, especially whole grains, should make up about 45% to 65% of daily intake as a general recommendation.
[Chapter 4 RM]

96–D. Large muscle group activity performed in rhythmic fashion over prolonged periods facilitates the greatest improvements in aerobic fitness. Walking, running, cycling, swimming, stair climbing, aerobic dance, rowing, and cross-country skiing are examples of these types of activities. Weight training should not be considered an appropriate activity for enhancing aerobic fitness, but should be part of in a comprehensive exercise program to improve muscular strength and muscular endurance. The mode(s) of activity should be selected based on the principle of specificity—that is, with attention to the desired outcomes—and to maintain the participation and enjoyment of the individual.
[Chapter 7 GETP]

97–D. Different types of health screenings are used for various purposes. In commercial settings, clients should be screened more extensively for potential health risks. At minimum, a personal medical history should be taken. In addition, present medical status should be examined and questions asked regarding the use of medications (both prescription and over-the-counter).
[Chapter 2 GETP]

98–C. The number of times per day or per week that a person exercises is interrelated with both the intensity and the duration of activity. Generally, sedentary persons or those with poor fitness may benefit from multiple short-duration, low-intensity exercise sessions per day. Individual goals, preferences, limitations, and time constraints also will determine frequency and the relationship between duration, frequency, and intensity.
[Chapter 7 GETP]

99–B. The strategic plan addresses strategic decisions of the organization in defining short-and long-term goals and serves as the overarching planning tool. Health and fitness programs, financial plans, risk management efforts and marketing plans only address subsegments within the overall strategic plan.
[Chapter 46 RM; Chapter 48 RM]

APPENDIX

B Clinical Comprehensive Examination

DIRECTIONS: Each of the numbered items or incomplete statements in this section is followed by answers or by completions of the statement. Select the ONE lettered answer or completion that is BEST in each case.

1. During a medical emergency, which of the following medications is an endogenous catecholamine that can be used to increase blood flow to the heart and brain?
   A) Lidocaine.
   B) Oxygen.
   C) Atropine.
   D) Epinephrine.

2. If a healthy young man who weighs 80 kg exercises at an intensity of 45 $mL \cdot kg^{-1} \cdot min^{-1}$ for 30 minutes, five times per week, how long would it take him to lose 10 pounds of fat?
   A) 9 weeks.
   B) 11 weeks.
   C) 13 weeks.
   D) 15 weeks.

3. Which of the following techniques can be used to diagnose coronary artery disease and assess heart wall motion abnormalities, ejection fraction, and cardiac output?
   A) Electrocardiography.
   B) Radionuclide imaging.
   C) Echocardiography.
   D) Cardiac spirometry.

4. During mild to moderate exercise, what is the primary cause of changes in minute ventilation?
   A) Increased tidal volume.
   B) Decreased respiratory rate.
   C) Decreased forced expiratory volume.
   D) Increased forced inspiratory volume.

5. Which of the following would be an adequate exercise prescription for a patient who has had a heart transplant?
   A) High intensity, short duration, small muscle groups, and high frequency.
   B) High intensity, long duration, small muscle groups, and high frequency.
   C) Moderate intensity, 6 days per week, large muscle groups, and moderate duration.
   D) Low intensity, 3 days per week, large muscle groups, and moderate duration.

6. Individuals with diabetes should follow exercise guidelines to avoid unnecessary risks. The following list of recommendations should include all of the following EXCEPT
   A) Avoiding injection of insulin into an exercising muscle.
   B) Exercising with a partner.
   C) Exercising only when temperature and humidity are moderate.
   D) Avoiding exercise during peak insulin activity.

7. Which of the following is a reversible pulmonary condition caused by some type of irritant (e.g., dust, pollen) and characterized by bronchial airway narrowing, dyspnea, and, possibly hypoxia and hypercapnia?
   A) Emphysema.
   B) Bronchitis.
   C) Asthma.
   D) Pulmonary vascular disease.

8. A supraventricular ectopic rhythm that results from a focus of automaticity located in the bundle of His is an example of
   A) Ventricular arrhythmia.
   B) Junctional arrhythmia.
   C) Atrioventricular block.
   D) Premature ventricular contraction.

9. Which of the following statements regarding contraindications to graded exercise testing are accurate?
   A) Some individuals have risk factors that outweigh the potential benefits from exercise testing and the information that may be obtained.
   B) Absolute contraindications refer to individuals for whom exercise testing should not be performed until the situation or condition has stabilized.
   C) Relative contraindications include patients who might be tested if the potential benefit from exercise testing outweighs the relative risk.
   D) All of the above statements are true.

10. Cardiac impulses originating in the sinoatrial node and then spreading to both atria, causing atrial depolarization, is represented on the electrocardiogram as a
    A) P wave.
    B) QRS complex.
    C) ST segment.
    D) T wave.

11. Which plane divides the body into symmetric right and left halves?
    A) Frontal.
    B) Transverse.
    C) Sagittal.
    D) Medial.

12. For previously sedentary individuals, a 20% to 30% reduction in all-cause mortality can be obtained from physical activity with a daily energy expenditure of
    A) 50 to 80 kcal/day.
    B) 80 to 100 kcal/day.
    C) 150 to 200 kcal/day.
    D) >400 kcal/day.

13. Exercise has been shown to reduce mortality in people with coronary artery disease. Which of the following mechanisms is NOT responsible?
    A) The effect of exercise on other risk factors.
    B) Reduced myocardial oxygen demand at rest and at submaximal workloads.
    C) Reduced platelet aggregation.
    D) Decreased endothelial-mediated vasomotor tone.

14. The degradation of carbohydrate to either pyruvate or lactate occurs during
    A) The adenosine triphosphate system.
    B) Anaerobic glycolysis.
    C) Aerobic glycolysis.
    D) Oxidative phosphorylation.

15. Which of the following is an INAPPROPRIATE strategy for permanent weight loss?
    A) Dietary changes.
    B) Increased exercise.
    C) Rapid weight loss.
    D) Dietary changes and exercise.

16. Which of the following treatment strategies are most commonly used in patients with multiple-vessel disease who are not responding to other treatments?
    A) Percutaneous transluminal coronary angioplasty.
    B) Coronary artery stent.
    C) Coronary artery bypass graft surgery.
    D) Pharmacologic therapy.

17. Which of the following statements BEST describes the exercise precautions for patients with an automatic implantable cardioverter defibrillator (AICD)?
    A) Persons with AICD must be monitored closely during exercise to avoid the level of the activation rate and trigger a shock.
    B) Persons with AICD are not at risk for an inappropriate shock because most AICDs are set to a heart rate of 300 bpm.
    C) Persons with AICD can inactivate the AICD before high-intensity exercise to avoid the risk of shock.
    D) Persons with an AICD can exercise at or above the cutoff heart rate but only if monitored by instantaneous ECG telemetry.

18. Which of the following is an example of physical activity requiring anaerobic glycolysis to produce energy in the form of adenosine triphosphate (ATP)?
    A) 400-m sprint.
    B) 2-mile run.
    C) 100-m sprint.
    D) All of the above.

19. Healthy, untrained individuals have an anaerobic threshold at approximately what percentage of their maximal oxygen consumption ($\dot{V}O_2$ max)?
    A) 25%.
    B) 55%.
    C) 75%.
    D) 95%.

20. Which of the following medications reduces myocardial ischemia by lowering myocardial oxygen demand, is used to treat typical and variant angina, but has NOT been shown to reduce postmyocardial infarction mortality?
    A) β-adrenergic blockers.
    B) Niacin.
    C) Aspirin.
    D) Nitrates.

21. Which of the following structures is located in the posterior wall of the right atrium, just inferior to the opening of the superior vena cava?
    A) Sinoatrial node.
    B) Atrioventricular node.
    C) Bundle of His.
    D) Purkinje fibers.

22. A 35-year-old female client asks the Exercise Specialist to estimate her energy expenditure. She weighs 110 lb and pedals the cycle ergometer at 50 rpm with a resistance of 2.5 kp for 60 minutes. The Specialist should report which of the following caloric values?
    A) 250 calories.
    B) 510 calories.
    C) 770 calories.
    D) 1,700 calories.

23. The cardiac rehabilitation's Medical Director orders a prerehabilitation electrocardiogram on a 50-year-old man. The Exercise Specialist performing the ECG notes the machine error message reads artifact in the precordial lead V_4. To correct the artifact, an Exercise Specialist would check which of the following lead positions for adhesive contact?
A) Fourth intercostal space, left sternal border.
B) Fourth intercostal space, right sternal border.
C) Midaxillary line, fifth intercostal space.
D) Midclavicular line, fifth intercostal space.

24. Which of the following cardiac indices increases curvilinearly with the work rate until it reaches near maximum at a level equivalent to approximately 50% of aerobic capacity, increasing only slightly thereafter?
A) Stroke volume.
B) Heart rate.
C) Cardiac output.
D) Systolic blood pressure.

25. A 55-year-old cardiac rehabilitation patient returned from vacation with the following complaints: elevation in blood pressure, slight chest pain, shortness of breath with chest wheezing, and dryness and burning of the mouth and throat. Based on this information, the Exercise Specialist would suspect the patient was exposed to which of the following environments?
A) Extreme cold.
B) Extreme heat.
C) High altitude.
D) High humidity.

26. What is the total caloric equivalent of 3.0 lb (1.36 kg) of fat?
A) 1,000 kcal.
B) 5,500 kcal.
C) 10,500 kcal.
D) 15,000 kcal.

27. All of the following are major signs and symptoms suggestive of cardiac or metabolic disease, EXCEPT?
A) Ankle edema.
B) Claudication.
C) Orthopnea.
D) Bronchitis.

28. Which of the following best describes an irreversible necrosis of the heart muscle resulting from prolonged coronary artery blockage.
A) Thrombosis.
B) Ischemia.
C) Infarction.
D) Thrombolysis.

29. An exercise specialist monitoring the ECG of a cardiac rehabilitation patient observes QT-interval shortening and ST-segment scooping during exercise. Based on the this observation, the specialist can suspect the patient is treated with which of the following medications?
A) β-blockers.
B) Calcium-channel blockers.
C) Potassium.
D) Digitalis.

30. The breakdown of______would be described as the energy used to perform physical work in a short time interval (5 to 10 seconds):
A) Testosterone.
B) Oxygen.
C) ATP.
D) Phosphocreatine.

31. The exercise specialist is orienting a 60-year-old patient entering cardiac rehabilitation after having coronary artery bypass grafting 3 weeks ago. All of the following statements are correct, EXCEPT?
A) The patient should avoid extreme tension on the upper body because of sternal and leg wounds for 2 to 4 months.
B) The clinician should observe for infection or discomfort along the incision.
C) The patient should be monitored for chest pain, dizziness, and dysrhythmias.
D) The patient should avoid high-intensity exercise early in the rehabilitation period.

32. All of the following are nonmodifiable risk factors for the development of coronary artery disease, EXCEPT?
A) Increasing age.
B) Male gender.
C) Family history.
D) Tobacco smoking.

33. An aerobic exercise prescription of 5 days per week at 50% to 85% of maximal oxygen consumption ($\dot{V}O2$ max) for 45 minutes, will most favorably affect which of the following blood lipid profiles?
A) Lipoprotein (a).
B) Triglycerides.
C) Total cholesterol.
D) Low-density lipoprotein cholesterol.

34. A______period redistributes blood flow from the trunk to peripheral areas, decreases resistance in the tissues, and increases tissue temperature and energy production?
A) Training.
B) Cool-down.
C) Warm-up.
D) Detraining.

35. The Exercise Specialist is asked to risk stratify a 65-year-old patient for exercise testing. The patient has shortness of breath with mild exertion, orthopnea,

smokes two packs of cigarettes a day and has a body mass index (BMI) of 32 $kg \cdot m^{-2}$. Based on this information, in which risk stratification category would this individual fall?
A) No risk.
B) Low risk.
C) Moderate risk.
D) High risk.

36. While monitoring the ECG of a cardiac rehabilitation patient, a progressive lengthening of the PR interval until a dropped QRS complex is observed. Based on this observation, what kind of AV block are you observing?
A) First-degree.
B) Mobitz type I.
C) Mobitz type II.
D) Third-degree.

37. Heart rate increases in a linear fashion with work rate and oxygen uptake during dynamic exercise. The magnitude of the heart rate response is mainly related to what factor?
A) Age.
B) Body position.
C) Medication use.
D) All of the above.

38. All of the following can be positively affected by regular exercise, EXCEPT?
A) Obesity.
B) Dyslipidemia.
C) Hypertension.
D) Cirrhosis.

39. You are asked to review an ECG strip for evidence of myocardial ischemia and/or injury. On what areas of the ECG should you focus?
A) Q wave.
B) PR interval.
C) ST segment.
D) T wave.

40. All of the following are classifications of obesity and result in an increased risk for coronary artery disease in males, EXCEPT?
A) BMI $\geq$30 $kg \cdot m^{-2}$.
B) Waist-to-hip ratio >0.95.
C) Body fat >25%.
D) Waist circumference >35 inches.

41. A balance between the energy required by the working muscles and the rate of ATP production during exercise is referred to as
A) Anaerobic cellular respiration.
B) Oxygen debt.
C) Oxygen deficit.
D) Steady state.

42. In an electrocardiogram recording, the presence of certain combinations of ST-segment abnormalities of significant Q waves or the absence of R waves may be suggestive of what condition?
A) Acute myocardial infarction.
B) Left ventricular hypertrophy.
C) Right bundle branch block.
D) Ventricular aneurysm.

43. What is the relative oxygen consumption rate for walking on a treadmill at 3.5 mph with a 10% grade?
A) 18.17 $mL \cdot kg^{-1} \cdot min^{-1}$.
B) 27.96 $mL \cdot kg^{-1} \cdot min^{-1}$.
C) 29.76 $mL \cdot kg^{-1} \cdot min^{-1}$.
D) 31.28 $mL \cdot kg^{-1} \cdot min^{-1}$.

44. Which of the following axes lies perpendicular to the frontal plane?
A) Anteroposterior.
B) Mediolateral.
C) Sagittal.
D) Transverse.

45. An expected benefit of regular exercise in patients with peripheral vascular disease is a(n)
A) Increased exercise tolerance.
B) Lower claudication pain tolerance.
C) Redistribution and reduced blood flow to the legs and skin.
D) Increased blood viscosity.

46. Which of the following individuals DO NOT need a physician's evaluation before initiating a vigorous exercise program?
A) Men >50 years of age with fewer than two risk factors.
B) Women <50 years of age with fewer than two risk factors.
C) Men <40 years of age with two risk factors.
D) Women <50 years of age with known disease.

47. Which of the following is a type of intraventricular conduction disturbance?
A) AV nodal reentrant tachycardia.
B) Premature ventricular contraction.
C) Right bundle branch block.
D) Sick sinus syndrome.

48. For persons free of absolute contraindications to exercise, the health and medical benefits of exercise clearly outweigh any associated risks. To ensure a safe environment during exercise testing and training, the clinical exercise specialist must be prepared to do all the following EXCEPT?
A) Explain the risks associated with exercise and exercise testing.
B) Implement preventive measures.
C) Perform emergency medical procedures.
D) Take care of an injury or medical emergency.

49. What is defined as a surplus of adipose tissue, resulting from excess energy intake relative to energy expenditure?
   A) Overweight.
   B) Android obesity.
   C) Obesity.
   D) Morbid obesity.

50. Although certification of clinical exercise rehabilitation programs is a relatively new concept, it involves many already established components of the exercise program. Which of the following is NOT an important component of a clinical exercise rehabilitation program certification?
   A) A policies and procedures manual.
   B) Program health outcomes and quality measures.
   C) Staff certification and/or licensure.
   D) Adherence to insurance codes for billing.

51. To what does preload of the left ventricle refer?
   A) Contractility.
   B) Diastolic filling.
   C) Systole.
   D) Ventricular outflow.

52. A burning, constricting, heavy, or squeezing sensation of the chest, neck, shoulders, or arms, provoked by physical work or stress, is characteristic of which of the following?
   A) Angina.
   B) Aortic aneurysms.
   C) Exercise-induced asthma.
   D) Atherosclerosis.

53. Health screening before participation in a graded exercise test is indicated for all of the following reasons EXCEPT
   A) To determine the presence of disease.
   B) To evaluate contraindications for exercise testing or training.
   C) To determine the need for referral to a medically supervised exercise program.
   D) To evaluate aerobic capacity.

54. Which of the following is the proper emergency response for a patient who has experienced a cardiac arrest but now is breathing and has a palpable pulse?
   A) Continue the exercise test to determine why the patient had this response.
   B) Place the patient in the recovery position with the head to the side to prevent airway obstruction.
   C) Place the patient in a comfortable seated position.
   D) Start phase I cardiac rehabilitation.

55. A patient weighing 200 lb sets the treadmill at 4.0 mph with a 5% grade. At peak exercise his blood pressure is 150/90 mm Hg, heart rate is 150 bpm, and respiratory quotient is 1.0. What is his estimated absolute energy expenditure?
   A) 1.07 L/min.
   B) 2.17 L/min.
   C) 4.28 L/min.
   D) 8.56 L/min.

56. Advanced aging causes a progressive decline in which of the following?
   A) Bone density.
   B) Bone distensibility.
   C) Bone fractures.
   D) None of the above.

57. Which of the following procedures provides the LEAST sensitivity and specificity in the diagnosis of coronary artery disease?
   A) Coronary angiography.
   B) Echocardiography.
   C) Electrocardiography.
   D) Radionuclide imaging.

58. Which of the following represents an electrical impulse generated in a particular area of the heart, where the outside of the cells in this area become negatively charged and the inside of the cells become positively charged?
   A) Depolarization.
   B) Polarization.
   C) Excitation.
   D) Repolarization.

59. At exercise intensities up to 50% of maximal oxygen consumption, what facilitates an increase in cardiac output?
   A) Heart rate and stroke volume.
   B) Heart rate only.
   C) Stroke volume only.
   D) Neither heart rate nor stroke volume.

60. What does flow-resistive training (a type of breathing retraining) teach patients with pulmonary disease?
   A) To effectively breathe through a progressively smaller airway.
   B) Coordinate breathing with activities of daily living.
   C) Increase respiratory muscle endurance and strength.
   D) Increase ventilatory threshold.

61. Which of the following refers to a muscular contraction sustained against a fixed load or resistance with no change in the joint angle?
   A) Eccentric load.
   B) Isokinetic contraction.
   C) Isometric contraction.
   D) Isotonic contraction.

62. Which of the following is a NONMODIFIABLE risk factor for the development of coronary artery disease?
   A) Tobacco use.
   B) Dyslipidemia.
   C) Family history.
   D) Hypertension.

63. Which of the following is NOT an example of a capital expense?
   A) Renovations.
   B) Staff salaries.
   C) Exercise equipment purchases.
   D) Furniture and fixtures.

64. Which of the following is a linear effect that can be defined as a push, pull, or tendency to distort?
   A) Drag.
   B) Torque.
   C) Vector.
   D) Force.

65. Which of the following is the thickest, middle layer of the artery wall that is composed predominantly of smooth muscle cells and is responsible for vasoconstriction and vasodilation?
   A) Endothelium.
   B) Intima.
   C) Media.
   D) Adventitia.

66. Which electrocardiographic electrode is positioned at the fourth intercostal space just to the left of the sternal border?
   A) V_1.
   B) V_2.
   C) V_3.
   D) V_4.

67. What is the total energy expenditure for a 70-kg man doing an exercise session composed of 5 minutes of warm-up at 2.0 METs, 20 minutes of treadmill running at 9 METs, 20 minutes of leg cycling at 8 METs, and 5 minutes of cool-down at 2.5 METs?
   A) 162 kcal.
   B) 868 kcal.
   C) 444 kcal.
   D) 1,256 kcal.

68. What is the cardiac output at maximal exercise with a heart rate of 200 beats/min and stroke volume of 100 mL/beat?
   A) 5 L/min.
   B) 10 L/min.
   C) 20 L/min.
   D) 20 mL/min.

69. How should the exercise prescription be initially altered for a patient exercising in the heat or in a humid environment?
   A) Increasing the intensity and increasing the duration.
   B) Decreasing the intensity and increasing the duration.
   C) Decreasing the intensity and decreasing the duration.
   D) Increasing the intensity and decreasing the duration.

70. Which of the following statements regarding an emergency plan is True?
   A) The emergency plan does not need to be written down as long as everyone understands it.
   B) As long as everyone knows his or her individual responsibilities during an emergency, a list of each staff member's responsibilities is not needed.
   C) All emergency situations must be documented with dates, times, actions, people involved, and outcomes.
   D) There is no need to practice emergencies as long as the staff members fully understand their responsibilities.

71. Which of the following is NOT considered to be an orthopedic condition that can lead to limitation of regular exercise (physical conditioning)?
   A) Osteoarthritis.
   B) Rheumatoid arthritis.
   C) Osteoporosis.
   D) Multiple sclerosis.

72. Which of the following is characterized by an inflammation and edema of the trachea and bronchial tubes; hypertrophy of the mucous glands that narrows the airway; arterial hypoxemia that leads to vasoconstriction of smooth muscle in the pulmonary arterioles and venules; and in the presence of continued vasoconstriction results in pulmonary hypertension?
   A) Emphysema.
   B) Bronchitis.
   C) Pulmonary hypertension.
   D) Asthma.

73. Which of the following would be prudent for any high-risk patient who wishes to exercise?
   A) Skip both the warm-up and the cool-down entirely.
   B) Increase the intensity of the warm-up, and decrease the intensity of the cool-down.
   C) Decrease the intensity of the warm-up, and increase the intensity of the cool-down.
   D) Prolong both the warm-up and the cool-down.

74. Which of the following methods CANNOT measure oxygen consumption?
   A) Direct calorimetry.
   B) Indirect calorimetry.
   C) Estimation from workload.
   D) Pulmonary function testing.

75. Which of the following is a symptom of a stroke (cerebrovascular accident)?
   A) Fatigue or weakness that occurs **only** late in the day.
   B) Altered sensation.
   C) Ventricular fibrillation.
   D) Pain in the chest that radiates to jaw or neck.

76. What is the sum of the oxygen cost of physical activity and the resting energy expenditure called?
   A) Relative oxygen consumption.
   B) Absolute oxygen consumption.
   C) Net oxygen consumption.
   D) Gross oxygen consumption.

77. Which of the following is NOT characteristic of ventricular tachycardia?
   A) Wide QRS complex (≥120 ms).
   B) AV dissociation (P waves and QRS complexes have no relationship).
   C) Flutter waves at a rate of 250 to 350 atrial depolarizations per minute.
   D) Three or more consecutive ventricular beats at 100 beats/min.

78. In which of the following conditions does necrotic heart muscle fibers degenerate, causing the muscle wall to become very thin resulting in a paradoxical bulging in that area during ventricular contraction?
   A) Left ventricular hypertrophy.
   B) Pericarditis.
   C) Myocardial infarction.
   D) Ventricular aneurysm.

79. Which exercise intensity is used for training muscular endurance?
   A) 10% to 40% of one repetition maximum.
   B) 20% to 40% of one repetition maximum.
   C) 40% to 60% of one repetition maximum.
   D) 60% to 80% of one repetition maximum.

80. What is a slotted, stainless-steel tube that acts as a scaffold to hold the walls of a coronary artery open, thereby improving blood flow and relieving the symptoms of coronary artery disease called?
   A) Percutaneous transluminal coronary angioplasty (PTCA).
   B) Coronary artery stent.
   C) Laser angioplasty.
   D) Coronary artery bypass graft.

81. Which type of AV block occurs with a PR interval that progressively lengthens beyond 0.20 seconds until a P wave fails to conduct?
   A) First-degree.
   B) Second-degree, Mobitz type I.
   C) Second-degree, Mobitz type II.
   D) Third-degree, AV block.

82. Which type of infarction is indicated if Q waves are detected by an electrocardiogram in leads V_1 and V_2, along with abnormal R waves?
   A) Anterolateral.
   B) Localized anterior.
   C) Posterior.
   D) High lateral.

83. What is an appropriate low-density lipoprotein (LDL) goal for a patient with a very high risk for coronary artery disease?
   A) <120 mg/dL.
   B) >100 mg/dL.
   C) <70 mg/dL.
   D) 100 to 120 mg/dL.

84. Which of the following graded exercise test protocols is NOT appropriate for previously sedentary individuals ?
   A) Cooper 12-minute test.
   B) Step test.
   C) Treadmill test.
   D) Cycle ergometer test.

85. For patients with congestive heart failure, which of the following statements is true?
   A) Patients may not exceed a workload of 5 METS.
   B) Warm-up and cool-down periods should be limited to 5 minutes.
   C) Patients should expect no significant improvement in exercise capacity.
   D) Peripheral adaptations are largely responsible for an increase in exercise tolerance.

86. Which of the following populations would benefit MOST from regular muscular strength and endurance training?
   A) Postmenopausal women.
   B) Athletes <14 years of age.
   C) Stroke survivors.
   D) Hypertensive adults.

87. Arterial oxygenation decreases despite increased ventilation at what altitude?
   A) >500 ft.
   B) <750 ft.
   C) >1,000 ft.
   D) >5,000 ft.

88. Which of the following electrocardiogram interpretations involves a QRS complex duration that exceeds

0.11 seconds and a P wave precedes the QRS complex if it is present?
A) AV conduction delay.
B) Normal cardiac function.
C) Supraventricular aberrant conduction.
D) Acute myocardial infarction.

89. What is the incidence of cardiac arrest during clinical exercise testing?
A) 1 in 10,000.
B) 1 in 2,500.
C) 1.4 in 10,000.
D) Minimal to nonexistent.

90. A regular exercise program will have what effect?
A) Increase myocardial oxygen cost for a given submaximal exercise intensity.
B) Increase serum high-density lipoprotein cholesterol; decrease serum triglycerides.
C) Reduce exercise threshold for the accumulation of lactate in the blood.
D) Increase total cholesterol:low-density cholesterol ratio.

91. In the "Readiness to Change Model," which stage can be achieved through the use of multiple resources to stress the importance of a desired change?
A) Precontemplation.
B) Contemplation.
C) Preparation.
D) Instruction.

92. Which should be lowered as an effective strategy in limiting the progression and promoting regression of atherosclerosis?
A) Low-density lipoprotein cholesterol.
B) High-density lipoprotein cholesterol.
C) Triglycerides.
D) Blood platelets.

93. Which of the following is a common type of "field test"?
A) Step test.
B) 1- and 6-minute walk test.
C) Cycle ergometer test.
D) Treadmill test.

94. A transmural myocardial infarction, marked by tissue necrosis in a full-thickness portion of the left ventricular wall, typically produces what initial changes on the electrocardiogram?
A) T-wave inversion.
B) P-wave inversion.
C) ST-segment depression.
D) ST-segment elevation.

95. Cardiorespiratory endurance, resistance, and flexibility programming are indicative of which phase of an exercise prescription?
A) Stimulus phase.
B) Warm-up.
C) Cool-down.
D) Resistance training.

96. Which of the following statements is TRUE?
A) A physician's approval should be required prior to all testing.
B) For all patients, the risks of testing and exercise outweigh the benefits.
C) For certain individuals, the risks of testing and exercise outweigh the potential benefits.
D) The potential benefits of testing and exercise always outweigh the risks.

97. Which of the following has a risk ratio in the development of coronary artery disease similar to that of hypertension, hypercholesterolemia, and cigarette smoking?
A) Type 2 diabetes mellitus.
B) Obesity.
C) Sedentary lifestyle.
D) Psychological stress.

98. Which of the following is the best example of physical activity requiring aerobic metabolism to produce ATP?
A) 40-yard dash.
B) 400-m sprint.
C) 5,000-m run.
D) Marathon run.

99. When determining the electrocardiogram mean axis, which of the following is more negative than $-30°$?
A) Normal.
B) Right-axis deviation.
C) Left-axis deviation.
D) Extreme left-axis deviation.

100. Which of the following medications does NOT affect exercise heart rate (HR) response?
A) Angiotensin-converting enzyme (ACE) inhibitors and angiotensin II blockers.
B) Calcium-channel blockers.
C) Thyroid medications.
D) β-blockers.

ANSWERS AND EXPLANATIONS

1–D. Epinephrine is an endogenous catecholamine that optimizes blood flow to the heart and brain by increasing aortic diastolic pressure and preferentially shunting blood to the internal carotid artery. Lidocaine is an antiarrhythmic agent that can decrease automaticity in the ventricular

myocardium as well as raise the fibrillation threshold. Supplemental oxygen ensures adequate arterial oxygen content and greatly enhances tissue oxygenation. Atropine is a parasympathetic blocking agent used to treat bradyarrhythmias.
[Chapter 7]

2–C. The steps are as follows:

a. Convert relative $\dot{V}O_2$ to absolute $\dot{V}O_2$ by multiplying relative $\dot{V}O_2$ ($mL \cdot kg^{-1} \cdot min^{-1}$) by his body weight.

b. The young man weights 80 kg. Therefore:

$$\begin{aligned} \text{absolute } \dot{V}O_2 &= \text{relative } \dot{V}O_2 \times \text{body weight} \\ &= 45\ mL \cdot kg^{-1} \cdot min^{-1} \times 80\ kg \\ &= 3{,}600\ mL \cdot min^{-1} \end{aligned}$$

c. To get $L \cdot min^{-1}$, divide $mL \cdot min^{-1}$ by 1,000:

$$3{,}600\ mL \cdot min^{-1} \div 1{,}000 = 3.60\ L \cdot min^{-1}$$

d. Multiply $3.60\ L \cdot min^{-1}$ by the constant 5.0 to get $kcal \cdot min^{-1}$:

$$3.60\ L \cdot min^{-1} \times 5.0 = 18.0\ kcal \cdot min^{-1}$$

e. Multiply $18.0\ kcal \cdot min^{-1}$ by the total number of minutes that he exercises (30 minutes × 5 times per week = 150 total minutes) to get the total caloric expenditure:

$$\begin{aligned} &18.0\ kcal \cdot min^{-1} \times 150 \text{ minutes} \\ &= 2{,}700 \text{ kcal per week} \end{aligned}$$

f. Divide by 3,500 to get pounds of fat:

$$\begin{aligned} &2{,}700 \text{ kcal/week} \div 3{,}500 \text{ kcal/pound of fat} \\ &= 0.7714 \text{ pound of fat/week} \end{aligned}$$

g. Divide 10 lb by 0.7714 to get how many weeks it will take him to lose 10 lb of fat:

$$10 \text{ lb of fat} \div 0.7714 = 12.96 \text{ weeks}$$

or approximately 13.0 weeks.
[Chapter 11]

3–C. In the diagnosis of coronary artery disease, electrocardiography, radionuclide imaging, and echocardiography are commonly used by themselves or with other tests. However, echocardiography uses sound waves to assess heart wall motion, abnormalities, ejection fraction, systolic and diastolic function, and cardiac output. Other important diagnostic studies for coronary artery disease include coronary angiography.
[Chapter 4]

4–A. During mild to moderate exercise, minute ventilation increases primarily through increased tidal volume. During vigorous exercise, minute ventilation is increased by greater values for tidal volume and respiratory rate.
[Chapter 2]

5–C. Patients who have had heart transplant should exercise at a rating of perceived exertion of between 11 and 15 (moderate), between 60% and 70% of maximal metabolic capacity (MET), or 40% to 75% of maximal oxygen consumption. Frequency should be 4 to 6 days per week. Duration should include a prolonged warm-up. In addition, resistance training can be used in moderation.
[Chapter 9 GETP]

6–C. Recommended precautions for the exercising patient with diabetes include wearing proper footwear, maintaining adequate hydration, monitoring blood glucose level regularly, always wearing a medical identification bracelet or other form of identification, avoiding injecting insulin into exercising muscles, always exercising with a partner, and avoiding exercise during peak insulin activity. There is no reason why a patient with diabetes cannot exercise at any time if proper precautions are followed.
[Chapter 8]

7–C. The only reversible pulmonary disease, asthma, is triggered by a mediator (e.g., dust, pollen) that increases calcium influx into mast cells, resulting in the release of chemical mediators (e.g., histamine). These mediators trigger bronchoconstriction (an increase in smooth muscle contraction of the bronchial tubes) and an inflammatory response. During asthma attacks, the individual becomes dyspneic and is likely to be hypoxic and hypercapnic. Attacks can last for hours or even days if they are not self-reversing or responsive to drug therapy.
[Chapter 4]

8–B. A junctional arrhythmia is a supraventricular ectopic rhythm that results from a focus of automaticity located in the bundle of His. A ventricular arrhythmia could be a premature ventricular complex (PVC) in which one of the ventricles depolarizes first and then spreads to the other ventricle or ventricular fibrillation, which is often triggered by the simultaneous conduction of ischemic ventricular cells within multiple locations of the ventricles. An atrioventricular (AV) block result when supraventricular impulses are delayed in the AV node. A premature ventricular contraction occurs when the ventricles are prematurely depolarized.
[Chapter 12]

9–D. All of these statements are true regarding contraindications to exercise testing.
[Chapter 6]

10–A. The cardiac impulse originating in the sinoatrial node that spreads to both atria causing atrial

depolarization is indicated on the electrocardiogram as a P wave. Atrial repolarization usually is not seen on the electrocardiogram, because it is obscured by the ventricular electrical potentials. Ventricular depolarization is represented on the electrocardiogram by the QRS complex. Ventricular repolarization is represented on the electrocardiogram by the ST segment, the T wave, and at times, the U wave.
[Chapter 12]

11–C. The sagittal plane divides the body into symmetric right and left halves. The frontal plane divides the body into front and back halves. The transverse plane divides the body in half superiorly and inferiorly. There is no medial plane.
[Chapter 1]

12–C. A minimal caloric threshold of 150 to 200 kcal of physical activity per day is associated with a significant 20% to 30% reduction in risk of all-cause mortality and this should be the initial goal for previously sedentary individuals.
[Chapter 7 GETP]

13–D. The mechanisms responsible for a reduction in deaths from coronary artery disease include its effect on other risk factors, reduced myocardial oxygen demand both at rest and at submaximal workloads (resulting in an increased ischemic and angina threshold), reduced platelet aggregation, and improved endothelial-mediated vasomotor tone.
[Chapter 4]

14–B. The degradation of carbohydrate (glucose or glycogen) to pyruvate or lactate occurs in a process termed **anaerobic glycolysis**. Because pyruvate can participate in the aerobic production of ATP, glycolysis also can be considered as the first step in the aerobic production of ATP. Anaerobic metabolism results in the accumulation of lactic acid in the blood, which can contribute to fatigue; lactic acid also can be used as a fuel both during and after exercise.
[Chapter 2]

15–C. Rapid weight loss is considered to be 3 lb per week for women and 3 to 5 lb per week for men after the first 2 weeks of the diet. Long-term maintenance usually is a problem with rapid weight loss; one study reported total recidivism within 3 to 5 years. Modifications in diet and exercise generally are associated with more permanent weight loss.
[Chapter 9]

16–C. Coronary artery bypass graft surgery usually is reserved for patients who have a poor prognosis for survival or are unresponsive to pharmacologic treatment, stents, or percutaneous transluminal coronary angioplasty. Such patients include those with angina, left main coronary artery stenosis, multiple-vessel disease, and left ventricular dysfunction.
[Chapter 4]

17–A. There are many benefits of chronic exercise for a patient with an AICD. Several precautions need to be taken, however, including monitoring the heart rate and knowing the rate at which the AICD is set to shock the patient. The rate for activation is preset and varies for each patient. Depending on the exercise prescription, it generally is safe to exercise a patient up to, but not at or above, the cut-off heart rate.
[Chapter 9 GETP]

18–A. A 400-meter sprint is an example of physical activity requiring anaerobic glycolysis to produce energy in the form of ATP. A 100-meter sprint requires rapid energy by transferring high-energy phosphate from creatine phosphate to rephosphorylate ATP. The 2-mile run will utilize oxidative phosphorylation for ATP production.
[Chapter 2]

19–B. A healthy, unconditioned person has an anaerobic threshold of approximately 55% of maximal oxygen consumption. A conditioned person can have an anaerobic threshold as high as 70% to 90% of maximal oxygen consumption. The onset of metabolic acidosis or anaerobic metabolism can be measured through serial measurements of blood lactate level or assessment of expired gases, specifically pulmonary ventilation and carbon dioxide production.
[Chapter 2]

20–D. Nitrates reduce ischemia by reducing myocardial oxygen demand, with some increase in oxygen supply; they are used in the treatment of typical and variant angina. Nitrates do not reduce the risk of postmyocardial infarction mortality. β-Adrenergic blockers reduce myocardial ischemia by lowering myocardial oxygen demand. These agents lower blood pressure, control ventricular arrhythmias, and significantly reduce first-year mortality rates in patients after myocardial infarction by 20% to 35%. Niacin lowers low-density lipids by inhibiting secretion of lipoproteins from the liver. Aspirin is a platelet inhibitor.
[Chapter 4]

21–A. Cardiac impulses normally arise in the sinoatrial or sinus node of the heart. The sinoatrial node is located in the right atrium (posterior wall), near the opening of the superior vena cava. From the sinoatrial node, impulses travel to the left atrium and to the AV node, through the bundle of His, and then to Purkinje fibers in the ventricles.
[Chapter 12]

22–B. The steps are as follows:

a. Choose the ACSM leg cycling formula.

b. Write down your knowns, and convert the values to the appropriate units:

$$110\ \text{lb} \div 2.2 = 50\ \text{kg}$$
$$50\ \text{rpm} \times 6\ \text{m} = 300\ \text{m} \cdot \text{min}^{-1}$$
$$2.5\ \text{kp} = 2.5\ \text{kg}$$
$$60\ \text{minutes of cycling}$$

c. Write down the ACSM leg cycling formula:

$$\begin{aligned}\text{Leg cycling } (\text{mL} \cdot \text{kg}^{-1} \cdot \text{min}^{-1}) &= (1.8 \times \text{work rate} \div \text{body weight})\\ &\quad + 3.5 + 3.5\ (\text{mL} \cdot \text{kg}^{-1} \cdot \text{min}^{-1})\end{aligned}$$

d. Calculate the work rate:

$$\begin{aligned}\text{Work rate} &= \text{kg} \cdot \text{m} \cdot \text{min}^{-1}\\ &= 2.5\ \text{kg} \cdot 300\ \text{m} \cdot \text{min}^{-1}\\ &= 750\ \text{kg} \cdot \text{m} \cdot \text{min}^{-1}\end{aligned}$$

e. Substitute the known values for the variable name:

$$\text{mL} \cdot \text{kg}^{-1} \cdot \text{min}^{-1} = (1.8 \times 750 \div 50) + 3.5 + 3.5$$

f. Solve for the unknown:

$$\text{mL} \cdot \text{kg}^{-1} \cdot \text{min}^{-1} = 27 + 3.5 + 3.5$$

$$\text{Gross leg cycling } \dot{V}O_2 = 34\ \text{mL} \cdot \text{kg}^{-1} \cdot \text{min}^{-1}$$

g. To find out how many calories she expends, we must first convert her oxygen consumption to absolute terms:

$$\begin{aligned}\text{Absolute } \dot{V}O_2 &= \text{relative } \dot{V}O_2 \times \text{body weight}\\ &= 34\ \text{mL} \cdot \text{kg}^{-1} \cdot \text{min}^{-1} \times 50\ \text{kg}\\ &= 1{,}700\ \text{mL} \cdot \text{min}^{-1}\end{aligned}$$

h. Convert $\text{mL} \cdot \text{min}^{-1}$ to $\text{L} \cdot \text{min}^{-1}$ by dividing by 1,000:

$$1{,}700\ \text{mL} \cdot \text{min}^{-1} \div 1{,}000 = 1.7\ \text{L} \cdot \text{min}^{-1}$$

i. Next, we must see how many calories she expends in 1 minute by multiplying her absolute $\dot{V}O_2$ (in $\text{L} \cdot \text{min}^{-1}$) by the constant 5.0:

$$1.7\ \text{L} \cdot \text{min}^{-1} \times 5.0 = 8.5\ \text{kcal} \cdot \text{min}^{-1}$$

j. Finally, multiply the number of calories she expends in 1 minute by the number of minutes that she cycles:

$$8.5\ \text{kcal} \cdot \text{min}^{-1} \times 60\ \text{minutes} = 510\ \text{total calories}$$

[Chapter 11]

23–D. The proper anatomic location of V_4 is the midclavicular line, fifth intercostal space. Precordial leads V_1 and V_2 are located at the fourth intercostal space, right and left sternal borders. There is no precordial lead site at the midaxillary line, fifth intercostal space.
[Chapter 12]

24–A. During exercise, stroke volume increases curvilinearly with work rate until it reaches near maximum at a level equivalent to approximately 50% of aerobic capacity, increasing only slightly thereafter. The left ventricle is able to contract with greater force during exercise because of a greater end-diastolic volume and enhanced mechanical ability of muscle fibers to produce force.
[Chapter 2]

25–A. Exposure to the cold causes vasoconstriction (higher blood pressure response), lowers the anginal threshold in patients with angina, can provoke angina at rest (variant or Prinzmetal's angina), and can induce asthma, general dehydration, and dryness or burning of the mouth and throat.
[Chapter 4]

26–C. To convert from pounds of fat to total kilocalories, multiply the fat weight (in pounds) by 3,500. The correct answer is 3 × 3,500 = 10,500 kcal.
[Chapter 11]

27–D. Bilateral ankle edema is a characteristic sign of heart failure, whereas unilateral edema of a limb often results from venous thrombosis or lymphatic blockage. Intermittent claudication, a condition caused by an inadequate blood supply, is an aching, crampy, and sometimes burning pain in the legs that typically occurs with exercise and disappears with rest. Orthopnea is characterized by the inability to breathe easily unless sitting up straight or standing erect and is a symptom of heart failure. Bronchitis, a pulmonary disorder, is characterized by inflammation and edema of the trachea and bronchial tubes. Classic symptoms of bronchitis include chronic cough, sputum production, and dyspnea.
[Chapter 4]

28–C. A thrombosis is a specific clot that may cause a myocardial infarction. Ischemia is insufficient blood flow to the heart muscle. Thrombolysis (thrombolytic therapy) uses a specific clot-dissolving agent administered during acute myocardial infarction to restore blood flow and to limit myocardial necrosis. Myocardial infarction is irreversible necrosis of the heart muscle resulting from prolonged coronary artery blockage.
[Chapter 4]

29–D. Digitalis is used to treat heart failure and certain arrhythmias. Shortening of the QT interval and a

"scooping" of the ST–T complex characterize the effects of digitalis on the electrocardiogram.
[Chapter 12]

30–C. The energy to perform physical work comes from the breakdown of ATP. The amount of directly available ATP is small, with action lasting only 5 to 10 seconds; thus, ATP must be resynthesized constantly.
[Chapter 2]

31–A. Avoiding tension on the upper body typically is recommended for 4 to 8 weeks, not for 2 to 4 months. All of the other precautions are appropriate.
[Chapter 8]

32–D. Aging, male gender, and family history of coronary artery disease are risk factors that cannot be controlled. Tobacco smoking can be modified or eliminated.
[Chapter 4]

33–B. Triglycerides are the only substance listed that has been proved to be directly affected by exercise. Lipoprotein (a) has not been shown to change favorably with exercise. Low-density lipoprotein cholesterol and total cholesterol are affected by diet and may be lowered indirectly from weight loss associated with exercise.
[Chapter 9]

34–C. Warm-up exercises tend to redistribute blood flow from the trunk to peripheral areas, decreases resistance in the tissues for movement, and increase tissue temperature and energy production. Cool-down has an opposite effect.
[Chapter 2]

35–D. Low-risk individuals are those men younger than 45 years and women younger than 55 years who are asymptomatic and meet no more than one risk factor. Moderate-risk individuals are those men ≥45 years and women ≥55 years of age or those who meet the threshold for two or more risk factors. High-risk individuals are those with one or more signs and symptoms or known cardiovascular, pulmonary, or metabolic disease.
[Chapter 2 GETP]

36–B. Second-degree AV block is subdivided into two types: Mobitz type I, and Mobitz type II. Mobitz type I also is known as the Wenckebach phenomenon. In this condition, the conduction of the impulse through the AV junction becomes increasingly more difficult, resulting in a progressively longer PR interval, until a QRS complex is dropped following a P wave. This indicates that the AV junction failed to conduct the impulse from the atria to the ventricles. This pause allows the AV node to recover, and the following P wave is conducted with a normal or slightly shorter PR interval.
[Chapter 12]

37–D. The magnitude of heart rate response is related to age, body position, fitness, type of activity, presence of heart disease, medications, blood volume, and the environment. In unconditioned persons, a proportionally greater increase in heart rate is observed at any fixed submaximal work rate compared with that seen in conditioned persons.
[Chapter 2]

38–D. Regular exercise increases caloric expenditure in an effort to reduce body weight for those who are obese; increases the activity of lipoprotein lipase, which alters blood fats (e.g., triglycerides); and lowers blood pressure. In addition to helping to reduce these risk factors for the development of coronary artery disease, exercise also can have positive benefits for those with diabetes mellitus, peripheral arterial disease, osteoporosis, and pulmonary disease.
[Chapter 4]

39–C. ST segments are considered to be sensitive indicators of myocardial ischemia or injury. A Q wave is a negative deflection of a QRS complex preceding an R wave. A "pathologic" Q wave is an indication of a old transmural myocardial infarction. The PR interval is the time that it takes from the initiation of an electrical impulse in the sinoatrial node to the initiation of electrical activity in the ventricles. The T wave indicates ventricular repolarization.
[Chapter 12]

40–D. The identification and classification of obesity and coronary artery disease risk has been somewhat discretionary, with a multitude of available techniques. Body mass index >30 kg · m^{-2}, waist-to-hip ratio >0.95, and body fat levels >25% are all objective measures of obesity for males. Waist circumference levels >35 inches is specific to women.
[Chapter 8]

41–D. At exercise a steady-state condition occurs when a balance exists between the energy required by the working muscles and the rate of ATP production through aerobic cellular respiration or aerobic metabolism. Anaerobic cellular respiration is a series of ATP-producing reactions that do not require oxygen. Oxygen debt is the oxygen consumption in excess of the resting oxygen consumption at the end of an exercise session. Oxygen deficit is the difference between total oxygen actually consumed and the amount that would have been consumed in a steady state.
[Chapter 2]

42–A. An electrocardiogram (ECG) is an excellent tool for detecting cardiac rhythm and conduction abnormalities, chamber enlargements, ischemia, and infarction. In an ECG recording ST-segment elevation with an absence of R waves that are replaced by Q waves is a sign of acute myocardial infarction.
[Chapter 4]

43–C. The steps are as follows:

a. Choose the ACSM walking formula.

b. Write down your knowns, and convert the values to the appropriate units:

$$3.5 \text{ mph} \times 26.8 = 93.8 \text{ m} \cdot \text{min}^{-1}$$
$$10\% \text{ grade} = 0.10$$

c. Write down the ACSM walking formula:

$$\text{walking } (\text{kg}^{-1} \cdot \text{min}^{-1}) = (0.1 \times \text{speed}) + (1.8 \times \text{speed} \times \text{ fractional grade}) + 3.5 \text{ } (\text{mL} \cdot \text{kg}^{-1} \cdot \text{min}^{-1})$$

d. Substitute the known values for the variable name:

$$\text{mL} \cdot \text{kg}^{-1} \cdot \text{min}^{-1} = (0.1 \times 93.8) + (1.8 \times 93.8 \times 0.1) + 3.5 \text{ mL} \cdot \text{kg}^{-1} \cdot \text{min}^{-1} = 9.38 + 16.884 + 3.5$$

e. Solve for the unknown:

$$\text{mL} \cdot \text{kg}^{-1} \cdot \text{min}^{-1} = 9.38 + 16.884 + 3.5$$
$$\text{gross walking } \dot{V}O_2 = 29.76 \text{ mL} \cdot \text{kg}^{-1} \cdot \text{min}^{-1}$$

[Chapter 11]

44–A. Segmental movements occur around an axis and in a plane. Each plane has an associated axis that is perpendicular to it. The mediolateral axis is perpendicular to the sagittal plane, and the anteroposterior axis is perpendicular to the frontal plane. There is only a transverse plane.
[Chapter 1]

45–A. The benefits of regular (endurance) exercise for patients with peripheral vascular disease include decreased blood viscosity, increased blood flow and redistribution to the legs, improved claudication pain tolerance, and increased exercise tolerance, especially walking.
[Chapter 8]

46–B. The purpose of health screening before engaging in vigorous exercise is to identify clients who require additional medical testing to determine the presence of disease, contraindications for exercise testing or training, or referral to a medically supervised exercise program. Men younger than 40 years and women younger than 50 years with fewer than two coronary artery disease risk factors do not require a physician's evaluation before initiating vigorous exercise.
[Chapter 6]

47–C. An intraventricular conduction disturbance is an abnormal conduction of an electrical impulse below the bundle of His. Intraventricular conduction disturbances include right and left bundle branch blocks as well as right and left anterior hemiblocks.
[Chapter 12]

48–C. Emergency plans must be created, practiced, and implemented in the event of a medical emergency. Clinical personnel must understand the risks associated with exercise and exercise testing, be able to implement preventive measures, and have knowledge regarding the care of an injury or medical emergency.
[Chapter 7]

49–C. Obesity is defined as a surplus of adipose tissue, resulting from excess energy intake relative to energy expenditure. Overweight is defined as a deviation in body weight from an "ideal" weight related to height standards. Android obesity describes fat accumulation over the chest and arms rather than the lower trunk (gynoid obesity). Morbid obesity is a clinically severe obesity defined as a body mass index (BMI) over 40 or a deviation of 100 lb over an ideal body weight standard.
[Chapter 9]

50–D. Program certification of clinical exercise rehabilitation programs, although a new concept, involves many components that have already been established as part of the exercise program, such as a clearly articulated mission statement, a defined organizational chart with methods to measure client health outcomes, a developed, implemented, and well-used policy and procedures manual, and so forth. The certification of a rehabilitation program is about the quality of the program as opposed to the financial operations (e.g., billing practices and use of insurance codes).
[Chapter 10]

51–B. Preload refers to diastolic filling (the amount of blood in the left ventricular prior to ejection). Contractility is the vigor of contraction and may be influenced by ventricular outflow (afterload). Systole refers to the phase of contraction in a cardiac cycle.
[Chapter 2]

52–A. Angina pectoris is the pain associated with myocardial ischemia. The pain often is felt in the chest, neck, cheeks, shoulder, or arms. It can be brought on by physical or psychological stress and is relieved after resting or by removing the

stressor. Angina can be either classic (typical) or vasospastic (Prinzmetal).
[Chapter 4]

53–D. The overall goal of health screening before participation in a graded exercise testing or an exercise program is to obtain essential information that will ensure the safety of the participant. Thus, health screening helps to determine the presence of disease, enables one to consider possible contraindications to exercise testing and training, and helps to determine whether referral to a medically supervised exercise program is needed.
[Chapter 6]

54–B. The proper response to a patient who has experienced a cardiac arrest yet is breathing and has a pulse is to call to the emergency medical system immediately; place the patient in the recovery position, with the head to the side to avoid an airway obstruction; and then stay with the patient and continue to monitor his or her vital signs.
[Chapter 7]

55–B. The steps are as follows:

a. Choose the ACSM walking formula.

b. Write down your knowns, and convert the values to the appropriate units:

5% grade = 0.05
4.0 mph = 107.2 m · min^{-1}
200 lb = 90.91 kg

c. Write down the ACSM walking formula: walking (kg^{-1}· min^{-1}) = (0.1× speed) + (1.8 × speed × fractional grade) + 3.5 (mL · kg^{-1} · min^{-1})

d. Substitute knowns

$$\dot{V}O_2 = (0.1 \times 107.2) + (1.8 \times 107.2 \times 0.05) + 3.5$$

e. Solve

$$\dot{V}O_2 = 23.87 \text{ mL} \cdot \text{kg}^{-1} \cdot \text{min}^{-1}$$
$$\dot{V}O_2 = 23.83 \times 90.01 \text{ kg}/1{,}000$$
$$\dot{V}O_2 = 2.17 \text{ L} \cdot \text{min}^{-1}$$

[Chapter 11]

56–A. Advanced aging brings a progressive decline in bone mineral density and calcium homeostasis. This loss accelerates in women immediately after menopause. As a result, older people, especially women, are at increased risk for bone fractures, which are a significant cause of morbidity and mortality. Hip fractures are the most common type and account for a large share of disabilities, death, and high medical costs associated with accidents and falls.
[Chapter 3]

57–C. Electrocardiography is the least sensitive and specific of all these tests. Directly visualizing the coronary arteries using coronary angiography provides the highest sensitivity and specificity. Radionuclide imaging and echocardiography have about the same sensitivity and specificity.
[Chapter 4]

58–A. In the resting period of the myocardial cell, the inside of the cell membrane is negatively charged, and the outside of the cell membrane is positively charged. As such, the term **polarized cell** is reserved for the normal "resting myocardial cell" and describes the presence of an electrical potential across the cell membrane caused by the separation of electrical charges. When an electrical impulse is generated in a particular area in the heart, the outside of the cell in an area becomes negative, whereas the inside of the cell in this same area becomes positive. This state of cell excitation (caused by a change in polarity) is called **depolarization**. The stimulated myocardial cells return to their resting state in a process called **repolarization**.
[Chapter 12]

59–A. At exercise intensities up to 50% of maximal oxygen consumption, the increase in cardiac output is facilitated by increases in heart rate and stroke volume. Thereafter, the increase results almost solely from the continued rise in heart rate.
[Chapter 2]

60–A. Flow-resistive training involves breathing through a progressively smaller airway or opening. Paced breathing helps to coordinate breathing with activities of daily living. Respiratory muscle training increases respiratory muscle endurance and strength. Ventilatory threshold is the breakpoint in ventilation during exercise and likely reflects a balance between lactate production and removal.
[Chapter 7 RM]

61–C. An isometric contraction occurs when a muscle group contracts against a fixed load with no apparent movement or no change in joint angle. An isotonic contraction makes a joint angle decrease or increase according to the movements and production of muscle forces. Isokinetic contractions refer to either a concentric or an eccentric contraction. An isokinetic contraction occurs at a fixed speed of movement and usually involves use of an isokinetic device that controls the speed of rotation along a joint's entire range of motion. An eccentric load is an amount of resistance applied directly to a muscle or muscle group during an eccentric contraction.
[Chapter 6]

62–C. **Nonmodifiable risk factors** include: age, male gender, family history of premature coronary heart disease. **Modifiable risk factors** include: hypertension, dyslipidemia, tobacco use, diabetes mellitus, overweight or obesity, physical inactivity.
[Chapter 11 RM]

63–B. **Staff salaries** are not capital expenses, but are grouped under variable costs. **Capital expense** is for large-scale purchases, such as renovations, expansions, furniture and fixtures.
[Chapter 48 RM]

64–D. A **force** is a linear effect that can be defined as a push, pull, or tendency to distort. **Torque** is a measure of the rotary effect of a force. **Vector** can represent forces and describe the magnitude (size) and direction of the force. **Drag** is the fluid force that acts parallel to the relative flow of fluid past an object.
[ACSM's Resource Manual for Guidelines for Exercise Testing and Prescription, 5th ed, Chapter 2, pp 34–35]

65–C. The **media** contains most of the smooth muscle cells, which maintain arterial tone. The **endothelium** comprises a single layer of cells that form a tight barrier between blood and the arterial wall to resist thrombosis, promote vasodilation, and inhibit smooth muscle cells from migration and proliferation into the intima. The **intima** is the very thin, innermost layer of the artery wall and is composed mainly of connective tissue with some smooth muscle cells. The **adventitia** is the outermost layer of the arterial wall and consists of connective tissue, fibroblasts, and a few smooth muscle cells. Adventitia is highly vascularized and provides the media and intima with oxygen and other nutrients.
[ACSM's Resource Manual for Guidelines for Exercise Testing and Prescription, 5th ed, Chapter 29, p 412]

66–B. V_2 electrode is located at the 4th intercostal space just to the left of the sternal border. **V_1** is at the fourth intercostal space just to the right of the sternal border. **V_3** is at the midpoint of a straight line between V_2 and V_4. **V_4** is at the midclavicular line onto the fifth intercostal space.
[ACSM's Guidelines for Exercise Testing and Prescription, 7th ed, 2006 p 279 Appendix C Table C-1]

67–C. First determine the MET level for each activity:
Warm-up is 2.0 MET × 5 minutes = 10 MET
Treadmill is 9.0 MET × 20 minutes = 180 MET
Cycle is 8.0 MET × 20 minutes = 160 MET
Cool-down is 2.50 MET × 5 minutes = 12.5 MET
Then determine the total number of METs for all activities: 10 + 180 + 160 + 12.5 = 362.5 MET.
Multiply 362.5 MET by 3.5 (because 1 MET $= 3.5\ mL \cdot kg^{-1} \cdot min^{-1}$), which equals 1,268.75 $mL \cdot kg^{-1}$.
Multiply 1,268.75 $mL \cdot kg^{-1}$ by body weight (70 kg), which equals 88,812.5 mL. Divide that number by 1,000 (because 1,000 mL = 1 L), which equals 88.81 L. Multiply 88.81 L by 5 (because 5 kcal equals 1 L of oxygen consumed), which equals 444 kcal
[ACSM's Metabolic Calculations Handbook, 2007 pp 7, 14]

68–C. **Cardiac output** (CO) is the product of stroke volume times heart rate.
$CO = (100\ mL \cdot beat^{-1}) \cdot (200\ beats \cdot min^{-1})$.
Convert mL to L divide by 1,000, which equals $20\ L \cdot min^{-1}$
[Chapter 3 RM]

69–C. High ambient temperature or relative humidity increases the risk of heat-related disorders, including heat cramps, heat syncope, dehydration, heat exhaustion, and heat stroke. In this type of environment, the exercise prescription should be altered by initially lowering the intensity and the duration of exercise to allow for acclimatation.
[Chapter 34 RM; pages 194–204 GETP]

70–C. The emergency plan must be written down and available in all testing and exercise areas. The plan should list the specific responsibilities of each staff member, required equipment, and predetermined contacts for an emergency response. All emergencies must be documented with dates, times, actions, people involved, and results. The plan should be practiced with both announced and unannounced drills periodically. All staff members, including nonclinical staff members, should be trained in the emergency plan.
[Chapter 50 RM]

71–D. **Osteoarthritis** is a degenerative joint disease that generally is localized first on an articular cartilage. **Rheumatoid arthritis** is an inflammatory disease affecting joints as well as organs. **Osteoporosis** involves the loss of bone density. Multiple sclerosis is a chronic inflammatory disorder with demyelination occurring in the central nervous system.
[Chapter 39 RM; Chapter 40 RM]

72–B. Signs and symptoms of **bronchitis** include chronic cough, mucous production, and mucous gland enlargement that involves the large airways. The body attempts to heal by depositing collagen in the airway walls. The effects includes further airway narrowing; an increase in airway resistance decreasing ventilation to the lung; increased perfusion resulting in ventilation-perfusion mismatch; arterial hypoxemia and

pulmonary arterial hypertension. Common clinical symptoms of **emphysema** are shortness of breath or coughing, sputum production notable in the morning, hypoxemia and eventual cor pulmonale. Emphysema primarily involves abnormalities of the lung parenchyma and smaller airways. **Asthma** is an episodic reversible condition that is characterized by increased airway reactivity to various stimuli resulting in widespread reversible narrowing of the airways. **Pulmonary hypertension** is a mean pulmonary artery pressure at rest >25 mm Hg or >30 mm Hg with exercise.
[Chapter 23 RM]

73–D. Warm-up may have preventative value, decreasing the occurrence of ischemic ST-segment depression, decreasing transient global left ventricular dysfunction following sudden strenuous exertion, and decreasing ventricular dysrhythmias. Cool-down provides a gradual recovery from exercising. It allows the return of heart rate and blood pressure close to resting levels, maintains venous return, and prevents postexercise hypotension, and facilitates dissipation of body heat.
[Chapter 7 GETP]

74–D. Oxygen consumption can be measured in the laboratory using techniques of direct and indirect calorimetry, or it can be estimated from the workload. Pulmonary function testing is used to identify pulmonary disorders, such as restrictive and obstructive pulmonary disease.
[Chapter 3 RM]

75–B. A cerebrovascular accident (CVA) or stroke results from compromised cerebral blood flow. CVA symptoms include variable loss of motor control and/or sensation, and impaired language and cognition.
[Chapter 38 RM]

76–D. Individuals require approximately 3.5 $mL \cdot kg^{-1} \cdot min^{-1}$ (1 MET) of oxygen at rest. Physical activity elevates oxygen consumption above resting levels. **Net oxygen consumption** is the difference between oxygen consumption value for exercise and the resting value. Net oxygen consumption is used to assess the caloric cost of exercise. **Gross oxygen consumption** is the sum of the oxygen cost of the physical activity and the resting component. Net and gross oxygen consumption can be expressed in relative or absolute terms.
[ACSM's Certification Review, 2nd ed, Chapter 11, p 210]

77–C. **Ventricular tachycardia** is characterized by three or more consecutive ventricular beats per minute or faster, a wide QRS complex (≥120 ms), AV dissociation (the P waves and QRS complexes have no relationship) and a QRS complex that does not have the morphology of bundle branch block. Atrial flutter is characterized by flutter waves at a rate of 250 to 350 atrial depolarizations per minute.
[Chapter 27 RM]

78–D. **Ventricular aneurysm** is a thinning of the ventricular wall resulting in paradoxical bulging in that area during ventricular contraction. **Pericarditis** is an infected or inflamed pericardium. **Left ventricular hypertrophy (LVH)** is associated with hypertrophy of the walls and dilation of the chambers and can be diagnosed on ECG by increased voltage owing to the increased mass of the myocardium. **Myocardial infarction** occurs when blood flow to a region of heart muscle is interrupted by total occlusion of a coronary artery.
[Chapter 27 RM]

79–C. Rapid strength gains will be achieved at higher resistance or weight (80% to 100% of one repetition maximum) and lower repetitions (six to eight). For muscular endurance, a lower weight is used (40% to 60% of one repetition maximum) with higher number of repetitions—usually 8 to 15.
[Pages 165–175 GETP]

80–B. **Coronary stent** is a mesh tube that acts as a scaffold to hold open the walls of the artery after **percutaneous transluminal coronary angioplasty (PTCA)**. In PTCA, a catheter with a deflated balloon is inserted into the narrowed portion of the coronary artery. The balloon is inflated and the plaque gets flattened to the walls of the artery. **Laser angioplasty** is similar to PTCA, where the end of the catheter emits pulses of photons that vaporizes the plaque. **Coronary artery bypass graft (CABG)** surgery involves attaching a large vein to the base of the aorta and/or any other area of stenosis of a coronary artery.
[ACSM's Certification Review, 2nd ed, Chapter 4, p 76]

81–B. Second-degree AV block: Mobitz I (Wenckebach). PR Interval lengthens until a P wave fails to conduct.
[Chapter 27 RM; Chapter 7 GETP Page 308]

82–C. V_1, V_2 based on abnormal Q waves except for true posterior myocardial, which is reflected by abnormal R waves.
[Chapter 27 RM; Table C.4 GETP Pages 304–305]

83–C. Since publication of ATP III major clinical trials question the treatment thresholds for LDL. In particular an LDL goal of <70 mg/dL appears to

be appropriate for those in a category of "very high risk."
[Chapter 3 GETP]

84–A. The advantages of field tests are that they all potentially could be maximal tests, and by their nature, are unmonitored for blood pressure and heart rate. An individual's level of motivation and pacing ability also can have a profound impact on test results. These all-out run tests may be inappropriate for sedentary individuals or individuals at increased risk for cardiovascular and musculoskeletal complications.
[Chapter 4 GETP]

85–D. Physical conditioning in patients with heart failure and moderate to severe left ventricular dysfunction results in improved functional capacity and quality of life and reduced symptoms. Peripheral adaptation (increased skeletal muscle oxidative enzymes and improved mitochondrial size and density) are responsible for the increase in exercise tolerance.
[Chapter 9 GETP]

86–A. A reduction in the risk of osteoporosis, low back pain, hypertension, and diabetes are associated with resistance training. In addition, the benefits of increased muscular strength, bone density, enhanced strength of connective tissue, and the increase or maintenance of lean body mass may also occur. These adaptations are beneficial for all ages, including middle-aged and older adults, and in particular postmenopausal women who may experience a more rapid loss of bone mineral density.
[Chapter 7 GETP]

87–D. Despite increased ventilation, arterial oxygenation (PaO_2 and SaO_2) usually falls when ascending to 5,000 feet above sea level or higher.
[Chapter 8 GETP]

88–C. Supraventricular aberrant conduction QRS complex $\geq$0.11 seconds; widened QRS usually with unchanged initial vector; P present or absent but with relationship to QRS.
[Chapter 27 RM; Table C.4 GETP Pages 304–305]

89–B. With the physical demands of exercise, emergency situations can occur, especially in a clinical setting where patients with disease are exercising. The incidence of a cardiac arrest during exercise testing is 0.4 in 10,000 (1/2,500).
[Chapter 6]

90–B. Regular physical activity and/or exercise reduces coronary artery disease risk by increasing serum high-density lipoprotein cholesterol and decreasing serum triglycerides.
[Chapter 1 GETP]

91–A. Precontemplation: Patients express lack of interest in making change. Moving patients through this stage involves use of multiple resources to stress the importance of the desired change. This can be achieved through written materials, educational classes, physician and family persuasion, and other means.
[Chapter 7 GETP]

92–A. Lowering total cholesterol and low-density lipoprotein cholesterol has proved to be effective in reducing and even reversing atherosclerosis. The goal is to reduce the availability of lipids to the injured endothelium. In primary-prevention trials, lowering total cholesterol and low-density lipoprotein cholesterol has been shown to reduce the incidence and mortality of coronary artery disease.
[Chapter 9]

93–B. Field tests consist of walking or running a certain distance in a given time (i.e., 12-minute and 1.5-mile run tests, and the 1- and 6-minute walk test).
[Chapter 4 GETP]

94–D. Transmural myocardial infarction produces changes in both the QRS complex and the ST segment. ST-segment elevation or tall, upright T waves are the earliest signs associated with transmural myocardial infarction. ST-segment elevation may persist for a few hours to a few days.
[Chapter 12]

95–A. The stimulus (conditioning phase) includes cardiorespiratory endurance, resistance, and flexibility programming.
[Chapter 7 GETP]

96–C. It is essential that clinicians be familiar with contraindications to exercise and exercise testing. For certain groups of patients, the risks of exercise testing (and of exercise in general) outweigh the benefits.
[Chapter 7]

97–C. Physical inactivity (sedentary lifestyle) has been determined to have a similar risk in the development of atherosclerosis as the other major risk factors (smoking, hypertension, and elevated cholesterol). Obesity, diabetes mellitus, and stress are important risk factors, but are not thought to be as significant as smoking, high blood pressure, or high cholesterol.
[Chapter 4]

98–D. The 400-m sprint is an example of physical activity requiring anaerobic glycolysis to produce energy in the form of ATP. Shorter sprints rely on ready stores of ATP and phosphocreatine. Longer runs require aerobic metabolism to produce ATP.
[Chapter 2]

99–C. A mean electrical axis between -30° and $+100^\circ$ is considered to be normal. An axis that is more negative than -30° is considered to be left-axis deviation; an axis greater than $+100^\circ$ is considered to be right-axis deviation until it reaches -180° and then is considered to be extreme right- or extreme left-axis deviation.
[Chapter 12]

100–A. Angiotensin-converting enzyme (ACE) inhibitor and angiotensin II receptor blockers ⇔ Heart Rate (R and E)
Calcium channel blockers: ⇑ or ⇑ or ⇔ Heart Rate (R and E)
β-blockers: ⇓ Heart Rate (R and E)
Thyroid medications: ⇑ Heart Rate (R and E)
[Appendix A GETP]

Index

Page numbers in *italics* denote figures; those followed by "t" denote tables

F

G

N

O

P